ENA
EMERGENCY NURSES ASSOCIATION

Core Curriculum for Pediatric Emergency Nursing

Editors

Donna Ojanen Thomas, RN, MSN
Director, Emergency Department and Rapid Treatment Unit
Primary Children's Medical Center
Salt Lake City, UT

Lisa Marie Bernardo, RN, PhD, MPH
Associate Professor
University of Pittsburgh School of Nursing
Pittsburgh, PA

Bruce Herman, MD
Assistant Professor, Pediatrics
University of Utah College of Medicine
Salt Lake City, UT
Attending Physician, Emergency Department
Primary Children's Medical Center
Salt Lake City, UT

JONES AND BARTLETT PUBLISHERS
Sudbury, Massachusetts
BOSTON TORONTO LONDON SINGAPORE

World Headquarters
Jones and Bartlett Publishers
40 Tall Pine Drive
Sudbury, MA 01776
978-443-5000
info@jbpub.com
www.jbpub.com

Jones and Bartlett Publishers Canada
6339 Ormindale Way
Mississauga, ON L5V 1J2
CANADA

Jones and Bartlett Publishers International
Barb House, Barb Mews
London W6 7PA
UK

Jones and Bartlett's books and products are available through most bookstores and online booksellers. To contact Jones and Bartlett Publishers directly, call 800-832-0034, fax 978-443-8000, or visit our website at www.jbpub.com.

Substantial discounts on bulk quantities of Jones and Bartlett's publications are available to corporations, professional associations, and other qualified organizations. For details and specific discount information, contact the special sales department at Jones and Bartlett via the above contact information or send an email to specialsales@jbpub.com.

Library of Congress Cataloging-in-Publication Data not available at time of printing.

ISBN-13: 978-0-7637-0176-5
ISBN-10: 0-7637-0176-9

Acquisitions Editor: Penny M. Glynn
Production Manager: Amy Rose
Associate Production Editor: Tara McCormick
Editorial Assistant: Karen Zuck
Production Assistant: Karen C. Ferreira
Senior Marketing Manager: Alisha Weisman
Marketing Associate: Joy Stark-Vancs
Manufacturing and Inventory Coordinator: Amy Bacus
Cover Design: Anne Spencer
Interior Design: Anne Flanagan
Composition: Northeast Compositors, Inc.
Printing and Binding: Courier Stoughton
Cover Printing: Courier Stoughton

6048

Printed in the United States of America
11 10 09 10 9 8 7 6 5

Dedication

For my husband, C. Richard Packer, whose love and support inspires and sustains me; our nieces Rachael, Kailey, and Tara and our nephew Kalen; and my nursing colleagues at Children's Hospital of Pittsburgh.

LMB

For my husband, Bruce M. Thomas, and our children, Kseniya, Dan, and Bill who believe in me, and keep me laughing; and for the nurses at Primary Children's Medical Center who never let me forget what is really important in nursing.

DRT

PREFACE

Children and adolescents use emergency services for a variety of injury and illness-related complaints. During the years from 1992 to 1994, there was a national average of 31,447,000 emergency department (ED) visits per year for patients 20 years of age or younger. This annual ED visit rate for the pediatric population is 41.2 ED visits per 100 persons. Therefore, a child or adolescent visits an ED once every second, which means 60 visits per minute, 3,600 visits per hour, 86,400 visits per day, and more than 31 million visits per year (Weiss, Mathers, Forjuoh, & Kinnane, 1997). These impressive statistics imply that emergency nurses are very likely to care for infants, children, and adolescents in their daily practice.

With changes in health care reimbursement, children presenting to EDs will be more acutely ill. Furthermore, children with congenital or acquired chronic health conditions are living longer, requiring technology for everyday living. Therefore, emergency nurses must have a core knowledge base of psychosocial and physiologic considerations to guide their practice.

The Core Curriculum for Pediatric Emergency Nursing (CCPEN) is a supplement for those nurses who desire comprehensive content on pediatric emergency nursing. The curriculum represents another landmark in the evolution of pediatric emergency nursing as a specialty within the Emergency Nurses Association (ENA). In 1991, the ENA convened the first pediatric committee, which was charged with charting a course for the development of pediatric-related projects within the organization. This group was the impetus for other projects, such as the EMSC/ENA Collaborative Curriculum.

The need for pediatric-specific knowledge intensified, and subsequently the Pediatric Committee was acknowledged as a standing committee. In 1993, the Emergency Nursing Pediatric Course (ENPC) was developed and tested; it is now in its second edition. This course is offered nationally and internationally. Over the years, numerous resolutions, policy statements, and guidelines have been created and disseminated. Pediatric-specific content was strengthened in existing courses and texts. Additional texts, such as the Comprehensive Care of the Pediatric Patient, demonstrated the ENA's leadership in the care of children throughout the continuum of health care.

The CCPEN evolved from a resolution approved at the 1996 General Assembly that charged the Emergency Nurses Association with developing a pediatric certification in emergency nursing examination. A core curriculum provides the necessary theoretical and practical knowledge required for creating and administering such an examination. This book represents the continued dedication to the emergency nursing care of children as professed by the ENA.

The CCPEN integrates the nursing process with pediatric physiology and psychosocial theories. Section 1 provides an overview of issues specific to pediatric emergency nursing in chapters on management, ethical and legal considerations, and future trends. Section 2 highlights developmental and psychosocial considerations, including health promotion, physical assessment and health history, triage and telephone triage, children with special health care needs, and transport. Section 3 addresses special problems in the ED pediatric population, including neonatal emergencies, common chief complaints, and pain assessment and management. In Section 4, neonatal and pediatric resuscitation are discussed. Section 5 delves into specific emergencies. It begins with a systems approach—respiratory, cardiovascular, neurologic, gastrointestinal, genitourinary, musculoskeletal, dermatologic, and eye, ear, nose, and throat emergencies—and concludes with a medical approach of endocrine, hematologic, oncologic, and infectious disease emergencies. Psychiatric emergencies and crisis intervention are presented as well. Section 6 is devoted to trauma and includes chapters on mechanisms of injury, initial assessment, and intervention. Section 7 covers specific traumatic conditions involving the head and spinal cord, maxillofacial, thoracic, abdominal, genitourinary, and musculoskeletal systems. Submersion, burn injuries, and shock complete the section. Section 8 details environment-related emergencies including heat- and cold-related injuries, bites and stings, toxicologic emergencies, and hazardous materials emergencies. Completing the text is Section 9, which covers abuse and neglect, and sexual abuse. Chapters follow an organized format for consistency of content that includes normal physiology, pathophysiology, the nursing process (assessment, planning, implementation, and evaluation), psychosocial considerations, and home care and prevention. References from current texts, clinical literature, and data-based publications form the CCPEN's and practitioners foundation. Tables and graphs enhance the text. All chapter authors are experienced pediatric and emergency nurses.

The CCPEN was written to assist emergency nurses in their assessment and treatment of ill and injured infants, children, and adolescents. When incorporating this text into daily practice, emergency nurses should review their state's Nurse Practice Act, as well as their ED's policies and procedures, to ensure quality care.

Reference

Weiss, B., Mathers, L., Forjuoh, S., & Kinnane, J. (1997). *Child and adolescent ED visit databook*, Pittsburgh Center for Violence and Injury Control, Allegheny University of the Health Sciences.

Contributors

Pam Baker, RN, BSN, CEN, CCRN
Director, Clinical Education
Rockford Health Systems
Rockford, IL
Chapter: *Pain Assessment and Management*

Lisa Marie Bernardo, RN, PhD, MPH
Associate Professor
University of Pittsburgh School of Nursing
Pittsburgh, PA
Chapters: *Management Issues; Ethical and Legal Issues; The Future of Pediatric Emergency Nursing; Oral and Maxillofacial Trauma*

Carol Bolinger, RN, MSN, CPNP, CPON
Primary Children's Medical Center
Salt Lake City, UT
Chapter: *Hematologic and Oncologic Emergencies*

Julie K. Briggs, RN, BSN, MHA
Administrative Director, Emergency Services
Good Samaritan Hospital
Puyallup, WA
Chapter: *Dermatologic Emergencies*

Laurel Campbell, RN, MSN, CEN
Quality Improvement Manager
Bozeman Deaconess Hospital
Bozeman, MT
Chapter: *Musculoskeletal Emergencies; Specific Injuries: Musculoskeletal Trauma*

Mary Jo Cerepani, MSN, CRNP, CEN
Family Nurse Practitioner
Emergency Department
Washington Hospital
Washington, PA
Chaper: *Burn Trauma*

Beth Cohen, RN, MSN, CRNP
Graduate Student Researcher
University of Pittsburgh School of Nursing
Pittsburgh, PA
Chapter: *Hematologic and Oncologic Emergencies*

Yvette Conley, PhD
Assistant Professor
University of Pittsburgh School of Nursing
Pittsburgh, PA
Chapter: *The Future of Pediatric Emergency Nursing*

Alice Conway, PhD, CRNP
Associate Professor
Department of Nursing
Edinboro University of Pennsylvania
Edinboro, PA
Chapter: *Developmental and Psychosocial Considerations*

Nancy Eckle, RN, MSN
Director of Emergency Services
Columbus Children's Hospital
Columbus, OH
Chapter: *Neurologic Emergencies*

Laurie Flaherty, RN, MS
Traffic Safety Consultant
U.S. Department of Transportation
National Highway Traffic Safety Administration
Washington, DC
Chapter: *Prevention of Illness and Injury*

Valerie G. A. Grossman, BSN, CEN
Nursing Director of Acute Services
Myers Community Hospital, Sodus, NY
Newark Community Hospital, Newark, NY
Chapter: *Telephone Triage*

Kathy Haley, RN, BSN
Trauma Coordinator
Columbus Children's Hospital
Columbus, OH
Chapters: *Mechanisms of Injury; Initial Assessment and Intervention; Head Trauma/ Traumatic Brain Injury; Spinal Cord Trauma; Thoracic Trauma; Abdominal Trauma; Genitourinary Trauma*

Bruce Herman, MD
Assistant Professor, Pediatrics
University of Utah College of Medicine
Attending Physician, Emergency Department
Primary Children's Medical Center
Salt Lake City, UT

Reneé S. Holleran RN, PhD, CEN, CCRN, CFRN
Chief Flight Nurse/Emergency Clinical Nurse
University Air Care
Cincinnati, OH
Chapters: *Triage; Transport*

Jackie Jardine RN, C
Nursing Director, Emergency Department
Arkansas Children's Hospital
Little Rock, AR
Chapters: *Respiratory Emergencies; Submersion Injuries*

Marilyn K. Johnson, RN
Safe and Healthy Families
Primary Children's Medical Center
Salt Lake City, UT
Chapter: *Child Sexual Abuse*

Tracy B. Karp, RNC, MS, NNP
Manager, NNP Service
Primary Children's Medical Center
Salt Lake City, UT
Chapters: *Neonatal Emergencies; Common Chief Complaints*

Roger K. Keddington, APRN, MSN, CEN, CCRN
Emergency Clinical Nurse Specialist
Intermountain Health Care Urban Central Region Hospitals
Salt Lake City, UT
Chapter: *Hazardous Material and Biochemical Emergencies*

Susan J. Kelley, RN, PhD, FAAN
Dean and Professor
College of Health and Human Sciences
Georgia State University
Atlanta, GA
Chapter: *Child Abuse and Neglect*

David C. LaCovey, NREMT-P
EMS Coordinator
Prehospital and Emergency Care Services
Children's Hospital of Pittsburgh
Pittsburgh, PA
Chapters: *Neonatal Resuscitation; Pediatric Resuscitation*

Deborah Lesniak, RN, MS
Director of Emergency Services
Children's Hospital of Pittsburgh
Pittsburgh, PA
Chapter: *Ethical and Legal Issues*

Robin Long, RN, MSN, PNP
Pediatric Nurse Practitioner
Richmond, VA
Chapter: *Respiratory Emergencies, Appendix A*

Sarah A. Martin, RN, MS, PCCNP, CPNP, CCRN
Teacher Practitioner
Pediatric Intensive Care Unit
Rush Children's Hospital
Rush-Presbyterian-St. Luke's Medical Center
Chicago, IL
Instructor
College of Nursing
Rush University
Chapters: *Pediatric Resuscitation; Cardiovascular Emergencies; Shock; Neonatal Resuscitation*

Nancy L. Mecham, APRN, FNP
Clinical Nurse Specialist
Primary Children's Medical Center
Emergency Department and Rapid Treatment Unit
Salt Lake City, UT
Chapters: *Mechanisms of Injury; Abdominal Trauma; Submersion Injuries*

Michelle R. Morfin, MS, RN, CNP, CS, CCRN
Cardiac Nurse Practitioner
The Heart Center
Children's Hospital Medical Center of Akron
Akron, OH
Chapter: *Cardiovascular Emergencies*

Christine Nelson, RNC, MS, PNP
Nurse Practitioner, Division of Emergency Medicine
Children's Hospital of Buffalo
Buffalo, NY
Chapters: *Genitourinary Emergencies; Endocrine Emergencies; Head Injuries; Spinal Cord Trauma*

Nancy A. Noonan, MS, APRN
Clinical Nurse Specialist, Blood and Marrow Transplant
Children's Hospital Oakland
Oakland, CA
Chapter: *Hematologic and Oncologic Emergencies*

Joan O'Connor, RN, MSN, CRNP
Pediatric Nurse Practitioner
Children's Community Care Center
Pittsburgh, PA
Chapter: *Health History and Physical Assessment*

Kathryn Puskar, RN, DrPH, CS, FAAN
Associate Professor
University of Pittsburgh School of Nursing
Pittsburgh, PA
Chapter: *Psychiatric Emergencies*

Cherie Jordan Revere RN, MSN, CEN, CRNP
Emergency Department Clinical Nurse Specialist
University of South Alabama Medical Center
Mobile, AL
Chapter: *Eye, Ear, Nose, and Throat Emergencies*

Cynde Rivers, RN, MN, CEN
EMS Coordinator
Mary Bridge Children's Hospital and Health Center
Tacoma, WA
Chapter: *Communicable and Infectious Diseases*

Rachael Rosenfield, RN, BSN
Staff Nurse
Magee-Women's Hospital
Pittsburgh, PA
Chapters: *Communicable and Infectious Diseases; Oral and Maxillofacial Trauma*

Kathleen Schenkel, RN, BSN, CEN
Manager
Emergency Department
Children's Hospital of Pittsburgh
Pittsburgh, PA
Chapter: *Thoracic Trauma*

Rose Ann Soloway, RN, BSN, MSEd, DABAT
Associate Director
American Association of Poison Control Centers
Washington, DC
Chapter: *Toxicologic Emergencies*

Treesa E. Soud, RN, BSN
Nurse Consultant
Jacksonville, FL
Chapters: *Gastrointestinal Emergencies; Common Chief Complaints*

Kathleen Sullivan, RN, PhD
Associate Professor
LaRoche College School of Nursing
Pittsburgh, PA
Chapter: *Psychiatric Emergencies*

Donna Ojanen Thomas, RN, MSN
Director, Emergency Department and Rapid Treatment Unit
Primary Children's Medical Center
Salt Lake City, UT
Chapters: *Management Issues; The Future of Pediatric Emergency Nursing; Common Chief Complaints; Crisis Intervention; Musculoskeletal Trauma; Eye, Ear, Nose and Throat Emergencies*

Jeanette H. Walker, RN, BSN
Nurse Manager, Emergency Department and Rapid Treatment Unit
Primary Children's Medical Center
Salt Lake City, UT
Chapters: *Heat-related Emergencies; Cold-related Emergencies; Bites and Stings*

Elizabeth M. Wertz, RN, FACMPE
Executive Director
Pediatric Alliance, PC
Pittsburgh, PA
Chapter: *Children with Special Healthcare Needs*

Reviewers

Connie Carter, RN
Nurse Manager, Behavioral Health Unit
Primary Children's Medical Center
Salt Lake City, UT

Kristyne Dalrymple, RN
Pediatric Emergency Department
Primary Children's Medical Center
Salt Lake City, UT

Nanette C. Dudley, MD
Associate Professor, Pediatrics
University of Utah School of Medicine
Attending Physician, Emergency Department
Primary Children's Medical Center
Salt Lake City, UT

Ron Furnival, MD
Associate Professor, Pediatrics
University of Utah School of Medicine
Attending Physician, Emergency Department
Primary Children's Medical Center
Salt Lake City, UT

Paul J. Kapsar, Jr., RN, MSN, CRNP
MAJ AN USAR
Instructor of Nursing
University of Pittsburgh
Pittsburgh, PA

Lisa Maloney, RN, BSN
Community Outreach Nurse
Children's Hospital of Pittsburgh
Pittsburgh, PA

Mary Ann Maycock, RN, BSN
Pediatric Life Flight
Primary Children's Medical Center
Salt Lake City, UT

Julie A. Melini, RN, BSN, CEN
Safe and Healthy Families
Primary Children's Medical Center
Salt Lake City, UT

C. Richard Packer, MS, NREMT-P
Emergency Preparedness Coordinator
Southwest Districts
Pennsylvania Department of Health
Pittsburgh, PA

Mary Clyde Pierce, MD
Director, Child Advocacy Center
Children's Hospital of Pittsburgh
Pittsburgh, PA

Brenda Rines, RN, BSN
Charge Nurse, Emergency Department
Primary Children's Medical Center
Salt Lake City, UT

Sharon Smarto, RN, BSN
Logicare Coordinator
Children's Hospital of Pittsburgh
Pittsburgh, PA

Eva Vogeley, MD, JD
Assistant Professor of Pediatrics
University of Pittsburgh
Chairperson, Human Rights Committee
Children's Hospital of Pittsburgh
Pittsburgh, PA

CONTENTS

Section 2
Developmental Aspects of Pediatric Emergency Nursing

Section 3
Special Problems

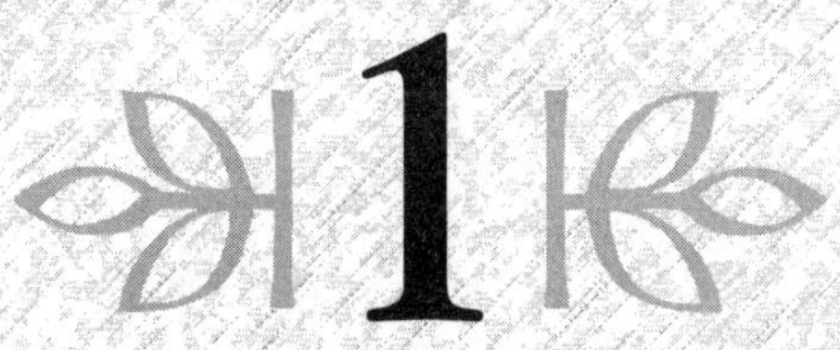

Management Issues

Donna Ojanen Thomas, RN, MSN
Lisa Marie Bernardo, RN, PhD, MPH

Introduction

Pediatric patients are seen in a variety of emergency department (ED) settings, from general EDs that deal with patients of all ages to pediatric EDs that exist within a pediatric specialty hospital. Pediatric patients represent more than 34% of all patients seen in the ED setting (Weiss, Mathers, Forjuoh, & Kinnane, 1997) (Table 1.1). Most often, the pediatric patient is integrated into the general ED, which has equipment and supplies to evaluate and care for children but no specific section or staff assigned to this care (Mellick & Asch, 1997). Increasingly, general EDs are recognizing that children require some special considerations not only for staffing, training, and equipment, but also in the design of the department.

Over the last several years, the types and numbers of pediatric patients seen in the ED are changing for many reasons, including (Eckle, Haley & Baker, 1998):

- Increased use for primary care. Many children lack health insurance and have no other place to go for care.
- More referrals by primary care physicians. Since the ED is open 24-hours per day, caregivers are often advised by their physician to come to the ED. In some hospitals, patients come to wait for an inpatient bed for admission to the hospital. Also, parents come seeking specialty care because it is quicker than waiting for an appointment.
- Higher survival rates and larger number of children with chronic illnesses. Because of advances in health care, many children are surviving what used to be fatal illnesses and injuries. They are also being sent home from the hospital sooner than they were in the past. Children also have "appliances," such as central lines, that require skill and training of ED staff to understand and manage.
- Increased violence against children.
- Infrequent use of emergency medical services (EMS) for emergencies. Because children can easily be transported, many families drive their children to an ED without involving EMS.
- Nonimmunized or underimmunized children. There has been an increase in the incidence of childhood diseases such as rubella because of the numbers of inadequately immunized children.

The emergence of pediatric emergency care as a separate and recognized discipline has significantly improved the care of infants, children, and adolescents in the ED (Eckle et al., 1998). The purpose of this chapter is to discuss management issues associated with treating children in the ED, including special considerations; staffing; orientation, continuing education, and resources; research; equipment; policies and procedures; disaster management; and quality management issues.

Special Considerations for Caring for the Child in the ED

In addition to the physiologic and psychosocial differences discussed throughout this book, the following points need to be considered, especially in planning pediatric care in a nonpediatric facility:

- Caring for children takes more resources. The younger the child, the more resources are needed to care for that child. Children are dependent on an adult for their care. They usually bring this adult and

TABLE 1.1 Epidemiology of Pediatric Emergency Care—Highlights of the National Hospital Ambulatory Medical Care Survey (NHAMCS) from 1992 and 1994

Total child and adolescent ED visits

- A total of 31,447,000 ED visits were made by children and adolescents (annual rate of 41.2 visits/100,000 persons). On average, a child or adolescent ED visit occurred every second.
- Children younger than 3 years of age composed the largest proportion of injury-related and medically related ED visits.
- The rate of pediatric and adolescent ED visits was greater in nonwhites (50.5/100,000) than in whites (38.9/100,000).
- Two-fifths of these ED visits were considered urgent or emergent.
- Six percent of the child and adolescent ED visits resulted in hospitalization.

Injury-related child and adolescent ED visits

- Of child and adolescent ED visits, 13,562,000 were injury-related (annual rate of 17.8/100,000).
- Sixty percent of injury-related ED visits were made by males.
- Falls were the leading mechanism of injury.
- Forty-four percent of the injuries occurred at home.
- About $4 billion per year was paid for injury-related ED visits.
- Twenty-eight percent of injury-related pediatric and adolescent ED visits were paid for in total or in part by government sources.

Medically related child and adolescent ED visits

- Of child and adolescent ED visits, 17,885,000 were medically related (annual rate of 23.4/100,000).
- Fifty-three percent of these medically related ED visits were made by females.
- Otitis media was the leading medically related diagnosis in children and adolescents.
- About $4.6 billion was paid for medically related diagnoses in children and adolescents.
- Forty-nine percent of medically related pediatric and adolescent ED visits were paid for in total or in part by government sources.

From: Weiss, H., Mathers, L., Forjuoh, S., & Kinnane, J. (1997). *Child and adolescent ED visit databook*. Pittsburgh: Center for Violence and Injury Control, Allegheny University of the Health Sciences. Single copies of the Databook are available at no cost from: Emergency Medical Services for Children (EMSC) Clearinghouse, 2070 Chain Bridge Road, Suite 450, Vienna, VA 22182-2536; Fax 703-821-8955. The Databook may be downloaded from the World Wide Web at www.pgh.auhs.edu/childed.

other family members with them to the hospital, which means that there are at least two persons with whom staff must interact. The family requires explanations and input on what needs to be done, and the child has to be convinced to cooperate with what will be done. Procedures such as catheterizations and intravenous insertions require two nurses, whereas in a cooperative, awake adult, only one nurse is needed.

- Caring for children takes more time. Preparing a child for a procedure and actually performing the procedure takes more time because a child generally will not be cooperative if something is perceived to be unpleasant or invasive. Many facilities have added child life professionals to the ED team to help assist the child and family during the ED visit.
- Children cannot communicate as effectively as adults, and often the effects of treatment are not readily apparent. Nurses need good assessment skills to notice subtle changes in the child's condition and must establish a relationship with the caregivers in a short time to develop trust in their assessment of the effects of treatment.
- Specialized equipment, such as airway management equipment, blood pressure cuffs, medications, and cribs (if patients are to be in the ED for extended times), is needed. This equipment is expensive, and its use requires training of staff, both of which add to the operating and capital budget of the department.
- A specialized area is needed to care for the child. Many general EDs have designated a pediatric area within the department, which may include a separate resuscitation area. This area usually has equipment and decor suitable for the child. Benefits of a

separate area include (Gausche, Rutherford, & Lewis, 1995):

- Isolation of patients most likely to have communicable disease, such as measles and chicken pox, may be needed.
- Medical equipment should be both age appropriate and easy to locate.
- Staffing can be modified to meet the needs of the pediatric patient in the ED.
- The patient care environment can be modified to better serve the pediatric patient.

- The serious illness, injury, or death of a child is very difficult for staff—even for those who routinely work with children. Child abuse, which has been on the increase over the years (Chapter 46) is especially hard, because staff must see first hand the often horrible injuries that people inflict on children. Often the hardest part of a pediatric resuscitation is to see the grief of the families. Staff need ways to cope with these events. Some methods for dealing with these situations are discussed in Chapter 28.
- Dealing with parents is often harder than dealing with the child. Parents who are worried about their child can become angry and confrontational. Staff need to understand that a parent's main concern is for his or her child and must learn how to deal with "difficult" families and help them without becoming defensive.

Staffing

Caring for pediatric patients takes more resources. Acuity systems that work for an adult patient will not be applicable to the pediatric patient. Separate acuity systems should be developed for pediatric patients. Patient acuity systems allow ED managers to determine the severity of patients' health conditions and to allocate resources appropriately (Bernardo, Smarto, & Henker, 1997). A system grounded in discharge diagnosis, using the depth of assessment, number of nursing diagnoses, and comprehensiveness of the plan of care, as well as its implementation and evaluation, can be predictive of severity of the health condition as well as hospital admissions (Bernardo et al., 1997). It will also allow the manager to plan staffing based on trends.

To assist with prediction of staffing needs, the following data have to be evaluated:

- Volume of pediatric patients. The age groups must be divided into appropriate categories, such as infant younger than 1 year, preschool-aged child (younger than 5 years), school-aged child (5 to 12 years), and the adolescent patient. The younger age groups generally are more dependent and take more time. They may also represent the largest volume of pediatric patients seen in the ED.
- Distribution of volume. The times of visits throughout the day and for specific seasons have to be evaluated. For example, many EDs see more children during the evening hours, when doctors' offices are closed. Lacerations, fractures, and other trauma are more common in the summer months, when school is out and there are more daylight hours. In the winter months, respiratory complaints may be more common. If volume distribution and seasonal trends are known, staffing can be planned based around this information.
- Types of illnesses and injuries seen in the pediatric population. These will vary according to the geographic location of the hospital. Injuries and severity of injuries differ in the general ED and the pediatric ED. The general ED treats a wide variety of pediatric patients but has a larger volume of minor trauma than does a pediatric ED (Nelson, Walsh, & Fleisher, 1992).

Time studies can be done to determine actual nursing time spent caring for children in different age groups and for different procedures. This process is tedious but will help to justify appropriate staffing. A good computerized database will be extremely useful in helping to collect some of the aforementioned information.

Other types of ancillary staff, such as child life specialist, may be helpful. A child life program in the ED can greatly assist in preparing children for procedures and providing age-appropriate diversional activities. Many EDs are beginning to provide this service, which has been shown to improve patient satisfaction and assist nursing staff in the ED (Christian & Thomas, 1998). This is an additional expense that more than pays for itself in the amount of goodwill it generates.

Orientation, Continuing Education, and Resources

The staff orientation and continuing education will depend on the types of illnesses and injuries seen in the pediatric population of the ED, including:

- Developmental and psychosocial considerations (Chapter 4). The Joint Commission on Accreditation of Healthcare Organizations (JCAHO) requires that staff receive training in age-related competencies. The Emergency Nurses Association (ENA) has developed educational strategies to meet these requirements (Emergency Nurses Association, 2000).
- Pediatric assessment. The ENA has developed the Emergency Nursing Pediatric Course (ENPC), which

covers all aspects of pediatric emergency nursing. Nurses working with children should be required to take this course as soon as possible after being hired.

- Pediatric triage. Triage categories are different for the pediatric patient. For example, fever may be a nonurgent condition in an adult. However, in a child younger than 2 months of age, this is an urgent condition. Triage is covered in the ENPC course and the ENA orientation program.
- Resuscitation and trauma. The Trauma Nursing Core Course (TNCC) includes content on pediatric trauma. An approved course in pediatric advanced life support should be taken by nurses who care for children. A plan for pediatric trauma should be developed, and agreements with pediatric tertiary care centers for the transfer of critically ill or injured children should be established (Chapter 10).

A core group of nurses who are specially trained in pediatric care could be developed so that at least one such nurse is on staff for each shift. Ideally, all nurses should be trained in pediatric emergency care. The ENA has additional pediatric-related education resources available to meet nurses' educational needs and to suggest standards of care (Table 1.2).

Another important resource is the Emergency Medical Services for Children (EMSC) model. An overview of this program is listed in Table 1.3.

TABLE 1.2 ENA Pediatric-Specific and Related Resources

- Point of View Series—CD-ROM
  - High-Risk Infants: ED Management of Preemies and Neonates
  - Prioritizing Pediatric Patients: Triage Decision-Making
- Comprehensive Care of the Pediatric Patient: Prehospital Rehabilitation
- Pediatric Pocket Guide
- Pediatric Emergency Nursing Manual
- Pediatric Emergency Nursing Resource Guide (Second Edition)
- Broselow Pediatric Resuscitation Tape
- Emergency Nursing Pediatric Course (ENPC)
  - Information Brochure
  - Teaching Resources
  - Pocket Review
- Presenting the Option for Family Presence
- Emergency Nurses Guide to Keeping Your Child Safe
- Age-Specific Competencies Resource Guide
- ENCARE Educational Materials
- ENA Position Statements
  - Care of the Pediatric Patient during Interfacility Transfer
  - Domestic Violence—Child Maltreatment and Human Neglect
  - Educational Recommendations for Nurses Providing Pediatric Emergency Care

(Contact 800-243-8362 for a resource guide and price list.)

TABLE 1.3 Overview of the Emergency Medical Services for Children (EMSC) Program

- Ensure state-of-the-art emergency medical care for ill or injured children and adolescents.
- Provide the integration of pediatric services into an emergency medical services system that is backed up by optimal resources.
- Ensure that the entire spectrum of emergency services, including prevention, acute care, and rehabilitation, is provided to all children and adolescents.

Emergency Medical Services for Children Program

Emergency Medical Services for Children (EMS-C) is specialized care for infants, children, and adolescents who have sustained a serious injury or illness. It is a comprehensive model that includes injury prevention strategies, emergency assessment and treatment, provider training, transportation, facilities, rehabilitation services, and contact with primary care physicians.

The federal EMS-C program promotes this comprehensive model to reduce pediatric deaths from injury and illness. Its goals are itemized in Table 1.3.

Federal EMS-C legislation was sponsored in 1984 and passed (Publ #98-555), and Congress approved a demonstration grant program for the states to expand access to and improve the quality of EMS-C in existing EMS systems.

The federal EMS-C program is administered jointly by the Maternal and Child Health Bureau in the Department of Health and Human Services and the National Highway Traffic Safety Administration (NHTSA) in the Department of Transportation. Grants are awarded to states for program planning and implementation of statewide EMS-C (state systems grants) and for specific activities to improve knowledge or develop and evaluate models or products (targeted issues grants). Almost all of the states and territories have received funding from the federal EMS-C program. Many states have enacted EMS-C laws, and others have created state offices or resource centers.

Educational products have been developed by many of the states and are available free or for a minimal cost through:

Emergency Medical Services for Children (EMS-C) Clearinghouse
2070 Chain Bridge Road, Suite 450
Vienna, VA 22182-2536
FAX 703-821-2098 Phone 703-821-8955
www.ems-c.org

The above data are adapted from *Emergency medical services for children*. Washington, DC: National Conference of State Legislatures (Perez, 1988).

Research

Nurses should be encouraged to participate and collaborate in research projects related to pediatric emergency care. Ways that emergency nurses can become involved in research include:

- Working with an established physician or nurse researcher to learn about the research process, from writing a proposal to entering data into the computer.
- Identifying problems or concerns. All research projects start with a simple question. It is important to ask a question that deserves an answer. Such questions may be epidemiologic ("How many newborns are being admitted for jaundice because of early hospital discharge?") or clinical ("Which topical analgesic is more effective in relieving pain during wound repair?"). Support should be garnered from the ED manager and staff.
- Reading the literature to learn more about the question. Other nurses or physicians may have answered the question or at least published a preliminary report. Textbooks, articles, and Internet resources are helpful in acquiring knowledge.
- Developing a plan for answering the question. It is helpful to collaborate with an established researcher, such as an ED nurse or physician or school of nursing faculty, to develop the research plan. This plan includes the methodology (e.g., randomized clinical trial or retrospective descriptive study) and data analysis.
- Writing the research plan in accordance with the hospital's institutional review board (IRB) guidelines (Chapter 2). Other nurses and physicians should be invited to read and critique the proposal. A mock intervention could be conducted, if needed, to identify any potential flaws or discrepancies.
- Revising the plan, as needed, and submitting it for IRB approval. The nurse should consider submitting the project to the ENA for funding.
- Moving forward with the research project once the proposal is approved. The researcher should expect delays and setbacks but must stay on track.
- Completing the study and writing up the results. The author should consider submitting the completed proposal for publication in the *Journal of Emergency Nursing* or the *International Journal of Trauma Nursing* and for presentation at Scientific Assembly or Leadership Challenge.

Many questions about clinical practice and ED usage in the pediatric population are raised, but few answers are offered. Emergency nurses are capable of becoming researchers through mentoring, a desire to seek new knowledge, and the search for answers to questions that will improve ED practice. Participation in interdisciplinary research allows health professionals to identify and study common issues in pediatric emergency care. This approach fosters communication and mutual respect, enhances collaborative practice, and adds to the knowledge of emergency care (Emergency Nurses Association, 1996).

Equipment

The National Emergency Medical Services for Children Resource Alliance has developed guidelines for pediatric equipment and supplies for ED (Committee on Pediatric Equipment and Supplies for Emergency Departments, National Emergency Medical Services for Children Resource Alliance, 1998). The guidelines contain lists of equipment that should be available at a minimum, and the committee recommends that this list be modified to meet the severity level of the patient population. These guidelines are shown in Table 1.4. The Committee also has made the following recommendations:

- Pediatric equipment and supplies should be organized separately and must be easily retrievable, either in a specific pediatric cart, pack, or section of the ED.
- When supplies and equipment are purchased, consideration should be given to the growing problem of latex sensitization of both patients and healthcare workers.
- ED staff members should be trained in the use of all equipment and supplies that are available for pediatric emergency care.
- Mock codes should be practiced to allow staff to find and use pediatric equipment.

Equipment is expensive. Small rural hospitals may be able to form buying cooperatives or even raise money through donations to purchase needed equipment. In some areas, pediatric hospitals may offer some supplies to hospital EDs that cannot purchase their own. A visit to a pediatric ED is often useful in determining equipment needs.

TABLE 1.4 Guidelines for Minimum Equipment and Supplies for Care of Pediatric Patients in EDs

Essential equipment and supplies

Monitoring

- Cardiorespiratory monitor with strip recorder
- Defibrillator (0 to 400 J capability) with pediatric and adult paddles (4.5 cm and 8 cm)
- Pediatric and adult monitor electrodes
- Pulse oximeter with sensors (sizes newborn through adult)
- Thermometer/rectal probe suitable for hypothermic and hyperthermic measurements with temperature capability from 25° to 44°C.
- Sphygmomanometer
- Doppler blood pressure device
- Blood pressure cuffs (neonatal, infant, child, adult, and thigh sizes)
- Method to monitor endotracheal tube and placement

Essential equipment and supplies

Vascular access

- Butterfly needles (19 to 25 gauge)
- Catheter-over-needle devices (14 to 24 gauge)
- Infusion device (to regulate rate and volume)
- Tubing for above
- Intraosseous needles (16 and 18 gauge; may be satisfied by standard bone marrow aspiration needles, 13 or 15 gauge)
- Arm boards (infant, child, and adult sizes)
- Intravenous fluid/blood warmers
- Umbilical vein catheters (sizes 3.5 French and 5 French; available within the hospital)
- Seldinger techniques vascular access kit (with pediatric sizes 3, 4, and 5, French catheters)

Airway management

- Clear oxygen masks (preterm, infant, child, and adult sizes)
- Nonrebreather masks (infant, child, and adult sizes)
- Oral airways (sizes 00 to 5)
- Nasopharyngeal airways (12 to 30 French)
- Bag-valve-mask resuscitator, self-inflating (450 and 1,000-mL sizes)
- Nasal cannulae (infant, child, and adult sizes)
- Endotracheal tubes, uncuffed (sizes 2.5 to 8.5) and cuffed (sizes 5.5 to 9)
- Stylets (pediatric and adult sizes)
- Laryngoscope handle (pediatric and adult)
- Magill forceps (pediatric and adult)
- Laryngoscope blades, curved (sizes 2.5 to 8.5) and straight (sizes 0 to 3)
- Nasogastric tubes (sizes 6 to 14 French)
- Suction catheters, flexible (sizes 5 to 16 French) and Yankauer suction tip
- Chest tube (sizes 8 to 40 French)
- Tracheostomy tubes (sizes 00 to 6); ensure availability within the hospital

Resuscitation medications (Chapters 14 and 15)

- Medication chart, tape, or other system to ensure ready access to information on proper per-kilogram doses for resuscitation drugs and equipment sizes
- System for estimating medication doses and supplies; may use the length-based method with color codes or another predetermined weight (kilogram/dose) method

TABLE 1.4 (continued)

Miscellaneous
- Infant and standard scales
- Infant formula and oral rehydrating solutions
- Heating source (may be met by infrared lamps or overhead warmer)
- Towel rolls, blanket rolls, or equivalent
- Pediatric restraining devices
- Resuscitation board
- Sterile linens (available within hospital for burn care)

Specialized pediatric trays
- Tube thoracostomy with water-seal drainage capability
- Lumbar puncture (spinal needle sizes 20, 22, and 25 gauge)
- Urinary catheterization with pediatric Foley catheters (size 5 to 16 French)
- Obstetric pack
- Newborn kit
  - Umbilical vessel cannulation supplies
  - Meconium aspirator
- Venous cut down
- Surgical airway kit (may include any of the following items: tracheotomy tray, cricothyrotomy tray, or endotracheal jet ventilation (needle jet)

Fracture management
- Cervical immobilization equipment (sizes child to adult). (Many types of cervical immobilization device are available. These include wedges and collars. The type of device chosen depends on local preferences, and policies and procedures. Whatever device is chosen should be stocked in sizes to fit infants, children, adolescents, and adults. The use of sandbags to meet this requirement is discouraged, because they may cause injury if the patient has to be turned.)
- Extremity splints
- Femur splints (child and adult sizes)

Desirable equipment and supplies

Medical photography equipment
- For documentation of injuries suspected to be caused by child maltreatment

From: Committee on Pediatric Equipment and Supplies for EDs, National Emergency Medical Services for Children Resource Alliance, 1998. Guidelines for pediatric equipment and supplies for EDs. *Annals of Emergency Medicine 31*(1), 56. Used with permission.

Policies and Procedures

Policies and procedures that apply to the adult patient do not always apply to the pediatric patient. Policies specific to pediatric patients must be developed for the following issues:

- Pediatric triage (Chapter 7).
- Frequency of vital signs and assessment.
- Administration of medications and the use of sedation.
- Parental presence during procedures.
- Child abuse and sexual assault protocols (Chapters 46 and 47).
- Follow-up visits and callbacks.
- Use of restraints.
- Transfer procedures and agreements.

Policies describing how certain procedures have to be performed also should be developed. There are many references to assist with this, including those listed in Table 1.2. Other pediatric hospitals are usually willing to share information, and national organizations, such as the ENA, are a great resource.

Evidence-Based Practice

Evidence-based practice is a method of incorporating research-based clinical decisions into practice (Cook &

Levy, 1998). This practice allows the critical evaluation of existing treatment recommendations prior to their implementation into practice (Smyth & Weindling, 1999). Evidence-based practice guidelines for pediatric emergency nursing care are being developed; one example is using evidence-based practice to treat hypothermia during pediatric trauma resuscitation (Bernardo, Henker, & O'Connor, 2000).

Practice guidelines can be useful in dealing with common pediatric complaints such as fever and respiratory distress. Some common conditions, such as croup, asthma, rule-out sepsis, and diabetic ketoacidosis, often fit well into care process models or clinical pathways. These practice guidelines provide a standard way of dealing with certain conditions and are easily measured for effectiveness. They may also expedite care of the child.

Disaster Management

A *disaster* is defined as any incident that results in multiple patients and an overload of either existing personnel or supplies and equipment, or that occurs in a situation where resources for backup or staff and equipment are not readily available in a reasonable amount of time. Disasters include natural occurrences, such as weather-related emergencies, or man-made acts, such as explosions and terrorist acts, as in the events of September 11. Pediatric considerations in disaster management include the following:

- Children's responses to disasters vary with their age and developmental status (Table 1.5). Early in the disaster, the children may experience denial, anger, guilt, or depression (Conway, Bernardo, & Tontala, 1990).
- More than one family member may be involved in a single incident, such as a hurricane or fire. When possible, the ED should accept all family members provided that the ED is prepared to provide the care they require (Augustine, 1995). This decision usually is made at the disaster site by the paramedics. If the family must be divided among institutions, communication must be assured among the family to afford proper information about the children's health history. Parental and family presence during a disaster is beneficial for children as they cope with the sudden changes of loss and destruction (Coffman, 1998). Plans to reunite the children and their families should be initiated as quickly as is feasible (Conway et al., 1990).
- Implied consent for evaluation and treatment must be evoked in cases of disasters or multi-incident scenarios (Augustine, 1995). Attempts to contact the parents and family are made accordingly.
- Healthcare professionals who can provide emotional support to children, such as child life specialists, child psychologists, and psychologists, should be included in the disaster response to help the children cope with the disaster situation (Conway et al., 1990). Provisions for follow-up counseling should be incorporated in the disaster plan; for example, the names and locations of qualified community mental health and other support agencies should be available.
- Decontamination following an exposure to hazardous materials may be necessary (Chapter 45).
- Debriefing may be required for the involved staff following a disaster that involves children (Chapter 28).
- Interventions for children and families following a disaster include individual, group, and family therapy; behavioral approaches; psychopharmacologic agents; and school-based programs (Pfefferbaum, 1998). Parents, teachers, nurses and others working closely with

TABLE 1.5 Children's Responses to Disasters

Age Group	*Responses*
Young children	Increased dependence on caregivers[1,3] Sleep disturbances[1,3] Developmental regression[1,2] Reexperiencing the event[2] Avoidance[2] Arousal
School age	Psychosomatic complaints[3] Depression/feelings of loss (if separated from peers)[3] Avoidance of previously enjoyed activities[4]
Adolescents	Stress-aggravated illness[3] Difficulty concentrating[4] Decreased interest in activities[4]

[1]American Academy of Pediatrics, 1999
[2]Gurwitch, Sullivan, & Long, 1998
[3]Coffman, 1998
[4]Garrison, Bryant, Addy, Spurrier, Freedy, & Kilpatrick, 1995

children should be taught to recognize and address children's responses to the disaster (Pfefferbaum, 1998).

Quality Management Issues

Emergency departments treating children should be involved in activities that evaluate the quality of care given to children. Most hospitals use separate indicators to monitor the care of pediatric patients in the ED (Gausche, Rutherford, & Lewis, 1995). This is necessary because adult indicators do not always fit pediatric patients. For example, chest pain is a common complaint monitored by quality management activities in the adult setting. In the pediatric patient, however, the care of an infant with fever is a more important indicator, because missed meningitis accounts for the largest financial loss in pediatric emergency medicine (Felter & Yama, 1992).

The development of indicators may be guided by the high-risk, problem-prone diagnoses seen in the pediatric population in a given area. A national survey showed the following to be typical indicators monitored (Gausche et al., 1995):

- Deaths occurring in the ED.
- Comparison of radiologist and ED physician reports. Missed fractures result in the highest numbers of lawsuits against emergency physicians (Felter & Yama, 1992).
- Cardiopulmonary resuscitation performed in the ED.
- The patient returned to ED within 48 hours for same complaint. Monitoring such repeat visits will help identify common problems that frequently result in return to the ED.
- The patient and caregiver left without being seen. A process should be in place to follow up with any patient who leaves prior to being seen or before care was completed.
- The patient was evaluated but vital signs were not documented.
- Child abuse or sexual abuse was suspected.
- Administration of antibiotics was delayed in a patient with a diagnosis of meningitis.

Parent complaints should also be monitored for trends. Typically, the following complaints are received in the pediatric ED (Burstein & Fleisher, 1991; Hanson, Clifton-Smith, & Fasher, 1994):

- Quality-of-care issues.
- Billing.
- Waiting times for nonurgent disorders.

Parents of children with more emergent complaints generally complain less than do those of children with urgent or nonurgent complaints (Chande, Bhende, & Davis, 1991; Hanson et al., 1994). This supports the development of programs that may expedite the care of patients with nonurgent complaints. Assessment of complaints is also useful to highlight areas of dissatisfaction and to develop plans to improve patient care.

The number of ED complaints can be reduced if good communication with patients and families is established while they are in the ED. Patients' perceptions of waiting and delays in attention or treatment have a significant effect on their satisfaction (Hall & Press, 1996). Some suggestions for good communication are listed below:

- Keep the family updated about how long they may have to wait.
- Communicate often with the family—each person who enters the room should let the family know what will happen next.
- Let the family know when specialists have been contacted and any delays that may occur.
- Give good follow-up instructions to the family.
- Apologize for delays and do not become defensive or make excuses; tell the truth.

Collection of Data

To facilitate quality improvement, research, and other patient information-related activities, the collection of uniform data elements is valuable. Standardized data elements, such as patient age and triage time, lend themselves to valid comparison among institutions and allow for the study and analysis of ED patient usage and trends.

Data Elements for Emergency Department Systems (DEEDS) is a recommended, standardized set of 156 data elements that EDs can use for patient record keeping. The DEEDS set was developed in collaboration with the Centers for Disease Control and Prevention and with public-private partnerships (including the Emergency Nurses Association). These data elements are organized into eight sections; the number of elements used to complete a patient's ED record will vary according to the complexity of the patient's health problem and the extent of ED care (DEEDS Writing Committee, 1998). A free copy of DEEDS can be obtained from the National Center for Injury Prevention and Control, Centers for Disease Control and Prevention, Atlanta, GA 30341-3724. It can be downloaded from the NCIPC web site: http://www.cdc.gov/ncipc/pubres/deedspage.htm.

Conclusion

Caring for children takes time, resources, and planning. The EMS-C Program has a new 5-year plan to promote ongoing efforts to improve and expand emergency medical services for children, from prehospital to rehabilitation to community integration. Emergency nurses can use this plan as a guide for promoting pediatric emergency care in their hospitals. An additional resource is the EMS-C Program's Resource Kit, a CD-ROM containing over 2,000 pages of information on injury and illness prevention, treatment, and rehabilitation. Both the 5-year plan and Resource Kit are available at www.ems-c.org.

General EDs must evaluate their pediatric populations and develop ways to educate staff to care for children and provide appropriate equipment. Additional staff may be necessary to meet the needs of the child. Having appropriate numbers of properly trained staff and the right equipment will improve both the comfort level of staff caring for children and the quality of care that is given.

References

American Academy of Pediatrics. (1999). How pediatricians can respond to the psychosocial implications of disasters (RE9813). *Pediatrics, 103*(2), 521-523.

Augustine, J. (1995). Pediatric trauma triage and major incident management. In A. Dietrich & S. Shaner (Eds.), *Pediatric basic trauma life support* (pp. 108-113). Oakbrook Terrace, IL: Basic Trauma Life Support International.

Bernardo, L., Henker, R., & O'Connor, J. (2000). Evidence based practice: Treatment of hypothermia during pediatric trauma resuscitation. *American Journal of Critical Care Nursing, 9*(4), 227-236.

Bernardo, L. M., Smarto, S., & Hencker, R. (1997). Validation of a patient acuity system for a pediatric ED [Abstract]. *Journal of Emergency Nursing 23*(2), 100.

Burstein, J., & Fleisher, G. R. (1991). Complaints and compliments in the pediatric ED. *Pediatric Emergency Care, 7*(3), 138-140.

Chande, V. T., Bhende, M. S., & Davis, H. W. (1991). Pediatric ED complaints: A three-year analysis of sources and trends. *Annals of Emergency Medicine, 20*(9), 1014-1020.

Christian, B., & Thomas, D. (1998). A child life program in one pediatric ED. *Journal of Emergency Nursing 24*(4), 359-361.

Coffman, S. (1998). Children's reactions to disaster. *Journal of Pediatric Nursing, 13*(6), 376-382.

Committee on Pediatric Equipment and Supplies for Emergency Departments, National Emergency Medical Services for Children Resource Alliance. (1998). Guidelines for pediatric equipment and supplies for EDs. *Annals of Emergency Medicine 31*(1), 54-57.

Conway, A., Bernardo, L., & Tontala, K. (1990). The effects of disasters on children: Implications for emergency nurses. *Journal of Emergency Nursing, 16*(6), 393-395.

Cook, D., & Levy, M. (1998). Evidence-based medicine: A tool for enhancing critical care practice. *Critical Care Clinics, 14*(3), 353-358.

DEEDS Writing Committee. (1998). Data elements for ED systems, Release 1.0 (DEEDS): A summary report. *Journal of Emergency Nursing, 24*(1), 36-44.

Eckle, N., Haley, K., & Baker, P. (Eds.) (1998). *Emergency nursing pediatric course, provider manual* (2nd ed.) Park Ridge, IL: Emergency Nurses Association.

Emergency Nurses Association (1996). *Collaborative and Interdisciplinary Research*. Des Plaines, IL: Author.

Emergency Nurses Association (2000). *Age-Specific Competencies Resource Guide*. Des Plaines, IL: Author.

Felter, R. A., & Yama, J. (1992). Quality improvement. In R. M. Barkin (Ed.), *Pediatric emergency medicine. Concepts and clinical practice* (pp. 66-70). St. Louis, Mosby.

Garrison, C., Bryant, E., Addy, C., Spurrier, P., Freedy, J., & Kilpatrick, D. (1995). Posttraumatic stress disorder in adolescents after Hurricane Andrew. *Journal of the American Academy of Child and Adolescent Psychiatry, 34*(9), 1193-1201.

Gausche, M., Rutherford, M., & Lewis, R. (1995). Emergency department quality assurance/improvement practices for the pediatric patient. *Annals of Emergency Medicine 25*(6), 804-808.

Gurwitch, R., Sullivan, M., & Long, P. (1998). The impact of trauma and disaster on young children. *Child and Adolescent Psychiatric Clinics of North America, 7*(1), 19-32.

Hall, M. F., & Press, I. (1996). Keys to patient satisfaction in the ED: Results of a multiple facility study. *Hospital and Health Services Administration 41*(4), 515-532.

Hanson, R., Clifton-Smith, B., & Fasher, B. (1994). Patient dissatisfaction in a pediatric accident emergency department. *Journal of Quality Clinical Practice, 14*(3), 137-143.

Mellick, L. B., & Asch, S. M. (1997). Pediatric ED environment. In R. M. Barkin (Ed.), *Pediatric emergency medicine. Concepts and clinical practice* (2nd ed., pp. 8-14). St. Louis: Mosby.

Nelson, D. S., Walsh, K., & Fleisher, G. R. (1992). Spectrum and frequency of pediatric illness presenting to a general community hospital ED. *Pediatrics 90*(1, Pt. 1):5-10.

Pfefferbaum, B. (1998). Caring for children affected by disaster. *Child and Adolescent Psychiatric Clinics of North America, 7*(3), 579-597.

Smyth, R., & Weindling, A. (1999). Research in children: Ethical and scientific aspects. *Lancet, 354* (suppl II), SII21-24.

Weiss, H., Mathers, L., Forjuoh, S., & Kinnane, J. (1997). *Child and adolescent ED visit databook*. Pittsburgh: Center for Violence and Injury Control, Allegheny University of the Health Sciences.

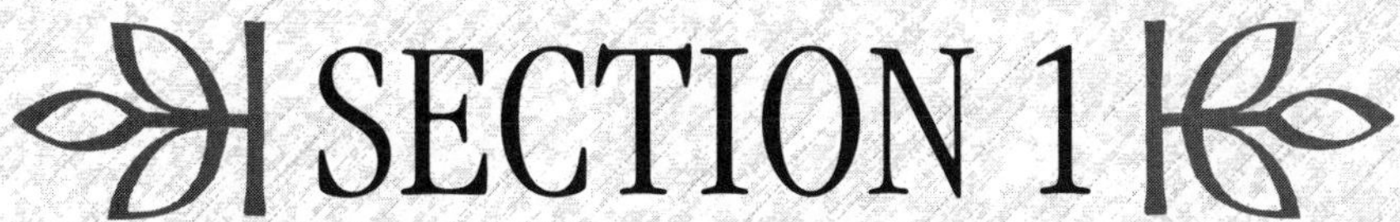

SECTION 1

Overview of Pediatric Emergency Nursing

2

Ethical and Legal Issues

Lisa Marie Bernardo, RN, PhD, MPH
Deborah Lesniak, RN, MS

Introduction

Emergency nurses face ethical and legal issues when caring for infants, children, and adolescents. These issues relate to assent and consent for treatment or research protocols, as well as legal requirements for transferring and transporting patients from the emergency department (ED). The purpose of this chapter is to highlight pertinent ethical and legal issues and to describe factors that nurses should consider when faced with such issues.

Under EMTALA (Emergency Medical Treatment and Active Labor Act), all patients, including pediatric patients, must receive a medical screening examination (Mitchner & Yeh, 2002, Guertler, 1997). This examination takes place with or without parental presence or consent. Therefore, any pediatric patient presenting to the ED for treatment is triaged and evaluated to determine if an emergency exists. After this evaluation, the ED physician determines if waiting for parental consent is appropriate; it would be negligent to delay care while trying to obtain parental consent if the patient requires emergency care (Guertler, 1997, p. 311).

Ethical Issues

Informed Consent

Consent is an individual's approval of or compliance with a proposed plan of action. Only patients who have appropriate decisional capacity and legal empowerment can give their informed consent to medical care. In all other situations, parents or other surrogates provide informed permission (Table 2.1) for diagnosis and treatment of children, with the assent of the child whenever appropriate (Committee on Bioethics, 1995, p. 314). In particular,

- Infants cannot provide consent for proposed treatment.
- Young children are unable to give definitive direction or an informed consent about their treatment; their values and desires may not be well articulated, and their appreciation of the consequences of treatment options may be lacking (Fleischman et al., 1994).
- School-aged children can give assent for treatment, along with their parents' informed permission.
- Adolescents can give consent for treatment if they are emancipated or mature minors (Table 2.2).

The law always implies parental consent and permission for a child's treatment in the event of an emergency; the child's life and health should never be compromised by a delay in treatment to obtain a parent's consent (Sullivan, 1993, p. 841; Guertler, 1997). Although the definition of an emergency has not been agreed on legally, it is safe to assume that an emergency

TABLE 2.1 Elements of Informed Permission

Information and explanations appropriate to the parents' level of understanding regarding the nature of their child's health condition.
The proposed diagnostic and treatment plans and their probability for success.
The potential risks and benefits of the proposed treatment.
The existence, benefits, and risks of alternative treatments, including no treatment.
An assessment of the parents' understanding of the above information.
An assessment of the parents' ability to make an informed decision/give informed permission.
An assurance that the decision is made without coercion or manipulation.

From: Committee on Bioethics. (1995). Informed consent, parental permission, and assent in pediatric practice. *Pediatrics, 95*(2) 315.

TABLE 2.2 Consent Situations with Families and Minors

Situation	*Consent Considerations*
Emancipated minors—minors who are self-supporting; not subject to parental control; not living at home; married; pregnant or a parent; or in the military (Committee on Bioethics, 1995; Sullivan, 1993; Fleischman et al., 1994; Guertler, 1997)	Able to give consent for medical treatment (Guertler, 1997). Initiate ED medical screening and treatment.
Mature minors (age range of 14–18 years, which varies among the states); unemancipated minors who understand the nature and risks of treatment; if the treatment is for their benefit; serious risk is not involved; and the ED physician believes the minor can make an informed decision (Committee on Bioethics, 1995; Guertler, 1997)	Able to seek or refuse emergency and nonemergency treatment. Statutes on treatment of minors vary among the states. These statutes allow minors to consent for treatment without parental involvement for such health conditions as sexually transmitted diseases, pregnancy, drug or alcohol abuse, and psychiatric problems (Sullivan, 1993; Committee on Bioethics, 1995; Guertler, 1997). Initiate ED medical screening and treatment.
Divorced or separated parents—parent with custodial authority	The custodial parent has the duty to obtain treatment and give consent/permission; permission does not need to be obtained from the noncustodial parent (Sullivan, 1993). Initiate ED medical screening and treatment.
Divorced parents—parent without custodial authority	Assume that the accompanying parent has authority to give consent/permission for treatment; while the parent may not retain the right or duty to provide treatment, the emergency care is provided as necessary (Sullivan, 1993). Initiate ED medical screening and treatment.
Divorced parents—joint custody	Assume parental authority to give consent/permission for treatment (Sullivan, 1993). Initiate ED medical screening and treatment.
Minors with a nonparental adult (guardianship or legal custody *in loco parentis*)	Other care can be initiated if the adult has guardianship or legal custody for the minor's health needs (Sullivan, 1993). Document the situation in the medical record, including attempts to contact the parents (Committee on Pediatric Emergency Medicine, 1993). Initiate ED medical screening and treatment.
Minors residing in foster care	Some states may allow for the individual or institution with custody to give consent/permission for treatment. For high-risk or elective procedures, parental consent/permission may need to be obtained (Sullivan, 1993; Committee on Pediatric Emergency Medicine, 1993). Initiate ED medical screening and treatment.
Minors in detention facilities	Parental consent/permission for routine health care is not needed. For high-risk or elective procedures, parental consent/permission may need to be obtained (Sullivan, 1993). Parental consent for low-risk emergency treatment may not be needed (Billittier, Lillis, & Lerner, 1996). Initiate ED medical screening and treatment.
Minors in camp, boarding school, and other locations	Parents usually sign a notarized, blanket consent (*in loco parentis*) for camp or school officials to consent for routine medical care (Billittier, Lillis, & Lerner, 1996). Parents must give consent/permission for high-risk or elective treatment (Sullivan, 1993). Initiate ED medical screening and treatment.
Runaway minors	Attempt to contact parents. If the minor refuses to identify the parents and the health care is routine, initiate the care. Contact legal counsel for high-risk or elective treatments (Sullivan, 1993). Initiate ED medical screening and treatment.

exists when immediate treatment is necessary to preserve a child's life or to prevent permanent disability, alleviate pain and suffering, and avoid eventual harm (Sullivan, 1993; Guertler, 1997). Similarly, immediate treatment to alleviate pain and suffering can be determined to be an emergency (Sullivan, 1993). If the child needs immediate assessment and treatment, and the treatment would have to be delayed to obtain parental consent, the emergency care professionals should initiate care (Sullivan, 1993). No emergency evaluation should be delayed because of inability to obtain parental consent or authorization for payment (Committee on Pediatric Emergency Medicine, 1993; Guertler, 1997). These guidelines apply to out-of-hospital pediatric emergency care as well (Billittier et al., 1996).

Assent

Assent is obtained from the child 7 years of age and older to help the child achieve a developmentally appropriate awareness of the health condition. Assent includes (Committee on Bioethics, 1995, p. 315):

- Telling the child what to expect during the proposed tests and procedures.
- Assessing the child's understanding of the situation, as well as any circumstances that may be influencing the child's response.
- Soliciting the child's willingness to participate in the proposed care.

In certain situations, the child's agreement to participate in the treatment plan is not obtained because of the severity of the situation or the best interests of the child (i.e., a 4-year-old, afraid of "shots," refuses an intravenous infusion for dehydration). The emergency care team still involves the child in discussions about his or her health care, though, by offering the child choices ("In which hand do you want your IV?"), which may foster the child's trust of healthcare professionals (Committee on Bioethics, 1995). The older the child, the more the child should be permitted to participate in the decisions affecting his or her health (Thewes, FitzGerald, & Sulmasy, 1996).

Nursing Considerations in Consent and Assent for Treatment

Because emergency treatment is never withheld until parental consent is obtained, interventions to save a child's life or to alleviate pain and suffering are initiated.

- Another staff member, such as a nurse, physician, or social worker, initiates efforts to locate the parents and obtain consent for treatment. These attempts are documented on the emergency record (Sullivan, 1993).
- Even though fear of legal repercussions surrounding treatment of adolescents without parental consent may arise, no cases in which a parent has successfully sued a physician for the care of an adolescent have been reported in the past 30 years (Sullivan, 1993).
- Emergency nurses should consult with their hospital's legal counsel to determine what their state's laws or legislation deem to be an emergency.

Parents should be encouraged to provide a written consent statement for nonelective health care for the child when the parents may not be available, such as when the child is in a child care setting, at camp, or with noncustodial relatives (Committee on Pediatric Emergency Medicine, 1993). They also should be encouraged to complete the emergency information cards provided in schools and camps. Necessary information includes the parents' home and work telephone numbers, immunizations, allergies, chronic health problems, and the primary healthcare provider's name and telephone number (Committee on Pediatric Emergency Medicine, 1993). Electronic mail (e-mail) addresses and cellular phone numbers should be included when available.

Children should be taught their home addresses, their telephone numbers, and the names of their parents' workplaces in the event of an unexpected visit to the ED (Committee on Pediatric Emergency Medicine, 1993).

Refusal of Treatment, Leaving without Being Seen, Elopement, Leaving against Medical Advice

Children are not considered cognitively or legally capable of refusing emergency care because they cannot fully understand the long-term consequences of such a refusal. However, the child's reluctance or refusal to participate should be respected when the proposed procedure is not essential to the child's welfare and/or can be deferred without a substantial risk to the child's health (Committee on Bioethics, 1995, p. 316). Adolescents may refuse care if they are (Sullivan, 1993):

- Emancipated (Table 2.2).
- A mature minor (Table 2.2).
- Meet one of the minor treatment statutes.

Adolescents and older children may refuse to participate in treatment plans, presenting the emergency professionals with an ethical or legal quandary. Up to the age of legal majority (18 years in most states), no specific criteria of chronologic ages, developmental levels, or physical maturity exist whereby all adolescents can be permitted to independently make healthcare decisions, such as refusing care (Fleischman et al., 1994). Such situations may arise in the adolescent in the end stages of a terminal disease—the adolescent does not want treatment to progress, while the family wishes otherwise. The patient's refusal should be accepted under the "mature minor" exception or may be covered by statutes concerning substance abuse or sexually transmitted diseases (Guertler, 1997, p. 311). Emergency professionals must collaborate with the adolescent and family to propose an acceptable plan of care.

Emergency professionals may encounter situations in which the parents refuse emergency treatment for their child. "Parents do not have the authority to forbid saving their child's life" (Sullivan, 1993, p. 847). In a life-threatening situation, when parents refuse emergency intervention, temporary protective custody measures are initiated based on child neglect (Sullivan, 1993; Guertler, 1997).

Parents may refuse treatment based on religious freedom; however, it has been determined that denying treatment to a child is not within the parents' First Amendment right of freedom of religion (Sullivan, 1993, p. 847; Guertler, 1997). Again, temporary protective custody measures may be initiated. When the child's life is not threatened and there is no serious risk to the child's health, the parents' refusal is respected and documented (Sullivan, 1993). This refusal is an informed one, meaning that the parents understand the risks or refusal, have asked questions, and are prepared to leave against medical advice (AMA). This situation differs from that of adolescents or parents who leave the ED prior to being evaluated by a physician (leaving without being seen) and from that of adolescents or parents who leave the ED prior to hospitalization or transfer to another facility (elopement). A comparison of these issues is outlined in Table 2.3.

Nursing Considerations in Refusal-of-Treatment Issues

Children demonstrate their refusal of treatment through physical means (kicking or screaming) or by attempting to leave the ED. Efforts to calm the child and to ascertain the reasons for the refusal should ensue. The child may have a misunderstanding about the treatment plan, or the plan may not have been explained properly. It is inadvisable to proceed against the child's wishes until such time that all explanations have been exhausted. If the treatment must ensue despite the child's refusal, the child should be informed of that fact (Committee on Bioethics, 1995).

Adolescents' refusal of treatment, if not reconciled through mediation with an ethics consultant, social worker, or other healthcare professional, should be respected; parents should be informed by the health professionals that they cannot morally accept surrogate (parents') decision making for a patient who is autonomous (Fleischman et al., 1994, p. 437).

Parents, too, may need extra time to fully understand the proposed treatment plan for their child. Including a social worker or patient advocate in the discussion may help parents understand the gravity of the situation. Contacting the family healthcare provider may also be of benefit. If parents leave before their child has been seen, the triage nurse's documentation should be reviewed to determine the urgency of the child's health condition. If the illness or injury is deemed serious, an attempt should be made to contact the family by telephone. All families who leave without being seen should be contacted within a specified time period (e.g., 48 hours) by an ED staff member to ascertain the patient's health status and to promote positive customer service.

When adolescents or parents choose to leave AMA, the ED should have a specific form for the adolescent or parent to sign that demonstrates their understanding of the child's health condition and the consequences of refusing proper treatment. If the ED staff believe that it is not in the child's best interest to leave the ED, a court order may be obtained to prevent the parents from removing the child from the hospital. For patients who

TABLE 2.3 Comparison of Treatment Refusals

Refusal	*Description*
Leaving without being seen by a physician (LWOT)	The child and family arrive in the ED, are evaluated by the triage nurse, and then leave prior to a physician evaluation. Often they tell no one of their intentions; their absence is detected when they are called to enter an examination room.
Leaving against medical advice (LAMA)	The child and family arrive in the ED and receive an examination from the ED physician. The physician recommends a specific treatment that the parent chooses not to accept, such as a diagnostic procedure or hospital admission.
Elopement	The child and family arrive in the ED and receive an examination from the ED physician. While the course of treatment is planned, or after the treatment has been decided, the child and family are missing, presumably having left the ED. No further treatment can be made.

elope, depending on their health condition, hospital police or other legal officers may have to become involved to bring the child and family back to the ED.

EDs should have policies and procedures in place for parents and adolescents who refuse ED treatment.

Consent to Research

Research in emergency care is an important process that allows the development of beneficial treatments and procedures. Emergency care research is subject to the review process of the hospital's institutional review board (IRB), as outlined by the Department of Health and Human Services (DHHS). The IRB assures that the proposed research is sound and that the risks to the patients and families are minimized (Spivey, Abramson, Iserson, MacKay, & Cohen, 1991). Because children requiring emergency care are a vulnerable population, the IRB assures that appropriate safeguards are in place to minimize research-associated risks.

The National Institutes of Health (NIH) has a policy and guidelines for including children as participants in research involving human subjects (NIH, 1998). The NIH states that "children (individuals < 21 years of age) must be included in all human subjects research conducted or supported by the NIH unless there are scientific and ethical reasons not to include them" (NIH, 1998, p. 2). Reasons for not including children in human subjects research are (NIH, 1998, p. 3):

- The research topic is irrelevant to children.
- Existing laws or regulations bar the inclusion of children in the research, such as projects that would require a higher level of risk.
- The knowledge to be gained from having children participate in the study is available, and an additional study would be redundant.
- A separate age-specific study is warranted.
- Insufficient data from adult subjects are available to judge the benefits and risks of the proposed intervention in children.
- The study involves a longitudinal design that collects data on pre-enrolled adult subjects.
- Other special cases not outlined above are described by the NIH (1998).

Prior to their children's participation in research, parents are required to give their informed consent (permission). Elements of informed consent for research, as outlined by the DHHS Regulations for the Protection of Human Research Subjects, are found in Table 2.4. These elements must be detailed in a consent form that is signed by the parent and researcher. Research has shown that such consent forms for pediatric research are written at a graduate-school reading level (Tarnowski, Allen, Mayhall, & Kelly, 1990), whereas the readability of consent forms in emergency medicine required a 10th grade education (Mader & Playe, 1997). Thus, the investigator must ensure that parents understand the research protocol prior to their child's enrollment.

TABLE 2.4 Elements of Informed Consent for Research

An explanation of the research study's purpose
The expected length of participation
A description of the study protocol or procedures
The identification of experimental procedures
An explanation of the potential risks or discomfort and measures to modify the risks
A description of benefits to the subject or to others
An explanation of any alternative treatments or procedures that might be advantageous
A description of confidentiality and/or anonymity methods for protecting the subjects and notice that the U.S. Food and Drug Administration may inspect the research records (in drug research)
An explanation of compensation for treatment should injury occur and where further information could be obtained
The name of a person to contact for answers to pertinent research-related questions, a description of the subject's research-related rights, and the name of a person to contact if a research-related injury is sustained
A statement that the consent is voluntary and that refusal or withdrawal involves no penalty or loss of entitled benefits

Adapted from: Tarnowski, Allen, Mayhall, & Kelly, 1990; Committee on Drugs, 1995; Department of Health and Human Services, Food and Drug Administration, 1993, pp. 2-30.

Prior to their participation in research, children are required to give their assent. Assent is "a cooperative process between children and researchers involving disclosure and discussion of the research project" (Lindeke, Hauck, & Tanner, 2000). Assent gives children an opportunity to discuss their views and concerns about the proposed research and indicates that the researcher respects children's rights and responsibilities as a research subject (Lindeke et al., 2000). Since 1983, children aged 7–18 years have been required to give their assent for research participation, and research protocols must have a process for obtaining and documenting this assent (Lindeke et al., 2000). The age of 7 years is used because Piagetian theory purports that by this age children can understand concrete explanations given to them (Thurber, Deatrick, and Grey, 1992). Assent includes the study's purpose, expectations, and risks and benefits, explained in age-appropriate language and methods.

Such methods include videotapes, peer discussions, and written materials (Broome, 1999). Children need to sign the assent form and take a copy with them, similar to informed consent forms signed and retained by parents.

Dissent is children's refusal to participate in a research study. Exploring children's fears and concerns about the research may help them understand their participation in the study. However, researchers must be careful not to coerce the child's participation. Because children are taught to obey and respect those in authority, they may submit to the researcher's or parents' desires to participate, even if they do not wish to participate. Researchers must remind children and families that their care will not be affected by their decision to not participate in the study (Lindeke et al., 2000). Children's dissent must be considered binding, especially in nontherapeutic research (Broome, 1999). Dissent may be overruled by parental consent in a situation where the children's research participation is of clear benefit (Lindeke et al., 2000). If children's dissent is overruled, the surrounding circumstances are recorded and explained to the children and families (Committee on Bioethics, 1995).

Nursing Considerations in Research Consent and Assent

Children should be given ample time to ask questions and to be informed of the expectations of participating in the research study (Thurber et al., 1992). In one study examining the capacity of children, adolescents, and young adults to assent and consent to research participation, most of the subjects knew the benefits to themselves for participating, the length of the research, their role, their freedom to ask questions, and the voluntary nature of their participation (Susman, Dorn, & Fletcher, 1992). Fewer than half of the subjects understood the research purpose, the benefits to others, alternative treatments, their freedom to withdraw, the procedures, and the risks of the study protocol (Susman et al., 1992). Therefore, research subjects' understanding of the research protocol and their participation should be ascertained.

Resuscitation Research

Conducting research in children who require resuscitation (i.e., trauma arrest) presents a unique problem because of the vulnerability of this population. These patients cannot give their assent or consent, and parents may not be available to give their consent or permission because they may be unavailable, delayed, or involved in the trauma themselves. These patients are not only vulnerable to research risks but are vulnerable to being denied potentially beneficial treatment when no known effective treatment for their life-threatening condition exists (Biros, Lewis, Olson, Runge, Cumins, & Frost, 1995).

The Food and Drug Administration (FDA) published the "Informed Consent and Waiver of Informed Consent Requirements in Certain Emergency Research Rule" (the Final Rule) on November 1, 1996, to assure proper protection of human subjects during resuscitation research (Table 2.5).

To effectively enact the Final Rule, safeguards must be in place to protect enrolled patients (Biros, Runge, Lewis, & Doherty, 1998):

- Public disclosure must occur before and after the study.
- An Investigational New Drug (IND) application or Investigational Device Exemption (IDE) must be filed with the FDA.
- The community must be consulted.
- An independent monitoring committee must be established and approved by the IRB.
- The investigators must inform the patient or family as soon as possible to obtain consent for the patient to continue in the protocol.

Nursing Considerations in Resuscitation Research

Emergency nurses can serve as members of their hospital's IRB to advocate for children and families involved in research. Becoming involved in their hospital's ethics committee and being acquainted with the hospital's

TABLE 2.5 Guidelines for Resuscitation Research

The health condition must be life-threatening.
Standard or available treatments are unproven or unsatisfactory.
The proposed research cannot be practically conducted otherwise.
The proposed research is necessary to determine the effectiveness of the study intervention.
It is not feasible to obtain informed consent from the patient or the patient's family.
The risks and benefits of the proposed treatment are reasonable compared to those risks and benefits associated with the standard or usual treatment.

Adapted from: *ACEP News*, (November, 1996), 15(10), 10, 11, 15; Department of Health and Human Services, 1996, Food and Drug Administration. *Federal Register, 61*(192), 21 CFR Parts 50, 56, 312, 314, 601, 812, 814).

legal counsel are ways in which emergency nurses can serve as patient advocates.

Pharmaceutical Research

Drugs must be studied in children to determine their safety and efficacy because growth and maturation can alter the kinetics, organ responses, and toxicities of drugs in neonates, infants, children, and adolescents (Committee on Drugs, 1995). Generally, drug studies in children are undertaken once initial adult clinical trials have been completed. There are four phases of drug studies: Phase I: clinical pharmacology (initial introduction into the human population); Phase II: clinical investigation (demonstration of drug effectiveness and safety); Phase III: clinical trials (effectiveness and drug-related adverse effects); Phase IV: postmarketing clinical trials (larger-scale trials). Drug studies must include measures to protect children's rights, as in other clinical investigations, and must follow the same procedures for informed consent and assent. Numerous safeguards must be in place for vulnerable pediatric patients, such as children with disabilities, children living in institutions, those requiring emergency care, dying children, children with chronically progressive or potentially fatal disease, and the newly dead (e.g., brain death) (Committee on Drugs, 1995).

Nursing Considerations in Pharmaceutical Research

Emergency nurses may care for patients who are enrolled in drug studies involving chemotherapeutic agents, vaccine combinations, or other adjunctive therapies. The emergency physician will need to contact the researcher during ED treatment to inform the researcher about the patient's condition. Generally, in double-blinded randomized clinical trials, the blinding will not need to be broken. The researcher will have to decide if the patient's ED visit is related to the study treatment, which would be considered a serious adverse event. The researcher will follow up with the patient after ED treatment.

Emergency nurses may be asked to administer drugs to patients enrolled in pharmaceutical research. Because this research often involves randomized clinical trials, the study drugs will be "blinded" to the nurses. Nurses, then, will not know if they are administering a drug or a placebo. Emergency nurses should share any concerns about their participation in randomized clinical trials with the study's investigators. Nurses' and investigators' financial relationships with the sponsoring drug company must be disclosed to avoid a conflict of interest. Nurses may receive a "bonus" for enrolling study patients; any rewards must be commensurate with the investigator's efforts to avoid bias or undue influence on reported results (Committee on Drugs, 1995).

Legal Issues

Numerous legal considerations confront emergency nurses as they care for children and families. These legal issues range from appropriate screening and assessment to end-of-life decisions. This section outlines the basic legal ramifications faced by emergency nurses as they care for children and families.

Consolidated Omnibus Reconciliation Act (COBRA)

The Consolidated Omnius Reconciliation Act (COBRA) was enacted by Congress in 1986 (42 U.S.C. 1395(dd)) to prevent the inappropriate transfer of patients based on their inability to pay for treatment. This law applies only to hospitals that have a provider agreement with Medicare and Medicaid. Medicaid coverage is for children; Medicare coverage is for adults. Although this law applies only to hospitals that receive Medicare and Medicaid patients, it applies to all patients, regardless of their insurance coverage.

Hospitals must state in their institutional bylaws that a medical screening examination will be conducted on all patients presenting to the ED for treatment. These bylaws specify:

- Those healthcare providers who can conduct the screening, such as a nurse or physician. It is important to determine who can provide the screening examinations, because such a formal determination assures that the hospital's governing body recognizes the hospital's capability and assumes proper accountability for this function (Hospital Association of Pennsylvania, 1996).
- The components of the screening, such as a cursory or comprehensive approach. *Medical screening examination* is defined by the institution as it deems appropriate. One recommendation for the medical screening examination is (Frew Consulting Group, 1996):
  - Log entry with disposition.
  - Triage record.
  - Recorded ongoing vital signs.
  - Oral patient history.
  - Physical assessment of the affected body systems.
  - Physical assessment of potentially affected body systems and known chronic health conditions.
  - Any testing necessary to rule out the presence of legally defined emergency health conditions.

- Use of on-call personnel to complete the above assessment.
- Use of on-call physicians to diagnose and stabilize patients.
- Discharge/transfer of vital signs.
- Adequate documentation of these points.

Medical screening is *not* equivalent to *triage* (Mitchner & Yeh, 2002) (Chapter 6). The Health Care Financing Administration posits that patients presenting to the ED must receive a medical screening examination beyond triage; the hospital must provide the appropriate medical screening examination with its capability, including the use of ancillary services routinely available to the ED (Frew Consulting Group, 1996; Mallon & Bukata, 1999; Mitchner & Yeh, 2002). This medical screening is documented, and this documentation becomes part of the patient's permanent medical record (Hodge, 1999). Triage only designates the order in which the patients are taken for the medical screening examination; triage is not a substitute for the medical screening examination. Therefore, medical screening examinations must be more comprehensive than a triage assessment that determines acuity and must be able to rule out the possibility of a legally defined emergency healthcare condition (Frew Consulting Group, 1996; Mallon & Bukata, 1999).

- Patient disposition following the screening. Examples of common dispositions are:
  - Remain in the ED for treatment.
  - Transfer to another area of the hospital.
  - Transfer to a different healthcare facility.
- Common violations of COBRA by hospitals include (Frew Consulting Group, 1996, p.1):
  - Referring patients to the proper provider without a medical screening examination.
  - Referring patients to the gatekeeper physician.
  - Forcing patients to call their insurance provider or gatekeeper for preauthorization.
  - Sending patients away based on a managed care or insurance denial of coverage for a visit.

Penalties for COBRA violations may include fines up to $50,000 and termination from Medicare participation (Comer, 1997).

Nursing Considerations with COBRA

Emergency nurses should work closely with their hospital legal department to create meaningful bylaws that meet COBRA requirements. It is important to avoid asking children and families about their insurance status prior to their medical screening because the families may believe that their treatment is being based on their ability to pay. This questioning is in violation of COBRA. If families believe their treatment was in violation of COBRA requirements, they can register a complaint with the government, and the hospital will be investigated. Violations can be expensive (up to $50,000); nurses can be terminated from their jobs for failing to adhere to EMTALA regulations (Mitchner & Yeh, 2002, p. 32).

Emergency Medical Treatment and Active Labor Act (EMTALA)

Within the COBRA mandate, EMTALA was enacted to prevent hospitals from refusing emergency health care or transferring patients before their health was stabilized. However, this act is not exclusive to ED treatment. As with the COBRA act, EMTALA applies to hospitals that receive Medicare and Medicaid funding, and hospitals can be fined for violations of these laws. The act requires that hospitals:

- Provide appropriate medical screening examinations to determine if an emergency health decision exists (42 USC. 1395(dd)(b)(1).
- Stabilize the patient's health condition and/or transfer the patient to another healthcare facility.

Every employee, from the registration clerk to the nurse and physician, needs to be educated about EMTALA requirements. Each of the employees has the potential to violate EMTALA.

Emergency nurses must initiate a departmental competency program in which emergency nurses can identify core competencies and develop performance objectives. Included in these core competencies can be scenarios related to medical screening examinations.

To meet EMTALA requirements, all patients must have a medical screening, as outlined under COBRA. Unfortunately, the *Federal Register* guidelines do not define what constitutes a medical screening examination, making it difficult for hospitals to enact the legislation. Under EMTALA an emergency medical condition is one with acute symptoms of severity or severe pain for which a medical condition manifesting itself by acute symptoms of sufficient severity (including severe pain) such that absence of immediate medical attention could reasonably be expected to result in serious jeopardy of health, serious impairment to or dysfunction of bodily functions, or other serious medical consequences (Comer, 1997, p. 99).

Other requirements under EMTALA include (Frank, 2000):

- Posting of EMTALA signs that alert patients and families of their rights to a screening exam.

- Reporting of inappropriate transfers from hospitals.
- Maintaining records of transfers to or from other departments for 5 years.
- Maintaining a central log of patients seeking assistance at the department and outcome of each.
- Maintaining an on-call list.
- Establishing protocols for the handling of individuals with potential emergency medical conditions at off-campus departments.

Under EMTALA, unstable patients include (Frew Consulting Group, 1996):

- Pregnant women with contractions.
- Patients with psychiatric conditions.
- Patients with substance abuse.
- Patients with undiagnosed acute pain.

Stabilization of the patient's emergency health condition requires that the hospital provide either (Comer, 1997)

- staff and facilities at the hospital for further evaluation and treatment needed to stabilize the patient's condition or
- transfer to another facility.

Transfer to another facility occurs after the patient's condition has been stabilized. The ED is not permitted to discharge or transfer the patient without stabilization unless the patient requests transfer in writing and the physician signs a certificate that the benefits of transfer outweigh the transfer risk (Comer, 1997). The transfer must include assurances that:

- Treatment provided by the transferring hospital minimizes the risk of transfer.
- The receiving facility has the space, qualified personnel, and agreement to accept and treat the patient.
- The transferring hospital will send the patients' records and informed consent for transfer.
- Transfer will be facilitated with qualified personnel and equipment.

One caveat to EMTALA is its authority during a biomedical or bioterrorism attack. EMTALA does not allow communities to separate hospitals into those that are clean and those that are exposed (Bentley, 2001). All hospitals must see, stabilize, and treat all patients presenting on their property. This rule may impede communities' abilities to make decisions related to hospital care during a bioterrorism event.

Nursing Considerations with EMTALA

In addition to working with the hospital's legal department to develop medical screening guidelines, emergency nurses should work with the hospital to develop guidelines for transport and transfer (Chapter 9). Transfer agreements should be in place among hospitals to facilitate the transfer and transport of pediatric patients requiring specialized treatment, such as burn care, intensive care, psychiatric care, or obstetric care. Some Web sites on EMTALA include www.EMTALA.com; www.MEDLAW.com; and www.ACEP.org.

Guidelines for Persons with Limited English Skills

The U.S. Department of Health and Human Services, Office of Civil Rights, recently issued guidelines to assist healthcare providers in ensuring that persons with limited English proficiency (LEP) or skills can effectively access needed health services. These guidelines apply to all state-administered private and nonprofit facilities, including prehospital and emergency care services that receive Medicare and Medicaid payments. A copy of the guidelines can be downloaded at www.hhs.gov/ocr. EDs can enhance their compliance with these guidelines by taking the following steps (Anonymous, 2000):

- Having policies and procedures for identifying and assessing the language needs of patients and families.
- Posting notices to LEP persons of their right to free language assistance.
- Holding staff training sessions and monitoring programs.
- Having available a range of oral language assistance options pertinent to each EDs population.
- Providing written materials in languages other than English when a significant proportion of the ED population requires services or information in another language to effectively communicate.

Reportable Health Conditions

Reportable pediatric health conditions in general include:

- Infectious diseases.
- Communicable diseases.
- Trauma-related injuries of a specific nature (e.g., fireworks injuries or gunshot wounds).
- Suspected or documented domestic violence and child maltreatment.

Table 2.6 outlines health conditions that must be reported to the health department. The reporting of these conditions serves the purpose of determining incidence (number of new cases of a disease within a population for a given time period) and prevalence (number of current or ongoing cases of a disease within a population for a given time period). Accuracy in reporting

TABLE 2-6 Reportable Health Conditions

Acquired immuno-deficiency syndrome	Food poisoning	Kawasaki disease	Plague	Toxic shock syndrome
Amebiasis	Giardiasis	Legionnaires' disease	Poliomyelitis	Toxoplasmosis
Animal bite	Gonococcal infections	Leptospirosis	Psittacosis	Trachoma
Anthrax	Guillain-Barre syndrome	Lyme disease	Rabies	Trichinosis
Botulism	Hemophilus influenza type B	Lymphogranuloma venereum	Reye's syndrome	Tuberculosis, all forms
Brucellosis	Hepatitis, non-A, non-B	Malaria	Rickettsial diseases	Tularemia
Campylo-bacteriosis	Hepatitis, viral, including types A and B	Measles	Rubella and congenital rubella syndrome	Typhoid
Cancer	Histoplasmosis	Meningitis, all types	Salmonellosis	Yellow fever
Chlamydia		Meningococcal disease	Shigellosis	Other conditions, as required
Cholera		Mumps	Syphilis (all stages)	
Diptheria		Pertussis	Tetanus	
Encephalitis				

From: Pennsylvania Code, Title 28, Chapter 27.

allows for the calculation of endemic (normal occurrence within the population) disease rates for the population. Failure to report these health conditions may lead to underestimation of the health condition. State health departments regulate which health conditions are reportable; these conditions are subject to change as needed. Local jurisdictions may require the reporting of additional conditions.

Nursing Considerations in Reportable Health Conditions

Emergency nurses should check with their local health department for reportable health conditions. Reporting forms should be kept on file in the ED to allow for the timely and accurate reporting of health conditions. Inviting local health department officials to the ED to review reported data from the hospital's community may help emergency nurses to understand the occurrence of disease and other health conditions within their locale.

Patient Self-Determination Act

The Patient Self-Determination Act (advance directives) was passed by Congress in 1990 and was put into effect in 1991. This act requires health maintenance organizations, home health agencies, and others who receive Medicare reimbursement to inform patients about their right to direct decisions about their healthcare treatment (including cardiopulmonary resuscitation, ventilatory assistance, artificial feeding, and hydration) when they might become terminally ill or permanently unconscious and unable to communicate. These agencies are required by law to:

- Inform patients about advance directives.
- Ask patients if they have advance directives.
- Educate the community (including employees) about advance directives.

Advance directives are written instructions that inform healthcare (including emergency care) personnel about an individual patient's choices of life-sustaining treatment in the event that the individual could not speak or decide for him or herself. Two types of advance directives are:

- Living will—a written document that describes those healthcare treatments a person would accept or refuse when that person is no longer capable of making those decisions or is in a permanently unconscious state.
- Durable power of attorney—a legal document that specifies the appointment of another person to make healthcare decisions for an individual when that individual is no longer able to make those decisions. The living will and durable power of attorney complement each other.

Advance directives pertain to adults; the definition of adult may vary from state to state but generally includes individuals who are 18 years of age or older, are married or have been previously married, and/or have graduated from high school.

Advance directives should be created before a crisis situation occurs. They are designed to encourage open dialogue among family members to prevent family, friends, and healthcare providers from having to make difficult decisions without the benefit of knowing the patient's wishes. The advance directives may be written on a declaration form available from the hospital. The form requires the signature of two witnesses, is simple to complete, and does not require notarization. Patients wanting to complete a declaration form should discuss the decisions with their physicians and families and should provide copies of the declaration to healthcare providers, including emergency personnel, when necessary.

The enactment of advance directives in the ED is very difficult because the emergency staff may have no prior relationship with the family forced to make end-of-life decisions. Although it is difficult to enact or ask families about advance directives, such difficulty does not diminish the emergency team's responsibilities to uphold the Patient Self-Determination Act.

Nursing Considerations in Advance Directives

Emergency nurses should work with the hospital legal department to identify methods for incorporating advance directives into ED care. For example, a process should be identified where every eligible patient is queried as to the presence of advance directives. This could occur at triage, at the registration desk, or upon initial treatment. Emergency nurses could role-play with other staff in asking about advance directives. Once they are comfortable in talking with each other about this topic, they may feel more comfortable discussing it with patients and families. Reassuring patients that the advance directives come into effect only when they are unable to express their wishes about their health care or are in a permanent unconscious state offers them confidence that their advance directives do not affect the course of their ED treatment.

Withdrawing and Withholding Treatment

Withdrawing treatment is the cessation of treatment once it has been initiated. Hospital EDs generally establish guidelines for such treatment, such as a specified time or specified number of medication "rounds" administered during cardiopulmonary resuscitation. Such guidelines may evolve from established guidelines or research literature.

Withholding treatment is when treatment never is initiated. For example, a patient with a terminal illness may not receive cardiopulmonary resuscitation measures upon ED presentation.

Nursing Considerations in Withdrawing and Withholding Treatment

When in doubt about withholding or withdrawing treatment, the ED staff should initiate measures until a legal guardian or representative speaks on behalf of the child. Contacting the child's primary care provider and discussing the situation with the provider may be beneficial. Emergency nurses should participate in the development of protocols and policies for withdrawing and withholding life support (Emergency Nurses Association, 1998a).

Do Not Resuscitate Orders

Do not resuscitate (DNR) orders are found in children with terminal illnesses. In some states, children with DNR orders attend school and other activities. Generally, these children wear a bracelet that must be updated and signed on a regular interval by the physician. School nurses, prehospital providers, and hospital personnel should uphold the DNR order. Upon presentation to the ED, the emergency personnel should follow the DNR order while providing comfort measures in conjunction with family wishes.

The DNR order can be overridden by the family members who bring the child to the ED and "want everything done" to prolong their child's life. In this circumstance, it may be wise to initiate the treatment while working with the child's physician and other support persons.

Nursing Considerations with DNR Orders

Emergency nurses can be prepared for the treatment of children in the ED with DNR orders by having policies and procedures in place that outline the steps emergency care providers should take when such a situation arises. The parents should be queried as to the enactment of the DNR order; that is, parents may want to resuscitate the child and void the original order. Parents should bring a copy of the DNR order with them to the ED. The emergency staff should contact the child's primary care physician for confirmation of the DNR order; the emergency team can collaborate with the physician and parents on how to proceed. At the time of impending death, parents may panic and bring the child to the ED; the family may require support and understanding from the staff as the child dies.

Organ Donation

Every state has requirements for asking families for organ donations through an adoption of the Uniform Anatomic Gift Act (ENA, 1998b). This is a very difficult request for an ED nurse to make, especially when dying children are involved. Many times, children may be resuscitated and admitted to the intensive care unit, where organ donation requests may be initiated. Most hospitals have access to an organ recovery team; members of the team come to the ED to speak with the family about organ donation.

Nursing Considerations in Organ Donation

Emergency nurses should play an active role in organ and tissue donation for transplantation in accordance with the Uniform Anatomical Gift Act (ENA, 1998b). EDs should have guidelines for emergency nurses' roles in organ and tissue procurement in collaboration with local organ and tissue recovery agencies (ENA, 1998b). Emergency nurses should receive continuing education in donor identification and management, including cultural, ethical, religious, and social issues affecting the donation process (ENA, 1998b). Continuous exploration and evaluation of one's individual values and beliefs regarding organ and tissue donation is important as well (ENA, 1998b).

Conclusion

Ethical and legal issues arise in the emergency nursing care of children. Emergency nurses should be prepared to work through these issues by having policies and procedures in place for guidance. Having access to the hospital's ethics and human rights committees is helpful as well. Incorporating the services of social workers, child life specialists, and patient-family advocates in the emergency treatment of children may help to prevent problems.

References

Anonymous. (2000). Facilities accepting Medicare, Medicaid get new guidelines for helping persons with limited English skills. *EMSC News, 13*(4), 5.

Bentley, J. (2001). Hospital preparedness for bioterrorism. *Public Health Reports, 116, Supplement 2*, 36-39.

Billittier, A., Lillis, K., & Lerner, E. (1996). Out-of-hospital care of the pediatric patients. *Topics in Emergency Medicine, 18*(2), 1-14.

Biros, M., Lewis, R., Olson, C., Runge, J., Cummins, R., & Fost, N. (1995). Informed consent in emergency research. *Journal of the American Medical Association, 273*(16), 1283-1287.

Biros, M., Runge, J., Lewis, R., & Doherty, C. (1998). Emergency medicine and the development of the Food and Drug Administration's final rule on informed consent and waiver of informed consent in emergency research circumstances. *Academic Emergency Medicine, 5*(4), 359-368.

Broome, M. (1999). Consent (assent) for research with pediatric patients. *Seminars in Oncology Nursing, 15*(2), 96-103.

Comer, R. (1997). COBRA: How to avoid being bitten by the snake. Pittsburgh, PA: Author.

Committee on Bioethics. (1995). Informed consent, parental permission, and assent in pediatric practice. *Pediatrics, 95*(2), 314-317.

Committee on Drugs. (1995). Guidelines for the ethical conduct of studies to evaluate drugs in pediatric populations. *Pediatrics, 95*, 286-294.

Committee on Pediatric Emergency Medicine. (1993). Consent for medical services for children and adolescents. *Pediatrics, 92*, 290-291.

Department of Health and Human Services, Food and Drug Administration. (1993, April 1). Part 50—Protection of Human Subjects. 45 C.F.R. Subtitle A.

Department of Health and Human Services. (1996, October 2). Food and Drug Administration Protection of human subjects; informed consent. *Federal Register, 61*(192), 51498-51524. 21 C.F.R. pp. 34, 50, 312, 601, 812, 814.

Emergency Nurses Association (1998a). Resuscitative decisions. Des Plaines, IL: Author.

Emergency Nurses Association. (1998b). Role of the emergency nurse in tissue and organ donation. Des Plaines, IL: Author.

Fleischman, A., Nolan, K., Dubler, N., Epstein, M., Gerben, M., Jellinek, M., Litt, I., Miles, M., Oppenheimer, S., Shaw, A., Eys, J., & Vaughan, V. (1994). Caring for gravely ill children. *Pediatrics, 94*, 433-439.

Frank, G. (2000). I was born a rambling law. Complying with EMTALA when coming to the emergency department may not actually mean "coming to the emergency department." *Journal of Emergency Nursing, 26*(4), 360-362.

Frew Consulting Group. (1996, Spring). Managed care leads COBRA risk list. *Risk Manager*.

Guertler, A. (1997). The clinical practice of emergency medicine. *Emergency Medicine Clinics of North America, 15*(2), 303-313.

Hodge, D. (1999). Managed care and the pediatric emergency department. *Pediatric Clinics of North America, 46*(6), 1329-1340.

Hospital Association of Pennsylvania. (1996). Guidelines on the use of nurse triage in a hospital emergency setting. Harrisburg, PA: Author.

Lindeke, L., Hauck, M., & Tanner, M. (2000). Practical issues in obtaining child assent for research. *Journal of Pediatric Nursing, 15*(2), 99-104.

Mader, T., & Playe, S. (1997). Emergency medicine research consent form readability assessment. *Annals of Emergency Medicine, 29*, 534-539.

Mallon, W. & Bukata, R. (1999). COBRA/OBRA and EMTALA. *Topics on Emergency Medicine, 21*(21), 17-27.

Mitchner, J. & Yeh, C. (2002). The emergency medical treatment and active labor act: What emergency nurses need to know. *Nursing Clinics of North America, 37*(1), 19-34.

National Institutes of Health. (1998). NIH policy and guidelines on the inclusion of children as participants in research involving human subjects. Bethesda, MD: Author.

Spivey, W., Abramson, N., Iserson, K., MacKay, C., & Cohen, M. (1991). Informed consent for biomedical research in acute care medicine. *Annals of Emergency Medicine, 20*, 1251-1265.

Sullivan, D. (1993). Minors and emergency medicine. *Emergency Medicine Clinics of North America, 11*, 841-851.

Susman, E., Dorn, L., & Fletcher, J. (1992). Participation in biomedical research: The consent process as viewed by children, adolescents, young adults, and physicians. *Journal of Pediatrics, 121*, 547-552.

Tarnowski, K., Allen, D., Mayhall, C., & Kelly, P. (1990). Readability of pediatric biomedical research informed consent forms. *Pediatrics, 85*, 58-92.

Thewes, J., FitzGerald, D., & Sulmasy, D. (1996). Informed consent in emergency medicine. *Emergency Medicine Clinics of North America, 14*, 245-254.

Thurber, F., Deatrick, J., & Grey, M. (1992). Children's participation in research: Their right to consent. *Journal of Pediatric Nursing, 7*, 165-170.

3

The Future of Pediatric Emergency Nursing

Lisa Marie Bernardo, RN, PhD, MPH
Donna Ojanen Thomas, RN, MSN
Yvette Conley, PhD

Introduction

As a subspecialty within emergency nursing, pediatric emergency nursing has evolved rapidly in the past decade. The future for our subspecialty is filled with possibilities in the clinical, education, research, and administration arenas. The purpose of this chapter is to describe current and future factors influencing pediatric and emergency care, and to articulate how these factors will affect our practice as pediatric emergency nurses.

Clinical

Genetic Testing and Therapy

The human genetic code is almost entirely deciphered due to the Human Genome project. Data collected through the Human Genome project will be utilized to determine the gene(s) involved with human genetic disorders, from rare to complex, from infrequent to frequent disorders of public health concern. Information about the Human Genome project is available at www.ornl.gov/hgmis.

Along with knowledge about the genetic causes of disease comes the potential for genetic testing and genetic-based therapeutics. Information on available genetic tests and laboratories equipped to perform these tests is available at www.genetests.org.

New discoveries of mutations for genetic disorders and gene-mapping efforts are quickly occurring; up-to-date information is available through the Online Mendelian Inheritance in Man (OMIM) at www.ncbi.nlm.nih.gov (select OMIM from the directory).

Implications for Pediatric Emergency Nurses

Throughout this core curriculum, embryologic and genetic considerations for various pediatric diseases are discussed. In the future, emergency nurses will need to know available and yet-to-be-developed genetic tests and genetic-based therapeutics for these and other diseases or chronic conditions.

Genetic testing is known to us in the context of forensic and sexual assault evidence. In addition, genetic technologies are becoming the "gold standard" for detecting viral infections such as influenza and chlamydia, even if present at low titer (VanElder, Nijhhuis, Schipper, Schuurman, & VanLoon, 2001; Wilcox, Reynolds, Hoy, & Brayson, 2000). Future genetic testing may be conducted in the Emergency Department (ED) to determine a patient's genotype prior to administering a particular intervention or medication. For example, studies are underway in adults to determine whether certain genotypes have a protective effect following severe traumatic brain injury (Kerr, Kraus, Marion, & Kamboh, 1999). In addition, certain genotypes have been associated with the rate of various drug metabolism and extent of side effects, some of which are potentially life threatening, such as in the case of malignant hyperthermia (Davies & Hanna, 1999). Conceivably, a patient will receive testing for a particular genotype in the emergency department, and an individualized treatment plan may be initiated.

Genetic-based therapeutics will be the future of pediatric emergency nursing. Treatment may no longer be a "one size fits all" approach, where every patient with reactive airway disease receives a standardized dose of bronchodilators for a predetermined time period. In the future, based on the patient's genotype, the type and dose of medications, as well as the duration of medication administration, will be individualized for each patient.

The route for medications will change as well. For chronic diseases, such as cystic fibrosis, genetic therapy will be the treatment of choice and will be administered through an inhaler whose actions are targeted toward the affected gene. Such genetic therapy may ameliorate or reduce the mutation's effect on the body. As with any treatments or medications, pediatric emergency nurses will have to be knowledgeable about the indications, contraindications, and side effects of genetic therapies.

Emerging Infectious Diseases

"Emerging (newly defined) and re-emerging (previously recognized) infectious diseases are infections which are increasing or, when prior incidence in specific human populations is uncertain, appear to be increasing or threaten to do so" (Stephens, Moxon, Adams, Altizer, Antonovics, Aral, Berkelman, Bond, Bull, Cauthen, Farley, Glasgow, Glasser, Katner, Kelley, Mittler, Nahmias, Nichol, Perrot, Pinner, Schrag, Small, & Thrall, 1998). Those most often affected by emerging infectious diseases are those with chronic illnesses or impaired immune systems, the elderly, and immigrants from countries where infectious diseases are widespread (Jackson, Rickman, & Pugliese, 2000). These diseases are clustered as follows (Stephens et al., 1998; Jackson et al., 2000; Fawal & Steele, 1998):

- Infections with unusual clinical features or unexpected virulence. Examples are Ebola hemorrhagic fever and hantavirus-induced pulmonary syndrome.
- Discovery of infectious agents for known illnesses (peptic ulcer disease, hepatitis C virus).
- Increased incidence of emerging infections in certain populations. There is a resurgence of tuberculosis in the United States in people who are homeless, HIV-infected, newly arrived immigrants, substance abusers, minorities, and institutionalized persons. Also, increases are reported in hepatitis C in people who are injection drug users.
- Bacterial infections that are resistant to antibiotics. Two examples are methicillin-resistant *staphylococcus aureus* (MRSA), found in hospitals and communities, and vancomycin-resistant *enterococcus* (VRE), which can cause life-threatening illness in hospitalized or immunocompromised patients.
- Food-borne illnesses. *Escherichia coli* 0157:H7 has been found in bacteria-contaminated ground beef and poultry that were improperly cooked, causing hemolytic uremic syndrome. *Campylobacter jejuni* has been reported in contaminated poultry that was improperly cooked, causing Guilain-Barre syndrome. Other food-borne illnesses include the Norwalk virus, *Toxoplasma gondii*, and newly discovered strains of enterotoxigenic *E. coli*.
- Animal-to-human transmission of disease. Bovine spongiform encephalopathy in cattle (mad cow disease) is possibly linked to infected meat.
- Protozoan infections. *Plas odiu* protozoan causes malaria; *Plas odiu falciparu* leads to central nervous system dysfunction, coma, renal failure, and death. Malaria is the second-leading cause of infectious disease-related deaths; 3,000 children under the age of 5 years die each day from malaria.

Implications for Pediatric Emergency Nurses

Patients with acute infectious diseases, especially those from at-risk populations, such as the homeless, uninsured, and recent immigrants, are frequently treated in the Emergency Department; as such, it is the ED staff who will have the first contact with patients suffering from emerging infectious diseases (Talan, Moran, Mower, Newdow, Ong, Slutsker, Jarvis, Conn, Pinner, & the EMERGEncy ID NET Study Group, 1998). Therefore, the ED staff have the potential to identify sentinel (original) cases of patients with these diseases. The EMERGEncy ID NET is an interdisciplinary, multicenter ED-based network for research on emerging infectious diseases. This network can help public and hospital workers rapidly respond to new diseases or epidemics.

Pediatric emergency nurses need to include questions, such as about recent international travel or contact with international travelers, when caring for ill children who present with unusual symptoms. Taking a careful history of food intake, symptoms in other family members, and past health history also may give clues to the possibility of an emerging infectious disease. Early consultation with infectious disease specialists, state health departments, and the Centers for Disease Control and Prevention are warranted in such patients.

Bioterrorism

Bioterrorism is the deliberate use of microorganisms and toxins as weapons (Christopher, Cieslak, Pavlin, & Eitzen, 1997). Bioterrorist agents include infectious (smallpox) and chemical (sarin gas) modalities (Chapter 45). For example, such agents can be dispersed among visitors to a recreation area, who then return to their homes and spread the agent to others; or a school could be targeted and children could be injured. Children's physical and psychosocial responses to bioterrorism are different from adults'.

- Children's faster respiratory rates result in greater dosage exposure following the inhalation of toxic agents (Bearer, 1995).
- Infants and children have permeable skin, leading to increased absorption of toxic agents (American Academy of Pediatrics, 2000); their increased ratio of body surface area to weight causes loss of body heat through convection and conduction during decontamination procedures, leading to hypothermia (Bernardo, 2001).
- Young children have limited motor and cognitive skills, so they cannot recognize danger or protect themselves from harm during a bioterrorist event.
- Children of all ages can experience post-traumatic stress disorder due to the bioterrorist event, fear and anxiety during treatment, separation from their families, and sustained illness or injury (Rosenbaum, 1993).

Implications for Pediatric Emergency Nurses

Pediatric emergency nurses need to be aware of the special needs of infants and children exposed to bioterrorist agents. The early identification and treatment of illness/injury in infants, children, and adolescents exposed to such agents is paramount. Emergency departments should conduct disaster drills with mock scenarios while wearing special protective equipment and avoiding contamination of others (American Academy of Pediatrics, 2000). Collaborating with local public safety, health department, and community agencies will heighten awareness and provide a coordinated response in such an event.

Tele-health and Tele-medicine

Recent technologic advances make it possible for physicians and nurses to treat patients without the patients being physically present in the same room. Tele-medicine is the practice of medicine via television and computer where physicians and nurses assess patients using video cameras and other equipment. Surgery also has been performed using this technique, and home health nurses use this technology for in-home patient monitoring. Patients benefiting from tele-medicine include those living in rural and frontier areas, those living in health professional shortage areas, or those having no access to healthcare services.

Implications for Pediatric Emergency Nurses

In the future, emergency nurses employed in tertiary care centers may be able to assess patients or serve as consultants to emergency nurses in rural or frontier areas. Such Emergency Departments may have transmitting and receiving equipment placed in patient rooms that allows emergency physicians and nurses to assess and intervene with patients prior to transport or to recommend treatment as needed. Robotics may allow lifesaving procedures to be performed over hundreds of miles. Legal issues, such as practicing nursing without a license in the receiving state, will have to be addressed.

Administration

Pediatric ED Visits

Pediatric visits to both pediatric and adult Emergency Departments will continue to increase in volume and acuity for many reasons, including:

- Children are returning home on ventilators, internal venous access devices, and other equipment generally used only for hospitalized patients.
- Continued lack of health coverage exists for children, leading to the provision of primary and acute care in the ED. Newborns discharged to home soon after birth may become symptomatic due to an undiagnosed congenital heart defect.
- EMTALA (Chapter 2) regulations dictate that all patients require a screening examination prior to being transferred to pediatric facilities. Because the screening examination can be extensive, many pediatric patients stay at the general emergency departments.
- Expense continues to be involved in creating separate trauma centers for children and adults. Children will be cared for more frequently in adult trauma centers.
- Pediatric hospitals are closing in some parts of the country for financial reasons, and the trend may be one center that treats both children and adults. This configuration will have an impact on educational requirements, equipment needs, and staffing patterns. The availability of outcomes data to support the finding that patients cared for by pediatric trained personnel have better outcomes than those treated by nontrained personnel will further encourage specific training for pediatric trauma, but not necessarily separate facilities.

Configuration of Emergency Services and Staffing

The change in the expectation of ED customers has resulted in changes to the ED process and environment. All EDs, but especially those that are for children, will need to become more consumer friendly. EDs are and will continue to be inundated with new technology that may trap nurses into taking care of the machine and not the patient. The needs of patients go far beyond the solutions offered by technology. Increasingly, patients are demanding care that is holistic and humanistic, something they have deserved all along (Proehl, 1999).

The challenge for all EDs will be to provide operational processes that are supported by appropriate technology and physical space (McKay, 1999). Many departments are examining their processes in order to get the patient into a room quicker, to be evaluated sooner, and to be discharged earlier, thus decreasing the overall length of ED stay. In-room registration will become the standard, with an abbreviated triage or in-room triage. The paper chart will be replaced with computerized charting, which will improve flow and decrease time searching for and retrieving medical records.

Parents will expect individualized treatment and attention throughout the ED visit, from triage through discharge. The concept of holistic medicine is advocated in pediatrics (Kemper, 2000) and should be incorporated into our nursing practice as well. Holistic medicine involves "caring for the whole child in the context of that child's values, their family's beliefs, their family system, and their culture in the larger community; and considering a range of therapies based on the evidence of their benefits and cost" (Kemper, 2000, p. 214).

Extrapolating this idea into pediatric emergency nursing practice is advocated throughout this core curriculum, with attention to culture, development issues, and children's special needs. To this end, emergency departments need to have resources available to patients and families. Child life specialists will be more common in the outpatient areas, such as the ED. Currently, very few hospitals offer this service because it is an additional expense to the hospital and it cannot be billed to patients' insurance carriers; however, families will demand it (Christian & Thomas, 1998). Interpreters, which are required; pastoral care services; social services; home care services; public health services and agencies, and other resources will need to be available to the ED population.

With the current and predicted nursing shortage, it will be difficult to find skilled emergency nurses, let alone skilled pediatric emergency nurses. Staffing an ED is difficult because the busiest times are generally nights, weekends, and holidays, which are not desirable working hours. Caring for children, especially those who are critically ill or injured, takes its toll on the staff. With the availability of employment options in the pediatric population (clinics, physicians' offices, and so on), nurses may not be willing to work in the ED. It will be necessary to hire new graduates in the ED, or delegate more tasks to ED technicians. There will be an increase in cross training of professionals. Respiratory care personnel are trained and skilled in many areas that are not used for patient care in the ED, other than respiratory care. A respiratory care professional paired with a pediatric registered nurse would provide a higher skill level than that of an unlicensed person such as a technician. The higher acuity of patients, coupled with the current and worsening nursing shortage, will require creative partnering options such as this.

Because of the high volume of pediatric ED visits and the trend toward more outpatient care, observation-type units may be created to care for children who are generally cared for in the ED for extended periods of time due to the unavailability of in-patient beds. These units will be flexible to serve many different needs, including observation for those children with minor head injuries and other minor trauma, respiratory illnesses, and those requiring minor procedures. One idea is to create a Rapid Treatment Unit adjacent to the ED, which will meet the needs of a variety of patients, such as those described above; will provide staffing backup for the ED; and will eliminate the "boarding" of patients in the ED (Thomas, 2000). The challenges will be in the billing process, as Medicare/Medicaid regulations continue to change how hospital care, including observational care, is reimbursed.

Violence in the Pediatric Emergency Department

The incidence of violence is increasing in the pediatric population. In the past, pediatric hospitals may have enjoyed a false sense of security, because violent acts in the ED seemed limited to the adult setting. With the increasing number of children in gangs, parents themselves being gang members, and intimate partner and domestic violence, pediatric EDs need to continuously evaluate their security system and not wait for a tragedy to provide better protection for staff and patients. Nurses need to demand protection if it is not provided.

Implications for Pediatric Emergency Nurses

Pediatric emergency nurses will be in demand in the general hospital setting and will need to be skilled in caring for children and families. The educational requirements for both pediatric and general ED nurses will increase, which may lead to decreased job satisfaction. Hospitals will need to find ways to pay for increasing educational requirements, as such requirements will be mandated by the Joint Commission on the Accreditation of Healthcare Organizations, national and state accrediting bodies, and other medical and health agencies and professional organizations who define standards for EDs and trauma centers. This will be difficult because most hospitals currently are looking for ways to decrease expenses, and educational benefits are the first to be eliminated. The key phrase for emergency nurses will be "more flexibility," an existing characteristic of emergency nurses.

Pediatric facilities are not and will not be exempt from caring for victims of bioterrorism or patients contaminated by hazardous material. Emergency nurses will need to be trained and to have a plan for caring for these patients. With the increase in methamphetamine laboratories, many children arrive in the ED contaminated with this substance. Emergency nurses need to be aware of the prevalence of methamphetamine in their communities and know how to care for contaminated children. Courses focused on the care of patients exposed to hazardous and bioterrorism media will need to be developed by ENA and other nursing organizations.

Education

Advances in Healthcare Education

Although the breadth of knowledge needed to treat ill and injured children is steadily increasing, the time available to nurses to extend their knowledge is declining. Longer work days, less staff to provide coverage, and elimination of nurse educator positions have an impact on pediatric emergency nurses' efforts to keep abreast of current trends in pediatric emergency care. Patients and parents, though, with the advent of home computers and Internet access, are increasing their knowledge of healthcare and treatment options. Many present to the Emergency Department with printouts downloaded from Web sites about their child's health condition or new therapies. Therefore, emergency nurses must be afforded the opportunities to receive education in recommended treatment modalities.

Implications for Pediatric Emergency Nurses

The methods for educating emergency nurses must be flexible in terms of time, cost, and availability. In the future, paper and pencil self-learning modules will be replaced with interactive education through computer-based services and Internet activities. Traditional lecture/discussion teaching methods will be enhanced with distance learning, whereby an education session is broadcast through a computer or through a television monitor. Such learning can incorporate national and international sites and enhance collaboration with national and international nursing colleagues. Both of these resources can be effective for reducing travel time and speaker costs. Psychomotor skill practice and testing may be enhanced through interactive tele-health or software programs. Many universities and major health care centers have these activities; hospitals can collaborate with these agencies to share in these important resources.

EDs should consider establishing programs with their schools of nursing to have senior nursing students precepted by experienced pediatric emergency nurses; these students are willing to learn and are future colleagues. Hiring patient care technicians who are nursing students also increases students' exposure to emergency nursing and helps them identify our specialty as a viable career option.

Research

Evidence-Based Practice

Evidence-based practice is the provision of patient care based on research findings. In emergency nursing, such practice is slowly growing. In evidence-based practice, a clinical question is asked, the literature is searched, and then best practices are examined and tested. Even though this process is lengthy, the reward comes in knowing that the nursing care rendered is based on facts and outcomes.

Implications for Pediatric Emergency Nurses

In the future, evidence-based practice will be the hallmark of excellence in nursing care. Evidence-based practice guidelines will be developed for triage, trauma care, surgical care, and disease management. Pediatric emergency nurses will collaborate with physicians, surgeons, and others to develop and test these practice guidelines.

Conclusion

The future of pediatric emergency nursing is challenging but secure. Pediatric emergency nursing is recognized as a specialty and will continue to be in the future. Pediatric emergency nurses will be welcomed into the general ED as specialists. Regardless of the setting, all nurses will need to be flexible, recognize their role as mentors and teachers, and learn to work and cooperate with nurses from different settings. Because the nursing shortage will continue and worsen, pediatric emergency nurses will need to work collaboratively with other specialties, such as respiratory therapists, to provide care to the increasingly high-acuity patients. Pediatric emergency nurses will need to work hard to provide the family-centered, humanistic care that our patients deserve.

References

American Academy of Pediatrics. Committee on Environmental Health and Committee on Infectious Diseases. (2000). Chemical-biological terrorism and its impact on children: A subject review. *Pediatrics, 105*, 662-670.

Bearer, C. (1995). How are children different from adults? *Environmental Health Perspective, 103*, 7-12.

Bernardo, L. (2001). Pediatric implications in bioterrorism, part 1: Physiologic and psychosocial differences. *International Journal of Trauma Nursing, 7*, 14-16.

Christian, B., & Thomas, D. (1998). A child life program in one pediatric emergency department. *Journal of Emergency Nursing, 24*(4), 359-361.

Christopher, G., Cieslak, T., Pavlin, J., & Eitzen, E. (1997). Biological warfare: A historical perspective. *Journal of the American Medical Association, 278*, 412-417.

Davies, N., & Hanna, M. (1999). Neurological channelopathies: diagnosis and therapy in the new millenennium. *Annals of Medicine, 31*, 406-420.

Fawal, H., & Steele, L. (1998). Emerging infectious diseases: Can we meet the challenge? *American Journal of Infection Control, 26*, 215-216.

Jackson, M., Rickman, L., & Pugliese, G. (2000). Emerging infectious diseases. *American Journal of Nursing, 100*, 66-71.

Kemper, K. (2000). Holistic pediatrics = good medicine. *Pediatrics, 105*(1) supplement, 214-218.

Kerr, M., Kraus, M., Marion, D., & Kamboh, I. (1999). Evaluation of apolipoprotein E genotypes on cerebral blood flow and metabolism following traumatic brain injury. *Advances in Experimental Medicine and Biology, 471*, 117-124.

McKay, J. (1999). The emergency department of the future—the challenge is changing how we operate! *Journal of Emergency Nursing, 25*(6), 480-488.

Proehl, J. (1999). Chaos and complexity: Preparing for the future of emergency nursing. *Journal of Emergency Nursing, 25*(6), 437-438.

Rosenbaum, C. (1993). Chemical warfare: Disaster preparation in an Israeli hospital. *Social Work and Health Care, 18*, 137-145.

Stephens, D., Moxon, E., Adams, J., Altizer, S., Antonovics, J., Aral, S., Berkelman, R., Bond, E., Bull, J., Cauthen, G., Farley, M., Glasgow, A., Glasser, J., Katner, H., Kelley, S., Mittler, J., Nahmias, A., Nichol, S., Perrot, V., Pinner, R., Schrag, S., Small, P., & Thrall, P. (1998). Emerging and reemerging infectious diseases: A multidisciplinary perspective. *American Journal of Medical Science, 315*(2), 64-75.

Talan, D., Moran, G., Mower, W., Newdow, M., Ong, S., Slutsker, L., Jarvis, W., Conn, L., Pinner, R. & The EMERGEncy ID NET Study Group. (1998). EMERGEncy ID NET: An emergency department-based emerging infections sentinel network. *Annals of Emergency Medicine, 32*, 703-711.

Thomas, D. (2000). Our new rapid treatment unit: An innovative adaptation of the "less than 24-hour stay" holding unit. *Journal of Emergency Nursing, 26*(5), 507-513.

VanElden, L., Nijhuis, M., Schipper, P., Schuurman, R., & VanLoon, A. (2001). Simultaneous detection of influenza viruses A and B using real-time quantitative PCR. *Journal of Clinical Microbiology, 39*, 196-200.

Wilcox, M., Reynolds, M., Hoy, C., & Brayson, J. (2000). Combined cervical swab and urine specimens for PCR diagnosis of genital *chlamydia trachomatis* infection. *Sexually Transmitted Infections, 76*, 177-178.

SECTION 2

Developmental Aspects of Pediatric Emergency Nursing

4

Developmental and Psychosocial Considerations

Alice E. Conway, PhD, CRNP

Introduction

To the child of any age, a visit to the emergency department (ED) can be, at best, a frightening event and, at worst, a traumatizing experience. In a brief amount of time, under stressful circumstances, emergency nurses must create and establish a trusting relationship with the child and family (Table 4.1).

Emergency nurses use principles of psychosocial development to facilitate family-centered care and coping among infants, children, and adolescents before, during, and after ED treatment. A working knowledge of these developmental stages allows the emergency nurse to anticipate the child's stage of psychosocial development and expected reactions to emergency care. Emergency nurses recognize that each child develops at his or her own pace (Table 4.2) and is influenced by many factors, including temperament, family relations, culture, experience, and perception of the current situation.

The purpose of this chapter is to demonstrate the integration of psychosocial principles into emergency nursing care and the implementation of approaches to family-centered care. This integration supports the Joint Commission on Accreditation of Health Care Organization's recommendation for age-specific competencies in the provision of emergency care.

Cultural Influences

Healthcare decisions are affected by a family's degree of acculturation, language barriers, educational opportunities, economic barriers to care, experiences of prejudice in the larger society and in the healthcare setting, and child-rearing practices (MacDonald, 2000). In an increasingly culturally diverse society, emergency nurses must appreciate each child's and family's sociocultural background. It is too easy to inadvertently insult a child and caregiver when "nurses act only on what they feel is correct, which is usually based only on their own values and education" (Lipson, Dibble, & Minarik, 1996, p. 2).

Cultural competence is a complex combination of knowledge, attitudes, and skills (Spector, 2000) that nurses attain through education and experience. Although it is impossible for the emergency nurse to be an expert about all cultures and ethnic groups who present to the ED, emergency nurses can:

- Have access to a cultural handbook (e.g., Lipson et al., 2000; Spector, 2000) for reference and clarification.
- Attend educational offerings on specific cultural and ethnic groups to enhance the nurse's sensitivity to specific cultural and ethnic beliefs and concerns.
- Invite representatives of local cultural and ethnic groups to the ED to share their experiences and collaborate with emergency nurses on how to provide culturally sensitive nursing care.
- Know which cultures and ethnic groups are prevalent in the ED's service area.
- Learn another language.
- Attend local cultural and ethnic events.

TABLE 4.1 General Guidelines to Create a Trusting Relationship with the Child and Family during ED Treatment

Nursing Intervention	*Rationale*
Call the child by name.	Demonstrates respect for each child's individuality.
Establish a working relationship with the child's parents or caregivers.	A child's anxiety level often mirrors the parents' anxiety level. Gaining the parents' trust and cooperation allays their anxiety and calms the child, thus breaking the cycle of anxiety (Lamontagne, Hepworth, Byington, & Chang, 1997; Newton, 2000).
Speak in simple, nonmedical terms.	Helps facilitate communication and promote comfort in a stressful environment.
Be direct and honest; tell the child and caregiver what they can or need to do to facilitate the ED treatment.	Promotes cooperation and increases the family's and child's sense of control.
Keep child and family informed about their treatment.	Lack of information is considered by many caregivers to be the most stressful factor in visiting the ED (Seidel & Henderson, 1997). Frequent updates on why families are waiting, what events are going to occur, and other information minimizes surprises.
Have the parent and child participate in care, as appropriate.	Giving the child and caregiver something to do helps to provide distraction and gives them a sense of control. For example, have the child hold a bandage or 4" by 4" package. Have the caregiver stroke the child's head, speak softly in the child's ear, softly sing the child's favorite song, or hold the child's hand. This reduces the child's fear of separation and abandonment (Melnyk, 2000).
Describe procedures and sensations.	Minimize the usage of words such as *pinch*, *bee sting*, and so on, until moments before the painful procedure, thus eliminating the anxiety of participation. Describe the sensations the child will feel (e.g., "I'm going to wipe your leg. It's going to feel wet and cool.").
Avoid separating the child and caregiver.	Keep the child and caregiver together to promote comfort and security. However, if the caregiver is extremely anxious, temporary separation of the child from the parent may help the child. In addition, the adolescent patient may want to be separate from the parent. Offer the adolescent a choice about having a support person present during treatment.
Assign one nurse to remain with the child who does not have family members present.	Provides the child with an advocate and support person until the family's arrival.
Assign a consistent emergency nurse to the child and family, if possible.	Continuity lessens confusion and helps build trust among the nurse, child, and family.
Make as many observations as possible without touching the child.	Provides important information about both the child and the parent-child interaction.
Avoid using the words *good* or *bad* to denote a child's health status.	Children perceive these words as descriptions of themselves, not as general comments. These words can also reinforce their misconceptions about the cause of the problem (Stanford, 1991).
Provide feedback and reassurance.	Children appreciate reassurance; rewards such as a sticker and praise are especially valued and remembered after a painful procedure. All children do their best to cooperate with the emergency staff.
Consult other healthcare professionals, such as child life specialists, social workers, and spiritual counselors.	Provides specialized care to the child.
Stay confident and calm.	A calm, soft voice, gentle assertiveness, and confidence help the nurse to maintain control of a difficult situation.

TABLE 4.2 Summary of Psychosocial, Cognitive, Moral, and Spiritual Development Theories

Developmental Theory/Age	*Infancy Birth–1 year*	*Toddlerhood 1–3 years*	*Preschool 4–6 years*	*School Age 7–12 years*	*Adolescence 13–18 years*
Psychosocial Development (Erikson, 1963)	Trust vs Mistrust "I am what I am given."	Autonomy vs Shame and Doubt "I am what I will."	Initiative vs Guilt "I am what I can imagine I will be."	Industry vs Inferiority "I am what I learn."	Identity vs Role Confusion "I am who I decide to be."
Positive outcome:	Hope; can delay gratification	Will, positive self-esteem	Purposeful, self-starter	Competence, perseverance	Fidelity, optimism
Negative outcome:	Suspicion, withdrawal	Compulsion, impulsivity	Inhibition	Inadequacy, gives up easily	Defiance, diffidence
Cognitive Development (Piaget, & Helder, 1969)	Sensorimotor (birth to 2 years)	Preoperational thought (transducive reasoning, 2 to 4 years of age)	Preoperational thought (intuitive phase, 4 to 7 years of age)	Concrete operations (inductive reasoning and beginning logic)	Formal operations (deductive and abstract reasoning)
Theme:	Object permanence	Egocentrism—cannot understand another person's point of view	Two events occur together	Conservation, reversibility	Logical conclusions
Moral Development (Kohlberg, 1969; Coles, 1997)	N/A	Preconventional (premoral) level	Preconventional (premoral) level	Conventional level	Postconventional level
Theme:	N/A	Punishment and obedience orientation	Naive instrumental orientation; child follows rules as he or she desires	Social system and conscience. "Good boy/nice girl" orientation. Law and order orientation	Social-contract orientation. Universal ethical principle
Spiritual Development (Coles, 1991)	Undifferentiated	Initiative-projective	Initiative-projective	Mythical-literal	Synthetic-convention
		Imitate behavior of others	Follow parental values and beliefs, especially about good and bad	Strong interest in religion; existence of deity usually accepted	Early adolescence—begin to question beliefs. Individuating—reflective, searching, and accepts uncertainty

Culturally Sensitive Nursing Assessment

Although a thorough cultural assessment in the ED is not feasible or practical, an abbreviated assessment is warranted to provide culturally sensitive care (Spector, 2000). This assessment is incorporated in the health history and physical assessment (Chapter 6) and includes the following information:

- Country of origin.
- Length of time the family has resided in the United States, if the child and family are immigrants.
- Child's and family's first and second languages.
- Information the family would like to share about themselves that would facilitate their ED care.
- Information on the use of home remedies or home prescriptions or treatments (type of remedy, when it was last used, for how long it was used, why it was used).
- Available social and economic resources.

Culturally Sensitive Nursing Interventions

Selected culturally sensitive nursing interventions that emergency nurses can incorporate into their practice include:

- Focusing on the family's attitudes and values while initiating emergency nursing interventions. Asking about the family's healthcare practices acknowledges the heterogeneity of such practices within cultural groups (MacDonald, 2000). Any generalizations about the family's ethnic group may not apply to certain groups or individuals. However, in general, families of Hispanic origin are insulted if the nurse doesn't touch the head of a young child. Conversely, it is considered a major insult if a person touches an Asian child's head without permission (Spector, 2000).

- Avoiding criticism of the family's cultural beliefs and related health practices. Such attacks may lead the family to mistrust the ED staff and may affect their compliance with treatment regimens.
- Collaborating with the family to blend traditional and cultural approaches to health care. This approach recognizes the family's values and provides an opportunity for teaching about traditional health care (e.g., the importance of childhood immunizations).
- Identifying the family's key members, such as a family elder. Failure to include these significant individuals in teaching and decision making can seriously hinder adherence to the plan of care (Ahammn, 1994).

Psychosocial Considerations by Age Group

Infants

The major developmental task of infancy is the attainment of trust (Erikson, 1963). *Trust* is established gradually and is facilitated when needs (feeding, comfort, and social interaction) are met in a consistent manner by a primary caregiver. If given inconsistent care, infants develop a sense of *mistrust* because they are not sure that their needs will be met. The following are key characteristics of infants:

- Infants pick up their emotional cues from the caregiver and become anxious if the caregiver is anxious.
- As infants grow, their motor skills increase and they use active withdrawal as a coping mechanism.
- Crying is the infant's major form of communicating distress, and the infant's cry is very stressful to the caregiver (Chapter 12).
- Infants feel pain and need appropriate analgesia (Chapter 13).
- Stranger anxiety and separation anxiety are major cognitive accomplishments in infancy, beginning around 7 or 8 months and peaking at 12 to 18 months (Santrock, 1999).

Specific interventions to facilitate infant coping and promote development are outlined in Table 4.3.

Toddlers

Upright locomotion and increasing language skills allow toddlers to be active explorers of self, others, and the environment. The toddler's developing sense of *autonomy* leads to a need for control ("Me do it.") and a differentiation of self from others ("No."). Failure to achieve autonomy can produce *shame* and *doubt*; the toddler may withdraw and be unable to test limits and learn about the environment (Erikson, 1963). The following are key characteristics of toddlers:

- Separation is necessary for autonomy, but this separation causes fears. Methods of coping with these fears include behaviors such as withdrawing, clinging, being aggressive, regressing, and using a transitional object (security blanket).
- Toddlers only understand time in terms of a daily schedule ("We'll see daddy after dinner.").
- Between 18 and 24 months, toddlers are capable of determining a cause after observing an effect, but only within the limits of their prior experiences (Piaget & Helder, 1969; Dixon & Stein, 2000) (e.g., a visit to the ED may mean a hurtful injection).
- Toddlers have limited expressive language skills, understanding more than they can verbalize. Toddlers focus their attention for a short time period.
- As toddlers learn to control their bodies, they also become fearful of being hurt and will use motor activities (e.g., hitting, kicking, or biting) when hurt.
- Toddlers can tell you where they hurt ("arm hurts") but cannot describe the pain (Franck, Greenberg, & Stevens, 2000).
- Toddlers are developing a body image and perceive body boundaries but have fears about bodily injury.
- Regressive behaviors, such as temper tantrums and refusal to obey, are often seen as a response to crisis situations and are adaptive (Dixon & Stein, 2000).

Specific interventions to facilitate toddler coping and promote development are outlined in Table 4.4.

Preschoolers

During the preschool period, the child believes, "I am what I can imagine I will be" (Erikson, 1967). This is a period of *initiative* where children are ready to try new activities and experiences. Preschoolers have very active imaginations that work to their benefit when fantasy is used as a distraction technique. Their imaginations can also increase their fears, and what they imagine is often worse than reality. The development of a sense of *guilt* is possible because so much of what they would like to

TABLE 4.3 Specific Interventions to Facilitate Infant Coping and Promote Development

Specific Intervention	*Rationale*
Offer self-comforting measures, such as the use of pacifiers; allow the infant access to the preferred hand for sucking.	Sucking provides oral comfort.
Keep the young infant, when possible, in a flexed position, with knees to chest and arms midline.	This position helps the young infant to retain or regain physiologic and behavioral functioning (Dixon & Stein, 2000).
Allow rest periods between procedures and treatments.	Helps the infant to restore energy. Overwhelmed infants will withdraw into sleep. They may also become hypothermic or hypoxic.
Help caregiver to stay calm when comforting the infant.	Infants are able to sense their caregiver's distress cognitively, even though they are not able to understand cause and effect.
Rock, swaddle, and sing softly to the infant.	Provides comfort to a stressed infant. Allowing the caregiver to comfort and hold the infant fosters the infant's body image, which is at a feeling level.
Reunite the infant and caregiver as soon as possible following treatments or procedures. Keep the parent in the infant's sight as much as possible.	Visual contact with the mother promotes maternal attachment and provides security and comfort (Deloian, 2000).
Release the infant from a restrained or held position as soon as possible following a procedure or treatment.	Infants diffuse stress and frustration through motor activity (Bernardo, Conway, & Bove, 1990); promotes coping.
Provide pharmacologic and nonpharmacologic pain control as needed (Chapter 13).	Newborns and infants have all of the physiologic mechanisms necessary to perceive pain (Franck, Greenberg, & Stevens, 2000).
Use warm hands, equipment, and room when caring for the infant.	Infants have a large body surface-to-weight area, and they quickly lose body heat; promotes comfort.
Maintain a safe environment.	Infants easily roll from tables, and older infants put objects into their mouths as they explore their environment.
Distract infants with brightly colored toys, hand puppets, or a human face talking to them.	Provides a diversion or distraction from the task at hand.

do is either forbidden or beyond their psychomotor capabilities. During this period, the child is very active, progressing rapidly in motor abilities, cognitive function, and language development. The following are key characteristics of preschoolers:

- Preschoolers are able to communicate their hurts and fears because of their increased language skills.
- Although preschoolers have a separate identity from that of their parents, they need their parents to reassure, to set limits, and to prevent loss of control.
- Because of their rich imaginations and the beginnings of conscience and preoperational cognition, preschoolers often interpret injury or illness as a result of something they did wrong.
- Preschoolers are egocentric and need to have procedures explained in terms of what they will feel, smell, and taste. They also believe that everyone sees the world the way they do.
- By the age of 4 years, children have a well-defined concept of their external bodies and the relationships among their body parts; however, their concept of the inner body is primitive (Vessey, Braithwaite, & Wiedmann, 1990).
- Sex-typing and sex-role identification are major tasks; preschoolers need to know that even brave boys and girls cry.
- Preschoolers possess an enhanced repertoire of coping skills. Although they continue to use language and motor activity as coping strategies, they also can use distraction, story telling, and simple information to cope with a stressful event.
- Body intrusions, such as rectal temperature measurement, otoscopic examinations, and sutures, are major fears. Separation anxiety remains a concern.
- Preschool children want to cooperate and please adults.
- Preschoolers believe that pain is punishment for "bad" or angry thoughts or actions. Thus, the preschooler whose inquisitiveness led to an injury and ED visit believes that he or she is being punished for this inquisitiveness.

Specific interventions to facilitate preschooler coping and promote development are outlined in Table 4.5.

TABLE 4.4 Specific Interventions to Facilitate Toddler Coping and Promote Development

Interventions	*Rationale*
Approach the toddler slowly; talk with the caregiver while the child becomes accustomed to the nurse's presence.	Minimizes fear and decreases stranger anxiety. If the caregiver trusts the nurse, then the child will trust as well.
Keep on the child's level—sit down or bend. Be alert to how the ED environment looks from the child's vantage point.	A new environment reminds children of their own smallness and lack of control (Grover, 2000).
Encourage the child to examine equipment and perform a procedure on a doll or caregiver. For example, allow the toddler to listen to the nurse's heart first.	Rehearsal helps the child feel a sense of control.
Give choices whenever possible (e.g., "Do you want your mom or dad to hold you while I listen to your heart?").	Gives the child some control and makes the child feel less threatened.
Use simple, concrete terms when explaining to the toddler what the toddler will feel during the procedure immediately before the procedure occurs.	Avoids undue fear or anxiety because the toddler's concept of time is not well developed.
Tolerate a moderate amount of verbal and motor protesting.	Mobility is the child's best avenue for expressing anger (Erikson, 1967); helps the child safely release energy through motor activity (Bernardo et al., 1990).
Give the child something to do (e.g., hold a bandage).	Provides the child with a sense of control, autonomy, and self-respect (Pridham, Adelson, & Hanson, 1987)
Tell the child, "I will help you to hold still."	Helps the child to gain control; accepting help is a means of coping (Ritchie, Caty, & Ellerton, 1988).
Have the caregiver involve the child in an interactive story (e.g., "We're going on a trip. Where shall we go? Who should we take with us? What should we bring along?").	Becomes an excellent distraction technique for both child and caregiver (Zelter, Bush, & Chen, 1997).
If separation for a treatment or procedure is necessary, allow the toddler to bring a security object (blanket, toy, or stuffed animal) or a parent's personal possession (scarf or hat).	Provides comfort for the child and decreases the child's sense of separation (Wear, 1974).
If a cast or large bandage is applied, reassure the toddler that the covered body part remains intact.	Promotes a positive body image because toddlers perceive body boundaries as indefinite (Bernardo et al., 1990).
Provide pharmacologic and nonpharmacologic pain control as needed (Chapter 13).	Decreases pain and anxiety.
Praise and reward the child frequently with a sticker or drink of juice; avoid implying that the child was bad.	Praise enhances the child's self-esteem and minimizes the older toddler's tendency to perceive pain as punishment for wrongdoing (Pridham et al., 1987).
Release any restraint as quickly as possible.	Avoids prolonged anxiety.
Reunite the toddler and the caregiver as soon as possible.	Decreases anxiety resulting from separation; promotes comfort.

TABLE 4.5 Specific Interventions to Facilitate Preschooler Coping and Promote Development

Interventions	*Rationale*
Encourage verbal expression of fears. Ask about any previous hospital experiences.	Permits the nurse to clarify any misconceptions. Egocentric thinking leads the child to believe he or she is being punished for a real or imagined wrong-doing (Goldberger, Gaynard, & Wolfer, 1990). The preschool child believes that events closely following one another have a cause–effect relationship (Bibace & Walsh, 1980). Guilt combined with fantasy creates erroneous impressions and causes generalized fears (Erikson, 1963).
Allow the preschooler to explore or use equipment. Demonstrate how the equipment works. Role play with the child. Use puppets for teaching and communication.	Facilitates communication and decreases fear and anxiety. Decreases the child's reported fantasies; direct action is a means of coping (Ritchie et al, 1988).
Use nonthreatening language such as *repair*, *make better*, *uncomfortable*, or *sore*.	Minimizes children's fear of invasive procedures. These words are descriptive and arouse more manageable feelings than such words as *cut* or *opening* (Goldberger et al., 1990).
Explain in simple, concrete words the need for the procedure or treatment; include sensations that the child may experience, such as *cold*, *wet*, *pinch* (Pridham et al., 1987).	Minimizes the child's fears. Avoids any unexpected sensations that might otherwise increase anxiety and cause the child to lose trust. When the child is told what sensations he or she may feel, the amount of distress associated with pain decreases (Pridham et al., 1987).
Acknowledge the child's feelings, and reassure the child that it is okay to be scared. Give the child suggestions to help master these feelings, such as, "Hold my hand," "Say ouch," "Take deep breaths," "Let's tell a story together," "Tell me about your favorite place." Have the child blow on a party blower or pinwheel; use soap bubbles as well.	These techniques increase the child's control and promote a sense of mastery; decreases the child's sense of guilt.
Encourage the child to participate in treatments or procedures by holding a bandage or tape.	Promotes cooperation, a sense of control, and self-respect.
Offer choices whenever possible.	Helps the child to feel less threatened.
Use pharmacologic and nonpharmacologic measures for pain control and relief. Use a pain rating scale (see Chapter 13).	Pain rating scales provide a subjective measure of pain.
Reinforce the child's coping behaviors ("You're such a big help.").	Avoids instilling a sense of failure in the child and promotes the child's emotional growth.
Actively involve the child with how the child can help during a treatment or procedure; use storytelling that involves the child.	Minimizes stalling techniques (Ott, 1996).
Observe for stalling techniques that would delay the onset of a procedure or treatment, such as crying, clinging, fighting, making excuses, and bargaining.	Stalling techniques are direct coping mechanisms used by preschool children (Ritchie et al., 1988).
Allow a minimal time lag (1 to 2 minutes) between explaining a procedure and performing the procedure.	Longer time lags cause preschoolers to frighten themselves with imagined horrors (Goldberger et al., 1990).
Use analogies when describing how the body works (e.g., the brain acts like the "boss" of the body and the heart keeps the body running like a car "motor.") (Burke, 1995, p. 46).	Preschoolers understand explanations if familiar words are used. Young children tend to be quite literal in their interpretation of information.
Reward the child frequently with praise, juice, or stickers.	Allows for mastery.
Reunite the child with the caregivers as soon as possible.	Avoids prolonged anxiety.
Use bandages liberally; use draping and gowns during examination and treatment.	Recognizes the child's concern for body intactness and vulnerability Respects the child's modesty. (Erickson, 1967).
Use rehearsal to prepare children for an ED visit.	Invite children 4 to 7 years of age to the ED for a field trip experience. Have them bring a stuffed animal or doll and describe symptoms as they act as the caregivers. This activity decreases their fear of the ED and allows them to perceive the emergency nurses as helpful and the ED as less frightening. Those children who participated in such a visit were found to be cooperative during an actual ED encounter (Zimmerman & Santen, 1997).

School-Aged Children

During this age span, children expand their world as they move into school and the world of teachers and peers. They enter the psychosocial stage of *industry* ("I am what I learn and do") and eagerly engage in tasks that will win approval (Erikson, 1967). If they experience repeated rejection and failure, a sense of *inferiority* develops; this can stunt further psychosocial growth. They understand the "rules" of health behavior but also need fairly concrete rewards for following the rules. The following are key characteristics of school-aged children:

- Children younger than 7 years of age are able to reason on the basis of only one characteristic at a time. They can recognize the relationships between cause of illness (e.g., virus) and getting sick (Dixon & Stein, 2000).
- Between 7 and 11 years of age, children can take note of several features and their interrelationship. They now can understand the reversible nature of cause and effect. Prevention of illness and injury is understood ("Playing with matches can cause fire. Fire can be prevented by not playing with matches.").
- School-aged children have an expanding vocabulary. Although they understand the concept of internal organs, they become confused about their function, especially when ill.
- Young school-aged children may consider illness as punishment for their actions.
- Bodily injury, loss of bodily function, loss of control, and loss of status are major worries and fears of this age group (Pridham et al., 1987). They need to have their modesty maintained and their questions answered honestly.
- School-aged children have increasing coping strategies but may need prompting to ask questions.
- School-aged children shift from a family-oriented environment to a peer-dominated society (Billings & Burns, 2000). Older children may wish to cope without their parents present; however, if stressed, these children may need to have their parents available. When feeling threatened, as in an emergency situation, school-aged children may withdraw and become reserved instead of seeking information.

Specific interventions used to facilitate coping in school-aged children and promote psychosocial development are outlined in Table 4.6.

Adolescents

Adolescence is a period of rapid growth, characterized by myriad interacting biologic, emotional, and social challenges. Early adolescents are still in the world of children, while later adolescents join the adult world. The adolescent experiences conflicts associated with a search for personal *identity*, separation from the family, peer-group relationships, management of sexual changes and feelings, and future career choices (Manning, 1990). Principal to these experiences is the effort to develop a personal identity that the adolescent carries into adulthood (Erikson, 1963). If a personal identity is not achieved, *role confusion* or *diffusion* occurs, leading to an excessive identification with and persistent dependence on others and a lack of self-confidence. The following are key characteristics of adolescents:

- Adolescents are able to take into account all variables within a situation because they are now capable of abstract thought.
- Adolescents understand causes of health and illness in physiologic terms. They are able to understand risks and consequences associated with certain behavior, but they generally believe that nothing will happen to them. Some of these risk-taking behaviors, such as active experimentation with alcohol and other drugs, may impair the adolescent's ability to make wise choices about his or her health (Manning, 1990). Respect for the adolescents' independence and values will increase chances of cooperation.
- Peers are important, and emancipation from parents is critical. However, when injured or ill, adolescents will often want a caregiver present; this is an individualized choice.
- Ill or injured adolescents fear loss of autonomy, privacy, being "different" from their peers, death, loss of peer acceptance, and disfigurement.
- Adolescents become idealistic and are egocentric when considering their ideals in relation to those of others in the world (Maier, 1978). Because of this idealism and their introspection, they are very critical of their own appearance and behavior, and they think that others are equally focused on them.
- Because of their rapidly changing bodies, they are very focused on their bodies and need reassurance that they are normal.
- Adolescents have many coping strategies and may need help in asking questions and in making choices to gain a sense of control.
- Adolescents can have rapid mood swings.

Specific interventions to facilitate adolescent coping and promote development are outlined in Table 4.7.

TABLE 4-6 Specific Interventions Used to Facilitate School-Aged Children's Coping and Promote Development

Interventions	*Rationale*
Use anatomic models and equipment to explain the child's health condition and the treatment that will ensue.	Takes advantage of the child's concrete thinking abilities by making body organs and processes "real" (Pidgeon, 1977).
Use a Gellert model; have the child draw and label the internal body organs.	Helps to clarify any misconceptions; provides a basis for teaching about the child's health condition and ED treatment.
Prepare for ED procedures with enough time for the child to think of questions and for the nurse to answer them.	Allows time for cognitive processing and mental preparation. Because school-aged children have a concept of time, the approximate length of time for the procedure may be offered, if it is known. Asking questions is a means of coping (Ritchie et al., 1988).
Provide specific instructions about the child's behavior (e.g., "You may make as much noise as you want if you hold your hand still.") (Seidel & Henderson, 1997).	Gives the child a sense of control; sets limits for acceptable behavior.
Offer an open-ended statement to draw out the concerns of the child who appears to be anxious but does not ask questions. For example, "Some children want to know about getting stitches. Would you like to know about getting stitches, too?"	Allows the child to know that his or her questions or fears are normal and that other children have had similar experiences. Provides a means for the child to turn an inhibition-or-action mechanism into a direct-action mechanism, thereby increasing his or her ability to cope (Ritchie et al., 1988).
State the approximate length of the treatment or procedure, but be as accurate as possible. "Five more minutes" should not turn into 15 minutes.	School-aged children have a concept of past, present, and future (Pridham et al., 1987).
Offer specific choices during treatment, if possible.	Helps the child to feel in control.
Encourage the child to participate in care, as feasible.	Conveys a sense of control and decreases the child's feelings of dependence on others.
Ask the child and family about specific techniques that helped the child cope with a previous stressful event (Lutz, 1986); allow time for the child and family to practice that technique. If no successful techniques are identified, offer concrete examples of coping strategies (e.g., deep breathing, relaxation techniques, self-talk, storytelling, describing a favorite place or event) (Brennan, 1994). Practice the techniques, if possible.	Helps the child to feel in control; helps the child to master the situation. Enhances the child's emotional and developmental growth (sense of industry). Direct-action techniques minimize passive resistance, such as clenched fists or teeth and body rigidity (Lutz, 1986).
Use pharmacologic and nonpharmacologic interventions for pain relief; assess for pain with pain rating scales (Chapter 13).	Provides for adequate analgesia. School-aged children can use visual analog scales because they understand the concept of numbering.
Praise the child's efforts to maintain control; offer suggestions and minimize attention to loss of control.	School-aged children's locus of control is becoming more internal than external. They have overly high and sometimes unrealistic expectations of themselves (Billings & Burns, 2000)).
Use draping and gowns during examinations and treatment.	Respects the child's modesty.
Allow caregiver to be with the child if the child wants this support; permit siblings or friends to visit, if appropriate.	Gives the child a sense of control in having a support person present.

(continued)

TABLE 4-6 (continued)

Interventions	*Rationale*
Maintain a positive manner regardless of the child's reaction; project a positive outcome of ED treatment.	Prevents feelings of inferiority and decreased self-esteem. Minimizes school-aged children's fears of disfigurement and responds to their incomplete understanding of death (Selbst & Henretig, 1989).
Encourage the child to talk about the ED experience.	The child's verbalization of thoughts and feelings allows the nurse to clarify any misconceptions.
Include older children in conversations regarding treatment and discharge instructions.	Allows the child to be involved with the decision-making process and treatment plan, which may increase compliance; increases the child's self-esteem.

TABLE 4.7 Specific Interventions to Facilitate Adolescent Coping and Promote Development

Intervention	*Rationale*
Talk with the adolescent first before talking with the parents.	Demonstrates respect for the adolescent as an individual with a developing sense of self-identity. Also, adolescents want to be part of the decision making about their own bodies and health care.
Ensure and maintain privacy during treatment; use gowns and drapes during examinations and treatments.	Promotes modesty. Recognizes that body image concerns are heightened during adolescence because of increased hormonal, physical, and emotional changes, resulting in increased sensitivity about personal appearance. Respecting physical modesty and autonomy and allowing choices and control facilitates cooperation (Widey, 2000).
Explain to the adolescent what to expect before touching him or her.	Demonstrates respect for the adolescent as an individual; allows the adolescent to prepare for the treatment.
Allow the adolescent to choose a support person for examinations and treatment.	Promotes autonomy.
Incorporate the adolescent in decision making.	Decreases the adolescent's loss of autonomy; increases the chances for compliance with the treatment regimen.
Allow for the verbalization of fear and anger, but provide coping strategies such as use of music, deep breathing, or guided imagery.	Acknowledges the adolescent's feelings and provides alternative means of expression.
Use pharmacologic and nonpharmacologic interventions for pain relief; use pain rating scales; observe for signs of masked pain behavior (Chapter 13).	Provides for adequate analgesia.
Give realistic and truthful explanations.	Promotes trust. Recognizes that adolescents can use reason and logical thinking and that information seeking is a major way of coping (Ritchie et al., 1988). Shows sensitivity to the adolescent's more advanced understanding of bodily functions and ability to use abstract thought (Pridham et al., 1987). Acknowledges that adolescents are curious about anything that affects them and that they need reassurance that they are normal (Manning, 1990).
Use diagrams of the human body or models to explain procedures; use correct terminology.	Shows sensitivity to the adolescent's more advanced understanding of bodily functions and ability to use abstract thought.
Encourage the adolescent to participate in care.	Demonstrates to the adolescent a sense of responsibility for his or her health.
Allow for privacy with the emergency nurse.	Gives the adolescent an opportunity to ask questions and discuss concerns.
Stress normalcy whenever possible.	Body image and concerns are heightened during adolescence, and personal appearance is of critical importance.
Reunite the adolescent with the support person as soon as possible; answer any questions.	Provides support to the adolescent.
Be honest about possible outcomes, but reassure the adolescent that he or she will get better, as appropriate.	Builds trust between the adolescent and the ED staff.

Psychosocial Considerations of the Family

Families today are diverse, complex, and self-defined. All family configurations, such as single families, step families, blended families, intergenerational families, foster families, or adopted families, have common concerns and needs when their child receives emergency treatment, including (Colizza, Prior, & Green, 1996):

- Accurate, timely, frequent, and truthful information about their child's condition, treatment, and prognosis.
- Assurance that all treatment is appropriate.
- Assurance that treatment is rendered in a competent, caring manner.
- The ability to trust their child's caregivers.
- The ability to be with their child.

Family-centered care is "an approach to care characterized by mutually beneficial collaboration between patient, family, and health professional. This approach is a direct reflection "of the expectation that consumers will be involved in their own care and in the design and modification of health care systems" (Johnson, Thomas, & Williams, 1997, p. 3). Even in the ED setting, family-centered care involves respecting and supporting families during resuscitation, episodic, and acute care. Selected concepts related to family-centered care include (Johnson et al., 1997):

- Respecting each family's human dignity, expertise, values, and culture.
- Sharing information that allows families to make informed decisions about their child's emergency care. Such sharing is communicated via methods appropriate to that family, including the use of translators and sign language interpreters.
- Collaborating with families in the enactment of an emergency treatment plan. Caregivers know their child best, because they care for their child on a daily basis. Therefore, collaborating with families early in the treatment process helps to assure compliance with subsequent home care or follow-up regimens.

Family-centered care and family presence during invasive procedures are advocated by the Emergency Nurses Association (1998). This participation is guided by a number of factors, including (Conway, 1993):

- The urgency of the situation.
- The invasiveness of the procedure.
- The staff's comfort in performing the procedure or treatment in the family's presence.
- The availability of a healthcare professional to stay with the family exclusively during the procedure or treatment.
- The availability of written hospital policies, procedures, or standards of care addressing parental participation.
- The family's ability to support and comfort the child during the procedure or treatment.

Siblings are important family members and should be included as much as is desired, feasible, and practical, based on (Conway, 1993):

- The siblings' ages and developmental abilities.
- The urgency of the situation.
- The invasiveness of the procedure or treatment.
- The staff's comfort in performing the treatment or procedure in the siblings' presence.
- The availability of a healthcare professional and family member to stay with the sibling exclusively during the treatment or procedure.
- The availability of written hospital policies, procedures, or standards of care addressing sibling participation.

Specific interventions to facilitate family coping are outlined in Table 4.8.

Conclusion

Emergency nurses treat each child and family as unique individuals, taking into consideration their developmental, ethnic, cultural, and racial diversity (Bernardo & Schenkel, 1995). The application of developmental principles and the initiation of family-centered care are the crux of pediatric emergency nursing. Emergency nurses should consider including parents and older children on their ED teams for system design, communications development, and community outreach (Johnson et al., 1997). The book by Johnson et al. (1997) includes self-assessment inventories to help emergency medical services and EDs to determine their readiness to enact family-centered care. The text can be obtained from the Emergency Medical Services for Children National Resource Center (www.ems-c.org).

TABLE 4.8 Specific Interventions to Facilitate Family Coping

Intervention	*Rationale*
Maintain a calm, nonjudgmental approach.	Instills the family with a sense of trust and acceptance; enhances the family's confidence in the ED staff.
Prepare family for the child's appearance (e.g., bandages, casts).	Parents may feel anxious and shocked by their child's appearance; preparation can lessen this shock (Broome, 2000).
Ask the family about child's previous healthcare experiences and how child responded, including successful coping strategies.	Demonstrates respect for the child's individual needs.
Reunite the child and the family as soon as possible following examinations and treatment.	Family's fantasies and fears seldom match reality; decreases the child's and the family's anxiety and provides reassurance and comfort.
Provide specific instructions as to how the parent can assist the child (e.g., "I want you to sit by your child's head, stroke your child's forehead, and softly sing your child's favorite song, or talk quietly to your child.").	Parents want to help their child and need to know how to participate. Caring for an ill or injured child may be a new role for the family.
Provide factual information simply and clearly.	In crisis situations, families have a reduced ability to comprehend information and to initiate problem solving.
Have the family identify a support person for themselves or provide one for them, if possible.	Assists the family to maintain emotional stability.
Have a family member give a personal object for the child to hold if the family member cannot or does not want to be with the child during a procedure or treatment.	Respects the family's wishes; gives the child a sense of trust that the family will not desert the child.
Tell the parents, prior to their participation in a treatment or procedure, that they may be asked to leave depending on how the child is responding or how they themselves are responding.	Establishes an honest relationship and informs the parents that their child's best interest is the priority.
Describe to the family what they can do to support their child during a treatment or procedure, if the parent wants to be present during a procedure. If a family member has difficulty coping during the procedure, the nurse should have the family member take a short break.	Children sense the family's anxiety, which heightens their own anxiety, which in turn increases the family's anxiety (emotional contagion theory). Taking a short break restores the family member's psychosocial strength.
If the parents make statements that seem to demonstrate unrealistic expectations of the child, provide a realistic explanation of what a child of that age might be expected to do. Suggest to parents some positive approaches to assisting the child; serve as a role model.	Provides appropriate information about child development and about how children may respond to stressful events. Prevents censure of the child. Actively incorporating parents in the care of their child helps them to maintain their parenting role and focuses the parents' energies on their strengths and maximizes their positive adaptation to the situation.
Offer respite care to the family member during lengthy procedures or treatments; have another family member or staff member serve as the child's support person.	Respects the family's need for self-care.
Collaborate and consult with additional healthcare professionals as needed (e.g., social worker, spiritual advisor, translator, or child life specialist).	Recognizes the family's unique needs.
Keep the family informed about their child's condition and the course of treatment. Acknowledge the difficulty in waiting. Suggest a short walk or a visit to the cafeteria, or offer a telephone.	Families in stressful situations often neglect themselves.
Respect the family's decisions and acknowledge their contributions to caring for and comforting their child.	Acknowledges the family's contribution to the child's treatment; recognizes the family as the child's source of support (Newton, 2000).

(continued)

TABLE 4.8 (continued)

Intervention	*Rationale*
Provide follow-up as needed. In addition to specific treatment regimens, discuss possible post discharge behaviors the child might exhibit, such as temporary sleeping and feeding difficulties; clinging behavior; temporary loss of recently acquired developmental milestones, such as staying dry at night or talking in sentences; and rebellious behavior in older children (Fletcher, 1981). The child may also play out his or her emergency experience. Tell parents to remain calm, reassure the child, and discuss the emergency experience in simple, honest terms to clarify the child's misconceptions (Association for the Care of Children's Health, 1989).	Prepares family for adequate healthcare followup. Allows family to anticipate their children's behavior. Children use play to master stressful experiences; role playing the emergency treatment with dolls or siblings helps the child to understand what happened and allows the child to incorporate the experience into his or her development. These behaviors are generally temporary and short-lived. If the behaviors continue, the parents should discuss them with their primary healthcare professional.

References

Ahammn, E. (1994). "Chunky Stew." Appreciating cultural diversity while providing health care for children. *Pediatric Nursing, 20*, 320–324.

Association for the Care of Children's Health. (1989). *Caring for your child in the emergency room*. Washington, DC: Author.

Bernardo, L., & Schenkel, K. (1995). Pediatric medical emergencies. In S. Kitt, J. Selfridge-Thomas, J. Proehl, & J. Kaiser (Eds.), *Emergency nursing: A physiologic and clinical perspective* (2nd ed., pp. 407–427). Philadelphia: Saunders.

Bernardo, L., Conway, A., & Bove, M. (1990). The ABC method of emotional assessment and intervention: A new approach in pediatric emergency care. *Journal of Emergency Nursing, 16*(2), 70–76.

Bibace, R., & Walsh, M. (1980). Children's conceptions of illness. In R. Bibace, & M. Walsh (Eds.). *Children's conceptions of health, illness, and bodily functions* (pp. 31–48). San Francisco: Jossey-Bass.

Billings, P., & Burns, C. (2000). Developmental management of school-age children. In C. Burns, N. Barber, M. Brady, & A. Dunn (Eds.), *Pediatric Primary Care: A handbook for nurse practitioners* (2nd ed., pp. 123–137). Philadelphia: W. B. Saunders.

Brennan, A. (1994). Caring for children during procedures: A review of the Literature. *Pediatric Nursing, 20*, 451–547.

Broome. (2000). Helping parents support their child in pain. *Pediatric Nursing, 26*(26), 315–119.

Burke, P. (1995). Developmental considerations. In S. Kelley (Ed.), *Pediatric emergency nursing* (2nd ed., pp. 39–51). Norwalk, CT: Appleton & Lange.

Coles, R. (1991). *The spiritual life of children*. New York: Random House.

Coles, R. (1997). *The moral intelligence of children*. New York: Random House.

Colizza, D., Prior, M., & Green, P. (1996). The ED experience: The development and psychosocial needs of children. *Topics in Emergency Medicine, 18*, (3), 27–40.

Conway, A. (1993). Psychosocial considerations for the child and family. In L. Bernardo, & M. Bove (Eds.), *Pediatric emergency nursing procedures* (pp. 11–27). Boston: Jones & Bartlett.

Deloian, B. (2000). Developmental management of infants. In C. Burns, N. Barber, M. Brady, & A. Dunn, *Pediatric primary care: A handbook for nurse practitioners* (pp. 82–99). Philadelphia: Saunders.

Dixon, S., & Stein, M. (2000). *Encounters with children: Pediatric behavior and development* (3rd ed.). St. Louis, MO: Mosby.

Emergency Nurses Association. (1998). Family presence at the bedside during invasive procedures and/or resuscitation. Des Plaines, IL: Author.

Erikson, E. (1963). *Childhood and society* (2nd ed.). New York: Norton.

Erikson, E. (1967, January). Identity and the life cycle: Selected papers. *Psychological Issues Monograph*.

Fletcher, B. (1981). Psychological upset in posthospitalized children: A review of the literature. *Mature Child Nursing Journal, 10*, 186–189.

Frank, L., Greenberg, C., & Stevens, B. (2000). Pain assessment in infants and children. *Pediatric Clinics of North America, 47*, 487–511.

Goldberger, J., Gaynard, L., & Wolfer, J. (1990). Helping children cope with healthcare procedures. *Contemporary Pediatrics, 7*, 141–162.

Grover, G. (2000). Talking to children. In C. Berkowitz, *Pediatrics: A primary care approach*. (pp. 7-9) Philadelphia: W. B. Saunders.

Johnson, B., Thomas, J., & Williams, K. (1997). *Working with families to enhance emergency medical services for children*. Washington, DC: Emergency Medical Services for Children National Resource Center.

Kohlberg, L. (1969). *Stages in the development of moral thought and action*. New York: Holt, Reinhart & Winston.

Lamontagne, L., Hepworth, J., Byington, K., & Chang, C. (1997). Child and parent responses during hospitalization for orthopedic surgery. *Maternal Child Nursing, 22*, 299-303.

Lipson, J., Dibble, S., & Minarik, P. (1996). *Culture and nursing care: A pocketguide*. San Francisco: UCSF Nursing Press.

Lutz, W. (1986). Helping hospitalized children and their parents cope with painful procedures. *Journal of Pediatric Nursing, 1*, 25-26, 28, 30.

MacDonald, M. (2000). Cultural perspectives for primary health care. In C. Burns, M. Brady, & A. Dunn (Eds.), *Pediatric primary care: A handbook for nurse practitioners*. pp. 53-60. Philadelphia: W. B. Saunders.

Maier, H. (1978). *Three theories of child development*. New York: Harper & Row.

Manning, M. (1990). Health assessment of the early adolescent. *Nursing Clinics of North America, 25*, 827-829.

Melnyk B. (2000). Intervention studies involving parents of hospitalized young children. An analysis of the past and future recommendations. *Journal of Pediatric Nursing, 15*(1), 4-13.

Newton, M. (2000). Family-centered care: Current realities in parent participation. *Pediatric Nursing, 26*, 164-168.

Ott, M. (1996). Imagine the possibilities! Guided imagery with toddlers and preschoolers. *Pediatric Nursing, 22*, 34-38.

Piaget, J., & Helder, S. (1969). *The psychology of the child*. New York: Basic Books.

Pidgeon, V. (1977). Characteristics of children's thinking and implications for health teaching. *Maternal Child Nursing Journal, 6*, 6.

Pridham, K., Adelson, F., & Hanson, M. (1987). Helping children deal with procedures in a clinic setting: A developmental approach. *Journal of Pediatric Nursing, 2*, 15-21.

Ritchie, J., Caty, S., & Ellerton, M. (1988). Coping behaviors of hospitalized preschool children. *Maternal Child Nursing Journal, 17*, 153-172.

Santrock, J. (1999). *Life span development* (7th ed.). Madison, WI: Brown & Benchmark.

Seidel, J., & Henderson, D. (1997). Approach to the pediatric patient in the ED. In R. Barkin (Ed.), *Pediatric Emergency Medicine* (pp. 4-10). St. Louis, MO: Mosby-Year Book.

Selbst, S., & Henretig, F. (1989). The treatment of pain in the ED. *Pediatric Clinics of North America, 36*, 968-969.

Spector, R. (2000). *Cultural diversity in health and illness* (5th ed.). Stamford, CT: Appleton & Lange.

Stanford, G. (1991). Beyond honesty: Choosing language for talking to children about pain and procedure. *Children's Health Care, 20*, 261-262.

Vessey, J., Braithwaite, K., & Wiedmann, M. (1990). Teaching children about their internal body. *Pediatric Nursing, 16*, 29-33.

Wear, R. (1974). Separation anxiety reconsidered: Nursing complications. *Maternal and Child Health Nursing Journal, 3*, 14-18.

Widey, L. (2000). Developmental management of adolescents. In C. Burns, N. Barber, M. Brady, & A. Dunn, *Pediatric primary care: A handbook for nurse practitioners*. (pp. 139-158). Philadelphia: W. B. Saunders.

Zelter, L., Bush, J. & Chen, E. (1997). A psychobiologic approach to pediatric pain: Part II: Prevention and treatment. *Current Problems in Pediatrics, 27*, 264-284.

Zimmerman, P., & Santen, L. (1997). Teddy says "Hi!": Teddy bear clinics revisited. *Journal of Emergency Nursing, 23*, 41-44.

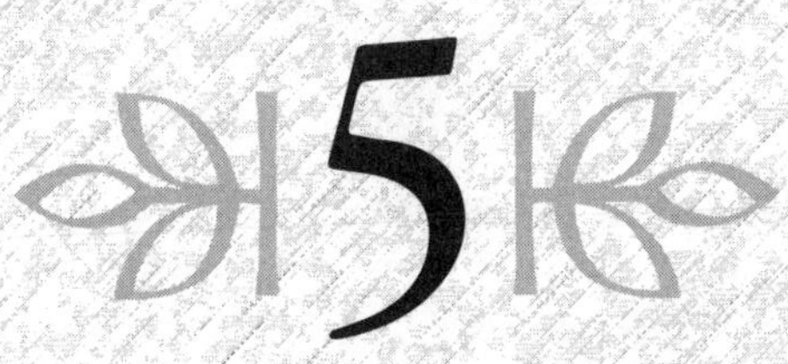

5 Prevention of Illness and Injury

Laurie Flaherty, RN, MS

Introduction

Childhood is a time of wonder and excitement. It is also a time of learning and experimentation. There may be no other time in life when the potential for the future is more appreciated or acted upon. The active promotion of behaviors that optimize health and minimize the risks of illness and injury should be incorporated into the health care of every child, whether the child is treated in a physician's office, clinic, or emergency department (ED). During ED visits, emergency nurses have opportunities for "teachable moments" with patients and families. Knowledge of selected health promotion issues allows emergency nurses to optimize these teachable moments.

Strategies for health promotion education are outlined in Table 5.1. To promote health and prevent illness and injury, emergency nurses employ primary, secondary, and tertiary prevention (Table 5.2). The purpose of this chapter is to outline primary prevention activities related to illness and injury prevention. Additional health promotion resources are provided.

Wellness and Illness Prevention

Primary prevention of illness involves the provision of adequate nutrition, the promotion of oral hygiene, and the administration of immunizations. Other strategies for illness prevention and health promotion are listed in Table 5.3.

Emergency nurses should be familiar with the endemic (baseline) diseases in their geographic location so that appropriate teaching and screening measures can be initiated. For example, children living in low-income housing may be exposed to lead, and homeless children may be exposed to tuberculosis. Knowing the community's risk factors can help emergency nurses to anticipate specific health risks and to intervene accordingly. The local health department may assist with additional resources for screening and education.

Nutrition

"Food and nutrition are not the same thing" (Hardin Gookin, 1995). *Food* is what is eaten, and *nutrition* is what results. Eating is an activity in which a child spends a lot of time. Food preparation and choices are grounded in cultural, ethnic, and personal beliefs. Parents may be concerned about their child's eating habits and may have questions such as "When should solid foods be started?", "How much food should a 2-year-old child eat?", "How does one encourage a child to eat?".

Children's uniqueness extends to their eating preferences and habits as well as to any other activity or attribute. Chances are, most children's eating habits will not follow any rule or match any chart. These habits may change from day to day and certainly may change over time. Recommendations for promoting healthy eating habits and nutrition begin in infancy and extend throughout the life span.

Several of the Healthy People 2010 goals center around nutrition. There is much concern about the increasing prevalence of obesity in children and adolescents. Patterns of healthy eating behavior need to begin in childhood and be maintained through adult life.

TABLE 5.1 Selected Strategies for Health Promotion Education

Strategy	*Rationale*
Match the teaching to the patient's and family's perceptions, beliefs, and concerns.	Identifying the family's health beliefs, as well as cultural, religious, and ethnic influences, allows the nurse to move forward with teaching.
Tell the patient and family the purposes and the expected effects of the health recommendations and when the results should be anticipated.	Most health-related behaviors require time before any noticeable changes or improvements are noted.
Suggest small changes at first.	Small, measurable goals for which results are obvious can encourage patients and families to continue with the health promotion activities.
Link new behaviors to current behaviors.	Linking allows the patient and family to incorporate changes more readily into their daily routine. For example, medications may be taken before bathing at bedtime.
Use a combination of teaching strategies.	The distribution of written education materials in the ED waiting area and treatment rooms, the use of audiovisual materials, and one-on-one counseling are methods emergency nurses can use for patient and family education.

From: U.S. Preventive Services Task Force (1996).

TABLE 5.2 Levels of Prevention

Level of Prevention	*Description*	*Examples*
Primary	Actions taken to prevent disease development in well individuals (Gordis, 1996, p. 5).	*Illness prevention:* Immunizations *Injury prevention:* Use of car safety restraints
Secondary	Identification of individuals who have a disease at an early stage in the disease's natural history, through screening and early intervention (Gordis, 1996, p. 6).	*Illness prevention:* Breast and testicular self-examination in adolescents *Injury prevention:* Home assessment for availability of phone number of poison control center
Tertiary	Prevention of disability or further injury once an illness or injury has occurred.	*Illness prevention:* Administration of antibiotics to prevent systemic infection *Injury prevention:* Application of spinal immobilization to prevent spinal cord injury

TABLE 5-3 Strategies for Illness Prevention

Strategy	*Earliest Age for Practicing the Strategy*	*Examples*
Handwashing	Preschool	Demonstrations on how to wash hands and when to wash hands; apply glitter ("germs") to the child's hands and observe the child wash off the "germs"
Personal hygiene	Grade school	Discussions on germs and body odors; demonstration of the use of deodorants (older grade school to middle school)
Tobacco use	Grade school	Discussions on the health risks of tobacco use; demonstrations on the effects of tobacco smoke and use
Alcohol/illicit drug use/intravenous drug use	Grade school	Discussions on the health risks of alcohol and illicit drug use
Exercise/regular physical activity	Grade school	Discussions on the need for proper exercise; demonstration of simple exercise activities
Sexually transmitted diseases and pregnancy	Late grade/middle school	Discussions on sexuality; discussions on the transmission of sexually related diseases; discussion on and demonstrations of methods to prevent sexually transmitted diseases and pregnancy (e.g., abstinence and application of condoms)
Breast and testicular cancer	Middle school/high school	Discussions on the causes of breast and testicular cancers; demonstration of breast and testicular self-examinations
Infectious diseases (acquired immunodeficiency syndrome, hepatitis)	Grade school	Discussion on disease transmission; discussion on preventing disease transmission
Eating disorders	Grade/middle school	Discussion on the importance of proper nutrition; discussion about appearance and self-esteem; discussion on the warning signs of eating disorders
Basic emergency life-saving skills	Grade school	Introduction, acquisition, and reinforcement of basic emergency life-saving skills

Healthy People 2010 also includes goals for specific kinds of nutritional and weight improvement:

- Goal 19-3: Reduce the proportion of children and adolescents who are overweight or obese. As of 1988–1994 baseline data, 11 percent of children age 6 to 11 years of age were overweight or obese, defined as at or above the gender and age-specific 95th percentile of BMI. 2010 target: 5 percent.
- Goal 19-5: Increase the proportion of persons aged 2 and older who consume at least 2 daily servings of fruit. At present, only 28 percent of persons age 2 and older consumed 2 servings in 1994–1996. 2010 target: 75 percent.
- Goal 19-6: Increase the proportion of persons aged 2 and older who consume at least 3 daily servings of vegetables. As of 1994–96, only 3 percent consumed 3 daily servings. 2010 target: 50 percent.
- Goal 19-7: Increase the proportion of persons aged 2 and older who consume at least 6 daily servings of grain products. Only 7 percent did so in the 1994–96 year period. 2010 target: 50 percent.
- Goal 19-9: Increase the proportion of persons aged 2 and older who consume no more than 30 percent of daily calories from fat. During the 1994–96 year period, 33 percent of persons age 2 and older consumed no more than 30 percent of daily calories from fat. 2010 target: 75 percent.

Although these targets are ambitious, even partial achievement will vastly improve health, as nutritional or dietary factors contribute substantially to the burden of preventable diseases in later life, such as coronary heart disease and diabetes.

Infants

Solid foods generally are introduced sometime between 4 and 6 months of age depending on the infant's:

- Weight gain (too much, too little).
- Frequency of feeding and signs of hunger (e.g., satisfaction or signs of hunger after formula or breast-feeding).
- Interest in the parents' food and eating patterns.
- Chances for allergies, according to the family's history of allergies.

The Food Guide Pyramid, introduced in 1992, is an educational tool that conveys recommendations about the number of daily servings from different food groups. It can offer healthy choices for meals and snacks. Free copies are available at www.usda.gov/cnpp.

In most cases, rice cereal is the first solid, because it is easier to digest than other cereals. To introduce cereal, feed it twice a day, with a thin rather than thick consistency. Once rice cereal is accepted by the infant, other foods, such as vegetables and fruits, can be introduced. New foods are introduced one at a time, for approximately 1 week at a time, to allow easier detection of food allergies. A balanced diet for infants is summarized in Table 5.4.

Toddlers

Toddlers are known for their highly selective (i.e., picky) food preferences. Many times, a toddler may only eat one food for days; this situation may be distressing to the parent. If the child is gaining weight and appears healthy, then the toddler's sometimes peculiar eating habits are satisfactory and not cause for alarm. Toddlers are mastering coordination skills and enjoy finger foods. Consequently, meal times may be messy. A balanced diet for toddlers is outlined in Table 5.5.

TABLE 5.4 Recommended Infant Diet

Component	*Daily Recommendation*
Calories	Not necessary to count. Rate of weight gain is an indicator of sufficient intake.
Protein	Two or three tablespoons a day of meat, chicken, cottage cheese, egg yolk, or yogurt; or 1 oz. of cheese; or 2 oz. of tofu.
Calcium	Two cups of whole milk or the equivalent of breast milk or formula. As these are decreased and solids are increased, cheese, yogurt, and other calcium foods are added.
Complex carbohydrates and whole grains	Two to four servings of grain foods (e.g., cereal, bread, pasta), legumes, or dried peas.
Green leafy and yellow vegetables and yellow fruits	Two to three tablespoons of winter squash, sweet potato, carrots, broccoli, kale, apricots, yellow peaches, cantaloupe, mango, or peaches.
Vitamin C foods	One-fourth cup of orange juice, cantaloupe cubes, mango cubes, broccoli, or cauliflower.
Other fruits and vegetables	One daily serving of applesauce, banana, peas, beans, or potatoes.
High-fat foods	Dairy byproducts should be full fat.
Iron-rich foods	One daily serving of meat, egg yolk, wheat germ, whole-grain bread, dried peas, and other legumes, or iron-fortified cereal.
Salty foods	Infant kidneys cannot process large amounts of salt, so baby's foods should not contain added salt.
Fluids	In first 4 to 5 months, will be supplied totally by formula or breast milk. As the infant grows older, add whole milk, fruit juices, and water. Increase in hot weather or when fever or diarrhea occurs.
Vitamin supplements	Use only as recommended by physician.

From: Eisenberg, Murkoff, & Hathaway (1989).

TABLE 5.5 Recommended Toddler Diet

Component	*Daily Recommendation*
Calories	900 to 1700 calories.
Protein	Four servings. One serving equals 3/4 cup milk, 1/2 cup yogurt, 3 tablespoons cottage cheese, 3/4 oz. hard cheese, 1 whole egg, 1 oz. poultry or meat, 2 oz. tofu, 1 1/2 tablespoons peanut butter, 1 oz. high-protein pasta.
Calcium	Four servings. One serving equals 2/3 cup milk, 1/2 cup yogurt, 1 1/3 oz. full fat cheese, 4 oz. calcium-fortified orange juice.
Vitamin C foods	Two or more servings. One serving equals 1/2 small orange, 1/4 medium grapefruit, 1/4 cup strawberries, 1/8 cantaloupe, 1/4 cup orange juice, 1/4 cup broccoli, 1 small tomato, 1/2 cup green pepper, 1/2 cup tomato sauce.
Green leafy or yellow vegetables and yellow fruits	One serving equals 1 apricot, 1 cup cubed cantaloupe, 1 nectarine, 1/2 yellow peach, 6 asparagus spears, 1/2 cup cooked broccoli, 3/4 cup peas, 1/4 carrot, 1 tablespoons cooked winter squash, 1 tablespoon sweet potato.
Other fruits and vegetables	One or two servings. One serving equals 1/2 apple, pear, or banana, 1/4 cup applesauce, 1/3 cup cherries, berries, or grapes, 2 or 3 asparagus spears, 3/8 cup green beans, 1/4 cup sliced mushrooms, yellow squash, or zucchini, 1/2 ear of small corn.
Whole grains and complex carbohydrates	Six or more servings. One serving equals 1/2 slice whole-grain bread, 1/4 bagel or English muffin, 2 to 3 crackers or bread sticks, 1/2 serving breakfast cereal, 1/2 oz. high-protein pasta, 1/4 cup cooked beans.
Iron-rich foods	Some every day.
High-fat foods	Five to eight servings a day. One serving equals 1/2 tablespoon oil, butter, margarine or mayonnaise, 1 1/2 tablespoon cream cheese, 1 tablespoon peanut butter, 1 egg, 3/4 cup whole milk, 3/4 cup yogurt, 2/3 oz. hard cheese, 9 French fries.
Salty foods	No added salt needed.
Fluids	Four to six cups daily.
Vitamin supplements	Only as recommended by physician.

From: Eisenberg, Murkoff, & Hathaway (1994), pp. 500–538.

Preschoolers and Older Children/Adolescents

Children, adolescents and adults should maximize their nutrition by eating the following foods every day:

- One serving of vitamin A foods, such as apricots, cantaloupe, carrots, spinach, or sweet potatoes.
- One serving of vitamin C foods, such as oranges, grapefruit, or tomatoes.
- One serving of high-fiber foods, such as apples, bananas, figs, plums, pears, strawberries, peas, potatoes, or spinach.
- One cruciferous vegetable several times a week, such as broccoli, cauliflower, Brussels sprouts, or cabbage.

Foods to avoid or minimize are:

- Refined sugar. When sugars combine with naturally occurring bacteria in the mouth, acids are produced. These acids eat into tooth enamel, beginning the tooth decay process.
- Corn, rice, and refined wheats. These are relatively low in valuable proteins compared with oats, rye, and whole wheat. Refining removes much of the vitamins, minerals, and roughage of foods.
- Caffeine. One cola drink for a child is equivalent to 4 cups of coffee for an adult (Hardin Gookin, 1995).
- Fried foods. These are not healthy for anyone in large amounts:
    - Best fats (monounsaturated): avocado oil, olive oil, canola oil, safflower oil, sunflower oil, corn oil, and soy oil.

- Bad fats (saturated): palm oil, coconut oil, vegetable fat or shortening, suet, lard, and butter.

- Low-nutrition juices. Intake of these should be limited to 4 to 8 ounces a day. They may replace milk intake, making the child feel full, and thereby reducing intake of healthy foods (Eisenberg et al., 1994).

Emergency nurses can apply this information in their health teaching to parents and children and can incorporate it into posters, pamphlets, or other media appropriate for teaching. Obtaining the child's weight and comparing it with age-adjusted norms may be a strategy for opening up discussion about a child's weight and growth.

Oral Hygiene

Oral hygiene usually is associated with the development of teeth, but good oral hygiene includes tooth and gum care as well as a diet that supports oral structure health and development. Oral hygiene should start simply and early and be maintained as a part of the daily routine. It is recommended that a child's first visit to a dentist be at age 3 years. Children with poor oral hygiene may refuse to eat because of pain from tooth decay or because food is not tasty, thereby compromising their nutrition. Parents should follow these recommendations for promoting oral hygiene:

- Clean the infant's gums daily with a wet baby washcloth or gauze.
- Remove the bottle from the infant's mouth prior to bedtime to avoid depositing milk and sugars onto the teeth.
- Encourage water consumption, because it is a simple, effective way to clean the mouth.
- Begin gentle toothbrushing with a soft toothbrush as soon as the infant's teeth erupt (generally at 6 to 7 months of age with a range of 2 to 12 months of age).
- Apply small amounts of toothpaste to a child-sized toothbrush. Large amounts of fluoride can stain teeth, and many water supplies already contain fluoride supplements. A pediatric-sized toothbrush is easier for the child to manage and to use consistently.
- Assist the child with toothbrushing until he or she is 7 or 8 years old. Brushing together after meals and before bedtime sets a schedule for the child and parent to follow.
- Encourage proper rinsing after brushing because it eliminates loosened food and generally cleans the mouth.
- Encourage adequate calcium intake, and limit intake of refined sugar.
- Consider eating a piece of cheese after eating sweets or high-carbohydrate foods between meals. The cheese will block the action of tooth-decaying acids produced by the bacteria in plaque.

Emergency nurses can incorporate this information into their patient assessments. Nurses can note the child's oral hygiene and offer suggestions for promoting oral hygiene. Company representatives from toothpaste and toothbrush companies may be willing to donate these items for emergency nurses to distribute to needy children and families.

Infectious Diseases/Immunizations

Illness is a part of life. Illnesses are likely to occur in those children who have increased exposure to other children, such as those in school or day care, and in children with siblings. Several simple measures to minimize and perhaps prevent infectious disease transmission in children of all ages include:

- Handwashing properly after using the bathroom, touching pets, sneezing or coughing, and before eating.
- Using only one's own personal hygiene items, such as towels, eating utensils, cups, and toothbrushes.
- Maintaining a clean environment.

Immunizations protect infants and children from potentially dangerous and life-threatening diseases. Before these vaccines were widely available, not only were infectious diseases common, but also many of them were deadly. Diphtheria outbreaks, for example, killed thousands of Americans every year, mostly children (Raskin, 1998).

Vaccines are a weakened, killed, or partial form of a disease-causing organism. When administered to the child, the vaccine prompts the body to produce antibodies against it. Subsequent exposures to the same organism prompt the body to recognize the organism and produce antibodies to ward off infection. Several doses of a vaccine may be required to produce and maintain adequate antibodies, which is why "booster" shots are needed.

Reactions to vaccines are rare and include fever, a mild rash, swelling in the neck or joints, and pain in the arms and legs. In only 7 per 70 million doses do children develop severe symptoms, such as dyspnea, hypotension, or anaphylaxis (Raskin, 1998). Most commonly, children experience discomfort at the vaccine site, which is usually relieved by administration of an age- and weight-appropriate dose of acetaminophen or ibuprofen.

Day care centers and schools may require proof of immunization prior to admission. The current immunization schedule, approved by the Centers for Disease Control, the American Academy of Pediatrics, the American Academy of Family Physicians, and the American Medical Association, is found in Table 5.6 along with information about each vaccine.

Given this complicated schedule, parents may not know whether their child is "up to date" on immunizations. Parents should be encouraged to carry written documentation of vaccinations to all healthcare visits. A copy of Table 5.6 should be available for reference in the triage area of the ED.

TABLE 5.6 Vaccine-Related Information

Vaccine	*Dose Schedule*	*Reactions/Side Effects*
Hepatitis B (Hep B or HBV)	3 doses 1) birth to 2 months of age 2) 1 to 4 months of age 3) 6 to 18 months of age	Site swelling and fever occur in 1-3% of recipients. Anaphylactic shock in one of every 600,000 doses.
Diphtheria, tetanus, and acellular pertussis	5 doses 1) 2 months of age 2) 4 months of age 3) 6 months of age 4) 15-18 months of age 5) 4-6 years of age Tetanus booster at 11-16 years of age	Until recently, the standard DTP vaccine contained the whole pertussis bacterium, causing site pain and vomiting in up to 50% of children and, in rare cases, seizures. The new DtaP vaccine uses only components of the bacterium and causes fewer side effects. About 25% of children experience site pain and fever.
Influenza type B (Hib)	3 or 4 doses 1) 2 months of age 2) 4 months of age 3) 6 months of age 4) 12-15 months of age	
Polio (OPV)	4 doses 1) 2 months of age 2) 4 months of age 3) 6-18 months of age 4) 4-6 years of age	Low-grade fever.
Measles, mumps, and rubella (MMR)	2 doses 1) 12-15 months of age 2) 4-6 years or 11-12 years of age	Fever, mild rash, swelling of neck and joints, and pain in the arms and legs. Anaphylactic reactions in 7 per 70 million doses (Raskin, 1998).
Varicella (VZV)	1 dose 1) 12-18 months of age Possible booster at 11-12 years of age	In 7% of recipients, a mild rash appears; in 20%, fever and site pain occur.

The American College of Emergency Physicians (1995) recently revised its policy statement on the immunization of pediatric patients in the ED to encourage a more active role of ED staff in the immunization process. ED physicians and nurses can identify underimmunized children and refer them to private healthcare providers or public health clinics for vaccine administration, or they can provide the immunizations in the ED (Robinson et al., 1996). EDs should have policies and procedures in place for administration of immunizations or for referral of children for immunizations.

Safety and Injury Prevention

Unintentional injury is the leading cause of death for people between the ages of 1 and 34 years (National Center for Injury Prevention and Control, 2000). Most of these injuries are preventable. Analyses of contributing factors leading to injuries reveal that very few are "accidents," but, rather, they are "accidents waiting to happen." There are many ways to teach children and their parents how to avoid injuries or at least to minimize their severity. Many small businesses exist solely to childproof or promote home safety, and many national organizations and government agencies provide products, resources, and guidance to parents looking for help in improving their children's home environment.

Injury prevention involves *education, enforcement*, and *engineering/environment*. Table 5.7 suggests ways for emergency nurses to become involved in these injury prevention strategies for selected mechanisms of injury.

Safety for Children with Special Needs

Injury prevention strategies can be adapted for children with special healthcare needs. Examples for such modifications include (Injury Prevention for Children with Special Health Care Needs Work Group, 1999):

Motor vehicle safety

- Distribute special child safety seats/booster seats to children with special healthcare needs.
- Check car seat temperature during hot weather to prevent burns.

TABLE 5.7 Sample Injury Prevention Strategies

Injury Mechanism	*Education/Behavior Change*	*Enforcement/Legislation*	*Environment/Engineering*
Motor vehicle	Establish hospital car seat expert to perform car seat safety checks. Implement a media campaign about the correct use of restraints and safety seats. Provide motor vehicle safety literature in the ED waiting area.	Testify for the establishment of vehicle restraint laws. Monitor and report results of ED parking lot child safety restraint usage. Publicly demonstrate support for enforcement of child passenger safety laws.	Support research that identifies potentially dangerous adaptations made to allow children to use adult seat belts prematurely, as with seat belt positioners.
Pedestrian	Encourage ED staff to educate patients and families about traffic dangers. Provide pedestrian safety programs at elementary schools.	Identify high-risk areas for pedestrian collisions. Report them to law enforcement agencies. Support enforcement of laws protecting pedestrians.	Distribute reflector tape products.
Bicycle	Provide bicycle safety rodeos at schools and community fairs. Provide safety literature in the ED waiting area.	Promote bicycle helmet legislation. Avoid participating in parades unless there is a bicycle helmet rule.	Support development of dedicated bike paths and bike lanes. Provide free bicycle safety checkups.
Firearms	Educate patients and families about firearm safety. Develop and provide a media campaign to promote the use of trigger locks and lock boxes.	Provide ED data on penetrating trauma to law enforcement officials to enhance firearm laws. Testify for safer firearm laws. Establish a hospital position statement on firearms.	Support product design modifications that require personal identification of gun owner before firearm can be discharged.

Adapted from: Allen, K. (1997). *Preventing childhood emergencies: A guide to developing effective injury initiatives*, (pp. 11–12). Washington, DC: Emergency Medical Services for Children National Resource Center.

- Assure proper positioning of child safety seats and booster seats.

Pedestrian safety

- Install curb cuts at crosswalks and audible crosswalk signals.
- Install surfaces to differentiate the street from the sidewalk.
- Mark safe places to stand while waiting for the school or public bus.
- Identify children who need constant supervision when crossing streets.

Bicycle safety

- Teach safe riding practices, including using properly designed bicycles, following the rules of the road, and wearing a helmet.
- Enforce helmet use when operating a racing wheelchair, rowcycle, or hand cycle.
- Advocate for production of smaller bicycle helmets.

Home safety

- Develop evacuation plans with appropriate exits in the event of a house fire.
- Install fire alarms that have flashing lights for children who are hearing impaired.
- Develop individualized evacuation plans for children who may have difficulty with changes in their environment or who may have special equipment.

Playground safety

- Install soft surfaces and accessible play space.
- Schedule individual or small group times on equipment.

Sports safety

- Enhance individual skill development.
- Match sports activities to the child's ability.
- Enforce the use of protective gear and follow appropriate game rules.
- Provide special protection for children who need to use assistive technology.

Water safety

- Use supervision when children are in and around water.
- Teach swimming skills and water safety.
- Swim with a buddy and only in areas with lifeguards on duty.
- Protect skin from rough surfaces (wear socks).

Safety in and around the Home

The home is one of the most common sites of injury for infants and young children. To gain perspective on the child's view of the home and potential hazards, parents may be encouraged to obtain a "child's-eye-view" of the home environment by crawling on the floor and seeing the home from the child's perspective. Inspecting the home area by crawling and reaching allows the parent to anticipate dangers to the mobile infant and young child. Potential dangers include:

- Ungated staircases.
- Uncovered electrical outlets.
- Uncovered doorknobs.
- Unlocked cabinets and drawers.
- Easy access to poisonous plants, chemicals, and sharp or breakable objects.
- Unsteady tables, lamps, and bookshelves.
- Hot ovens and stoves.
- Television stands.

Home inspections should be repeated periodically because, as children grow, their mobility increases, and the home safety plan requires modification. Specific aspects of home safety are discussed further.

Furniture safety

The following are factors for optimal crib safety:

- Place infants to sleep in a crib on a firm, flat mattress. Do not place a baby on a waterbed, sofa, soft mattress, pillow, or other soft surface to sleep.
- Do not place soft, fluffy products, such as pillows, comforters, quilts, or sheepskins under infants while they sleep or nap.
- Consider using a sleeper as an alternative to blankets. If using a blanket, place baby with feet at the foot of the crib. Tuck the blanket around the foot of the crib mattress, only as far as the baby's chest, and make sure the baby's head remains uncovered during sleep.
- Never place a child's crib within reach of a window blind or its cords.
- Slats should be no more than 2 3/8 inches apart, to prevent the infant's head from getting stuck between them.
- Mattress should be flush against the crib sides. If two fingers can fit between the mattress and the side of the crib, the crib should not be used.
- Fluffy pads, pillows, or toys inside a crib may cause suffocation and should be removed.
- Bumper pads should be used around the entire crib until the infant begins to stand. Then the pads should be removed so that they are not used as steps.

- The crib mattress should be lowered before the baby can sit alone. The mattress should be at its lowest point before the baby can stand.
- Young children should be taken out of a crib when they reach 35 inches in height or when they begin to climb out of the crib, whichever happens sooner.

The following are safety factors for other furniture:

- High chairs, strollers, and changing tables should have safety straps that are used routinely and are in working condition.
- Toy chests, trunks, freezers, or other large containers with lids should have locks, or the lid should be removed.
- Children should not be expected to sleep safely in the top bunk of a bunk bed until approximately 7 years of age.
- No child should be left unattended in a high chair, stroller, or changing table (Smith, 1997).

Home structure safety

Certain structures within the home are particularly dangerous, such as stairs, balconies, counter tops, windows, and chairs that can lead to falls. Simple actions can minimize the risk of injury:

- Keep stairs well lit and clear of clutter.
- Install window guards when appropriate. Keep furniture away from windows, and allow windows to be opened only 5 inches or less.
- Never leave children unattended on a porch or balcony.
- Repair loose railings or boards on stairs, porches, and balconies.
- Use nonslip safety mats under area rugs.
- Avoid placing electrical cords under rugs or across walking paths.
- Install garage door openers only if they have sensors, to prevent crush injuries.
- Do not place breakable dishes or hot liquids on countertop or table edges, where they might be within a child's reach.
- In the kitchen, latch all cabinets and drawers containing heavy, sharp, or poisonous objects. Allow access to one cabinet (e.g., those containing pot lids) to direct and divert the child's energy for exploration.
- Use back burners on the stove. When front burners must be used, turn pot handles toward the back of the stove.
- When possible, place chairs in "unclimbable" positions.
- Keep window-covering cords and chains permanently out of reach of children.
- Never knot or tie window-blind cords together because this creates a new loop in which a child could become entangled.

Pet safety

Pets enrich children's lives, especially when children and adults practice basic rules of pet safety (Smith, 1997):

- Introduce infants and pets slowly and cautiously.
- Do not tease pets or handle them roughly.
- Leave pets alone when they eat, drink, and sleep.
- Supervise children when they play with pets.
- Avoid stray or unfamiliar animals, and report strays to local Humane Society or Animal Control personnel.
- Consider obedience training and socialization training for pets.
- Keep pets' immunizations up to date.

Prevention of choking, suffocation, and strangulation

Choking prevention is necessary for everyone:

- Withhold round or hard foods, such as peanuts, popcorn, hard candies, hot dogs, grapes, and raisins, from children less than 4 years old.
- Cut food into bite-sized (child bite-sized) pieces, appropriate for the child's age and ability to chew and swallow.
- Avoid roughhousing, laughing, and playing during mealtimes.
- Keep small objects, such as safety pins, paper clips, pins, screws, nails, coins, jewelry, and small batteries, off the floor and away from accessible shelves or drawers.
- Keep marbles, small toys, and small toy parts away from very small children.
- A simple rule of thumb is that any small object or any toy that fits inside the cardboard tube of a roll of toilet paper is small enough to be a choking hazard (Smith, 1997). Alternatively, choke tubes can be purchased to test for choking hazards.
- Keep balloons away from children under 6 years. If the balloon pops while against a child's mouth, the child may startle, gasp, and aspirate the balloon. Consider using Mylar balloons as an alternative.

The following measures can be taken to prevent suffocation:

- The most obvious source of suffocation danger to a child is a plastic bag. These bags exist in many sizes in every home. Keep all dry cleaning, produce, grocery, and trash bags away from small children.

- At very young ages, when infants cannot support their weight with their arms, other objects may be hazardous. Never allow an infant to sleep with a soft pillow under the head. Fluffy pads, pillows, bean bag cushions, or toys inside a crib might also cause suffocation because the infant can roll onto the stomach but cannot lift the upper body and head with the arms.

Strangulation can occur if children have access to window dressing cords, belts, long necklaces, ribbons, or toys with long strings. The following measures may prevent strangulation:

- Avoid putting pacifiers on strings or cords around the child's neck.
- Do not place mobiles or hanging objects on string or elastic longer than 7 inches, or within reach above a child's crib, especially if the object has loops or openings greater than 14 inches.
- Avoid jackets with drawstrings because these strings can get caught on any number of items, such as playground equipment (Smith, 1997).

Safety in and around Water

The following measures should be taken to decrease the risks associated with swimming or playing in and around water:

- Never leave a child alone in the bathtub, or near any water, even if the telephone or the doorbell rings. Even a 5-gallon pail can cause drowning; as the small child falls in, the child falls head first into the bucket and is unable to extricate himself or herself from the pail.
- Whenever a child is in or around water, as in a large pool, an adult who can swim should be with that child. Children may not retain their swimming skills in an emergency. Even children who know how to swim are not "waterproof."
- Children who learn to swim reduce their risk of drowning. Enrollment in organized classes should be encouraged.
- Pools and hot tubs should be fenced in on all four sides, and a telephone should be placed within the fence. Hot tub covers should be locked.
- No one should dive or swim into any body of water (e.g., pond, back yard creek) until the depth and character of the water are known. Practice "feet first the first time."
- If the home is near or on a large body of water, personal flotation devices (PFDs) should be used whenever the child is near or in the water. They should be approved for the setting in which they are used, have an 11-digit United States Coast Guard approval number, and have a safety strap that fits under the crotch to prevent the PFD from sliding off, as well as handles on the collar that can be used to grab the child. The PFDs should not be used as cushions, because damage that can affect their flotation ability may occur (Smith, 1997).

Safety during Play

Play is the child's work. As children play, they learn, develop physical skills, hone eye–hand coordination, and, most of all, have fun! Unfortunately, many children are also injured as a result of their interactions with toys and playground equipment. In 2000, the Consumer Product Safety Commission reported approximately 191,000 toy-related injuries in the United States, and there were 16 toy-related deaths (CPSC, 2001a). Almost half of these deaths occurred when children choked on small objects or balloons; injuries resulted most frequently from use of riding toys (CPSC, 2000a). The following are measures to promote safe play with toys:

- Match toys to the child's skill and developmental level. Read toy labels to determine which toys are appropriate for the child's age, and keep older children's toys away from younger children.
- Inspect toys for potential hazards (e.g., button eyes, tags) before allowing small children to play with them.
- Teach older children to tell a grownup when small children have inappropriate toys.
- Check toys, clothes, and any other chewable objects, such as pacifiers, regularly (monthly) for loose or broken buttons, decorations, pieces, or rough edges.
- Check toys and furniture regularly (monthly) for loose decorations or hardware.
- Toy chests should have a strong lid with locking supports and safety hinges. The chest should stay open in any position and should have ventilation holes to prevent suffocation if a child becomes trapped inside.
- Avoid toys that are inherently dangerous, such as toys with exposed wires, toxic materials, lead paint, breakable or brittle parts, sharp points or edges, or toys that have springs or hinged parts that could pinch or trap fingers (American Academy of Pediatrics, 1994).

Safety on the Playground

Playground areas can bring hours of joy and exercise for children and can be safe with proper planning and construction. Injuries often result from falls, scrapes, cuts, sharp objects, and improper landing surfaces. Each year, approximately 200,000 children are treated in U.S. emergency rooms for playground equipment-related injuries; fractures are the most common injury (CPSC, 2000a). The following are guidelines for safe playground areas:

- Almost 60 percent of all injuries are caused by falls to the ground. Protective surfacing under all playground environment can reduce the risk of injury. Surfaces should have a minimum of 12 inches of a soft substance such as wood chips, mulch, sand, sawdust, or pea gravel. Existing surfaces, such as concrete or cement, should be covered with these materials. The use of safety mats is another alternative.

- Platforms should have guardrails and should be no more than 6 feet off the ground.
- "Fall zones" of at least 6 feet in all directions should be created around playground equipment.
- Play structures should be at least 12 feet apart.
- Eliminate "tripping" hazards, such as uneven surfaces, exposed cement, or ground surfaces.
- Carefully maintain all equipment. Check periodically for splinters or decayed wood components, deterioration or corrosion on structural components, or missing or damaged equipment components.
- Place swings away from other equipment to keep walking areas safe.
- Check for hot metal surfaces on equipment, such as slides, to prevent burns.
- An adult should be present whenever children play on playground equipment (Smith, 1997).
- Remove hood and neck drawstrings from all children's outerwear, and do not allow children to play on playground equipment with bicycle helmets on, as both drawstrings and helmets have been demonstrated to pose a strangulation hazard.

Firearm Safety

Americans possess nearly 200 million firearms, including 65 million handguns. An estimated 40 percent of all homes in the United States have some type of firearm, and one in four homes has a handgun. Each year, an estimated 1,500 children aged 14 and under are treated in emergency rooms for unintentional firearm-related injuries. Approximately 38 percent of these injuries are severe enough to require hospitalization. The unintentional firearm death rate among children aged 14 and under in the United States is nine times higher than in 25 other industrialized countries combined. Fifty percent of all childhood unintentional shooting deaths occur in or around the home of the victim, and nearly 40 percent occur in the home of a friend or relative (National SAFE KIDS Campaign, 1999).

The following safety measures are recommended to prevent gun-related injuries:

- Teach children to respect the potential danger of guns. Teach them to always assume a gun is loaded.
- Instruct children never to play with guns or to point them at anyone. Teach them that if they find a gun, they should not touch it and should tell an adult.
- Firearms should be kept unloaded, securely locked with trigger locks, and stored in a locked gun cabinet or vault. Bullets should be stored separately from the gun.
- Gun cabinet keys and ammunition keys should be stored in a separate location from frequently used keys.
- Discuss gun safety with the parents of children's friends. Children often play at each other's homes. If 1 of every 3 homes has a gun, it is not enough to make sure one's own firearm is securely stored (Smith, 1997).
- Parents should check with neighbors, friends, or relatives—or adults in any other homes where children may visit—to ensure they follow safe storage practices if firearms are kept in their homes.

Bicycle Safety

Each year, approximately 300 children aged 14 years and younger are killed in bicycle-related incidents. Of these 300 deaths, 90% are as a result of collisions with motor vehicles; 4 of 5 deaths result from head injuries (Consumer Product Safety Commission, 1997). An estimated 140,000 children are treated annually in the ED for bicycle-related head injuries (National Center for Injury Prevention and Control, 2001). Unfortunately, most of these children were not wearing bicycle helmets. Bicycle helmets have been shown to reduce the risk of head injury by 85% and the risk of brain injury by almost 90% (Thompson, Rivara, & Thompson, 1989). The following are measures to promote bicycle safety:

- Wear a helmet whenever riding a bicycle; this includes all family members, both children and adults. The four-step helmet-fit test, which requires little time to complete, is detailed in Table 5.8.
- Do not allow children to ride after dark.
- Make sure the bicycle has lights and reflectors.
- Limit or avoid riding bikes to school. Riding bikes to school involves riding during high commute times, making the ride more dangerous.
- Never ride with passengers on the bike.
- Bicycle seats for small children on adult bikes should be used only for children older than 1 year who can hold their head up and control their upper body with their arms. Children younger than 1 year should be placed in a bicycle-wagon carrier (Smith, 1997).
- Children should not grow into their bicycles; they should be able to straddle the bicycle comfortably with both feet firmly on the ground.
- Children should not ride in the street until they are 10 years old, demonstrate good riding skills, and are able to observe basic rules of the road.

TABLE 5.8 Four-Step Helmet Fit Test

Step	*Problem*	*Solution*
Press or push the *front* of the helmet with the heel of the hand.	Lifts the back of the helmet up and forward, covering the eyes.	Tighten front strap to junction. Adjust padding thickness, especially in the back. Ensure the chin strap is snug. If none of these solutions is effective, the helmet may be too big.
Press or push the *back* of the helmet with the heel of the hand.	Lifts the front of the helmet up and forward, uncovering the forehead.	Tighten back strap. Ensure the chin strap is snug. Protect the child's chin by shielding for possible skin pinching with your two fingers between the strap and the child's chin. Adjust padding thickness and/or position, especially in the front. Save extra padding for adjusting the helmet to the child's growth.
Ask the child to open his or her mouth as wide as possible, without moving the head. The top of the helmet should pull down.	Helmet does not pull down when opening the mouth.	Tighten chin strap. Ensure the front and back strap junction is under each ear.
Assess if the front edge of the helmet covers the forehead. The front helmet edge should not be more than one to two finger widths from the eyebrows.	Helmet does not cover the forehead.	Position the helmet no more than one to two finger widths above the eyebrows. Adjust so the helmet stays over the forehead. A sizing measurement tape, included in the helmet box, serves as a guide for helmet size selection.

Adapted from: National Highway Traffic Safety Administration, 1996, September. *Your bicycle helmet—A correct fit* (DOT Publication No. DOT HS 808 421) Washington, DC: Author.

- Learn the rules of the road and obey all traffic laws. Ride with the traffic, on the right side of the road. Use appropriate hand signals. Respect traffic signals, and stop and look both ways before entering a street (CDC, 2000).

Winter Safety

Winter sports and activities (sledding, snowboarding, skiing, ice-skating) are fun for children and families alike. These activities, though, can be dangerous for children. In one study of children admitted to trauma centers over a 5-year period, 224 children aged 2 to 18 years were injured while sledding; seven children died (Bernardo, Gardner, & Rogers, 1998). Measures to promote winter safety include:

- Dress in warm clothing to prevent hypothermia; wear layers of clothing to maximize body temperature.
- Ski and snowboard on marked, groomed trails to avoid avalanche risk; follow posted signs and obey the rules of the slopes.
- Sled in areas that are free of stationary obstructions, motor vehicle traffic, and large numbers of sledders; sled with only one person per sled.
- Avoid lakes and ponds that may not be completely frozen; obey all signs and warnings.
- Wear protective gear, such as helmets, when sledding, skiing, and snowboarding.
- Test all equipment prior to its use.

In-Line Skating, Roller Skating, Scooter, and Skateboard Safety

Wheeled recreational equipment is associated with more than one-third of all toy-related injuries (Consumer Product Safety Commission, 1996). Children aged 5 to 14 are particularly vulnerable, suffering more than 60,000 injuries per year (Consumer Product Safety Commission, 1996). Between 1993 and 1995, injuries associated with in-line skating rose from 37,000 to 105,000, a 184% increase (CPSC, 1996). Six of 10 skateboard injuries are to children younger than 15 years and those with skating experience of less than 1 week (CPSC, 1996). There are 26,000 injuries seen in EDs annually related to the use of skateboards (CPSC, 1996).

Data from the year 2000 collected by the U.S. Consumer Product Safety Commission show a dramatic increase in injuries related to scooter use, with more than 4,000 scooter-related injuries in hospital emergency rooms in the month of August alone.

Many of these injuries to young children reflect a lack of coordination, motor skills, and thinking ability needed to use scooter-related products safely. In older children, a general attitude of invincibility contributes to an increase in risk-taking behaviors and high rates of injury. Most injuries are to the wrists, arms, and legs, all of which could be protected with the use of proper equipment (CPSC, 1996). Children should take the following measures to prevent injuries (CPSC, 2001c):

- Wear protective clothing (helmet, gloves, wrist guards, elbow, knee, and shin pads) to avoid injuries while still enjoying "wheeled" activities.
- Skate on smooth, paved surfaces.
- Avoid auto traffic; consider skating in designated parks or other areas.
- Learn how to stop and how to fall.
- Curtail or avoid night nighttime skating because of decreased visibility.

Safety with Shopping Carts and Baby Walkers

In 1996, the Consumer Product Safety Commission reported an estimated 22,000 ED visits for children younger than 5 years of age who had fallen out of shopping carts and sustained head injuries. Baby walkers were associated with 14,300 injuries requiring emergency care during 1997 alone (CPSC, 2000). Baby walkers increase the mobility of infants and toddlers and allow them access to dangerous objects that would usually not be within their grasp. Parents and caretakers should be counseled to remove these devices from their home. Extreme care and caution must be used when considering the use of baby walkers and shopping carts (Smith, 1997):

Shopping-cart safety

- Use seatbelts to restrain children in the cart seat.
- Don't allow children to ride in the cart basket or stand in the shopping cart.
- Don't allow children to ride or climb the sides or front of the cart.
- Don't allow an older child to push the cart with another child in it.
- Consider bringing a harness or safety belt with you when shopping.
- Always stay close to the shopping cart.

Safety with walkers

- Close all doors and gates at the top of stairways.
- Use walkers only on smooth surfaces.
- Use only walkers that have a wide base that prevents tipping.
- Keep electrical and window dressing cords out of reach.
- Keep all objects away from table edges and avoid the use of tablecloths.
- Check the child's path for other hazardous items, such as potentially poisonous plants.
- As an alternative, use toys that allow children movement within a saucer, without a wheeled base.

Outdoor Safety

Pedestrian Safety

On average, a pedestrian is killed in traffic every 96 minutes. Darting out into the street from between intersections accounts for 50 to 70% of pedestrian injuries among children aged 9 years and younger. Children 15 years of age and younger account for 12% of all pedestrian fatalities and 32% of all nonfatal pedestrian injuries (National Center for Injury Prevention and Control, 2001). Children are also often injured in driveways and parking lots. Children are at a high risk for pedestrian injuries because of physiologic and developmental features:

- As pedestrians, children believe that if they can see a car, the car can see them.
- Children's ability to judge distances and localize sound is limited.
- Children's field of vision is one-third less than adults' vision, so they must turn their heads from side to side to see oncoming cars.
- Children believe cars can stop as quickly as they can.
- Children devote their attention to only one activity at a time.
- Children's concept of danger and understanding of death is different from that of adults'.
- Children cannot comprehend complicated traffic situations.
- Children tend to be impulsive and, often, motion exceeds caution.

To prevent pedestrian injuries:

- Children should not be allowed to cross the street or walk to school alone until they are at least 7 to 9 years old (American Academy of Pediatrics, 1994).
- Children should be taught to cross the street only at intersections.

- Children should be taught what traffic signals and markings mean and to obey all traffic rules.
- Children should be taught to stop at the curb or edge of the road, look left, look right, and look left again before crossing, and to continue looking as they cross the street.
- Children should not enter the street from between parked cars or from behind bushes or shrubs.
- Children should be taught to treat driveways like roadways, and to treat parking lots like intersections.
- Children should be taught to look for a sign that a car is about to move (e.g., rear lights, exhaust smoke, engine noise).
- Children should wear reflective clothing and materials that have fluorescent or Day-Glo colors.

Safety in Motor Vehicles

Of all the dangers facing children, the automobile poses the greatest threat to their safety. Motor vehicle crashes are the leading cause of death for children of every age from 6 to 14 years old. In the United States, an average of 7 children 0–14 years old were killed and 872 were injured every day during 1999. Among children fatally injured where restraint use was known, 61 percent were completely unrestrained (National Highway Traffic Safety Administration, 2000). Anatomic distinctions of children of children in motor vehicle crashes are outlined in Table 5.9.

Frontal impact (head-on collisions) and front-angle crashes are responsible for two-thirds of all crash fatalities (Stewart, 1997). Passenger restraint systems were designed to protect occupants in these crashes. The consequences of improper restraint are outlined in Table 5.10.

Motor vehicle-related passenger injuries can be prevented through the proper use of child safety devices, such as child safety seats for passengers and seat belts and air bags for adolescent drivers and front-seat passengers. Advantages of child safety seats are discussed in Table 5.11. While the present system of child auto restraint is not without challenges, it is well worth the family's effort to learn about child safety seats and how to use them properly. Emergency nurses play a role in promoting the safe vehicular transport of children by knowing how and when to use car safety devices and what information to teach parents about child passenger safety. The levels of safety seat use are itemized in Table 5.12.

Child passenger safety is a relatively new concept (Table 5.13). The Bunny Bear Company first produced car seats in 1933; in 1947, they manufactured two different child safety seats (Kuska, 2002). Before child safety seat laws, even *with* public education, the National use of child safety seats was only approximately 11% (Stewart, 1997). Although all 50 states have child passenger safety laws, most have large gaps because the law:

- Includes only children up to a certain age.
- Does not include children in all vehicle types.
- Does not hold nonparental drivers responsible.
- Covers only front-seat passengers.
- Does not cover out-of-state drivers.
- Does not cover taxis.
- Exempts emergency medical services and police vehicles, but holds them liable.

TABLE 5.9 Anatomic Distinctions of Children in Car Crashes

Anatomy	*Distinction*
Large, heavy head	The head acts as a missile, and the rest of the body follows.
Bone structure	
Infants:	
Shoulders are flexible, to fit through the birth canal (Stewart, 1997).	Infant seat belt systems are designed to spread crash impact forces across all of the infant's back and do not transfer impact to pelvic or shoulder girdles.
Hips are not fully developed until age 15 to 17 months (National Highway Transportation Safety Administration, 1992).	
Toddlers:	
Shoulders are much smaller.	Makes the chest clip (which holds shoulder harnesses together) essential in keeping the child in the safety seat in a crash.
Adults:	
Strongest bone groups are the pelvic girdle and shoulder girdle.	Adult lap and shoulder seat belts are designed to anchor across these bone groups.

TABLE 5.10 Consequences of Improper Car Safety Restraint

Improper Restraint Mechanism	*Outcome*
Holding child on adult lap.	Child is crushed between adult and dashboard, or ejected. To restrain child adequately, an adult holding the child would have to be able to restrain the weight of the child times mph at time of crash (e.g., 20-lb child × 30 mph = 600 lb). No adult could restrain that much weight (Flaherty, 1996).
Older child with adult shoulder belt behind back or under arm.	Child lunges forward from waist up, striking dashboard, or sustaining "lap belt syndrome"—trauma to intestines and lower spine. Airbag deploys as child moves forward into it.
Child too small for adult seat belt.	Child wears shoulder belt across neck, increasing risk of potential injury to neck in a crash or with sudden deceleration or swerving of vehicle.
Forward-facing infant seat.	In a frontal crash, infant is thrown forward. Infants' neck muscles are weak and head is large, increasing the risk of severe neck injury.
Not anchoring seat to car with seat belt.	On impact, seat becomes projectile with child in it.
Wrong size or type seat for child.	If seat is too small, it may not adequately protect child in crash. If seat is too large, child may slide out of the seat on crash impact.
Loose seat belt attachment points.	Seat belts are designed to "give" a few inches on crash impact, to decrease rate of sudden deceleration, thereby decreasing force of impact transferred to child's body. If seat belts are too loose, child safety seat will be allowed excessive movement on crash impact, increasing the risk of injury to its occupant. Child may submarine under the belt, causing hyperflexion and hyperextension of cervical spine.
Wrong angle of seat.	If infant seat is too upright or too flat, may occlude infant's airway.
Shoulder straps in wrong slots.	Child may be pulled out of seat upon crash impact.
Locking clip needed but not used.	Seat belt may not hold child safety seat securely on crash impact.
Child placed facing forward too soon.	In a frontal crash, infant is thrown forward. Infants' neck muscles are weak and head is large, increasing risk of severe neck injury. Infant should be at least 1 year of age *and* at least 20 lb to face forward.
Bulky liners, blankets, padding between child and restraining straps.	Build too much "give" into system, allowing too much body movement on crash impact, and increasing potential for injury. Maximum allowable "slack": one finger fitting between child and straps.
"After-market" devices, (e.g., those that reposition adult shoulder straps).	These devices are not crash tested or approved by U.S. Department of Transportation. They may not work in a crash or may cause injury.
Seats that are too old or recalled.	Seats manufactured before 1981 do not meet current federal motor vehicle safety standards. Recalled seats have particular defects not meeting current federal motor vehicle safety standards and must be fixed or replaced.
Cracked seats.	These seats may break on crash impact. Any child safety seat that has been in a crash should not be used again. Warm climates may crack plastic and decrease life of seat.
Two-point or lap belt.	Child's center of gravity is above the restraint, allowing child to jackknife forward on impact, causing flexion-distraction injuries to the lumbar spine, small-bowel contusion and perforation, degloving injuries to hollow viscus, pancreatic fracture, and external contusions.

TABLE 5.11 Advantages of Child Safety Seats

Child safety seats are designed primarily to protect the child's head and spinal cord (Stewart, 1997).
Child safety seats are designed to spread crash forces over a larger body area.
Properly used child safety seats come into contact with the body's strongest points during impact.
Secured child safety seats prevent vehicular ejection by restraining the child to the seat.
Properly restrained child occupants are prevented from crashing into each other on impact.
Child safety seat restraint straps give slightly, allowing the child's body to slow down gradually during sudden deceleration, thus reducing the force of impact.

TABLE 5.12 Levels of Vehicle Restraint Use

Age	*Use of restraints*
Infants <1 year	88% properly restrained
1–4 years	68% properly restrained
	11% not restrained
	21% in adult seat belts only
4–5 years	6% properly restrained
	19% not restrained
	75% in adult seat belts only
5–15 years	58% properly restrained
16–24 years	53% properly restrained

TABLE 5-13 History of Child Passenger Safety

Date	*Event*
1967	First manufactured child safety seat that protected child from crash forces rather than controlled child's movement.
1971	First Federal Motor Vehicle Safety Standard (FMVSS), written by National Highway Traffic Safety Administration (NHTSA).
	• Outlawed seats that hooked over adult seat.
	• Static testing only.
Late 1970s	First rear-facing infant seat.
1978	First child safety seat law passed in Tennessee.
1981	FMVSS 213 developed and revised previous NHTSA standard, including dynamic testing.
1985	All 50 states had child safety seat laws.
2000	National Child Passenger Safety Act of 2000 has provisions for improving child restraint performance.

From Kuska, 2002.

- Makes exceptions for "tending to child's needs."
- Makes exemptions for overcrowded vehicles.

As of August 2000, only 17 states had primary seat belt laws, which allow a law enforcement officer to pull over a driver purely for seat belt offenses; these states have seat belt usage rates 10 to 15% higher than do states with secondary laws (National Highway Traffic Safety Administration, 2000), where the officer must first pull over the driver for another offense. Despite child safety restraint laws, the appropriate use of child seats is extremely low (National Highway Traffic Safety Administration, 1996b).

Mechanics of car safety seats

Child safety seats are categorized as infant, convertible, toddler, and booster seats (Table 5.14). Each year, 7 million child safety seats are manufactured in the United States; there are more than 100 kinds of child safety seats. There are also hundreds of different makes and

TABLE 5.14 Categories and Features of Child Safety Seats

Infant	*Convertible*	*Toddler*	*Booster*
Used until infants are *both* 1 year old *and* at least 20 lb.	Used for either infant or toddler.	For children 20 to 40 lb., and *at least* 1 year of age.	For children 40 to 80 lb. and 4'9" tall.
Must be rear-facing, to spread crash forces safely.	Requires special adjustments to "convert" seat from toddler to infant mode.	Front facing.	Shield booster seat—used when only lap belt is available in vehicle.
Must be at 45-degree angle, to keep airway patent.	Ideal for children younger than 1 year of age who have surpassed the recommended weight limit for infant seats but still need to face rear (e.g., over 20 pounds, but younger than 1 year of age).	Should be in most upright position possible.	Shield booster does little to restrain upper body. In some models, shield may be removed, and adult lap and shoulder belt may be used to restrain child.
Top of shoulder harness straps should be at or below shoulder level.		Top of shoulder harness straps should be at or above shoulder level.	
Adequate until top of infant's head reaches past top of seat or child surpasses weight limit stated on labels. At this point, infant should ride in convertible seat, in rear-facing position, until infant is *both* 1 year-old *and* at least 20 lb.	Seat can be "converted" from infant to toddler seat when child reaches 1 year of age.	Used until child surpasses weight limit stated on labels or until child's ears reach above the top of the seat back, or shoulders reach above top strap slot.	Belt-positioning booster seat and high-backed seat. May have five-point harness that may be used with smaller children.
Designed to push baby into back of seat in a crash (toward front of car) and to rebound to almost stand baby up on feet. Shoulder harnesses and chest retainer clip prevent infant from sliding out of the top of the seat, and crotch strap prevents "submarining" out the bottom of the seat.	Seat use described in infant and toddler sections.	Designed to hold child in seat in a frontal crash with shoulder harness straps and chest clip. Top shoulder strap slot is directly above a metal bar designed to withstand crash impact. If shoulder straps are below top slot, child seat has only plastic shell to withstand impact and weight of child's body in a crash.	For larger children, five-point harness may be removed and adult lap and shoulder belt may be used to restrain child.

models of automobiles in the United States, with dozens of different seat belt systems, all of which are designed for adult passengers. Many of these seat belt systems do not restrain child safety seats well because they were not designed for this purpose. All child safety seats share the following features (Stewart, 1997):

- Shell—structure of the seat
- Shield/harness—to hold the child in the seat
- Belt path—for adult seat belt
- Labels (e.g., manufacture date, weight limits)
- Instructions

Children may use an adult lap and shoulder belt when all of the following criteria are met:

- The feet reach the floor.
- The knees bend over the edge of the seat.
- The back is against back of seat.
- The adult shoulder belt goes across shoulder instead of the neck. For most children, this does not occur until the child is approximately 80 pounds, or about 4 feet 9 inches.

Installation of a child safety seat should always follow the seat manufacturer's as well as the automobile manufacturer's instructions. The adequacy of installation can be inspected at child safety seat checkpoints sponsored by local fire departments, National Safe Kids Campaign Coalitions, or other reputable organization. Despite these instructions, challenges can impede families' compliance with installing and using child safety seats. Emergency nurses may offer possible solutions to these challenges (Table 5.15).

To rectify the problem of safety seat installation, NHTSA has implemented a new standardized system called LATCH (Lower Anchors and Tethers For Children). To meet this new standard, most forward-facing child seats will be equipped with a tether strap from the back of the child seat, which attaches to the vehicle. This strap will provide more head protection by allowing less forward motion by the seat and the child, and is the first step in a three-year phase-in that will also require two lower attachment points in vehicles and child safety seats. Neither the tether or attachment points will require the use of seat belts to install a child safety seat.

The lower anchorage points are small rods or bars located between the vehicle's seat cushion and seat

TABLE 5.15 Challenges with Child Safety Seats

Challenge	*Possible Solution*
There is often more than one seat belt system within the same vehicle. Each system works differently and may not secure the child seat adequately without some augmentation (e.g., locking clip).	Learn how to maneuver all seat belt systems within the vehicle. Determine the need for augmentation. Have seat checked by trained technician.
Some belts come out of the seat several inches ahead of the seat "crack," making it difficult to secure seats adequately.	Ensure that there is no more than 1 inch of movement in the child safety seat *base* when pushed or pulled. Place the safety seat in another seating position if the seat belts are as tight as possible and the child safety seat base moves more than 1 inch.
Auto seats themselves may be so deeply contoured that the child seat base may not fit in the seat.	Place the child safety seat in another seating position.
Some buckles are on long "stalks," building in several inches of slack and making secure installment difficult.	Assure that there is no more than 1 inch of movement in the child safety seat base when pushed or pulled. Place the safety seat in another seating position if seat belts are as tight as possible and the child safety seat *base* moves more than 1 inch.
Some auto seats come with large humps between seating positions, making secure attachment on this hump (without wobbling) difficult.	Avoid placing child safety seats on large seat humps.
Some seat belts are so close together that the child seat base will not fit between them.	Place the child safety seat in another seating position.
Some auto seats are severely tilted, making the angle of the child seat incorrect.	Place the seat at the correct angle by bolstering the child safety seat at the seat crack with rolled towels.
Some child seats extend beyond the front of the seat bottom.	Place the child safety seat in another seating position.
Some seat upholstery (e.g., leather) may be very slippery.	Place a plastic or rubber mat between the seat and upholstery.
Seat belts are loose and allow excessive movement of the child safety seat.	Push the child seat into the auto seat as much as possible, eliminating as much "cush" as possible from the seat cushion to decrease slack and potential seat movement. The child seat base should not move more than one inch when pulled or pushed.

back, allowing a child safety seat to be attached or snapped into the vehicle instead of being held secure by the vehicle's seat belt system. As of September 1, 2002, all child safety seats are required to have two attachment points that will connect to the vehicle's lower anchorage attachment points.

While this is the ideal system, it is notable that the average lifespan of a child safety seat is approximately 15 years, so it may be some time before the compatibility issue of child seat and vehicles is a thing of the past. Any of the new safety seats (with tethers and attachment points) can be used in older vehicles by installing them using the vehicle's safety belt system. In some cases, it may be possible to retrofit cars with tether anchors to allow use of the tether strap.

Compliance with child safety seat usage

Child behavior influences compliance with safety issues. For example, the parent may report that the child tries to get out of the safety seat or protests loudly while in the safety seat. Emergency nurses can recommend helpful strategies for enhancing compliance in car safety seat usage (Table 5.16).

TABLE 5.16 Strategies to Enhance Compliance with Car Safety Seats

Problem	*Strategy*
Screaming or crying rear-facing infant.	Pull over to determine the cause of the crying.
	Entertain a crying child by singing, talking, playing the radio, or providing distracting toys.
Concerns related to choking in the rear-facing infant.	Reduce choking risk by not feeding the infant immediately before or during vehicular travel.
Toddlers/older children who will not remain in the safety seat.	Compare traveling in a car to another dangerous situation in the home; use the same techniques to change the child's behavior.
	Avoid calling safety seats *baby seats*.
	Entertain the child by singing, talking, playing the car radio, and having distracting toys available.
	Add a second chest clip to prevent the child from getting out of the harness.

Air bags

Air bags are designed to protect the unrestrained adult passenger at speeds of 0.10 second during a frontal crash. The air bag must inflate quickly, at speeds of 140 to 200 mph, before the passenger impacts the dashboard or steering wheel. This inflation speed rate is in itself a significant source of energy, and a potential source of injury, if the passenger comes in contact with an inflating air bag.

It is estimated that as of 1999, more than 91 million air-bag-equipped passenger vehicles were on the road, including 65 million with dual air bags. At least one million new air-bag-equipped vehicles are sold each month. Air bags have saved 1,231 lives during 1999 alone, and from 1987 to 1999 saved a total of 4,969 lives.

As of October 1, 2000, 98 pediatric deaths have been reported from air bag deployment. These deaths were associated with children being unrestrained or improperly restrained ($n = 75$), an infant place in a rear-facing infant seat on the front passenger seat ($n = 18$), the child seat not restrained to the vehicle seat ($n = 2$), or the child being held in the lap of a passenger ($n = 3$). These deaths could have been prevented by:

- Using adult seat belts properly and only when the child is large enough to use adult seat belts—usually when the child weighs at least 80 pounds or is approximately 4 foot 9 inches tall.
- Properly restraining all children younger than 12 years old in the back seat.
- Moving the car seat as high as possible.

Conclusion

Health promotion and health protection are areas for emergency nurses to explore in their own practices. Many EDs have health and safety fairs to demonstrate positive health behaviors for children and adolescents. Some authors advocate hospital-based injury prevention programs that are activated at the time of an ED visit (Mulligan-Smith, Puranik, & Coffman, 1998), when children and families may be receptive to preventive education. Collaboration with other disciplines and with other agencies may lead to the incorporation of health promotion activities into ED care. While there are many hazards to children's health and safety, there are often simple, effective remedies, and numerous resources available to parents and care givers. By incorporating simple interventions and adopting healthy behaviors, children's health can be protected and promoted.

Resources

Air Bag and Safety Belt Safety Campaign
1019 19th Street, N.W., Suite 401

Washington, DC 20036
(202) 625-2570
Fax (202) 822-1399

American Academy of Pediatrics
141 Northwest Point Boulevard
P.O. Box 927
Elk Grove Village, IL 60009-0927
(800) 433-9016 or (847) 228-5005
<http://www.aap.org>

American College of Emergency Physicians
P.O. Box 619911
Dallas, TX 75261
(214) 550-0911 or (800) 798-1822
<http://www.acep.org>

American Dental Association
211 East Chicago Avenue
Chicago, IL 60611
(312) 440-2500
Fax (312) 440-7494

American Society of Dentistry for Children
875 North Michigan Avenue, Suite 4040
Chicago, IL 60611
(312) 943-1244
Fax (312) 943-5341

American Trauma Society
8903 Presidential Parkway, Suite 512
Upper Marlboro, MD 20772
(301) 420-4189 or (800) 556-7890
Fax (301) 420-0617
<http://www.amtrauma.org>

Bicycle Federation of America
1506 21st Street, N.W., Suite 200
Washington, DC 20036
(202) 463-6622

Center to Prevent Handgun Violence
125 Eye Street, N.W., Suite 1100
Washington, DC 20005
(202) 898-0792
Fax (202) 371-9615
<http://www.handguncontrol.org>

Children's Safety Network, Inc. (CSN)
1400 Eye Street, N.W.
Washington, DC 20005
(202) 842-4450

CSN: Rural Injury Prevention Assistance Center
National Farm Medicine Center
1000 North Oak Avenue
Marshfield, WI 54449-5790
(715) 389-4999

CSN: Injury Data Technical Assistance Center
San Diego State University
6505 Alvarado Road, Suite 205
San Diego, CA 92120
(619) 594-3691

CSN: Third-party Payers Injury Prevention Resource Center
National Center for Education in Maternal and Child Health
2000 15th Street, North, Suite 701
Arlington, VA 22201-2617
(703) 524-7802

CSN: Adolescent Violence Prevention Resource Center
Education Development Center, Inc.
55 Chapel Street
Newton, MA 02160
(617) 969-7100

Insurance Institute for Highway Safety
1005 North Glebe Road
Arlington, VA 22201
(703) 247-1500
Fax (703) 247-1678

National Center for Nutrition and Dietetics
American Dietetic Association
216 West Jackson Boulevard
Chicago, IL 60606
(312) 899-0040 or (800) 366-1655

National Dairy Council
O'Hare InterNational Center
10255 West Higgins Road, Suite 900
Rosemont, IL 60018
(800) 426-8271
Fax (847) 803-2077

National SAFE KIDS Campaign
1301 Pennsylvania Avenue, N.W., Suite 1000
Washington, DC 20004-1707
(202) 662-0600
Fax: (202) 393-2072
Info@safekids.org

National Safety Belt Coalition
1025 Connecticut Avenue, N.W., Suite 1200
Washington, DC 20036
(202) 296-6263
Fax (202) 293-0032

Pedestrian Federation
1506 21st Street, N.W., Suite 200
Washington, DC 20036
(202) 463-6622

U.S. Consumer Product Safety Commission (CPSC)
5401 Westbard Avenue, Room 625
Washington, DC 20207
(301) 504-0424 or (800) 638-2772
<http://www.cpsc.gov>

U.S. Department of Health and Human Services
Public Health Service
Centers for Disease Control and Prevention (CDC)
National Center for Injury Prevention and Control (NCIPC)
(Mail Stop F-41)
4770 Buford Highway, N.E.
Atlanta, GA 30341-3724
Unintentional Injuries (770) 488-4672
Violence-related Injuries (770) 488-4362
<http://www.cdc.gov>

Maternal and Child Health Bureau (MCHB)
5600 Fishers Lane, Room 18-A-39
Rockville, Maryland 20857
(301) 443-4026
<http://www.os.dhhs.gov/hrsa/mchb/>

National Maternal and Child Health Clearinghouse
2070 Chain Bridge Road, Suite 450
Vienna, VA 22182
(703) 356-1964
mchc@circsol.com

Emergency Medical Services for Children (EMSC)
111 Michigan Avenue, N.W.
Washington, DC 20010
(202) 884-4927
Fax (301) 650-8045
<http://www.ems-c.org>

U.S. Department of Transportation (DOT)
National Highway Traffic Safety Administration (NHTSA)
400 7th Street, S.W.
Washington, DC 20590
(202) 366-95880 or (800) 424-9393
<http://www.nhtsa.dot.gov>

References

American Academy of Pediatrics. (1994). *TIPP: The injury prevention program. A guide to safety counseling in office practice*. Elk Grove Village, IL: Author.

American College of Emergency Physicians. (1995). Policy statement: Immunization of the pediatric patient. *Annals of Emergency Medicine, 26*, 403–404.

Bernardo, L., Gardner, M., & Rogers, K. (1998). Pediatric sledding injuries in Pennsylvania. *Journal of Trauma Nursing, 5*(2), 34–40.

Centers for Disease Control and Prevention. (2000). *Recommended childhood immunization schedule—United States 2001.* Morbidity and Mortality Weekly 2001; 50(01): 7–10, 19.

Centers for Disease Control and Prevention. National Center for Injury Prevention and Control (January, 2000). *Preventing bicycle-related head injuries. Fact sheets.* Atlanta, GA: Author.

Eisenberg, A., Murkoff, H., & Hathaway, S. (1989). *What to expect the first year*. New York: Workman.

Eisenberg, A., Murkoff, H., & Hathaway, S. (1994). *What to expect the toddler years*. New York: Workman.

Flaherty, L. (Ed.). (1996). *A crash course in motor vehicle injury prevention*. Park Ridge, IL: Emergency Nurses Association.

Gordis, L. (1996). *Epidemiology*. Philadelphia: Saunders.

Hardin Gookin, S. (1995). *Parenting for dummies*. Foster City, CA: IDG Books Worldwide.

Injury Prevention for Children with Special Health Care Needs Work Group. (1999). *Injury prevention information for children with special health care needs*. Emergency Medical Services for Children Program. Washington, DC: Author.

Kuska, T. (2002). Child passenger protection: Then and now. *Journal of Emergency Nursing, 28*(1), 52–56.

Mulligan-Smith, D., Puranik, S., Coffman, S. (1998). Parental perception of injury prevention practices in a multicultural metropolitan area. *Pediatric Emergency Care, 14*(1), 10–14.

Murphy, Sherry L. (July 2000). *National vital statistics report. Deaths: Final data for 1998.* Department of Health and Human Services. Centers for Disease Control. National Center for Health Statistics. Division of Vital Statistics.

National Center for Injury Prevention and Control. (2000). *Injury prevention: Meeting the challenge*. New York: Oxford University Press.

National Center for Injury Prevention and Control. (2001). *Injury Fact Book 2001–2002.* Atlanta, GA: Centers for Disease Control and Prevention.

National Highway Traffic Safety Administration. (1992). *Child passenger safety resource manual*. Washington, DC: Author.

National Highway Traffic Safety Administration. (1996a). Traffic safety outlook: Child passenger safety. *Safe & Sober Quarterly Planner*. Washington, DC: Author.

National Highway Traffic Safety Administration. (September 1996). *Your bicycle helmet—A correct fit* (DOT Publication No. DOT HS 808 421). Washington, DC: Author.

National Highway Traffic Safety Administration. (1996b). *Patterns of misuse of child safety seats* (DOT Publication No. DOT HS 808 440). Washington, DC: Author.

National Highway Traffic Safety Administration. (1997). *Presidential initiative for increasing seat belt use nationwide*. Washington, DC: Author.

Nationa1 Highway Traffic Safety Administration. National Center for Statistics and Analysis. (2000). *Traffic safety facts 1999—Children.* Washington, DC: Author.

National SAFE KIDS Campaign. (1999). *Unintentional firearm injury.* 1999 fact sheets. Washington, DC: National SAFE KIDS Campaign.

Raskin, B. (1998). *The new mom's guide to immunizations*. Boulder, CO: Parenting Magazine.

Robinson, P., Gausche, M., Gerardi, M., Kim, J., Walkley, E., Santamaria, J., & Foltin, G. (1996). Immunization of the pediatric patient in the ED. *Annals of Emergency Medicine, 28*, 334-341.

Smith, T. (Ed.). (1997). *Child safety: Unintentional injury prevention and preparation*. Park Ridge, IL: Emergency Nurses Association.

Stewart, D. (1997). *Child passenger safety master trainer technical curriculum*. Washington, DC: National Highway Traffic Safety Administration.

Thompson, R., Rivara, F., & Thompson, D. (1989). A case-control study of the effectiveness of bicycle safety helmets. *New England Journal of Medicine, 320*, 1362-1367.

U.S. Consumer Product Safety Commission. (1996). *Accident facts 1996 edition*. Itasca, IL: Author.

U.S. Consumer Product Safety Commission. (1997). *Accident facts 1997 edition*. Itasca, IL: Author.

U.S. Consumer Product Safety Commission. (2001b). Home playground equipment-related deaths and injuries. Washington, DC: Author.

U.S. Consumer Product Safety Commission (2001c). Skate but skate safely—always wear safety gear. Washington, DC: Author.

U.S. Preventive Services Task Force. (1996). *Guide to clinical preventive services* (2nd ed.). Alexandria, VA: InterNational Medical Publishing.

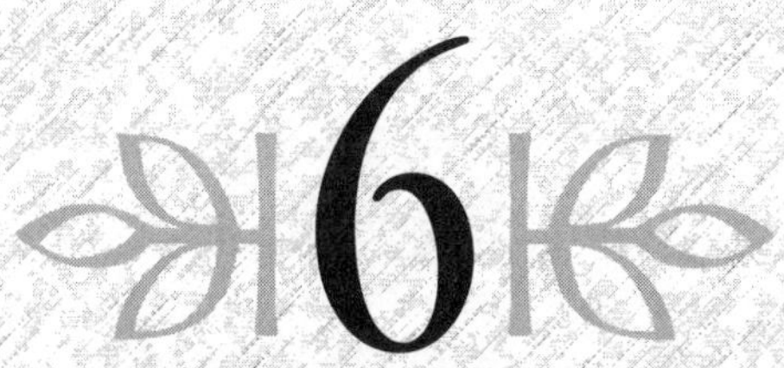

Health History and Physical Assessment

Joan O'Connor, RN, MSN, CRNP

Introduction

Obtaining a health history and performing a physical assessment of infants, children, and adolescents can be a challenge. In a busy emergency department (ED), where time is of the essence, the relationship among the patient, parent, and nurse must develop quickly. This relationship affects the quality and progress of the history taking and physical assessment process. Trust is an essential element throughout this process; if the parent and patient develop trust with the emergency nurse, their participation in the assessment may be enhanced.

The purpose of this chapter is to describe a history-taking and physical assessment process that emergency nurses can use with pediatric patients. Focused physical assessments of particular body systems are provided in their respective chapters. The history taking and physical assessment process discussed in this chapter is applied throughout this core curriculum.

Health History

The health history provides 85% of the information leading to a diagnosis (Gundy, 1997). There are three general goals of and interventions for preparation and completion of the pediatric health history (Conedera, 1993):

1. Gain the parents' trust. Address the parent by name to demonstrate the concern for the parent as an individual. Children sense the parent's distrust and fear and exhibit these qualities themselves. Engagement of the parent is an important key to a successful assessment.
2. Elicit a meaningful health history. Allow time for the parent to reveal the child's health problem; rushing into a history without listening to the parent may cause the parent to withhold important information.
3. Maintain the parent's and child's privacy. Elicit the health history in a private area because crowded waiting areas or busy hallways may create a feeling of vulnerability.

Various formats can be used by emergency nurses to obtain the information in the health history (Bates, 1999; Engel, 1997; Lissauer & Clauden, 1997). Each format elicits the same information. The Emergency Nurses Association (ENA) recommends the CIAMPEDS format (Table 6.1).

Physical Assessment

The pediatric physical assessment has the following four goals and interventions (Conedera, 1993):

1. Minimize stress and anxiety associated with the physical assessment. For the stable child, begin the assessment with those activities that can be presented as games and end with more traumatic procedures. A calm, unhurried approach engages even the most taciturn child.
2. Foster trust among the child, parent, and emergency nurse. Address the child by name. Show a genuine interest in the child; ask about hobbies, likes, dislikes, pets. Listen to what the child has to say. Examine the affected (i.e., painful or injured) body area last to minimize distress; focus on the healthy body areas first. Respect the need for privacy among children of all ages.
3. Prepare the child as much as possible for the physical assessment. Explain to the child and parent what the assessment entails and what to expect. Allow some time for the child to adjust to the ED environment before proceeding with the history and physical assessment. Some children will protest throughout the assessment despite the aforementioned

TABLE 6-1 CIAMPEDS Format for Obtaining a Health History

Historical Information	*Components and Rationale*
Chief complaint	Focus on the reason for the current ED visit. Identify the primary health problem and its duration.
Immunizations	Determine the child's immunization status and/or potential need for further immunization (e.g., tetanus booster). This helps to determine whether the child's current health problem may be related to inadequate immunization (e.g., respiratory illness in the young infant prior to the initial pertussis immunization).
Isolation	Recent exposure to a communicable disease (e.g., varicella) and assessment findings suggestive of that disease may require that the child be isolated from other ED patients. Isolate children who are immunosuppressed from chemotherapy or antirejection medications to prevent their exposure to other diseases.
Allergies	Known medication, food, and environmental allergies should be documented. Note the reactions to the allergens.
Medications	Elicit from the parent the names of prescribed and over-the-counter medications and herbal products that the child is taking.This will help to prevent duplication of medication administration and to determine the effectiveness of current medications. Note the medication's name, dosage, route, frequency, duration, and effectiveness.
Past health history	For children younger than 2 years of age and children with disabilities, the health history should include the birth history (maternal age, birth weight, discharge weight, gestational length, complications, and medications). For all children, the health history should include prior hospitalizations or illnesses, ongoing chronic illnesses or conditions (e.g., asthma, congenital heart disease), physical growth, attainment of developmental milestones, and family health patterns.
Parent's impression of the child's health condition	Elicit from the parent what is different about the child's health that prompted the ED visit. The parent is best able to judge improvement or worsening in the child's health condition. Include information about patterns such as sleeping and playing.
Events surrounding the illness or injury	For illness, obtain information about the onset (rapid or protracted), duration, and involvement of other family members. Determine whether recent travel to another state or a foreign country occurred. For injury, obtain information about the time of the injury, the mechanism of injury, and witnesses to the event.
Diet	Determine the child's normal eating patterns and how they are different with the onset of illness or injury. Elicit the time of the child's last oral intake in the event that surgery or a procedure is needed.
Diapers	Determine the child's normal urine and bowel elimination patterns. Elicit the time of the child's last urination and bowel movement and changes from the normal patterns.
Symptoms associated with the illness or injury	Symptomatology, together with a physical assessment, allows for the accurate diagnosis of the child's health condition. Include a description of the symptoms, the time of their onset, and interventions that alleviated or worsened the symptoms.

Adapted from: Emergency Nurses Association. (1995). *Policy statement on pediatric emergency nursing*. Park Ridge, IL: Author.

interventions. With these children, proceed calmly and confidently.

4. Maximize the accuracy and reliability of the physical assessment findings. Position the child as needed if he or she exhibits physical distress or anxiety, thus enabling completion of the assessment. Table 6.2 describes age-specific approaches for the pediatric physical assessment.

There are numerous examples of pediatric physical assessment techniques in the literature (e.g., Bates, 1999; Engel, 1997). The ENA (1998) recommends the *A* to *I* approach for this assessment process in the ED:

- *A*irway
- *B*reathing
- *C*irculation

TABLE 6.2 Age-Specific Approaches to Pediatric Physical Assessment

Age	*Position*	*Sequence*	*Preparation*
Young infant	Infant too young to sit unsupported: Seat the infant on the parent's lap or against the parent's shoulder.	If the infant is quiet or sleeping, auscultate heart, lungs, and abdomen, then palpate these areas as needed.	■ Undress to diaper but keep wrapped in a blanket. ■ Use distraction techniques (bright objects, rattles, soft talking) to gain cooperation (Chapter 4) ■ Smile; use a soft, gentle voice.
	Infant aged 4–6 months: Place the infant on the parent's lap or examination table.	Proceed in a head-toe direction: May assess skin, cardiovascular system, thorax, and lungs, proceed with abdomen, genitalia, lower extremities, and finish with the head. Elicit moro (startle) reflex last.	■ Pacify with a feeding (if permitted) or a pacifier. ■ Ask the parent to assist with assessment if he or she is able to do so. For example, have the parent palpate the affected area or perform passive range-of-motion exercises to elicit tenderness.
Older infant	Infant able to sit unsupported: Place the infant on the parent's lap whenever possible; if the infant is positioned on the examination table, keep parents in full view.	■ Perform the most intrusive aspects of the assessment last ■ Elicit reflexes as the body part is examined.	■ Avoid quick movements or prolonged eye contact (older infants) to prevent surprises and promote trust.
Toddler	Position sitting or standing on or by parent or sitting upright on parent's lap.	■ Inspect body areas through play (count fingers, tickle toes). ■ Use minimal contact initially. ■ Introduce equipment slowly. ■ Discuss the child's fears with the parent and order the examination sequence accordingly. ■ Auscultate, percuss, and palpate when the child is quiet. ■ Perform the most intrusive aspects of the assessment last.	■ Have the parent remove outer clothing; remove the underpants when that body area is examined. ■ Encourage inspection of equipment. ■ Allow the child to hold a transitional object or toy during the assessment. ■ Demonstrate the assessment on a toy, the parent, or self; create a story about the assessment. ■ Speak to the child in terms that a toddler can understand. ■ Keep the parent's face in the child's view. ■ If the child is uncooperative, perform the assessment quickly and efficiently. ■ Praise and reward cooperative behavior. ■ Elicit the parent's assistance if he or she is able to do so, as described in the infant section.

(continued)

TABLE 6.2 (continued)

Age	*Position*	*Sequence*	*Preparation*
Preschooler	▪ Position sitting, lying, or standing. ▪ May cooperate when prone or supine. ▪ Prefers parents nearby.	If cooperative: ▪ Proceed in head-to-toe fashion. If uncooperative: ▪ Proceed as with toddler. ▪ Perform the most intrusive aspects of the assessment last.	▪ Request self-undressing. ▪ Permit underpants to be worn and assure privacy. ▪ Offer equipment for inspection; demonstrate on the parent or a doll. ▪ Create a story about the procedure ("Let's see how strong your muscles are."). ▪ Offer choices when appropriate. ▪ Expect cooperation; elicit the child's help whenever possible ("Point to where it hurts."). ▪ Educate the child about his or her body ("I am going to listen to your heart; can you point to your heart?").
School-aged	▪ Prefers sitting. ▪ Cooperates when placed in most positions. ▪ Younger school-aged child usually prefers parental presence; older school-aged child may want privacy.	▪ Proceed head-to-toe. ▪ Examine genitalia last (may be deferred).	▪ Request self-undressing. ▪ Allow to wear underpants and assure privacy. ▪ Explain purpose of equipment and significance of procedure in terms the child can understand. ▪ Teach about body functioning and healthy habits. ▪ Tell the child it is permissible to cry. ▪ Offer choices when appropriate.
Adolescent	▪ Prefers sitting. ▪ Offer parental or peer presence for support. ▪ Speak with the adolescent first before talking with the parent.	▪ Proceed head-to-toe. ▪ Examine genitalia last (usually deferred).	▪ Have adolescent undress in private and maintain privacy. ▪ Expose only the body area to be examined. ▪ Explain assessment findings. ▪ Be matter of fact about sexual development; emphasize normalcy. ▪ If genital assessment is performed, examine the genitalia as any other body part; may leave until the end. ▪ Consider using a mirror during the genital examination to allow the adolescent to view the genital area.

From: Conedera, 1993; Wong, 1999.

- *D*isability
- *E*xposure and environmental control
- *F*ullset of vital signs
- *F*amily presence
- *G*ive comfort measures
- *H*ead-to-toe assessment
- *I*nspect posterior surfaces

Normal and abnormal assessment findings and selected nursing interventions will be summarized in Table 6.10.

Airway

- Observe for airway patency.
- Listen for sounds of airway obstruction (stridor).
- Observe the child's position for air entry (tripod, neck extended, or lowered jaw).
- Observe for airway obstruction (blood, mucous, oral edema, foreign body, secretions, carbonaecous sputum, or singed nasal hair).
- Note breath odor (e.g., ketones or alcohol).

Breathing

- Observe the child's work of breathing:
  - Nasal flaring.
  - Use of accessory muscles.
- Listen for audible adventitious sounds (wheezing).
- Observe the child's breathing pattern:
  - Regular versus irregular.
- Observe the depth of respirations.

Circulation

- Observe the color of the skin.
- Measure capillary refill:
  - Theoretically, a normal refill time is a measure of adequate peripheral perfusion and thus normal cardiac output and peripheral vascular resistance. In healthy, warm children a normal capillary refill value is approximately 2 seconds or less.
  - A low ambient temperature has a significant effect on capillary refill in both healthy and ill or injured children; thus, it is not used as a sole indicator for shock.
- Palpate the central and peripheral pulses for strength and equality.
- Palpate the skin with the back of the hand to determine skin temperature; compare the temperature of the upper and lower extremities.

Disability

- Observe the child's activity level.
- Note the child's level of consciousness; observe the child's ability to follow directions, respond to questions, and interact with the caregiver.
- Observe the child's response to the ED environment; note the child's level of consolability.
- Obtain a Glasgow Coma Scale score (Table 6.3) or AUPU assessment:
  - A = Alert.
  - V = Responds to verbal stimuli.
  - P = Responds to painful stimuli.
  - U = Unresponsive.
- Measure the pupillary equality and response.

TABLE 6.3 Glasgow Coma Scale

Parameter	*Score for Children > 2 Years*	*Score for Children < 2 Years*
Eye opening	4 Spontaneously	4 Spontaneously
	3 To verbal stimuli	3 To speech
	2 To pain	2 To pain
	1 No response	1 No response
Best verbal response	5 Oriented/uses appropriate words and phrases	5 Coos, babbles
	4 Confused	4 Irritable, cries
	3 Inappropriate words/screams/cries	3 Cries to pain
	2 Nonspecific sounds	2 Moans to pain
	1 No response	1 No response
Best motor response	6 Obeys commands	6 Normal spontaneous movement
	5 Localizes pain	5 Withdraws to touch
	4 Withdraws to pain	4 Withdraws to pain
	3 Flexion response to pain	3 Abnormal flexion
	2 Extension response	2 Abnormal extension to pain
	1 No response	1 No response
Total score	< 8 = Severe head injury	> 8 = Head injury moderate/minor

Exposure and environmental control

- Remove the child's clothing as needed to continue the assessment.
- Initiate measures to maintain a normothermic state or to warm the child.

Full set of vital signs

- Measure the respiratory rate:
  - Count the respiratory rate by auscultation for one full minute in children of all ages.
- Measure the heart/pulse rate:
  - Count the apical pulse for one full minute for greatest accuracy in children of all ages; an alternative is to count the brachial pulse.
  - Count the radial pulse in children older than 2 years.
  - Grade the pulse amplitude (Table 6.4).
- Measure the blood pressure:
  - Measure the blood pressure with a sphygmomanometer or electronic blood pressure device.
- Measure the temperature:
  - Select a route for temperature measurement. Table 6.5 compares the advantages and disadvantages of commonly used measurement routes.
- Obtain the child's weight with the appropriate-sized scale:
  - Compare these findings on the male or female growth chart. A child whose weight falls below the fifth percentile is underweight, whereas a child whose weight falls above the 95 percentile is overweight. Measure the child's weight to the nearest 10 g or 0.50 oz for infants and 100 g or 0.25 lb for older children.
  - When weighing infants, note whether the weight is measured with or without clothes; for infants and young children with questionable dehydration, measure with diaper or underclothes only.
  - Always weigh infants and children in kilograms to prevent errors in medication dosing. Medications are generally offered in mg/kg doses.

TABLE 6.4 Pulse Grading

Grade	*Description*
0	Not palpable
+1	Difficult to palpate, thready; easily obliterated with pressure
+2	Difficult to palpate; may obliterate with pressure
+3	Easy to palpate; not easily obliterated (normal)
+4	Strong, bounding; not obliterated with pressure

TABLE 6.5 Routes for Temperature Measurement

Route	*Indications*	*Method*
Oral	Useful in children who can follow directions and who can keep the thermometer probe under the tongue without biting (usually 5 years of age, maybe younger).	Insert the thermometer probe into the right or left posterior sublingual pocket; leave in place for approximately 2 to 3 minutes (depending on the model of thermometer used).
Axillary	Useful in children who will not tolerate a rectal temperature measurement and who are too young to keep the oral thermometer in place, such as toddlers; also used in neonates.	Place the thermometer probe in the axillary space, held firmly between the arm and the axilla; leave in place for approximately 5 minutes (depending on the model of thermometer used). Usually, this temperature measurement is 1 degree lower than an oral temperature measurement.
Tympanic	Useful in children of all ages, although use in infants may depend on the manufacturer's recommendations.	Position the thermometer in the external auditory canal and depress the thermometer "trigger." The temperature measurement requires a few seconds to obtain.
Rectal	Useful in infants and young children; considered to be the "gold standard" in temperature measurement in ill or injured infants and children. Rectal temperatures are contraindicated in children with immune disorders, bleeding disorders, and rectal abnormalities or trauma.	Insert the thermometer probe no more than 2.5 cm or 1 inch into the rectum; leave in place for approximately 3 minutes (depending on the model of thermometer used). The temperature measurement is usually considered 1 degree higher than an oral temperature measurement.

Family presence

- Assess needs of family, taking into consideration cultural variables.
- Support family's involvement of the child's care.
- Assign a healthcare professional to provide explanations to the family.
- Assign a staff member to provide support.

Give comfort measures

- Initiate comfort measures based on the chief complaint or obvious injury.
- Evaluate presence and level of pain (Chapter 13).
- Stabilize suspected fractures.

Head-to-toe assessment

The head-to-toe assessment is conducted using *observation*, *inspection*, *auscultation*, *palpation*, and *percussion* (Bates, 1999; Engel, 1997).

- General state of health:
    - Posture.
    - Gait.
    - Fine and gross motor activity.
    - Dress, grooming, and hygiene.
    - Odors.
    - Facial expressions.
    - Speech, state of awareness, and interaction among child, parent, and siblings.
- Head:
    - Observe and inspect the shape, symmetry, and hair distribution of the infant's and young toddler's head.
    - Palpate the suture lines in the infant's and young toddler's head. The suture lines may overlap in the newborn, but they usually flatten out by age 6 months.
    - Palpate the anterior and posterior fontanelles while the infant is in a sitting position; note bulging (indicative of increased intracranial pressure) and depressed (indicative of dehydration) fontanelles.
    - Observe and inspect the shape, symmetry, and hair distribution of the head of older children.
- Ears and eyes:
    - Observe and inspect the ears for normal external aural characteristics—ear alignment, size, and position. Observe for piercing or scars.
    - Test for gross hearing by talking with the child and listening to the responses; for the infant, ring a bell or shake a rattle near the infant's ear and observe the infant turn toward the noise.
    - Observe and inspect the pupils for size, equality, and response to light.
    - Test for gross vision by having the child point to an object or having an infant visually follow an object. The six cardinal gazes are assessed beginning at 5 to 6 months of age. Steady fixation and following an object are assessed beginning at 3 months of age.
- Face:
    - Observe and inspect the face for symmetric features that are well-proportioned.
    - Palpate the face to detect smooth contours, pain, or tenderness.
    - Observe and inspect the external nares for discharge, excoriation, and odor.
    - Observe and inspect the oral cavity and pharynx (tongue, lips, and tonsils) for a pink color with moist and intact mucous membranes. Inspect for primary and secondary dentition. By 24 months of age, all deciduous teeth have erupted. Beginning at age 5 to 6 years, deciduous teeth are lost. By age 12 years, all 32 teeth are in place.
- Neck:
    - Observe and inspect the neck for surface trauma or scars.
    - Palpate the lymph glands for enlargement; note their color, size, consistency, location, temperature, and tenderness.
- Chest:
    - Inspect and observe the chest's anterior-posterior diameter. Observe for symmetric chest expansion on inspiration. Observe for abdominal breathing in children younger than 7 years of age and thoracic breathing in children older than 7 years of age.
    - Auscultate breath sounds in all lung lobes, from the apex to the base.
    - Auscultate for the presence and location of adventitious sounds (Table 6.6).
- Heart and vascular system:
    - Observe the anterior chest for symmetry of chest movement, pulsations, and lifts or heaves.
    - Auscultate the heart at the apex and the lower sternal border with the bell of the stethoscope; listen at each auscultatory area with the diaphragm of the stethoscope.
    - In children younger than 7 years of age, the point of maximum intensity is lateral to the left mid-claviculas line and fourth intercostal space.

TABLE 6.6 Significance of Adventitious Sounds

Breath Sound	*Characteristics*	*Underlying Cause*
Rales		
Fine	Intermittent, high-pitched; heard during inspiration	Indicates alveolar fluid; pneumonia; congestive heart failure
Medium	Intermittent, wet, loud; heard during inspiration; clear with coughing	Indicates fluid in bronchioles and bronchi; pulmonary edema
Coarse	Loud, bubbling; heard during expiration; clear with coughing	Indicates fluid in bronchioles and bronchi; resolving pneumonia; bronchitis
Rhonchi		
Sonorous	Continuous, snoring, low pitched; heard during inspiration and expiration	Indicates involvement of large bronchi and trachea; bronchitis
Sibilant	Continuous, musical, high pitched; heard during expiration	Indicates edema and small airway obstruction; asthma
Wheezes		
Inspiratory	Sonorous, musical	Upper airway obstruction
Expiratory	Whistling, sighing	Lower airway obstruction

Adapted from Engle: J., 1997. *Pocket guide for pediatric assessment* (pp. 164). St. Louis: Mosby—Year Book.

- In children older than 7 years of age, the point of maximum intensity is at the mid-claviculas line and fifth intercostal space. Heart sounds should be clear, distinct, and synchronous with the radial pulse (Table 6.7).
- Abnormal heart sounds (auscultate for):
  - Clicks.
  - Murmurs (Table 6.8).
  - Precordial friction rubs–high-pitched, grating sounds that stop with breath holding.
- Peripheral pulses:
  - Palpate the peripheral pulses in both extremities. Compare their equality, rate and rhythm; note any discoloration and edema of the extremities.
- Lymph glands:
  - Palpate the lymph glands in the axillae for enlargement; note their color, size, consistency, location, temperature, and tenderness.
- Abdomen:
  - Inspect and observe the abdomen's contour; observe for protuberance (normal in toddlers; otherwise may indicate fluid retention, tumor, organomegaly, or ascites) and depression (dehydration or high abdominal obstruction).

TABLE 6.7 Auscultation of Heart Sounds

Heart Sound	*Anatomic Location for Auscultation*	*Significance of the Heart Sound*
S_1	Loudest in the mitral and tricuspid areas; "lub" from atrioventricular valve closure.	Intensified with fever, exercise and anemia; may indicate mitral stenosis; variability in intensity may indicate dysrhythmia.
S_2	Base of heart (aortic and pulmonic areas); loudest in these areas; "dub" from aortic and pulmonic valve closure.	Split S_1 or S_2: Occurs because left-sided valves close slightly before right-sided valves.
S_3	Lying on left side.	Rapid ventricular filling ("Ken-tuc-ky"); normal in children and young adults.
S_4	Lying on left side.	Atrial contraction at the end of diastole ("Ten-nes-see"); abnormal in most persons.

TABLE 6.8 Comparison of Innocent and Organic Heart Murmurs

Characteristic	*Innocent Heart Murmur**	*Organic Heart Murmur†*
Child's growth	Does not increase over time and does not affect the child's growth.	May worsen over time; may affect the child's growth.
Sound	Systolic; low-pitched; musical heard at the second and third left intercostal spaces.	Variable, depending on its associated lesion (harsh, rumbling, or blowing).
Presence	May disappear with a position change.	Always present.

*Nonpathologic

†Occurring before age 3 related to congenital defects; occurring after age 3 related to rheumatic heart disease.

- Inspect the skin for scars (surgery, child maltreatment), trauma, color (yellowness may indicate jaundice), striae (obesity or fluid retention), and dilated vessels.
- Observe for movement in the abdomen, such as visible peristaltic waves (obstruction or pyloric stenosis).
- Inspect the umbilicus for its color, presence of discharge, inflammation, and herniation.
- Observe the child's position during the assessment, such as splinting or guarding.
- Auscultate for bowel sounds in all four quadrants using both the bell and diaphragm of the stethoscope. Ideally, bowel sounds should be auscultated for 1 full minute in each quadrant; auscultate for a minimum of 5 minutes to determine if bowel sounds are absent.
- Palpate (lightly and then deeply) and percuss the abdomen in the absence of surgical disease. If the child is in pain or discomfort, defer palpation.

- Genitalia and anus (usually deferred):
  - Inspect the female genitalia (hymen, labia majora, labia minora) and anus for signs of trauma, irritation, or discharge.
  - Inspect the male genitalia (penis and scrotum) and anus for signs of trauma, irritation, and discharge.
  - Inspect the anal area for irritation, prolapse, or signs of itching (pinworms).
  - Palpate the lymph glands in the groin for enlargement; note their color, size, consistency, location, temperature, and tenderness.
  - Note Tanner staging (Chapter 20).
- Neuromuscular system:
  - Inspect and observe the upper and lower extremities for signs of trauma, deformities, and enlarged joints.
  - Palpate the upper extremities for pain and deformities.
  - Palpate the joints for pain.
  - Assess active and passive range of motion.
  - Test for upper extremity strength by having the child squeeze the nurse's fingers.
  - Test for lower extremity strength by having the child push against the nurse's hands with the soles of the feet.
  - Assess for congenital hip dislocation in children up to 2 years of age.
  - Observe the child's muscle tone and coordination.
  - Assess the cranial nerves (may be deferred; Chapter 18).
- Skin:
  - Observe and inspect the skin for odor; malodor indicates infection or poor hygiene.
  - Observe moistness of the exposed skin areas and mucous membranes; dryness indicates dehydration.
  - Observe color and pigmentation (Table 6.9).
- Lesions (Chapter 22):
  - Location.
  - Distribution.
  - Arrangement.
  - Type.
  - Color.
- Inspect the hair for distribution, color, texture, amount, and quality.
- Inspect the nails; note their characteristics—smooth, convex, pink, well groomed.
- Palpate the skin's texture; observe for scars, keloids, or hypertrophic scarring.
- Palpate for skin turgor and mobility. (Grasp a fold of skin on the upper arm or abdomen and quickly release it; note how quickly the skin returns to its normal position with residual marks.)

TABLE 6.9 Comparison of Skin Color

Color	*Suggestive Health Condition*	*Best Location to Detect*
Blue (cyanosis)	Peripheral—anxiety or cold; Central—decrease in the blood's oxygen-carrying capacity	Lips, mouth, and trunk
Jaundice	Liver disease, biliary obstruction, severe infection in infants	Sclerae, mucous membranes, and abdomen
Yellow	Carotenemia	Palms, soles, and face (mucous membranes and sclerae not involved)
Yellow	Chronic renal disease	Exposed skin (mucous membranes and sclerae not involved)
Pallor (lack of pink skin tones in caucasians; ash-gray color in African-Americans)	Syncope, fever, shock, anemia	Face, mouth, conjunctivae, and nails

Adapted from: Engle, 1997.

- Palpate for edema; compress a thumb into an area that appears to be swollen.
- Inspect posterior surfaces:
  - Inspect the back for surface trauma and vertebral alignment.
  - Observe for the spinal curves.
  - Observe for symmetric hip and shoulder alignment.

Interpretation of Assessment Findings

At the completion of the physical assessment, the normal and abnormal findings are noted and documented. These findings are considered in context with the child's health history, triage findings, and the nurse's observations of the child and parent during the assessment (Table 6.10).

Conclusion

The history and physical assessment provide a beginning understanding of the child's health condition on presentation to the ED and form the basis for the development of nursing diagnoses and a plan of care. Because health is a dynamic state, reassessment should occur at regular intervals, in accordance with the child's health condition and hospital policy. Assessment findings should be documented at regular intervals to demonstrate changes in the child's health condition and to allow for modification of the treatment plan. The prepared emergency nurse who has learned the nuances of physical assessment likely will have a successful outcome—a calm, trusting child—which is the utmost reward.

TABLE 6.10 Summary of Normal and Abnormal Pediatric Physical Assessment Findings and Nursing Interventions

Assessment Parameter	*Normal Findings*	*Abnormal Findings*	*Interventions*
Airway	▪ Patent. ▪ Clear. ▪ Odor-free breath.	▪ Inability to maintain own airway. ▪ Signs of airway obstruction. ▪ Malodorous breath.	▪ Maintain child in position of comfort. ▪ Position airway (jaw thrust/chin lift). ▪ Insert airway adjunct. ▪ Prepare for endotracheal intubation.
Breathing	▪ Respiratory rate within age-appropriate limits. ▪ Regular breathing pattern. ▪ Absence of audible adventitious sounds or use of accessory muscles.	▪ Bradypnea. ▪ Tachypnea. ▪ Nasal flaring. ▪ Abnormal breath sounds. ▪ Accessory muscle use. ▪ Abnormal breathing pattern.	▪ Administer supplemental oxygen. ▪ Initiate bag-valve-mask ventilation if spontaneous respirations absent or ineffective. ▪ Prepare for mechanical ventilation.
Circulation	▪ Heart rate within age-appropriate limits. ▪ Pink, warm, and dry skin. ▪ Strong and regular peripheral pulses. ▪ Capillary refill < 3 seconds.	▪ Bradycardia ▪ Tachycardia ▪ Mottled, pale, cool, or moist skin. ▪ Weak peripheral pulses. ▪ Capillary refill > 2 seconds.	▪ Initiate chest compressions if cardiac function absent or ineffective. ▪ Obtain vascular access. ▪ Initiate fluid volume replacement and/or medication therapy. ▪ Initiate cardiorespiratory and oxygen saturation monitoring. ▪ Prepare for cardiac defibrillation or synchronized cardioversion.
Disability	▪ Awake, alert, active. ▪ Round, equal pupils reactive to light and accommodation.	▪ Altered level of consciousness. ▪ Unequal, nonreactive pupils or sluggish pupillary responses.	▪ Treat the underlying cause. ▪ Monitor closely.
Exposure/ Environmental control	▪ Intact skin surfaces. ▪ Maintain normothermic environment.	▪ Surface trauma indicative of child maltreatment or child sexual abuse (Chapters 46 and 47). ▪ Hyperthermia. ▪ Hypothermia.	▪ Notify child protective services. ▪ Prepare for interview and examination (see Chapters 46 and 47). ▪ Employ supplemental warming or cooling measures.
Get full set of vital signs	▪ Vital signs and weight within age-appropriate limits.	▪ Fever (infection or poisoning). ▪ Hypothermia (sepsis, shock, or exposure). ▪ Bradycardia (hypoxia). ▪ Tachycardia (early sign of shock). ▪ Tachypnea ("quiet tachypnea"—ketoacidosis, dehydration, poisoning, fever, respiratory distress, congestive heart failure)	▪ Monitor vital signs in response to treatment.

(continued)

TABLE 6.10 (continued)

Assessment Parameter	*Normal Findings*	*Abnormal Findings*	*Interventions*
Get full set of vital signs *(continued)*		▪ Bradypnea (respiratory failure, shock, acidosis, hypothermia). ▪ Hypertension (increased intracranial pressure, renal disease, coarctation of the aorta, or ventriculoperitoneal shunt malfunction). ▪ Hypotension (late sign of shock or poisoning).	
Head-to-toe assessment			
General appearance	▪ Clean and age-appropriate physical appearance. ▪ Well nourished. ▪ Behavior appropriate for age and level of development. ▪ Healthy family interaction patterns.	▪ Unkempt appearance. ▪ Unseasonal clothing. ▪ Malnourished. ▪ Behavior not usual for the child. ▪ Unhealthy family interaction patterns.	▪ Elicit further family social information; prepare to consult social services. Monitor child's behavior and responses. ▪ Observe family dynamics; offer support for parenting.
Head	▪ Well-proportioned size. ▪ Symmetric features. ▪ Flat fontanelles in infants and young toddlers. ▪ Normal hair distribution.	▪ Bulging fontanelles (indicative of intracranial pressure). Depressed fontanelles (indicative of dehydration). ▪ Asymmetry ▪ Occipital bald spots in infants; bald spots in young toddlers. ▪ Bruises (indicative of child neglect or maltreatment; see Chapters 46 and 47).	▪ Monitor closely for changes in neurologic functioning.
Eyes	▪ External structures within normal limits (lids, lashes, and lacrimal ducts). ▪ Equal pupils reactive to light and accommodation. ▪ Intact extraocular movements. ▪ Visual acuity within normal limits or corrected with eyeglasses or contacts. ▪ Pink conjunctiva.	▪ Ptosis. ▪ Sty. ▪ Irregular pupil size. ▪ Nonreactive pupils or sluggish reaction to light. ▪ Strabismus. ▪ Scleral jaundice. ▪ Conjunctival injection or discharge.	▪ Monitor for pupillary changes. ▪ Document noted abnormalities.
Ears	▪ Gross hearing within normal limits or corrected with hearing aid devices. ▪ Ear size, alignment, and position within normal limits.	▪ Hearing loss. ▪ Red external ear canal. ▪ Pain or pulling at ears. ▪ Ear drainage. ▪ Mastoid tenderness. ▪ Tragus tenderness. ▪ Edema or trauma.	▪ Note abnormalities. ▪ Prepare for otoscopic examination.

(continued)

TABLE 6.10 (continued)

Assessment Parameter	*Normal Findings*	*Abnormal Findings*	*Interventions*
Face	■ Symmetric, well-proportioned features. ■ Absence of pain, tenderness, or edema. ■ Absence of nasal discharge. ■ Pink, moist, and intact oral cavity and pharynx. ■ Uvula midline. ■ Healthy dentition.	■ Asymmetries. ■ Low-set ears. ■ Edema. ■ Trauma. ■ Pain or tenderness on palpation of the frontal and maxillary sinuses. ■ Pain or tenderness on palpation of the temporomandibular joint, maxilla, or mandible. ■ Nasal discharge and odor. ■ Dental caries. ■ Missing teeth. ■ Malocclusion. ■ Enlarged tonsils with exudate. ■ Oral lesions or ulcerations. ■ Erythema or petechiae on the anterior or posterior pharynx.	■ Note abnormalities. ■ Prepare for diagnostic tests. ■ Prepare for medication administration.
Neck	■ Absence of surface trauma. ■ Nonpalpable lymph glands. ■ Flat neck veins. ■ Trachea midline.	■ Trauma. ■ Palpable lymph glands. ■ Distended neck veins. ■ Tracheal deviation.	■ Prepare for diagnostic or therapeutic interventions.
Chest	■ Age-appropriate anterior-posterior diameter. ■ Symmetric expansion. ■ Vesicular, bronchovesicular, and bronchotubular breath sounds within normal limits in all lung fields.	■ Thoracic deformity. ■ Adventitious sounds. ■ Retractions. ■ Chest pain. ■ Cough. ■ Bradypnea. ■ Tachypnea. ■ Enlarged axillary lymph nodes.	■ Administer oxygen. ■ Monitor cardiorespiratory and oxygen saturation. ■ Administer medications.
Heart and vascular system	■ Absence of pulsations, lifts, or heaves. ■ Absence of abnormal heart sounds. ■ Heart rate within normal limit for age. ■ Peripheral pulses equal in rate and rhythm. ■ Pink, warm, and dry skin.	■ Murmurs. ■ Tachycardia. ■ Bradycardia. ■ Diminished or unequal peripheral pulses. ■ Mottled, cool, or clammy skin.	■ Initiate cardiorespiratory and oxygen saturation monitoring. ■ Obtain venous access. ■ Prepare to administer intravenous fluids and/or medications. ■ Prepare to initiate cardiorespiratory resuscitation measures.

(continued)

TABLE 6.10 (continued)

Assessment Parameter	*Normal Findings*	*Abnormal Findings*	*Interventions*
Abdomen	▪ Age-appropriate contour. ▪ Bowel sounds within normal limits. ▪ Clean and intact umbilicus. ▪ Absence of pain or tenderness.	▪ Enlarged abdominal organs. ▪ Enlarged inguinal node. ▪ Abdominal distention. ▪ Splinting, guarding or tenderness. ▪ Dilated vessels. ▪ Umbilical, inguinal, or femoral hernia.	▪ Prepare for diagnostic testing. ▪ Prepare for medication administration.

Genitalia and anus	▪ Age-appropriate sexual development.
	▪ Secondary sex characteristics: Male
	  ▪ Presence or absence of foreskin.
	  ▪ Meatus/scrotum within normal limits.
	  ▪ Testes descended.
	▪ Secondary sex characteristics: Female
	  ▪ External structures within normal limits.
	  ▪ Onset of menses.
	▪ Absence of anal trauma or irritation.
		▪ Anal redness or itching.
		▪ Undescended testes.
		▪ Vaginal or penile irritation or discharge.
		▪ Signs of child sexual abuse (Chapters 46 and 47).
		▪ Enlarged lymph nodes.
			▪ Prepare for diagnostic tests.
			▪ Prepare for sexual abuse/assault examination (Chapters 46 and 47).

Neuromuscular system	▪ Alert and oriented for age. ▪ Intact deep tendon reflexes. ▪ Attainment of developmental milestones (Chapter 18). ▪ Age-appropriate behavior and vocabulary (Chapter 4). ▪ Appropriate social interaction (Chapter 4). ▪ Gross and fine motor abilities within normal limits. ▪ Joints with full range of motion symmetric, well-developed muscles with good tone and strength.	▪ Hypoactivity ▪ Hyperactivity ▪ Irritability. ▪ Disorientation. ▪ Abnormal cry. ▪ Convulsions. ▪ Nuchal rigidity. ▪ Red or tender joints. ▪ Spastic or flaccid muscles. ▪ Limp or unsteady gait. ▪ Fracture, pain, or limb deformity.	▪ Monitor neurologic and neurovascular status. ▪ Prepare to treat underlying health problems.
Skin	▪ Warm, dry, intact. ▪ Odor free. ▪ Clean and shiny hair with healthy texture. ▪ Smooth, convex, pink, well-groomed nails; capillary refill < 3 seconds. ▪ Absence of trauma or edema.	▪ Pallor or cyanosis. ▪ Jaundice. ▪ Erythema. ▪ Skin lesions. ▪ Bruises. ▪ Ulcerations. ▪ Scars. ▪ Edema.	▪ Prepare to treat underlying health conditions.

(continued)

TABLE 6.10 (continued)

Assessment Parameter	*Normal Findings*	*Abnormal Findings*	*Interventions*
Skin *(continued)*		▪ Dull, brittle hair. ▪ Unusual hair growth patterns. ▪ Alopecia. ▪ Infestations. ▪ Nail biting. ▪ Nail clubbing. ▪ Capillary refill > 2 seconds.	
Inspect the posterior surfaces	▪ Vertebral alignment within normal limits. ▪ Posture within normal limits ▪ Absence of trauma.	▪ Vertebral scoliosis. ▪ Poor posture. ▪ Pain or tenderness. ▪ Trauma.	▪ Suspect vertebral or spinal cord injury and initiate spinal immobilization. ▪ Note other spinal abnormalities.

Adapted from: Emergency Nurses Association, 1995.

References

Bates, B. (1999). *A guide to physical examination* (7th ed.). Philadelphia: Lippincott.

Conedera, J. (1993). Physical assessment and triage. In L. Bernardo & M. Bove (Eds.), *Pediatric emergency nursing procedures* (pp. 1-10). Boston: Jones & Bartlett.

Emergency Nurses Association. (1995). *Policy statement on pediatric emergency nursing*. Park Ridge, IL: Author.

Engel, J. (1997). *Pocket guide to pediatric assessment*. (3rd ed.). St. Louis: Mosby-Year Book.

Gundy, J. (1997). The pediatric physical examination. In R. A. Hoekelman, S. B. Friedman, N. M. Nelson, H. M. Sdidel, & M. L. Weitzman (Eds.), *Primary pediatric care* (pp. 55-97). St. Louis: Mosby—Year Book.

Lissauer, T., & Clauden, G. (1997). *Illustrated textbook of pediatrics*. St. Louis: Mosby—Year Book.

Wong, D. (1999). Physical and developmental assessment of the child. In D. Wong (Ed.), *Whaley and Wong's nursing care of infants and children* (6th ed., pp. 217-283). St. Louis: Mosby—Year Book.

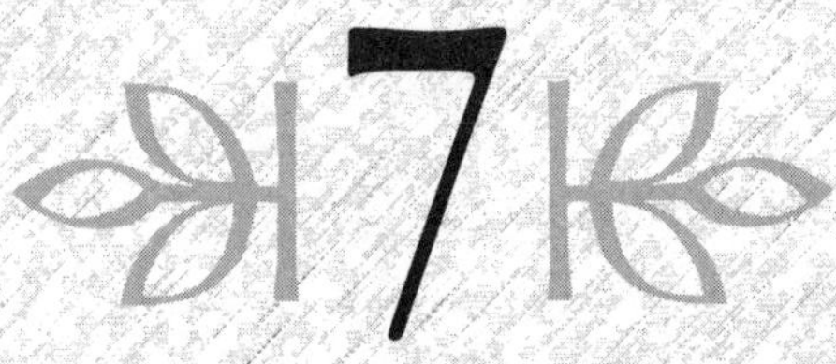

7 Triage

Reneé Semonin Holleran, RN, PhD, CEN, CCRN, CFRN

Introduction

Triage of the pediatric patient follows the same format as that of the adult. However, determining a triage acuity in a child is more difficult because physiologic and psychosocial differences make children harder to evaluate. Symptoms that may be nonurgent in the adult may be urgent or even emergent in the child. The purpose of this chapter is to define the pediatric triage process, the qualifications for triage personnel, and the triage assessment.

The word triage *is derived from the French word that means "to sort." In emergency care, triage is a process that encompasses the assignment of a priority for treatment, including the use of appropriate personnel and supplies. For the pediatric patient, triage may also include a decision as to whether the patient can be cared for in a facility that sees both children and adults or requires one that specializes in the care of ill or injured children.*

The triage area is usually near the general waiting area, allowing the triage nurse the ability to perform an "episodic" assessment, including the collection of historical data and a brief evaluation that focuses on the chief complaint. Ideally, the triage area should provide privacy, and the waiting area should be visible to the triage nurse.

Types of Triage

There are three types of triage systems involving different levels of staffing, assessment, and interventions (Emergency Nurses Association, 1992): (1) traffic director, (2) spot-check, and (3) comprehensive. These are described in Table 7.1.

Ideally, a registered nurse with pediatric emergency experience should be responsible for the triage of the pediatric patient. It is best that such nurses:

- Attend a formal triage course that addresses pediatric specific concerns. (Table 7.2 lists suggested content for a pediatric training program.)
- Have 6 months' to 1 year's experience as an emergency department nurse.
- Possess knowledge of growth and development principles (Chapter 4).
- Recognize a variety of pediatric-related patient problems.
- Possess excellent pediatric assessment and interaction skills.
- Have Advanced Cardiac Life Support (ACLS)/Pediatric Advanced Life Support (PALS) and Emergency Nursing Pediatric Course (ENPC) verification.
- Demonstrate competence in the process of pediatric triage; have the ability to perform the four components of pediatric triage (see the section on the triage process).

TABLE 7.1 Types of Triage Systems

Type	*Description and Staffing*
Traffic director	Directs flow of patients in and out of the department. Usually responsible for collecting and documenting demographic information about the patient. Usually staffed by an emergency department (ED) clerk, an emergency technician, or a nursing assistant. Usually located outside the department at a desk or enclosed space.
Spot-check	Takes "quick look" or "eyeballs" the child arriving in the ED. Generally done by a registered nurse or physician.
Comprehensive triage	Includes an episodic patient history and assessment, triage classification, documentation, and initiation of treatment or diagnostic procedures. Usually done by an experienced registered nurse.

From: Requirements to perform pediatric triage. In *Triage: Meeting the Challenge,* Emergency Nurses Association, 1992; Ramler & Mohammed, 1995; Grossman, 1999; Murphy, 1997).

TABLE 7.2 Suggested Content for a Pediatric Triage Training Program

Philosophy of pediatric triage
Creating a child-friendly environment
Approaching the child
Approaching the parents/caregivers
Emergency department policies and procedures
Triage admission procedures
Standing orders/protocols
Legal considerations
Emergency Medical Treatment and Active Labor Act (EMTALA) legislation/state laws
Documentation
Suspected child abuse or neglect
Dealing with violent or disruptive behavior
Use of the panic button (how to summon additional help)
Defusing anger
Infection control
Communicability of infectious diseases
Plan for isolation of contagious children
Review of child development
Characteristics of psychosocial development
Characteristics of physical development
Tips for gaining the child's cooperation
The pediatric assessment
Across-the-room assessment
Triage history
Triage physical
Triage vital signs
Pediatric red flags
The triage classification system
Categories of classification
Description of categories
Workshop
Triage case studies
Work with experienced triage nurse

From: Soud & Andry, 1998. Pediatric triage. In T. Soud & J. Rogers (Eds.), *Manual of pediatric emergency nursing* (p. 90). St. Louis: Mosby. Used with permission.

- Possess strong interpersonal communication skills.
- Collaborate with the child and family during the triage assessment.
- Trust their "sixth" sense.

Special Considerations for Pediatric Triage

The triage process sets the tone for the remainder of the emergency department visit. The triage nurse must be aware of how he or she approaches the parent and child. Table 7.3 outlines some considerations for interacting with the parent and child. Chapter 4 also contains information for approaching the child according to age and developmental level.

"Difficult" Parents

Because parents who bring their children to the ED are often under stress, worried about their child, or angry about the wait, they may become difficult. "Difficult" may describe those parents who are angry, confrontational, demanding, or hysterical. These parents must be handled in a calm manner to prevent them from disrupting the entire ED and patient care. Often the triage nurse may be able to deal with the situation quickly by recognizing the concern, but he or she may have to involve other staff members, including the physician or the charge nurse. The following tips may help when it is necessary to manage a crisis with a difficult parent (Walker & Joseph, 1997):

- *Intervene early.* Do not avoid the confrontation in hopes that it will go away. Deal with the problem as soon as it presents. Involve the charge nurse or the nursing supervisor if necessary. Take the parent into a private area if you need time to calm him or her.
- *Have one person take charge.* Allow one person to interact with the parent. This may have a calming effect; having to repeat the story to several different people may increase the parent's frustration and hostility.
- *Gather complete data.* Find out what the parent is upset about and listen without being judgmental.
- *Listen first.* Listen to the parent without arguing.
- *Be aware that information does not always solve the problem.* The situation may be exacerbated by an excess of facts because an angry or frightened parent may not be able to process what is being said.

TABLE 7.3 Approach to the Child and Family during the Triage Process

Concept	*Nursing Intervention/Considerations*
There is diversity in family composition, including single parent, divorced, and same-sex parents. The caregiver's or family's values will vary and may conflict with normal or accepted values.	Respect diversity. Do not assume anything. Observe and assess the family's strengths, weaknesses, and resources while conducting the interview. Be nonjudgmental in approach.
The anxiety of the caregiver or parent will affect the interaction.	Reassure the caregiver honestly with your triage findings: "I know your baby sounds like he is having trouble breathing, but he is moving air well and his color is good." Explain briefly what you are doing and what will happen next: "I am going to have you sit across from my desk where I can observe you. The nurse will come to take you to a room soon."
	Listen to the caregiver because he or she knows the child better than anyone else. Ask, "What do you think is the problem?"
The anxiety of the child will affect the examination.	Approach the child slowly. Sit down, if possible, and allow the parent to hold the child.
	Speak to the child directly, no matter the age.
	Anticipate that the child will be fearful and use distraction techniques, such as stickers and toys.

Data from: Engle, 1993; Seidel & Henderson, 1997.

- *Use plain language.* Avoid medical jargon and tailor the explanations to the perceived educational level of the parent.
- *Do not be repetitious.* Repeating what was said in a louder voice will not be effective and may only inflame the situation.
- *Be aware that the parent may have serious psychopathology.* Involve security if you suspect that the parent has an altered mental status or if the parent is behaving inappropriately.

Latex Allergies

An allergic reaction to latex may prove fatal to a pediatric patient. The triage nurse needs to be able to identify risk factors for latex allergy so that the child can be treated in a latex-safe environment. Risk factors for latex allergy include a positive history of a latex allergic reaction, patients with spine bifida, children who had frequent latex catheterizations, and children who have had frequent contact with natural rubber latex. Unexplained anaphylactic reactions to food should also raise suspicions of a latex allergy (Miller & Weed, 1998).

Once the potential for a latex allergy has been identified, the triage nurse should assure that patient assessment and care is performed using latex-safe precautions. These precautions include using products that are latex free (blood pressure cuffs) and covering latex portions of the equipment when the latex portion cannot be removed (Miller & Weed, 1998).

The Triage Process

Components of Pediatric Triage

Four components of triage include (1) the pediatric assessment triangle, (2) initial assessment, (3) pediatric triage history, and (4) triage decision or acuity (Eckle, Haley, & Baker, 1998).

1. The Pediatric Assessment Triangle

The pediatric assessment triangle is an "across-the-room assessment" or an "as-you-approach-the-child-assessment." The triangle looks at the overall *appearance* of the child, work of *breathing*, and *circulation* to the skin. It is done on the child's entry to the ED waiting area or the triage room. It consists of observation of the following.

- *Overall appearance,* including look or gaze, speech, cry, how the child is dressed, and hygiene.
- *Breathing,* including effort being used, rate.
- *Circulation to the skin* including color (e.g., cyanosis, pale, mottled).

2. Initial Assessment

In the triage setting, the initial assessment starts with a rapid primary assessment (Chapter 6). Generally, the assessment is focused on the chief complaint. Life-threatening problems identified during the initial assessment may require that the child be taken immediately to a treatment area. After the primary assessment, the secondary assessment is completed (Chapter 6). Modifications of this assessment may be necessary because of space and privacy, and many components of the secondary assessment will have to be completed after the child is taken to a room. The following signs and symptoms may be "red flags" or warnings of a serious illness or injury (Fredrickson, 1994):

- Apnea.
- Choking.
- Drooling.
- Stridor.
- Grunting.
- Retractions.
- Use of accessory muscles.
- Irregular respiratory pattern.
- Wheezing.
- Bradypnea.
- Tachypnea.
- Changes in color or skin temperature.
- Cyanosis.
- Diaphoresis.
- Hypotension.
- Tachycardia.
- Bradycardia.
- Decreased or absent peripheral pulses.
- Uncontrollable bleeding.
- Petechiae.
- Purpura.
- Changes in mental status.
- Unresponsiveness.
- New onset of seizure activity.
- Loss of consciousness.
- Irritability.
- Bruising or injuries suggestive of child abuse (Chapter 46).
- Contagious skin conditions (Chapter 22).
- Abnormal skin turgor.

3. Pediatric Triage History (Eckle, Haley, & Baker, 1998)

The CIAMPEDS mnemonic is a systematic way of obtaining important components of the triage history:

C = Chief Complaint
I = Immunizations or Isolation (exposure to communicable disease.
A = Allergies to food or medications
M = Medications
P = Past Medical History
E = Events surrounding the illness or injury
D = Diet or Diapers (bladder and bowel habits)
S = Symptoms associated with the illness or injury.

The history at triage should be brief but should allow enough information to make an accurate triage decision and to permit the patient care nurse to build on the information to care for the child (Thomas, 2002).

4. Triage Decision or Acuity

The triage decision is made at the completion of the triage process. The triage decision determines the priority for care based on the results of the child's assessment and the chief complaint. The most common triage classification contains three levels of acuity:

- *Emergent:* Requires immediate care; life or limb threatening (e.g., apnea, pulselessness, or uncontrolled bleeding, threatening to life or limb if not treated immediately).
- *Urgent:* Requires care within a few hours. Requires prompt care but is not life or limb threatening (e.g., respiratory distress or irregular pulse rate). May be life-threatening if not treated within 2 hours.
- *Nonurgent:* Does not require ED treatment. Requires evaluation and treatment, but time is not critical.

Internationally, national standardized five-level systems with proven reliability are being instituted. There is a growing interest in the United States to create such a standardized system, which would be more accurate and would allow comparison between hospitals and better care and standardized teaching (Thomas, 2002).

Triage Interventions

Some life-saving interventions may be done at triage, but if the child's condition is emergent, he or she is taken directly to a treatment area. Common interventions that may be initiated in the triage area include:

- Isolating the child if an infectious disease is suspected or if the child is immunosuppressed.

- Obtaining initial laboratory work based on individual hospital triage protocols:
    - Complete blood count.
    - Glucose.
    - Electrolytes.
    - Urinalysis.
    - *Beta-streptococcus* screen.
- Obtaining radiographic studies according to existing protocols. (Table 7.4 shows an example of a triage protocol for ordering X-rays for pediatric patients.)

TABLE 7.4 General Guidelines for Ordering X-Rays from Triage

1. X-rays should be ordered from triage only for those patients brought in for evaluation of isolated extremity injuries and suspected foreign-body ingestions.
2. X-rays should be ordered only when there is clear deformity of a limb or significant swelling accompanied by point tenderness. Whenever there is uncertainty as to whether an X-ray should be obtained or as to what specific films should be ordered, the triage nurse should consult either a resident or the attending physician. Specific guidelines will follow for injuries of various portions of both upper and lower extremities.
3. All potentially unstable fractures must be immobilized before X-rays are taken. A sling or a simple splint made using an arm board will be adequate in many cases; for grossly deformed fractures, a more substantial splint (e.g., using splinting material such as fiberglass) may be needed. Fractures that are causing neurovascular compromise or that are open must be seen immediately by the attending physician.
4. When a child with a suspected foreign-body ingestion or aspiration is in any way symptomatic, a physician must be promptly consulted prior to the ordering of X-rays.
5. A physician should be consulted before X-rays are ordered for any patients who could conceivably be pregnant (any menstruating female).
6. On the X-ray requisition, please include the following:
    - Specific study desired; make sure to clearly distinguish right from left.
    - Brief history of injury (e.g., crushed in car door or eversion injury playing basketball).
    - Brief description of physical findings (e.g., tenderness and swelling over distal radius).
    - Type of foreign body, nature of symptoms, and time of ingestion, if foreign-body ingestion is suspected.
    - Name of ED attending physician.

Table 7.5 lists specific guidelines for X-rays of the upper extremity.

- Obtaining a pulse oximetry reading.
- Beginning initial health education and/or preventive education (such as immunization schedules and wearing helmets, seat belts, and other protective gear).

Patient Disposition

On completion of triage, patients are transferred to:

- *An assigned area within the ED:* Based on the data collected and the acuity of the child's problem, the child is assigned an area within the department. If the child's problem is nonurgent and if a room is not available, the child may be sent to a specific place to wait. The triage nurse or another designated nurse should perform periodic reassessments of the child's condition to determine if the condition has changed from the initial assessment.
- *Another department within the hospital:* Triage protocols may allow the triage nurse to refer nonurgent problems to other areas within the hospital. For example, if the child needs a prescription refilled, a new prescription may be written and the family sent to the pharmacy without being seen within the department. Established and approved guidelines for doing this will prevent violations of the Emergency Medical Treatment and Active Labor Act (Chapter 2).
- *Another health care facility:* Based on guidelines, done when the child's needs may be better met in a different facility.

Documentation

Documentation of the triage assessment, interventions, and triage acuity is completed prior to the child's discharge from the triage area. Emergency departments should have protocols that describe the charting format to be followed. Typical documentation formats include:

- Charting by exception.
- Use of a checklist.
- Narrative.
- Computerized charting driven by chief complaints.

Whatever charting format is used, the following must be documented:

- Chief complaint.
- Assessment—may include vital signs.

TABLE 7.5 Specific Guidelines—Upper Extremity

Site of Injury	*X-ray Study*	*Comments*
Finger, including metacarpal-phalangeal joint.	Finger(s)	Request the specific finger(s) injured (e.g., right fourth finger). Note: thumb = first finger, little finger = fifth.
Hand, metacarpal bones.	Hand	Note on requisition which metacarpals are injured (number as above).
Wrist, includes distal one-fourth of forearm.	Wrist	If significant deformity is present, forearm may be better view; check with physician.
Forearm—injuries involving middle half.	Forearm	Immobilize if unstable.
Elbow—includes distal one-fourth of humerus, proximal one-fourth of forearm.	Elbow	Have physician assess first. Do not X-ray possible nursemaid's elbow.
Humerus.	Humerus	Humeral fractures are less common; have physician assess.
Shoulder, includes proximal one-fourth of humerus.	Shoulder	Dislocations rare prior to midteen years. Have physician assess first.
Clavicle.	Clavicle	If uncertain whether to order shoulder or clavicle, consult physician. Clavicular fractures are much more common. Slings are recommended.
Toe, including metatarsal-phalangeal joint.	Toe(s)	Request specific toe(s) injured. Note: big toe = first toe.
Foot, metatarsal bones.	Foot	Note on requisition which metatarsals are injured (number as above).
Ankle, includes distal one fourth of tibia and fibula.	Ankle	Order only if marked swelling and bruising are present. If deformity is present, tibia/fibula may be better view; check with physician.
Tibia/fibula, injuries involving middle half.	Tibia/fibula	Remember splinting prior to X-rays.
Knee—includes proximal one-fourth of tibia and very distal femur.	Knee	Order only if marked swelling and bruising are present.
Femur.	Femur	Must be seen by physician first.
Hip.	Hip	Must be seen by physician first.

Source: Primary Children's Medical Center Emergency Department, 1998. Salt Lake City, Utah. Used with permission.

- Triage classification.
- Any treatment initiated.

Conclusion

Triage is defined as the ability to "to sort." In the ED, this includes the skills to perform a rapid, focused assessment of the child's airway, breathing, circulation, and level of consciousness and to collect a focused patient history. Based on this initial examination, the triage nurse decides the child's disposition.

To perform triage, the emergency nurse needs experience, advanced assessment skills, and the willingness to listen to the "sixth sense." Triage is an important component in the care of the pediatric patient in the ED.

References

Eckle, N., Haley, K., & Baker, P. (1998). *Emergency nursing pediatric course provider manual* (2nd ed., pp. 82-85). Park Ridge, IL: Emergency Nurses Association.

Emergency Nurses Association. (1992). *Triage: Meeting the challenge.* Park Ridge, IL: Author.

Engel, J. (1993). *Pediatric assessment.* St. Louis: Mosby—Year Book.

Fredrickson, J. (1994). Triage. In S. Kelley (Ed.), *Pediatric emergency nursing* (pp. 11-16). Norwalk, CT: Appleton & Lange.

Grossman, V. (1999). Quick reference to triage (p. 5). Philadelphia: Lippincott.

Miller K. & Weed, P. (1998). The latex allergy triage or admission tool: An algorithm to identity which parents benefit from "latex-safe" precautions. *Journal of Emergency Nursing 24*(2): 145-152.

Murphy, K. (1997). *Pediatric triage guidelines* (pp. 316-323). St. Louis: Mosby-Year Book, Inc.

Haley, K., & Baker, P. (1993). *Emergency nursing pediatric course.* Park Ridge, IL: Emergency Nurses Association.

Ramler, C. L., & Mohammed, N. (1995). Triage. In S. Kitt, J. Selfridge-Thomas, J. Proehl, & J. Kaiser (Eds.), *Emergency nursing: A physiologic and clinical perspective* (pp. 19-27). Philadelphia: Saunders.

Seidel, J., & Henderson, D. (1997). Approach to the pediatric patient in the emergency department. In R. Barkin (Ed.), *Pediatric emergency medicine: Concepts and clinical practice* (2nd ed., pp. 1-7). St. Louis: Mosby—Year Book.

Soud, T., & Andry, C. (1998). Pediatric triage. In T. Soud & J. Rogers (Eds.), *Manual of pediatric emergency nursing* (pp. 89-106). St. Louis: Mosby.

Thomas, D. (2002). Special considerations for pediatric triage in the emergency department. *Nursing Clinics of North America* 37(1): 145-159.

Walker, A., & Joseph, J. (1997). The difficult parent. In E. Crain & J. Gershel (Eds.), *Clinical manual of emergency pediatrics* (3rd ed., pp. 675-676). New York: McGraw-Hill.

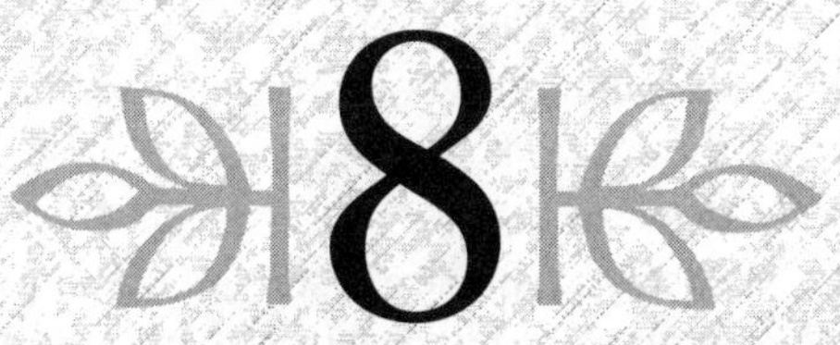

Telephone Triage

Valerie G. A. Grossman, BSN, CEN

Introduction

Telephone triage is the practice of conducting a verbal interview to assess a patient's health status and to offer recommendations for treatment and referral. The goal of telephone triage is timely patient referral to the appropriate level of care. Telephone triage systems originate from many settings, including emergency departments (EDs), health maintenance organizations (HMOs), private offices, and independent companies. Services offered vary as much as the settings and range from general helplines to subspecialty (e.g., cardiology or hematology/oncology) after-hours lines to organized services that assist callers with access to necessary health care.

The educational and clinical background required for the person performing the telephone triage role varies depending on the type of service to be delivered. Some calls are answered by physicians, nurse practitioners, or physicians assistants, but a majority of the calls are handled by highly skilled registered nurses (RNs). Some programs require RN certification in the specialty area (e.g., emergency nursing, telephone nursing, or nephrology nursing). In addition, some programs may use unlicensed assistive personnel to perform tasks delegated by the RN. These duties must be restricted to such tasks as documenting the patient's initial demographic data or obtaining the patient's medical records.

The purpose of this section is to describe the telephone triage process. Examples of telephone triage protocols are included at the end of the chapter in Appendices A and B.

History of Telephone Triage

Telephone triage has been occurring since the creation of the telephone; in fact, it is said that Alexander Graham Bell used his telephone to call for help when he spilled acid on himself. Health maintenance organizations began to establish "gatekeeper" or telephone advice services in the 1970s. In the 1980s, isolated programs were developed around the country to service after-hours calls regarding access to health care. By 1997, 35 million Americans had access to an established telephone triage system. It is estimated that by the year 2001, the number will grow to more than 100 million (Anders, 1997).

Telephone Triage Programs

Well-structured and systematic telephone triage programs use highly skilled RNs who confidently and consistently respond to parents' calls. Nurses assist parents in making informed healthcare decisions while strengthening the parent's perception of the healthcare provider, healthcare system, and their child's healthcare management. Programs may be operated by EDs, HMOs, private offices, or independent companies.

Emergency Departments

Emergency department nurses possess a broad knowledge base, are skilled in rapid patient assessment, and are accustomed to triaging children and families with a wide variety of problems, healthcare issues, and cultural differences. Many ED-based telephone triage programs require nurses to rotate through the ED to maintain their clinical skills.

Health Maintenance Organizations

Telephone triage is an integral part of many HMOs and provides an important service to the clients of these large systems. The call volume is often high, requiring that the nursing staff have optimal organizational and communication skills.

Private Offices

Telephone triage is a growing practice within physician's offices as managed care works to reduce unnecessary office visits (Marsden, 2000). Parents are more frequently calling their primary care provider for advice or

TABLE 8.1 Other Settings for Telephone Triage

Service	*Example*
Crisis line.	Poison control centers.
	Suicide prevention lines.
	Child abuse hot lines.
Health information.	Physician referral service.
	Recorded advice lines.
Hospital discharge follow-up.	Same-day surgery.
	Outpatient services.
	Emergency services.
Emergency medical dispatch.	911 centers.
	Air ambulance centers.
School district.	Off-site school nurses.
Military.	Off-base advice and referral lines.

counseling before requesting an appointment for their child. Office triage nurses must be knowledgeable, possess good interviewing skills, and have well-developed telephone assessment skills.

Independent Companies

Independent and/or community-based programs are available for use by private physicians and their patients. These programs are staffed with highly skilled RNs who follow established protocols in assessing a child's condition and making recommendations to the parent. This autonomous nursing role allows the RN to advise the parent on a variety of healthcare issues, from seeking emergent care for the child to appropriate home care.

Telephone triage is also used in other settings. Some of these settings are described in Table 8-1.

Benefits and Risks

Benefits

The benefits of quality telephone healthcare include:

- A link between parents seeking healthcare information and knowledgeable healthcare professionals.
- Parent satisfaction and good customer service. Parents are generally more comfortable caring for their own children when the stress associated with their sick or injured child is shared with the telephone nurse. They can have their questions answered and receive advice and/or a referral over the telephone. Advice calls generate good customer service for the program they represent (hospital, doctor's office, or other locations).
- Reduced cost. Patient care is streamlined during regular office hours and fewer patients are seen unnecessarily after hours. Referrals to appropriate care save the parents time and money.

Risks

There are risks associated with telephone triage, just as there are with every other area of health care. The risks of telephone triage stem from the incorrect assessment of the child's condition, usually because of an incomplete history, leading to:

- An incorrect or untimely referral decision.
- Inadequate advice.
- Misinterpretation of advice by the parent. Table 8.2 lists ways to avoid the risks associated with telephone triage.

Telephone Triage Process

Several steps are involved in the telephone triage process.

Introduce Self

The nurse begins the call by introducing herself or himself by name and title. This information provides the parent with the confidence that the advice is given by a warm, compassionate, and knowledgeable professional. Opening the communication between the nurse and the parent begins with this simple act of developing trust and allows for the establishment of a rapport. The nurse's caring voice and nonjudgmental manner set the tone for the entire call. The trust gained during the initial communication encourages the parent to reveal information, thus allowing the nurse to make informed decisions about the child's health.

Conduct the Interview and Assessment

When performing triage by telephone, the nurse relies on listening, intuition, and nursing knowledge. The telephone triage nurse listens to what the caller is saying, what the caller is *not* saying, and is alert for "aural cues." The parent's breathing pattern or the pauses in sentences may give important insights into the parent's anxiety level. Background sounds, conversations, or activity, such as a crying infant or a shouting family member, may provide the telephone triage nurse with a clue about the pressures the parent is facing at home. The

TABLE 8.2 Risks of Telephone Triage

Risk	*Ways to Avoid the Risk*
Wrong assessment, decision, or advice.	▪ Always follow established protocol. Never assume, never guess, and never compromise; be certain of the history, decision, or advice.
Incomplete history.	▪ Ask open-ended questions whenever possible, and offer suggestions that might spur the parent's memory. *Example:* "What type of past medical history does your child have, such as heart disease, liver disease, seizures, asthma, immune problems, and so forth?" *Example:* "What types of injuries has your child been treated for in the past?"
Incomplete assessment.	▪ Always address each possible system involved, including the social situation surrounding the parent. ▪ Follow guidelines carefully. ▪ Perform a focused assessment of the complaint. ▪ Restate questions if the parent's answer was ambiguous.
Parent mistrust of telephone program.	▪ Establish an excellent rapport with the caller immediately in the conversation. Remember that the parent is stressed, may have poor communication skills, or may be very frightened. ▪ The parent must know that the care of the child is of utmost importance to the telephone nurse. ▪ Always ask the caller if he or she is comfortable with the topics discussed and the advice given.
Parental misunderstanding.	▪ Ask parent to repeat instructions when given and suggest that the parent writes them down. ▪ Ask if the parent has any questions.
Poor documentation.	▪ Document precisely. This is necessary so that future readers understand exactly the dynamics of the call.

From: Briggs, 1997; Marsden, 2000.

telephone triage nurse may ask the parent to bring the child to the telephone and listen carefully for signs and symptoms such as coughing, wheezing, congestion, a muffled voice, shortness of breath, pain, fear, and other indicators of a problem. Whether listening to the respirations of an 18-month-old toddler or discussing an adolescent's abdominal pain, the telephone triage nurse relies solely on an ability to listen and interpret.

The interview follows many of the same guidelines used in any other patient setting. It provides data that form the basis for the nurse's assessment. Thus, the interview must be concise and focused. Information obtained from the parent includes demographic data, baseline health information, and current symptoms (Tables 8.3 and 8.4).

Make a Triage Decision Using the Established Protocol or Guideline

Once the assessment is completed, the appropriate triage protocol or guideline is selected. These protocols ensure that advice given to the parent is consistent and precise. The protocols can be generated from a com-

TABLE 8.3 Suggested Information to Obtain during the Parent Interview

Demographic Data	*Baseline Information*
Name	Weight
Date of birth	Birth weight (for neonates)
Telephone number	Birth history (for neonates)
Caller's name and relationship	Immunization state
Primary care physician	Medications (prescription and over the counter)
Today's date	Medication allergies
Type of insurance	Past medical/surgical history
Important times: ▪ When parent called service or hospital ▪ When triage nurse began speaking to the parent ▪ When call finished ▪ When 911, physicians, ED, and others were notified	

TABLE 8.4 Suggested Mnemonic for Obtaining Information about Symptoms: The PQRST Mnemonic

P	Provoking factors	What makes it (pain, breathing, or other symptoms) worse?
		What makes it better?
Q	Quality of pain	What does it feel like?
		Has the child ever experienced pain like this before?
R	Region/radiation	Where is the pain?
		Is it in one spot?
		Does it start in one spot and travel to another?
S	Severity of pain	Is this the worst pain ever experienced?
		If abdominal pain, is the pain worsened with movement, such as climbing stairs or jumping on one foot?
T	Time	When did it start?
		How long have the symptom(s) persisted?
		How long did the pain last?
		Has it ever happened before?
T	Treatment	Has the child been given any medication to treat this problem?
		What time was the last dose?
		Has the parent tried any home remedies for the child?
		What has or has not worked for the child?

puter-based system or a manual system of reference texts and paper reports. Following the protocol guidelines, the triage nurse advises the parent as to the type of care needed for the child. The ultimate decision regarding care rests with the caller.

There are times when a parent's description may not "fit" a particular protocol. The parent may communicate in a vague manner, or the concern or timing may seem inappropriate. The triage nurse must take special care with these parents, question precisely, and listen carefully to determine the parent's main concern. A good question to ask is "What worries you the most about your child at this time?". Once the concern is identified, the triage nurse should follow the protocol that most closely matches the child's symptoms and manage the call with a very conservative approach. If physician backup is available, the nurse may choose to review the call with the physician or call the parent back to follow up on the condition of the child. Appendix A, at the end of this chapter, provides an example of a protocol for fever control and Appendix B provides a protocol for respiratory difficulty.

Offer the Predetermined Advice

If advice is given, the telephone triage nurse must ensure that the parent clearly understands the advice by having the parent repeat the information. Whether the advice is to "Call 911 *now*" or how to manage vomiting at home, the nurse must be clear and use simple terms when giving directions and be certain that the parent understands the information. Encourage parents to write the home care advice on a piece of paper.

The nurse offers the parents positive reinforcement whenever possible to help alleviate apprehension and heighten their comfort level in caring for the sick or injured child. The nurse should consider health insurance and be knowledgeable of what insurance carriers will permit as a disposition, making sure to always put the welfare of the child first.

Conclude the Call and Follow Up as Needed

When concluding a call, the nurse always should encourage the parent to call back if symptoms persist, worsen, or change, if new symptoms develop, or if anything occurs that concerns the parent. Parents tend to be more comfortable with their telephone advice if they believe that the telephone triage nurse is easily accessible. The telephone triage nurse has the additional option of calling the parent back to follow up on the child's condition or the parent's understanding of any advice previously given.

Document the Call

Documentation of each call must be complete and follow the protocol used. The most comprehensive style of documentation is by inclusion. In this style, all pertinent negatives are listed. This creates a clearer picture of the patient scenario. Appendix C illustrates a sample documentation form.

Quality Improvement and Continuing Education

A quality improvement program should be established to monitor clinical performance and customer satisfaction. Each type of program will establish key indicators and the subsequent process to review and evaluate the program. Regular documentation reviews may be performed to evaluate protocol compliance and appropriate documentation for each nurse involved. This should also be done for any calls that resulted in a parent's complaint or physician's concern with how the call was handled.

Common trends should be reviewed and evaluated. These might include:

- Parent compliance with information recommended by the nurse
- Common patient complaints and protocols used.
- Nursing compliance to protocols.
- Call volume and staffing ratio.

The satisfaction of both the physicians using or otherwise involved with the service and of the parents calling the service should be evaluated on a regular basis. Regular continuing education on topics such as risk management, current medical and nursing trends, and subjects the nurses identify as areas of interest or concern should be provided for the nursing staff (Fulkner & Gary, 1999).

Conclusion

Telephone triage is an important aspect of pediatric health care. For telephone triage to be successful, these important features must be addressed:

- Established and approved protocols to provide consistency with an approved standard of care within the community.
- Accurate documentation to provide valuable resource information regarding the patient's triage and recommendations.
- Triage decisions, not differential diagnoses—to ensure the nurse is providing suggestions for symptoms and not a disease process.
- Necessary education if home care advice is recommended.
- Patient safety balanced with the efficient use of available resources.
- The role of the nurse as a patient advocate (American Academy of Ambulatory Care Nursing, 1997).

The Emergency Nurse Association has also developed a position statement concerning telephone advice calls (ENA, 1998). This can be obtained at www.ena.org or by writing to ENA at 915 Lee Street, Des Plaines, IL 60016-6569.

A

Protocol for Fever

Fever is defined as:

- Rectal temperature higher than 101.5°F (38.5°C). In infants younger than 3 months, 100.4°F (38.0°C).
- Oral temperature higher than 99.5°F (37.5°C).
- Axillary temperature higher than 99.0°F (37.2°C).

Obtain and record telephone triage assessment that includes:

Fever:

- Onset
- Duration
- Degree
- Method of measurement

Symptoms and behavior associated with fever:

- Feeding problems.
- Change in normal play behavior or lethargy.
- Normal cry.
- Respiratory symptoms.
- Irritability.
- Change in urination or stooling.
- Seizure.
- Limping or refusal to use an extremity.
- Rash.
- Localized swelling or erythema.
- Tugging at ears.
- Vomiting or diarrhea.
- Sore throat.
- Difficulty swallowing.
- Cough.
- Runny nose.
- Headache.
- Changes in urinary output in past 8 hours.

Use of antipyretics, including:

- Type.
- Time of last dose.
- Amount administered, rectally or orally
  - Have the caller read the concentration (i.e., mg/ml) from the label of the bottle.
  - Calculate accurate dose based on child's weight to ensure proper dosing by parent.

Risk factors that increase the acuity of a child with a fever:

Infants younger than 3 months of age:

- Exposed to organisms for which they have no immunity, placing them at higher risk of systemic infections.
- Passive immunity from birth decreases before the infant's own immune response is fully competent.

Immunosuppressed:

- Congenital (rare).
- Acquired (HIV/AIDS).
- Chemically induced (chemotherapy, corticosteroids).

Splenic dysfunction:

- Lack the ability to mount effective response if spleen has been removed or have developed functional asplenia (i.e., sickle cell anemia, splenectomy).

See immediately:

Triage nurse should advise using an ambulance when the child's current status is life-threatening or may deteriorate en route to hospital or when parental anxiety level is too high to safely drive child to closest ED.

- Temperature >101°F (38.3°C) with history of high-risk factors.
- Temperature >105°F (40.6°C) in any age.
- Rash with purple or red spots or dots.
- Seizure.
- Difficulty in breathing.
- Stiff neck.
- Behavior changes that sound to the nurse as if the child is very ill. Child is:
    - Lethargic or confused.
    - Difficult to arouse or unresponsive.
    - Crying inconsolably.
    - Limp, weak, or not moving.
- Dehydration (no urinary output for more than 8 hours, sunken eyes, crying without tears, etc.).
- Difficulty in swallowing or new drooling.
- Pain:
    - Abdominal pain.
    - Arm, leg, or joint pain with no known injury.

See within 24 hours:

- Pain (difficulty walking, urination, ear, throat, etc.).
- Fever for more than 24 hours with no other symptoms.
- Fever for more than 72 hours.
- Recurrent or intermittent fevers.
- Persistent cough with a fever.
- Acting sick.
- Past medical history of diabetes, steroid use, cystic fibrosis, asthma, or seizures.
- Vaginal or penile discharge.

Cross reference to other protocols as indicated:

- Abdominal pain, rash, respiratory distress.

Home care advice:

- Encourage fluids, especially calorie-containing liquids, such as popsicles, juice, etc.
- Dress lightly, cover with lightweight blanket for comfort, if desired (prevent shivering).
- Administer antipyretic:
    - Acetaminophen, 10 to 15 mg/kg, every 4 to 6 hours.
    - Ibuprofen, 10 mg/kg, every 6 to 8 hours for children older than 6 months.
    - Do *not* use aspirin.
- Lukewarm (85° to 90°F) tub bath for comfort or temperature higher than 104°F after antipyretic:
    - Do *not* use rubbing alcohol.
- Encourage quiet activity to avoid production of excess body heat.
- Reassure the caller:
    - Temperatures up to 104°F in children are uncomfortable but not harmful.
    - Use of antipyretic usually lowers the fever by 2 to 3°F.
- Monitor temperature every 2 to 4 hours.

Call back if:

- The temperature is greater than 105°F (40.6°C).
- The child looks worse.
- The child develops rash, difficulty breathing, seizure, headache, neck pain, or dehydration.
- The parent has increased concern, anxiety, or new questions.
- The child develops any new symptoms or if symptoms change.

From: Briggs, 1997; Schmitt, 1999.

B

Protocol for Respiratory Difficulty

Variety of presentations including (but not limited to):
"Common cold":

- Red eyes
- Fever
- Swollen glands
- Sore throat
- Cough
- Nasal congestion/discharge

Wheezing:

- High-pitched purring or whistling during expiration as a result of bronchospasm.
- Most common cause in children younger than 12 months of age is bronchiolitis.
- Most common cause in children older than 3 years is asthma.

Croup:

- Hoarseness.
- Tight, low-pitched cough resembling a barking seal.
- Wheezing may be heard during inspiration and expiration.
- Harsh, raspy inspirations (stridor) in severe croup.

Obtain and record telephone triage assessment that includes:

- Time of onset
- Rate and quality of respirations:
  - Instruct caller to put telephone to child's nose and mouth and listen carefully.

Assess symptoms and behavior associated with respiratory difficulty:

- Cough
- Exertional dyspnea
- Difficulty feeding
- Fever
- Position of comfort
- Ability to speak in sentences
- Drooling
- Chest pain
- Cough (short, wet, bark, etc.)
- Choking
- Vomiting
- Eye or nasal discharge (color?)
- Earache
- Wheezing

- Sore throat and/or hoarseness
- Headache
- Retractions
- Level of consciousness
- Rash
- Stridor
- Difficulty swallowing
- Cyanosis
- Hemoptysis
- Foreign-body aspiration
- Pallor
- Grunting
- Inability to bend neck forward

Risk factors that increase the acuity of the child:

- Infants or small children.
- Chronic or recent illnesses.
- Immunosuppressed.
- Recent trauma, surgery, or childbirth.
- Cardiac disease.

Activate emergency medical system for ambulance transport (call 911 *now!*):

- Severe difficulty in breathing.
- Decreased level of consciousness or syncope.
- Grunting respirations.
- Wheezing after ingestion of medication, allergenic food, or bee sting:
  - Use prescribed anaphylactic kit as directed for known allergies.
- Blue lips, tongue, face, or ears.
- Pale or gray face with clammy skin.
- Drooling or inability to swallow.
- Apnea (give instructions for mouth-to-mouth breathing).
- Apnea for more than 15 seconds but is now breathing.
- Inability to speak or cry.
- Need for sitting position or leaning-forward position.

See immediately:

Triage nurse should advise using an ambulance when the child's current status is life-threatening or may deteriorate en route to hospital or when parental anxiety level is too high to safely drive child to closest ED.

- Difficulty in breathing not relieved by cleaning nose (younger than 12 months of age).
- Difficulty in breathing when not coughing (older than 12 months of age).
- Facial cyanosis during coughing spasms.
- Younger than 12 weeks of age with temperature greater than 100.4°F rectally.
- Temperature greater than 105°F.
- Choked on foreign body or small object.
- Severe chest pain.
- Retractions with moderate or minimal difficulty in breathing.
- Stridor unresponsive to 20 minutes of steam mist.
- Inability to bend neck forward.
- Wheezing heard from across the room.
- Tachypnea:
  - Respirations more than 60 per minute in infants younger than 12 months of age.
  - Respirations more than 40 per minute in children older than 12 months of age.
- Appearance is similar to that in previous instance when child was hospitalized for difficulty breathing.
- Peak flow less than 50% of the personal-best baseline.
- Asthma and wheezing not improved after normal home management.
- Child younger than 3 months.
- Parent or caregiver extremely anxious regarding this episode.
- Sounds very ill to triage nurse.
- Has risk factor along with any of the above.

See within 4 hours:

- Continuous or nonstop coughing, unresponsive to:
  - Home care advice for general cough.
  - Mist treatments for croup.
  - Two asthma treatments with nebulizer or inhaler.
- Stridor that responds to mist but has occurred three or more times in past 24 hours.

See within 12 to 24 hours:

- Younger than 4 weeks of age with a cough or symptoms of croup.
- Younger than 3 months of age with a cough for more than 3 days.
- Fever for more than 3 days (those less than 2 months of age should be seen immediately).
- Earache with or without discharge from the ear canal.
- Mild or unexplained wheezing.
- Yellow or green nasal drainage for more than 3 days.
- Sinus pressure or headache.
- Blood-tinged sputum.

- Coughing-induced chest pain.
- Coughing-induced vomiting on more than three occasions.
- Has missed more than 3 days of school.
- Severe sore throat.

Cross reference to other protocols:

- Fever, abdominal pain.

Home care advice:

- Increase intake of clear fluids:
  - For coughing spasms, encourage warmed, clear fluids (apple juice, tea, etc.).
- Older child can suck on hard candy or cough drops.
- Clean nose with warm water or saline nose drops or spray, and then use bulb syringe.
- Use humidifier or cool-mist vaporizer in bedroom.
- Encourage small, frequent feedings.
- Encourage proper use of asthma medications, allergy medications, etc.
- Avoid known triggers of asthma and allergies (tobacco smoke, animals, etc.).
- If coughing induces vomiting, reduce feeding amounts.
- Avoid active or passive smoking.
- Use cough suppressant at bedtime for severe coughs as approved by physician.
- For croup, sleep in same room as child for a few nights.
- For stridor, croup, respiratory distress, or severe coughing:
  - Breath warm mist from a steamy bathroom for 15 to 20 minutes.
  - Bundle child, and go out into the cold night air for 15 to 20 minutes.

Call back if:

- There are signs of respiratory distress.
- Breathing is not improved 20 minutes after use of asthma nebulizer or inhaler.
- Fever lasts for more than 3 days.
- Fever goes away for more than 24 hours and then returns.
- Nasal discharge lasts for more than 10 days.
- There is no improvement after warm-mist treatment or cold air treatment.
- The child looks or seems worse.
- The parent has increased concern, anxiety, or new questions.
- Any of the above-mentioned symptoms appear, if current symptoms change, or new symptoms develop.

From: Briggs, 1997; Schmidt, 1999.

C

Telephone Consultation Documentation Form

Patient's name ______________________ Date ______________

Date of birth ______________________ Time call received ______________

Telephone number ______________________ Time call returned ______________

Primary provider ______________________ Time call finished ______________

Gender: M F Weight: kg - lb ______________ Attempted callbacks ______________

Meds ______________________ Caller's name ______________

Allergies ______________________ Relationship ______________

PMH ______________________ Immunizations ______________

______________________ LNMP ______________

Presenting symptom or concern: ______________________

Nursing assessment: ______________________

Fever ________ Oral ____ Rectal ____ Axillary ____ Other ____________ Fluid intake: ________

Urine output: ____________ Vomiting : ____________ Diarrhea : ____________

HEENT: ______________________

Neurologic/activity level: ______________________

Chest/lungs/heart: ______________________

GI/GU: ______________________

Musculoskeletal: ______________________

Skin ______________________

Disposition: EMS (911) See immediately See within 4 hrs See within 12–24 hours Home care

Call referred to: Poison Control Center Mental Health Crisis Center

Protocol(s) used for assessment: ______________________

Protocol(s) used for home care advice: ______________________

Additional comments or advice: ______________________

Parent/caller verbalizes understanding of instructions given? Yes No

Parent/caller agrees with action taken? Yes No

Caller agrees to call back if symptoms worsen or caregiver concern increases? Yes No

Caller disagrees with advice given, caller preference is: ______________________

Signature: ______________________ RN NP MD

References

American Academy of Ambulatory Care Nursing. (1997) *Telephone nursing practice administration and practice standards*. Pitman, NJ: Jannetti, Inc.

Anders, G. (1997, February 4). Telephone triage: How nurses take calls and control the care of patients from afar. *The Wall Street Journal*.

Briggs, J. (1997). *Telephone triage protocols for nurses*. Philadelphia, PA: Lippincott.

Emergency Nurses Association (1998). Position statement. Telephone advice. Des Plaines, IL: Author.

Fulkner & Gary (1999). *Directory of medical call centers 2000*. New York, NY: Faulkner & Gray, Inc.

Marsden, J. (2000). *Telephone triage in an ophthalmic A & E department*. Philadelphia, PA: Whurr Publishers Ltd.

Schmitt, B. (1999). *Pediatric telephone advice*. Philadelphia, PA: Lippincott—Raven Publishers.

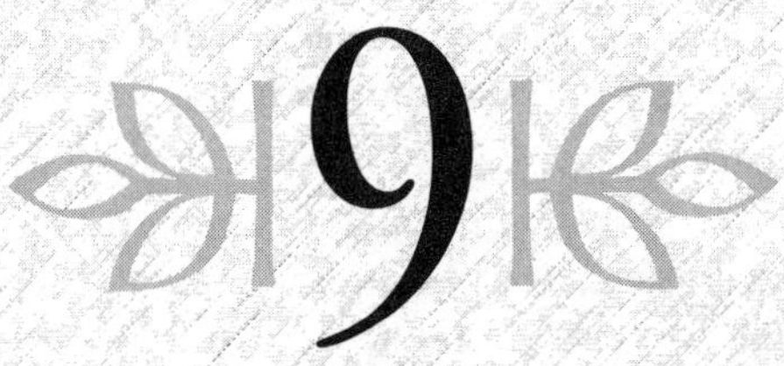

Children with Special Healthcare Needs

Elizabeth Wertz, RN, FACMPE

Introduction

As a result of the vast improvements in healthcare delivery and technology, children with congenital conditions or life-threatening illnesses and injuries survive to adulthood. These children are valuable members of their communities, but their health conditions pose life-long challenges that interfere with their growth and development.

Children with special health care needs are those who have or are at increased risk for a chronic physical, developmental, or emotional condition and who also require health and related services of a type or amount beyond that generally required by children (McPherson, 1998). These conditions include mental disabilities, physical disabilities, the need for technologic support, and chronic illnesses, of which there are approximately 200 (Wallace, Biehl, MacGreen, & Blackman, 1997) (Table 9.1). Although most of these conditions and disabilities are rare, others, such as asthma, respiratory ailments, and allergic reactions, are prevalent in the pediatric population. It is estimated that between 2 and 32% of children in the United States have some type of disability or chronic illness (Wallace et al., 1997). In 1988, it was estimated that 100,000 American children alone were dependent on medical technology (Wallace et al., 1997).

TABLE 9.1 Descriptions of Selected Special Healthcare Conditions

Body System	*Description*
Respiratory	*Congenital:* Laryngeal malacia; underdeveloped lungs; cystic fibrosis.
	Acquired: Pulmonary neoplasms; asthma; chronic bronchitis; bronchopulmonary dysplasia.
Cardiovascular	*Congenital:* Heart disease (Chapter 17).
	Acquired: Heart disease (Chapter 17).
Neurologic	*Congenital:* Spina bifida; Arnold-Chiari malformation; chromosomal anomalies; Dandy-Walker malformation; hydrocephalus.
	Perinatal: Infections; anoxic encephalopathy; birth trauma; cerebral palsy.
	Postnatal: Head and spinal cord trauma; neoplasms.
	Seizure disorders: Infantile spasms; Lennox-Gastaudt syndrome; epilepsy.
Immunologic	*Congenital:* Immune disorders.
	Acquired: Human immunodeficiency virus; hepatitis; carcinomas.
	Induced: Immunosuppression following solid organ or bone marrow transplants and chemotherapy for cancer treatment.
Mental retardation	*Physical appearance:* Well-proportioned physical features or characteristic features such as low-set ears, soft neurologic signs (e.g., microcephaly), poor fine and/or gross motor coordination.
	Cognitive function: Educable or needing assistance or total care.
Other	*Physical:* Limb deformities; craniofacial malformations; paralysis.
	Sensory: Alterations in hearing, vision, or tactile perceptabilities.
	Cognitive: Alterations in thinking abilities.

Adapted from Wertz, 2001a. The patient with special needs. In *The basic EMT-comprehensive prehospital patient care* (2nd ed., p. 770). St. Louis: Mosby—Year Book.

Children with special healthcare needs present to the emergency department (ED) for treatment related to their underlying health condition or for the usual childhood illnesses and injuries. The purposes of this chapter are to familiarize emergency nurses with the care of children with special healthcare needs and to recommend modifications in emergency nursing care for this patient population.

History

The history is obtained from the patient and parent as outlined in Chapter 6. Additional information is obtained related to the child's special healthcare needs (Wertz, 2001b):

- Ask the parent, "What is special about your child?" to promote trust and understanding. The question, "What is wrong with your child?" may create parental anger and resentment.
- Ascertain the child's communication patterns. Determine whether the child uses eye blinks, a communication board, sign language, or other nonverbal forms of communication. Learn and use the child's words for descriptions of pain, cold, and so forth.
- Ask the parent about the child's comprehension ability and what the child is able to do. This inquiry promotes self-esteem and a healthy self-image. Always assume that the child understands what is being said.
- Inquire as to dietary considerations that must be followed. For example, children on the ketogenic diet for severe seizures should receive intravenous fluid containing normal saline. Administration of dextrose will negate the ketosis and may potentiate breakthrough seizures.
- Encourage the parent to explain the child's medication regimen, because the medications and their dosages may be unfamiliar to emergency nurses. For example, children with cancer pain may receive very high doses of narcotics, and children with seizures may receive what appear to be inordinate doses of anticonvulsants.
- Elicit the child's and parent's assistance in explaining any technologic devices that accompany the child, such as a ventilator, gastrostomy tube, cardiopulmonary monitor, or central venous access device with "cycling" of total parenteral nutrition and lipids.

Assessment

Physical Assessment

The physical assessment of the child with special healthcare needs follows the same priorities as for all pediatric patients (Chapter 6), with a few exceptions:

- The neurologic (disability) assessment still refers to the child's neurologic status and not to the child's special needs or disabling condition.
- Determine the preexisting level of deficit prior to the ED visit: "Is this your child's usual behavior (or posture, color, etc.)?" This inquiry implies acceptance of the child's health condition and avoids the normal-abnormal dichotomy. Furthermore, by focusing on the child's ***abilities*** and not the ***disabilities***, the question helps to establish trust between the emergency nurse and parent.
- Seek parental assistance when removing braces or other adaptive devices while performing the physical assessment. Protect the devices carefully, because they usually are customized for the child and can be quite expensive. If the devices are removed, ensure that they leave the ED with the child and parent.
- Incorporate information about the technologic aid or device into the physical assessment. For example, state the condition of the tracheostomy site and the current ventilator settings.
- Note the presence of identifying jewelry, such as a Medic Alert™ bracelet or necklace. Older children may resist this identification, because they do not want to draw attention to their differences. Although the absence of such identification does not rule out a disability or chronic condition, its presence can be helpful during the physical assessment and subsequent treatment.

Psychosocial Assessment

The child's and family's coping strategies are assessed. Most families have positive coping strategies and have the emotional fortitude to care for their child. However, in cases where the child is in serious jeopardy or death is imminent, usual coping strategies may not be effective (Chapter 4). The following psychosocial considerations should be entertained (Schultz & Chalanick, 1998):

- Parents may experience an acute sense of anxiety during the ED visit.
- Parents may feel a loss of parental control. These families are familiar with their child's care and routines and may be at a loss in the ED when the staff intervene to treat the child. They may be concerned about staff being too assertive, which they may believe will adversely affect their child's ED treatment.
- Parents may perceive their child to be "vulnerable" and may overprotect the child.
- Family members may have an unrealistic perception or may fantasize about the child's health condition; they may have signs of grieving or chronic sorrow.

- Siblings of these children have psychosocial needs as well. Assessment of their roles and participation in family-centered care is important and should be done early in the treatment process.

Triage Decisions

Triage decisions for children with special healthcare needs should take into account the underlying condition because these children may be at a higher risk for developing complications than are children without these health conditions.

Nursing Interventions

Nursing interventions to promote comfort and security, such as addressing the child by name and offering praise and rewards, are outlined in Chapter 4 and are applied to children with special healthcare needs. Some nursing interventions may be modified based on the child's underlying health condition:

- Anticipate modifications in treatment based on the child's health condition. For example, the child with cerebral palsy typically may have profuse oral secretions that can interfere with airway maneuvers. Suction and high-concentration oxygen administration may be needed.
- Avoid cervical hyperextension in the child with Arnold-Chiari malformation because undue pressure may be placed on the brain stem and result in complications.
- Adapt equipment to meet the child's needs. For example, the child with cerebral palsy who has severe spinal curvatures may not be able to lie flat on a long backboard. Immobilization may be supplemented with padding from towel rolls or pillows. The child with physical disabilities, such as contractures or rigid body parts, may not be able to remain in a fixed position for procedures or treatments. The contractured limbs never should be forced into a particular position. Frequent rest periods may be necessary during lengthy procedures (Emergency Nurses Association, 1999).
- Use latex-free gloves and equipment. Many children with spina bifida have known latex allergies. Because not every child's latex allergy status is known, it is best to have latex-free gloves, at a minimum, in the ED.
- Limit exposure of the child's body with gowns and drapes as necessary. ED physicians and nurses may be tempted to show the child's disability to other staff members as a "learning experience." The child's modesty must be respected, and exposure or discussion of the child's disability should be limited to the rendered treatment.
- Ask the parent if he or she feels comfortable with performing procedures, such as tracheal suctioning, or if the emergency nurse can perform the procedures. At times, a homecare nurse or aid may accompany the child and family to the ED. Policies should be in place for determining the role of these nonhospital healthcare providers in the child's ED treatment.
- Initiate consultations with other healthcare professionals, such as pediatric emergency physicians and nurses, clinical nurse specialists, social services personnel, hospice workers, child life specialists, physical and occupational therapists, and nutritionists. Community organizations also provide family support. Families may be too proud to ask for assistance or may believe that they are not entitled to or cannot afford to use specialty services. Social services and community organizations can arrange for follow-up contacts and plans prior to discharge from the ED.

Home Care and Prevention

Children with special needs and their families should develop a written emergency care plan that is kept in easily accessible places in the children's home or other location where they frequently spend time (Emergency Medical Services for Children, National Task Force on Children with Special Health Care Needs, 1997). This emergency care plan should document any special training needed by emergency personnel, family members, and others who may be called on to provide emergency care to these children. Individuals and groups who should know about the emergency care plans are:

- Dispatchers for 911.
- Local emergency medical services agencies and fire departments.
- Education and health services of the children's school.
- ED, specialty, and primary care physicians.
- Family members.

To facilitate the emergency care of these children, it is recommended that a mechanism be available to identify the child with special healthcare needs when that child presents for emergency care (American College of Emergency Physicians, 1998). The child's special healthcare needs should be recorded, and this record should be accessible and usable (American College of Emergency Physicians, 1998). A standardized information form is available to prepare caregivers and healthcare professionals for emergencies in children with special healthcare needs.

Additionally, a discharge-planning guide that begins with the initial ED visit has been developed to assist in planning for children with special healthcare needs (Rushton & Witte, 1998). These guidelines are available from the Emergency Medical Services for Children National Resource Center at www.ems-c.org.

Conclusion

Emergency nurses are likely to encounter children with special health care needs. Table 9.2 offers guidelines for disability awareness. Written policies and procedures should be in place to facilitate the care of children with special healthcare needs. Collaboration with the child, family, and specialists throughout the ED treatment promotes family-centered care and expedites the child's return to the home environment.

TABLE 9.2 Guidelines for Disability Awareness

Use the word *disability* instead of the word *handicap*.

Refer first to the person and then to the particular disability.

Avoid calling a person *wheelchair bound* or saying that the person is *confined to a wheelchair*. In reality, people with disabilities are made more mobile by using a wheelchair.

Avoid using negative descriptions of people with disabilities, such as *invalid, mongoloid, epileptic, suffers from,* and *afflicted with*. Avoid referring to seizures as fits.

Do not use the "N" word—*normal*—when describing people without disabilities. Instead, use *typical* or *people without disabilities*.

Avoid making reference to a person's disability unless it is relevant.

Adapted from Coalition for Tennesseans with Disabilities, 1993. *Talking about disability: A guide to using appropriate language*. Nashville, TN: Author.

References

American College of Emergency Physicians. (1998). Emergency information form for children with special healthcare needs. Dallas, TX: Author.

Emergency Medical Services for Children, National Task Force on Children with Special Health Care Needs (1997). EMS for Children: Recommendations for coordinating care for children with special health care needs. *Annals of Emergency Medicine,* 30:274-280.

Emergency Nurses Association. (1999). Latex allergy. Des Plaines, IL: Author.

McPherson, M. (1998). A new definition of children with special healthcare needs. *Pediatrics, 102*(1), 137-139.

Rushton, D., & Witte, M. (1998). *Children with special healthcare needs—Technology-assisted children*. Salt Lake City, UT: Utah Department of Health, Bureau of Emergency Medical Services, Primary Children's Medical Center.

Schultz, A., & Chalanick, K. (1998). Children with special needs. In T. Soud & J. Rogers (Eds.), *Manual of pediatric emergency nursing* (pp. 712-726). St. Louis: Mosby—Year Book.

Wallace, H., Biehl, R., MacQueen, J., & Blackman, J. (1997). *Mosby's resource guide to children with disabilities and chronic illness*. St. Louis: Mosby—Year Book.

Wertz, E. (2001a). *The basic EMT—Comprehensive prehospital patient care* (2nd ed.). St. Louis: Mosby—Year Book.

Wertz, E. (2001b). *Emergency care for children*. Albany, NY: Delmar Thomson Publishing.

10

Transport

Reneé Semonin Holleran, RN, PhD, CEN, CCRN, CFRN

Introduction

The care of the ill or injured pediatric patient requires specialized skills and equipment. This care often extends beyond the emergency department (ED) to the operating room, intensive care unit, and other inpatient units. When the personnel and technology needed to afford the child with the best care possible are not available, transfer to another facility may be required.

Transfer of the pediatric patient began at the turn of the century, but much of the development of neonatal and pediatric transport did not occur until the 1960s. Discussion continues today concerning who is best suited to transfer the critically ill or injured pediatric patient. Table 10.1 highlights the important milestones in pediatric transport.

ENA has developed a position statement regarding care of the pediatric patient during interfacility transfer (ENA, 1996). ENA believes that:

- The goal of pediatric interfacility transfer is to decrease morbidity and mortality and improve patient outcomes.
- The composition of the transfer team and the mode of transport must be based on patient acuity, established and anticipated treatment needs, and special patient circumstances.
- Persons involved in the transport of the pediatric patient must have the knowledge and expertise to deliver the appropriate level of care to patients with a variety of illnesses and injuries. The configuration of the team caring for the critically ill or injured child must include a registered professional nurse with pediatric emergency or pediatric critical care expertise.
- The transfer team involved in the transport of the critical pediatric patient must complete a minimum of six hours of continuing education related to pediatric emergency and/or critical care on a yearly basis, maintain verification in the Emergency Nursing Pediatric Course, and complete a yearly age-specific competency evaluation.

TABLE 10.1 History of Pediatric Transport

Year	Event
1900	Newborns were transferred to Chicago Lying-in Hospital by ambulance.
1934	The first dedicated neonatal transport vehicle was in use in Chicago.
1960s	Children's Hospital in Denver developed neonatal regionalization, and ill newborns were transferred to specific hospitals to be cared for.
1960s	A transport incubator was developed. It was used in all modes of neonatal transport, including air and ground.
1970	Stanford University Hospital added an air medical component to their neonatal transport team.
1970s	Children's Hospital in Columbus, Ohio, reported the use of National Guard helicopters to transport critically ill and injured pediatric patients to their institution.
1980	Regional critical care for the pediatric patient began to emerge. Many pediatric centers developed critical care transport teams.

Data from: Carter, Couch, & O'Brien, 1988; Hackel, 1995.

- The appropriate equipment must be available to accommodate all pediatric patients regardless of age, weight, size, and acuity level.
- Transfer arrangements must consider family needs.

The purposes of this chapter are to discuss the personnel, skills, and equipment needed to transfer the pediatric patient and to review the indications for transport.

Indications for Transport

The indications for pediatric transport have been developed by consensus from pediatric experts and from other transport and critical care associations, such as the American College of Surgeons and the National Association of Emergency Medical Services (American Academy of Pediatrics, 1999). These indicators include:

- Serious injury to more than one system.
- Head injury involving the following:
  - Cerebro spinal fluid leak.
  - Altered mental status.
  - Deteriorating neurologic status.
  - Signs and symptoms of increasing intracranial pressure.
- Hypovolemic shock:
  - Requiring more than one transfusion.
  - Requiring operative management to stop the hemorrhage.
- Spinal cord injuries.
- Blunt abdominal trauma with hemodynamic instability.
- Thoracic injuries requiring advanced ventilatory support.
- Orthopedic injuries involving:
  - Two or more long-bone fractures.
  - Fractures of the thoracic cage.
  - Compromised neurovascular status.
  - Fracture of the axial skeleton.
  - Fractures that may require extensive rehabilitation.
- Extremity reimplantation.
- Respiratory distress:
  - Airway obstruction.
  - Respiratory failure.
  - Foreign-body aspiration.
- Septic shock.
- Status epilepticus.
- Multiple-organ failure.
- Near-drowning.
- Arrhythmia/dysrhythmia with impending hemodynamic implications.
- Burns.
- Specialty referrals:
  - Cardiology: Congenital anomalies requiring surgery.
  - Hematology: Need for a bone marrow transplant.
  - Oncology: Need for a pediatric oncologist.
  - Nephrology. Need for consultation for renal injury or disease.
  - Pulmonology: Need for specialized ventilation.
  - Specialized surgical procedures: Transplant.

Legal Implications

Comprehensive Omnibus Reconciliation Act (COBRA) and Emergency Medical Treatment and Active Labor Act (EMTALA) (Williams & Johnson, 1995; McCleary, 1997) (Chapter 2)

- Hospitals must examine all children who present to the ED and provide the necessary care for stabilization.
- Patients are not to be transferred until they have been assessed and stabilized.
- Patients should be transferred in a vehicle and with personnel comparable to the level of care that they require. Pediatric patients should be transported with personnel trained in the care of the ill or injured pediatric patient.

State and local regulations

- Regulations will vary among states and local areas.
- The referring facility and the transport team must be aware of regulations in different areas and adhere to these regulations.

Consent (Chapter 2)

- If possible, parental consent should be sought before the child is transported.
- The name of the receiving facility, and the person accepting for the facility, the method of transport, and the name of the team providing transport must be included on the consent form.
- A written order for the transport must be obtained from the physician.

Licensure

- Transport team members must be appropriately licensed and certified for their area of practice.
- Most transport team members are functioning members of the hospital in which they are based.
- State licensing may not be required, particularly because there are no federal regulations (other than for ambulances, but not specific to critical care or pediatric transport). The Commission for Accreditation of Medical Transport Systems (1999) offers a guideline for standards related to critical care transport by both air and ground for both pediatric and neonatal transport.

Transfer agreements

- Transfer agreements between facilities should be written.
- Agreements should reflect the levels of responsibility during the transport process.
- Agreements should reflect the local and state regulations that govern the transport process.

Specifications for Pediatric Transport

Team composition

- Registered nurse.
- Neonatal nurse practitioner.
- Neonatologist.
- Pediatrician.
- Respiratory therapist.

Essential Training for Transport (American Academy of Pediatrics, 1999)

- How a transport is initiated, including legal implications, transfer agreements, and receiving institutions.
- Communication skills, team interactions, referring-receiving facility personnel interactions.
- Communication equipment use (e.g., radios, cellular telephones).
- Public relations skills.
- Transport equipment and medications.
- Transport safety.
- Transport regulations.
- Patient care issues in the transport environment.
- Altitude physiology.
- Management of motion sickness:
  - Medications, ginger root.
  - Patient and crew positioning within the transport vehicle.
- Pediatric transport medicine.
- Advanced pediatric management skills including airway, breathing, circulation, and neurologic interventions.

Equipment for Pediatric Transport

See Table 10.2 for a summary of equipment.

TABLE 10.2 Equipment for Pediatric Transport

Airway and ventilation equipment

- Ambu bag (infant, child, and adult). (Include appropriate-sized masks for each age group.)
- Anesthesia bag.
- Oxygen masks in various sizes.
- Nasal cannula (infant, child, and adult).
- Intubation equipment for infant, child, and adult.
- Endotracheal tubes.
  - Uncuffed: 2.5 to 6.5
  - Cuffed: 6.0 to 8.0
- Magill forceps (pediatric and adult).
- Stylets.
- Tonsil suctions.
- Suction catheters (sizes 5/6, 8, 10, and 14).
- Oral airways.
- Cricothyrotomy trays.
- Tracheostomy tubes.
- Portable suction unit.
- Pulse oximeter with appropriate-sized probes.
- CO_2 detector/monitor.
- Benzoin, adhesive tape, and tracheostomy tape.
- Medications for intubation:
  - Sedation agents.
  - Neuromuscular blocking agents.
  - Lidocaine.
- Transport ventilator.
- Needle/chest decompression equipment, including chest tubes:
  - Heimlich valves.
  - 10 to 40 French chest tubes.

TABLE 10.2 (continued)

Circulatory equipment

- Cardiac monitor.
- Defibrillator (pediatric paddles).
- External pacer.
- Thoracostomy tray.
- Blood pressure monitor (various-sized cuffs).
- Umbilical catheters (3.5 and 5.0 French).

Nasogastric tubes

- Feeding tubes (5 to 8 French).
- Salem sumps (10 to 18 French).
- Syringes.

Intravenous equipment and medications

- Intravenous catheters (24 to 14 gauge).
- Conversion kits (7 French).
- Blood administration tubing.
- Stopcocks.
- Minidrippers.
- Syringes.
- Intraosseous needles.
- Extension tubing.
- Intravenous pumps and monitors.
- Pressure bags.
- O-negative blood.
- Blood cooler.
- Blood tubes.
- Intravenous starter packs.
- Advanced Cardiac Life Support/Pediatric Advanced Life Support medications.
- Vasopressor agents per protocols.
- Mannitol.
- Other medications as directed by protocols.

Additional equipment

- Transport isolette.
- Universal precaution equipment.
- Survival pack.
- Instant camera and film.
- Maps to the receiving facility.
- Measuring tapes.
- Drug and equipment calculation cards.
- Car seat.
- Pediatric transport board.
- Cervical collars.
- Soft restraints.
- Warming equipment.

Preparation for Transfer and Transport

- Identify the need for transport as listed in the section on indications, based on:
  - The child's illness or injury.
  - The need for additional interventions.
  - The request of the family.
- Contact the referring facility:
  - Determine bed availability.
  - Evaluate whether the necessary equipment and staff are available to care for the patient.
  - Identify the receiving physician and the person accepting the patient on behalf of the hospital (e.g., nursing supervisor).
- Designate the mode of transportation to be used for transport, based on:
  - The condition of the child.
  - The distance of the transport.
  - The weather and road conditions.
- Provide the initial care for the child, based on the referring facility's abilities:
  - Manage the child's airway, breathing, and circulation.
  - Obtain requested laboratory or other diagnostic tests.
  - Administer medications as indicated by the child's illness or injury.
  - Perform interventions to prevent further injury.
- Notify the child's family. The family needs the following information (Fultz, McKee, Zalaznik, & Kidd, 1993; Lewis, Holditch-Dorist, & Brunssen, 1997; Fultz, 1999):
  - Why the child has to be transported.
  - The mode of transportation and estimated time for transport.
  - Who will care for the child during transport.
  - Policy on who can accompany the child during transport. Allow the family to see the child before transfer, if possible, especially if the family will not be permitted to accompany the child during transport.
  - Reassurance of the safety of transport. Never promise the family that they may accompany the child during transport.
  - Directions to the referring hospital.
  - Where the child will be in the referring hospital and who will be caring for the child.
  - Insurance information.

Preparation of the Child for Transport

- Explain to the child what is happening and where he or she will be going.
- Secure any lines, tubes, or dressings after ensuring that they are patent.
- Remove any wet clothing and cover the patient with dry, warm blankets.
- Immobilize as indicated by the child's condition.
- Maintain cervical immobilization during transport of the injured child.
- Consider the use of soft restraints for safety. The smaller child may be secured on a papoose board.
- Consider sedation if the child's neurologic status is intact.
- Allow the child to keep security objects, such as a stuffed animal, pacifier, or blanket.
    - Administer medications as indicated by the child's illness or injury.
    - Assess security of tubes and patient equipment.
- Provide medication for sedation and pain management (Chapter 13).
- Keep the child warm:
    - Wrap the child in a transfer blanket.
    - Turn on vehicle heat.
    - Wrap the child's head for heat conservation, if appropriate.
- Establish communication:
    - Bring all transfer documents with the child.
    - Request that the referring facility provide a report to the receiving facility.
    - Provide an adequate report to the receiving facility on arrival.

Care during Transport

- Ensure safety:
    - Secure the child in the age-appropriate transport device.
    - Appropriately restrain all equipment and personnel.
    - Position the transport team for optimal safe patient care.
- Provide continuous assessment and management of the child's airway, breathing, and circulation:
    - Monitor vital signs.
    - Maintain tube placement.
    - Monitor effectiveness of ventilation.
    - Monitor patency of intravenous lines.

Conclusion

The transfer and transport of the ill or injured child requires that the appropriate personnel and vehicle be used. Personnel should be competent in providing emergent care for any emergency they may encounter during transport. The transport vehicle has to be outfitted with equipment that is essential to the care of the ill or injured pediatric patient, including equipment to maintain airway, breathing, and circulation.

The family is an important part of the care of the pediatric patient and should be included in the transport process when possible or, at a minimum, be provided with information to make their journey to the receiving facility as easy as possible. Transfer and transport of the pediatric patient should be a life-saving, not a life-threatening, process.

References

American Academy of Pediatrics. (1999). *Guidelines for air and ground transport of neonatal and pediatric patients.* Elk Grove Village, IL: Author.

Carter, G., Couch, R., & O'Brien, M. (1988). The evolution of air transport systems: A pictorial review. *Journal of Emergency Medicine*, 6: 499-504.

Commission on Accreditation of Medical Transport Systems. (1999.) *Guidelines for air medical transport systems.* Anderson, SC: Author.

Emergency Nurses Association. (1996). Position statement. Care of the pediatric patient during interfacility transfer DesPlaines, IL: Author.

Fultz, J. (1999). Tips for helping families of patients transported by helicopter. *Journal of Emergency Nursing, 25*(2): 132-134.

Fultz, J., McKee, J., Zalaznik, F., & Kidd, P. (1993, November/December). Air medical transport: What the family wants to know. *Air Medical Journal*, pp. 431-435.

Hackel, A. (1995). History of medical transport systems: Air, ground, and pediatric. In K. McCloskey & R. Orr (Eds.), *Pediatric transport medicine* (pp. 5-14). St. Louis: Mosby—Year Book.

Lewis, M., Holditch-Davis, D., & Brunssen, S. (1997). Parents as passengers during pediatric transport. *Air Medical Journal, 16*(2): 38-43.

McCleary, N. (1997). Air medical transfers: Are you COBRA compliant? *Air Medical Journal, 16*(4): 113-116.

Williams, M., & Johnson, K. (1995). Transport regulations. In K. McCloskey & R. Orr (Eds.), *Pediatric transport medicine* (pp. 15-32). St. Louis: Mosby—Year Book.

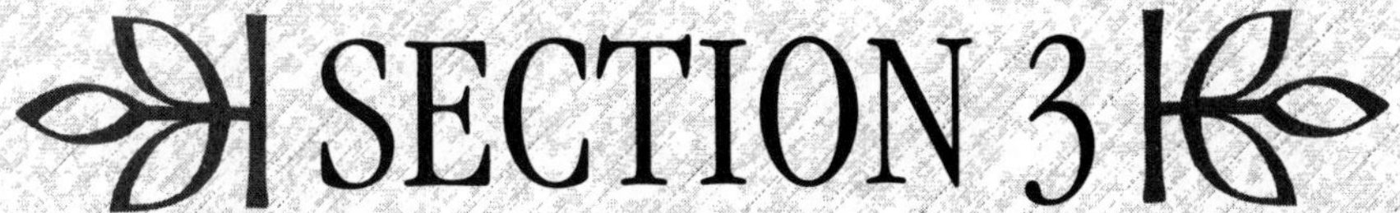

Special Problems

11

Neonatal Emergencies

Tracy Karp, RNC, MS, NNP

Introduction

While most neonates are born in organized perinatal service settings, some are born at home or in the emergency department (ED). Those born at home or in the ED may require more care than can be provided in their birth setting (Burchfield, 1997). Changes in healthcare insurance and reimbursement have resulted in earlier discharge of neonates from their birth settings before serious or life-threatening health conditions are detected. In addition, advances in neonatal intensive care therapies save the lives of many premature neonates and infants, many of whom are discharged home with complex health needs. For these reasons, neonates and premature infants are presenting to EDs in significant numbers. Therefore, emergency nurses must be prepared for delivery, resuscitation, and transfer and transport of these newborns.

Standardized courses, such as the Neonatal Resuscitation Program, provide education on the delivery and resuscitation of the neonate. Chapter 14 reviews principles of neonatal resuscitation. The purpose of this chapter is to discuss the assessment and treatment of selected neonatal conditions.

In general, the neonatal ED patient is one who presents within the period of time from birth to 28 days of age. Because of advances in neonatal intensive care, many neonatal patients may still be premature or have a postnatal age greater than 28 days. Emergency department nurses must be aware of the definitions that describe infants, depending on the factors that include chronologic age as well as gestational age. These definitions are listed in Table 11.1.

Embryologic Development

From conception to birth, dramatic developmental and physiologic changes take place in the fetus and neonate. A brief review of embryology of the newborn is provided in Table 11.2 (Moore & Persaud, 1993b).

Neonatal Considerations

Physiologic Transitions

At birth, the neonate continues to undergo dramatic physiologic transitions.

Respiratory transitions

The organ of respiration changes from the placenta to the lungs:

- Effective respirations must be established.
- Lung liquid must be replaced by air.

TABLE 11.1 Common Definitions of Neonatal Terminology

Term	*Definition*
Neonate	Infants from birth to 28 days.
Neonatal period	Postconceptual age of 42 to 46 weeks.
Term infants	Those born at 38 to 42 weeks' gestation.
Premature infants	Those born before 38 weeks' gestation.
Corrected age	Amount of time postdelivery added to birth age. For example, a neonate presents to the ED 4 weeks' postdelivery. The neonate was born at 32 weeks' gestation. The neonate's corrected age is 36 weeks. The infant is not as well developed as a term infant of 4 weeks and may appear and act like an infant of 36 weeks' gestation.

Data from: Flaherty, 1996; O'Toole, 1992.

TABLE 11.2 An Embryology Primer

Week of Gestation	*Development*
12 Weeks	Basic systems are formed, but fetus is not capable of survival. Heart is beating by day 22; all chambers and vessels are completely formed by day 50. Lungs resemble exocrine gland, but most structures are present except air exchange units. Major organs in the gastrointestinal system are formed. Intestines have herniated out and returned. Anus is patent. Brain and spinal cord are formed. Interim kidneys are formed and urine is produced.
24 Weeks	Basic systems are refined and remodeled. With specialized care, infant could survive at 24 weeks. Growth of the cardiac system continues, and vascular shunts develop. Primitive air exchange units are developed in the lungs. Surfactant may be present, but in limited amounts. However, surfactant production can be induced. Pulmonary capillaries begin to grow closer to saccule. Maturation of organ in the gastrointestinal system with elongation of intestines occurs. Some enzymes are present. Central nervous system is active and responsive; brain is fragile, especially to bleeding. Permanent kidneys are formed; urine is produced, which is majority of amniotic fluid. Poor ability to concentrate or dilute urine.
Term	Basic systems are refined and functional, but some are still immature. Heart has right-sided hypertrophy and vascular shunts. Full complement of airways; primitive alveoli limited in number (one-eighth of the eventual total). Surfactant system is functional; good network of pulmonary capillaries. Gastrointestinal system is functional and full of meconium (intestinal and amniotic debris and bile). Central nervous system is mature and less susceptible to bleeding. Kidneys continue to produce urine, but still with limited function.

Data from: Moore & Persaud, 1993b.

- Surfactant, a combination of phospholipids and proteins that lower surface tension, must be present in sufficient quantities at the air-liquid interface.

Circulatory transitions

Circulation must convert from the fetal parallel pathways to the postnatal series pathway (Moore & Persaud, 1993a):

- When respirations begin, pulmonary blood flow increases because of the rapid drop in pulmonary vascular resistance.
- Systemic vascular resistance dramatically increases with loss (clamping) of the low-resistance placenta.
- The fetal shunts of the ductus venous, ductus arteriosus, and foramen ovale functionally close, converting blood flow across these shunts from right to left to none or left to right.
- Cardiac output goes from right ventricular predominance to equal output. Although the neonatal heart has a limited ability to increase output in response to stress (Lott, 1998), it can increase cardiac output, predominantly by an increase in heart rate.

Thermoregulatory transitions

The neonate transitions from the relatively stable temperature of the womb to the cooler external environment.

Nutritional transitions

Neonates transition from the relatively stable and supportive nutritional and fluid intake provided by the placenta to the need to "go it on their own."

Anatomic and Physiologic Differences

Just as children are not small adults, neonates are not just small children (Flaherty, 1996). The following anatomic and physiologic differences in neonatal body systems have an impact on ED nursing care.

Respiratory system

The neonate has only 24 to 50 million alveoli, while the adult has 300 to 400 million (Burke, 1998). When oxygen requirements increase because of illness or cold stress, the neonate has a limited ability to increase gas exchange, and hypoxia can rapidly develop. Even minor illnesses that place demand on the respiratory system can produce respiratory distress in the neonate.

Cardiovascular system

The neonate has a limited ability to increase stroke volume during cardiovascular compromise because the heart of the neonate has limited compliance. To maintain cardiac output, the neonate relies mostly on an increase in the heart rate. Bradycardia is an emergent sign in a neonate, because it indicates an inability to compensate, as cardiac output is rate dependent.

Fluids and electrolytes

Neonates have proportionately more total body water and extracellular fluid than do adults. Total body water is approximately 75% in the neonate and 60 to 70% in the adult (Hazinski, 1999). Extracellular fluid constitutes up to 40% of the of the total body water in the newborn but 20% of the total body water in the adult (Wong, 1999). Neonates can lose bodily fluids more rapidly from normal processes, such as insensible and renal losses, as well as from vomiting and diarrhea. The infant also has limited glucose stores, which can easily be depleted with cold stress or infection.

Immune system

The neonate, especially the premature infant, has an immature immune system. All three levels of the neonatal immune system are at a disadvantage in fighting infection (Flaherty, 1996). At the first level of protection, physical barriers such as the skin are much thinner. The mucous membrane junctions are looser, allowing larger molecules and larger pathogens to cross. Chemical barriers, such as tears, are not produced in sufficient quantity to adequately fight infection. Deficiency in immunoglobulin and polymorphonuclear leukocyte stores and lack of previous exposure to antigens increase the neonate's susceptibility to infection (Burke, 1998). An inability to localize infections makes neonates harder to assess because they may have few signs and symptoms.

Thermoregulatory system

Neonates have a limited ability to make or conserve heat, putting them at a higher risk for cold stress than other age groups (Perlstein, 1997). Keeping the infant warm must be a high priority. Heat loss is facilitated by a high surface-to-mass ratio and reduced ability to regulate skin flow. The head is the largest source of heat loss. Vasoconstriction shunts blood to the core, leading to reduced peripheral perfusion. Once vasoconstriction is reversed, large amounts of acid may enter the central circulation. Adverse effects of cold stress are multisystemic but lead to metabolic acidosis because of the burning of brown fat (Karlsen, 2000).

Heat by-production is limited. Shivering is an ineffective heat-producing mechanism in the neonate. Neonates and premature infants respond to cold by burning brown fat to generate heat. The hypothermic infant releases norepinephrine, which increases the metabolic rate, making the infant susceptible to hypoxia, hypoglycemia, and metabolic acidosis.

Gastrointestinal system

Most of the metabolic functions of the fetal liver are performed by the maternal placenta, which conjugates most of the fetal bilirubin (Flaherty, 1996). The neonatal liver is immature and cannot efficiently conjugate bilirubin. During the first several days of life, the increased by-production of bilirubin from the normal hemolysis of red blood cells can overwhelm the liver's ability to excrete bilirubin, resulting in physiologic jaundice (Burke, 1998).

The neonate also has a relaxed lower esophageal sphincter and rapid peristalsis, which result in frequent "spitting up." Variation in stool pattern is common. Almost all neonates pass their first stool by 24 hours of age.

Vital signs

In neonates, the temperature should be obtained by axillary or rectal measurement. Tympanic temperatures are not reliable because correct placement in the ear canal is difficult. It is important to obtain an accurate temperature, because neonates may have infections without fever, but the neonate with a fever generally has an infection of greater severity than an older child with the same temperature (Chapter 12). This is because a higher level of Interleukin 1 is needed to "flip the switch" on the hypothalamus and cause a fever (Flaherty, 1996).

Resting heart rate and respiratory rate are most meaningful in the neonate. Blood pressure is not a reliable indicator of serious illness because it varies with age and activity. Low blood pressure is a late sign of compromised circulation in neonates.

Special Equipment

Proper equipment is necessary to care for the neonate in the ED. This equipment includes:

- Heating sources (usually radiant) with a temperature feedback control device and warm blankets.
- Manual ventilation devices with both preterm and term-sized masks and endotracheal tubes.
- Medications (Chapter 14).
- Intravenous access devices: umbilical catheters (3.5 to 5 French) and small-gauge (22 to 24) intravenous catheters.

Focused History

The care and assessment of the neonate are guided by the history (Carey, 1996).

Birth history

- Maternal history (Chapter 14).
- The maternal history provides many clues to neonatal illness (Cloherty Scott, Feinberg, & Reke, 1998).

Table 11.3 discusses maternal disorders and the resultant fetal and neonatal effects.

TABLE 11.3 Maternal Disorders and Fetal/Neonatal Effects

Disorder	*Fetal/Neonatal Effects*
Antepartum period	
Liver disease	Preterm birth
Congenital heart disease	Small for gestational age
Diabetes mellitus	Large for gestational age
Hypertension	Small for gestational age
Immune thrombocytopenia	Thrombocytopenia; bleeding
Pregnancy-induced hypertension	Small for gestational age
Renal disease	Small for gestational age
Sickle cell anemia	Small for gestational age
Systemic lupus erythematosus	Heart block; bone marrow depression
Graves' disease	Thyrotoxicosis; congestive heart failure
Obesity	Large for gestational age; hypoglycemia
Infections:	
▪ Viral	Preterm birth; hepatic, hematologic, and birth defects
▪ Bacterial	As above; pneumonia (especially Group B beta-hemolytic *streptococci* and *E. coli*)
Intrapartum period	
Preterm contractions	Preterm birth
Prolonged rupture of membranes (> 18 hours prior to birth)	Infection
Bleeding	Asphyxia
Rapid delivery	Asphyxia; trauma
Fever	Infection
Meconium-stained amniotic fluid	Asphyxia
Multiple births	Asphyxia; trauma

Data from: Cloherty et al., 1998.

Delivery and immediately postpartum history

- Apgar score (Chapter 14).
- Other indicators of distress, such as meconium staining or abnormal fetal heart tones.
- Gestational age at birth.
- Congenital anomalies, conditions, or illnesses.
- Surgical procedures performed on the neonate.

Risk factors for being ill at birth or in the neonatal period (Behrman & Shiono, 1997)

- Being preterm or postterm.
- Having a birth weight of less than 2.5 kg or more than 4.0 kg.
- Being large or small for gestational age.
- The need for resuscitation at birth.
- Maternal infection, illness, lack of prenatal care, or social issues.
- Multiple gestation or short period between pregnancies.
- Obstetric complication requiring cesarean section birth.
- Congenital malformations.
- A history of fetal problems.
- Home oxygen and percent administered (may be less than 1 L)
- Maternal age. Younger (< 15 years) or older (> 40 years) mothers have an increased risk for problems.

Behavioral history

- Changes in feeding behavior, such as decreased intake or vomiting.
- Changes in activity, such as lethargy, irritability, or both.

Sibling history

- Fetal death.
- Neonatal illnesses, such as infection, respiratory distress syndrome, and hyperbilirubinemia.
- Inherited disorders, such as bleeding.

Paternal history

- Inherited disorders.
- Congenital syndromes or anomalies.

Focused Assessment

Physical Assessment

For many infants who are born at home, the first examination of life may be in the emergency department. The focused nursing assessment for the neonate is described in Chapter 14. Considerations in the assessment of the neonate include:

- Keep the infant warm during the examination.
- Auscultate before palpating. (This is true for examinations of any patient.)
- Redress the infant after the examination to prevent hypothermia.

After the initial examination of airway, breathing, and circulation, the examination should be systematic from head to toe. Because the patient cannot verbalize complaints, observation of signs and symptoms is one of the most important assessment tools. Table 11.4 provides observation guidelines for the physical assessment of the neonate.

Other considerations in the head-to-toe assessment of the neonate include:

- Auscultation:
  - Heart and breath sounds are usually more rapid and difficult to hear.

TABLE 11.4
Observation Guidelines for Physical Assessment

To Assess	*Observe*
Distress	Facial expression; respiratory effort; activity; tone
Color	Tongue; mucous membranes (centrally pink vs. cyanotic); nailbeds; hands; feet (peripherally pink vs. cyanotic); skin (jaundice, pallor, ruddiness, mottling); perfusion, meconium staining
Nutritional status	Subcutaneous fat; muscle mass
Hydration status	Skin turgor; anterior fontanelle
Neurologic status	Posture; tone; activity; response to stimuli; cry; state; state transition; reflexes
Respiratory/chest	Respiratory rate and effort, retractions; nasal flaring; grunting; audible stridor or wheezing; chest shape; nipples (number and position); skin color.
Cardiovascular status	Precordial activity; visible point of maximal intensity; skin perfusion and color
Abdomen	Size full (distended, taut, shiny); shape (round, concave); distension (generalized or localized); visible peristaltic waves; visible bowel loops; muscular development/tone; umbilical cord; umbilical vessels; drainage from cord; periumbilical erythema
Head	Size, shape, anterior fontanel, hair distribution, and condition
Eyes and ears	Shape; position; external auditory canal; response to sound
Nose	Shape; nares; flaring; nasal bridge
Mouth	Shape; symmetry; movement; philtrum; tongue; palate; natal teeth; gums; jaw size
Neck	Shape; range of motion; webbing
Genitalia (male)	Scrotum; descent of testes; rugae; inguinal canals; foreskin; penile size; urine stream; meatus; perineum; anus; color (hyperpigmented)
Genitalia (female)	Labia majora; labia minora; clitoris; vagina; perineum; inguinal canals; anus
Skin	Color; texture; firmness; vernix caseosa; masses; lanugo; lesions (pigmented, vascular, trauma-related infections)
Extremities	Posture; range of motion (involuntary movement); digits; palmar creases; soles of feet; nails

From: Honeyfield, 1996. Principles of physical assessment. In E. P. & M. E. Honeyfield (Eds.), *Physical assessment of the newborn* (2nd ed., p. 2). Petaluma, CA: NICU. Used with permission.

TABLE 11.5 Gestational Age and Risk Assessment

Gestational Age and Description	*Risks to Infant*
Term infant: Developmentally mature; can maintain nutrition and thermoregulation. Requires limited observation period.	At risk for delayed disorders of transition, infection, or congenital anomalies or conditions not diagnosed at early discharge.
Preterm infants: 35–37 weeks' gestation May have had only short hospitalization until they demonstrated maturity. Look and act like term infant.	At risk for the same problems as term infants, but have limited reserve and so, when stressed by environment or illness, can decompensate easily.
Preterm infants: Less than 35 weeks' gestation Usually have varied length of initial hospitalization.	In addition to above, at risk of reoccurrence or exacerbation of any illness or condition. Especially sensitive to infection, fluid imbalances, and alterations in respiratory control.

- Soft murmurs are common (in about 50% of neonates) in the first 48 hours of life. The murmurs are usually systolic ejection (flow across a pulmonary valve) or continuous systolic (closing ductus arteriosus) (Vargo, 1996).

- Palpation:
  - Make sure your fingers are warm.
  - Assess fontanelle and pulses when the infant is in a quiet state.
  - Save deep palpation (liver, masses) for last. The legs of the neonate may have to be flexed at the knees to relax abdominal muscles. The normal liver may be 2 cm below the right costal margin.
  - Percussion is of limited value, because it is difficult to localize sounds.
- Gestational age assessment. Gestational age assessment is the process of estimating the postconceptual age of the infant. It provides risk assessment and anticipatory guidance for care needs. The gestational age should be assessed for all newly born infants within the first few hours of life. The parents should be asked about the gestational age of other neonates. Table 11.5 compares gestational age and risks to the infant. There are three general groups:
  - Preterm: less than 37 weeks' completed gestation.
  - Term: 38 to 42 weeks' gestation.
  - Postterm: greater than 42 weeks' gestation.

Several methods for evaluating gestational age are available; however, this evaluation is generally not performed in the ED.

Psychosocial Assessment

Parents of neonates are almost always nervous, especially if this child is their first. Even a minor illness can cause great concern. The nurse needs to assess the family's support system as well as the parent–infant interaction to identify any high-risk social situations that may have an impact on the infant's health. Parents who have poor attachment behaviors will limit contact and communication with the infant and not respond to his or her cry. Social services or other support systems may be necessary to help the family.

Nursing Diagnoses

- Actual or potential infection, related to immature immune system.
- Risk for altered body temperature (hypothermia), related to immature thermoregulation.
- Altered tissue perfusion (cardiopulmonary, cerebral, renal, gastrointestinal, and peripheral), related to infection, hypothermia, or shock.

Expected Outcomes

- The potential for infection will be minimized by preventing exposure of the neonate to other ED patients. Existing infection will be recognized and treated promptly.
- Body temperature will be maintained by using a radiant warmer, keeping the infant covered as much as possible, and preventing heat loss.
- Tissue perfusion will be restored to normal by proper treatment of underlying condition.

Interventions to support the family

- Explain all procedures and the rationale for the treatments.
- Allow the family to ask questions.
- Reassure the family that everything possible is being done.
- If the mother is breast-feeding, make sure that a breast pump is provided if she is unable to feed the baby. She should pump as often as she was nursing.
- Evaluate the need for and provide necessary referrals to outside agencies.

Triage Decisions

Emergent

- Signs and symptoms of sepsis (see the following discussion on neonatal sepsis).
- Cyanosis.
- Respiratory distress (grunting, rapid respirations, gasping).
- Inconsolable crying with other symptoms, such as bloody stool.
- Fever or decreased temperature.
- Preexisting congenital condition (cardiac or respiratory).
- Total body jaundice; abnormal neurologic examination.
- Vomiting bile (suspect volvulus (Chapter 19) until proven otherwise).

Urgent

- Crying, but consolable.
- Awake, alert, and taking fluids.
- Younger than 72 hours old; examination normal but jaundice to lower body.

Nonurgent

- Neonatal complaints are rarely classified as nonurgent, because complaints are usually nonspecific with few symptoms and an examination must be done to rule out any serious condition.

Nursing Interventions

As with all patients, initial interventions are focused on the airway, breathing, and circulation. It may be difficult to determine if cyanosis in an infant is caused by a respiratory or a cardiac problem, but the child's behavior and response to treatment may be useful. The condition of a cyanotic child with a respiratory problem who receives oxygen could be expected to improve, in terms of color and oxygen saturation. In a child with a congenital heart disease, blood would continue to bypass the lungs, and there would be little improvement after administration of oxygen (Flaherty, 1996). Also, a child with a respiratory condition increases air movement and gas exchange when crying, and color and oxygen may improve. A child with congenital heart disease will increase the workload of the heart with crying, and color and oxygen saturation may worsen.

Specific interventions are discussed in the following sections under each condition. General nursing interventions for the neonate are discussed in Chapter 14.

Specific Neonatal Conditions

Neonatal Sepsis

Sepsis continues to be a major cause of morbidity and mortality in the neonatal age group. Bacterial infections are commonly divided into two onset periods (Greij & McCracken, 1999):

- *Early:* Usually occurs within the first 24 hours of life (range: 0 to 6 days). Early sepsis is associated with a higher mortality and morbidity rate than is late-onset sepsis and is usually caused by bacteria acquired from the maternal genital tract either in utero or during delivery (Burke, 1998).
- *Late:* Usually occurs at 3 to 4 weeks of age (range: 7 days to 3 months). After 3 to 4 days of age, sepsis is more often associated with focal disease, such as meningitis (Burke, 1998).

Sepsis can also result from bacteria acquired perinatally with a delay in onset of symptoms, nosocomially from contaminated equipment or human contact, or through the umbilical cord, especially if hygiene is poor.

Sepsis affects 1 to 811,000 live births. The risk for sepsis increases with lower birth weight, rupture of membranes greater than 24 hours prior to birth, and the presence of maternal fever (Guerina, 1998). Postnatal susceptibility to infection is increased with neonatal intensive care admissions, invasive procedures, or artificial ventilation. Meningitis sepsis is more common in the first month of life than at any other time, affecting 0.4 to 1 infant per 1,000 births (Wiswell, Baumgart, Gannon, & Spitzer, 1995). Common causes of sepsis in the neonate are listed in Table 11.6.

Respiratory syncytial virus is the most important respiratory pathogen in infants and children (in terms of morbidity and mortality), especially in those children younger than 2 years of age. The highest risk group includes those younger than 2 months of age, preterm infants, and those with bronchopulmonary dysplasia. Respiratory syncytial virus can rapidly

TABLE 11.6 Common Causes of Neonatal Infections

Bacterial	Group B *streptococcus* (GBS)
	Escherichia coli type K1 (*E. coli*)
	Coagulase-negative *staphylococcus*
Fungal	*Candida albicans*
Viral	Cytomegalovirus (CMV)
	Herpes simplex virus (HSV)
	Respiratory syncytial virus (RSV)
	Rotavirus

Data from: Burchett, 1998; Guerina, 1998.

progress to a lower respiratory infection and respiratory failure in these at risk populations. Respiratory syncytial virus is discussed in detail in Chapter 16.

Group B streptococcal infections have a 13 to 50% mortality rate. The mortality rate is higher in preterm babies. Meningitis has a general fatality rate of 20 to 25% and is also more likely to be fatal in preterm infants. Neurologic side effects of sepsis, especially high-tone hearing loss, are present in 20 to 60% of affected infants.

Pathophysiology

Neonates, especially those who are premature, have an immature immune system and decreased levels and functions of immunoglobulins, complement, and white blood cells. They have a less functional barrier protection (skin, mucous membranes, and intestinal tract) and also unusual portals for infection, such as the umbilicus and circumcision site.

The pathophysiology of sepsis is the same as it is for older children, but the onset is more rapid and severe. Systemic infections can rapidly progress to septic shock. Septic shock is caused by a systematic activation of the inflammatory response as a result of the infection, which, in turn, results in profound vasodilation and disturbances in cardiovascular and other organ system functioning.

Focused History

- Onset of symptoms, especially changes in infant's behavior (lethargy or irritability). Parents may simply say, "He isn't acting normal."
- Maternal history:
    - Group B streptococcus carrier.
    - Perinatal fever.
    - Rupture of membranes (amount of time prior to birth of baby).
    - Herpes simplex virus.
- Exposure to viruses.
- Cord care practices (Cleaning with plain water is acceptable) (Krebs, 1998; Medves & O'Brien, 1997).
- Circumcision surgical site (rare) (Cleary & Kohl, 1979).

Focused Assessment

Nonspecific signs and symptoms

- Fever or subnormal temperature.
- Tachypnea.
- Feeding difficulties.
- Lethargy.
- Vomiting and/or diarrhea.
- Abdominal distention.
- Jaundice.
- Petechiae.
- Apnea spells.

Signs of meningitis (may be present along with above symptoms)

- Bulging anterior fontanelle.
- Irritability.
- Seizures.

Signs of shock (these are all emergent symptoms that must be treated immediately)

- Tachycardia (early sign).
- Bradycardia (late sign).
- Delayed capillary refill (greater than 2 seconds).
- Weak or absent peripheral pulses.
- Pallor, cyanosis, or mottling.
- Altered level of consciousness.
- Hypotension.

Signs and symptoms of respiratory distress may indicate a respiratory pathology, but may also be indicative of heart disease, especially left-sided obstruction. Other disorders that can mimic sepsis include endocrine, metabolic, gastrointestinal, and neurologic disorders, and the effects of child abuse.

Nursing Interventions

Suspected sepsis

- Perform rapid triage and immediate laboratory workup:
  - Lumbar puncture to evaluate cerebrospinal fluid (Wiswell et al., 1995).
  - Blood and urine cultures; culture of umbilicus (if draining).
  - Viral cultures.
  - Complete blood count and electrolytes.
- Administer intravenous antibiotics after all cultures are obtained.
- Provide vasopressor support as necessary.
- Prepare for admission.

Prevention

- Treat mothers who are infected or colonized with *group B streptococcus* with antibiotics during labor.
- Prepare for operative delivery for infants whose mothers have active primary herpes lesions.
- Administer respiratory syncytial antibody.
- Avoid exposure of infants to crowds, other children, and anyone with an infectious disease.

Congestive Heart Failure

Congestive heart failure (CHF) is a condition in which the heart is unable to provide adequate cardiac output or regional blood flow to meet the circulatory and metabolic requirements of the body (Callow, Suddaby, & Slota, 1998). The most common cause of CHF in infants is congenital heart disease (CHD) (Chapter 17).

Pathophysiology

Congestive heart failure can be described as high-output failure or low-output failure (Redfearn, 1998).

High-output failure

A congenital heart defect is usually present at the ventricular or great vessel level, causing left-to-right shunting, which increases pulmonary blood flow and volume overload of the right and left sides of the heart. Severe anemia will also produce high cardiac output because high levels are needed to maintain oxygenation.

Low-output failure

This is seen in association with CHD that results in left-sided heart or aortic obstruction, cardiomyopathies, and dysrhythmias. These conditions impair the pumping ability of the heart, resulting in venous congestion. Several compensatory mechanisms take over, including dilation and hypertrophy of the left ventricle; vasoconstriction of the arterioles of the skin, skeletal muscles, gut, and kidneys; and retention of sodium and water.

Focused History

The following history should be obtained:

- Feeding behavior:
  - Increased time to feed.
  - Tachypnea and or diaphoresis during feeding.
- Poor weight gain.
- Postnatal age at deterioration:
  - Sudden deterioration in health, especially soon after birth, may be caused by closing of a patent ductus arteriosus in a child with a ductal-dependent lesion.
  - Congestive heart failure from pulmonary overperfusion (left-to-right shunting) usually occurs later in the neonatal period.

Focused Assessment

Signs and symptoms of CHF include the following:

- Tachypnea (most sensitive sign for CHF), usually with a respiratory rate greater than 60 breaths per minute.
- Retractions and nasal flaring.
- Hepatomegaly.
- Cyanosis—mild or severe. Severe cyanosis may be related to closure of the patent ductus in a ductal-dependent lesion that has not been diagnosed.
- "Grayness" or poor perfusion. The child may present in profound shock and with impending cardiac collapse.
- Edema. Periorbital edema is often present.
- Absent femoral pulses.

Nursing Interventions

Stabilize airway, breathing, and circulation

Oxygen is usually provided. However, oxygen may increase the distress of the infants with left-to-right shunts because it is a potent vasodilator and will cause increased pulmonary blood flow. If the infant's condition worsens with the administration of oxygen, a ductal-dependent lesion should be suspected and the child will need prostaglandin E to keep the ductus open. Mechanical ventilation may also be necessary.

Perform the following additional interventions:

- Administer diagnostic tests, including:
  - Chest X-ray—usually reveals cardiomegaly.

- Blood and urine studies to evaluate for sepsis or infection.
- Electrocardiogram.
- Echocardiogram (if available).

- Administer medications:
  - Prostaglandin E, to maintain patency or reopen the ductus arteriosus. A continuous infusion is necessary because of its short half-life. Observe the neonate for apnea.
  - Inotropic agents, such as dopamine, dobutamine, or digoxin, to increase both the force and velocity of ventricular contractions.
  - Diuretics.

Home Care and Prevention

Early recognition of congenital heart defects is the best means of preventing congestive heart failure in neonates. ED nurses must be able to recognize signs and symptoms of CHF to prevent deterioration of the infant's condition.

Apnea

Apnea is the cessation of breathing for 20 seconds or any respiratory pause that leads to bradycardia or cyanosis (desaturation). It is a sign of significant illness or immaturity of the respiratory control system (Goodwin, 1999).

The etiology is dependent on the gestational and postnatal age of the child. For most neonates, apnea must be considered a sign of a serious illness or condition, such as:

- Hypoxemia caused by respiratory distress, anemia, or airway obstruction.
- Infection—bacterial or viral (respiratory syncytial virus is a common cause of apnea in the neonate).
- Severe congestive heart failure.
- Inborn errors of metabolism caused by the lack of an enzyme allowing the accumulation of toxic by-products or by-products of metabolism or the inability to make necessary substances. Inborn errors of metabolism are rare and include phenylketonuria, galactosemia, fructose intolerance, and urea cycle defects.
- Metabolic abnormalities:
  - Hypoglycemia (discussed later in this chapter).
  - Hypocalcemia.
  - Hyponatremia.
- Ingestion of narcotics:
  - Direct (intentional or accidental).
  - Indirect via breast milk.
- Gastroesophageal reflux.
- Child abuse.
- Hypothermia.
- Post immunization in a former preterm infant.

Pathophysiology

Apnea is a diagnosis of exclusion and can be the result of respiratory immaturity. Breathing control, both centrally and peripherally, is immature at birth but develops rapidly over the first year of life. Neonates may respond to hypoxemia with a brief increase in respiratory rate, followed by apnea. Hypoxemia also decreases the response to arterial carbon dioxide tension and further depresses the respiratory drive. The infant is more vulnerable during sleep because of the decrease in oxygen tension. Apnea can be potentiated by exposure to anesthesia in premature infants up to 52 weeks' postconceptual age, or by systemic illness in post-term infants, especially those with apnea at discharge from the hospital.

Focused History

- Gestational age and birth history.
- Previous apnea spells and treatment given.
- Current and family illnesses (viral; history of inborn errors of metabolism).
- Feeding difficulties.
- Use of apnea monitor at home.
- Immunizations—Apnea can worsen or reappear within 24 hours after immunizations.

Focused Assessment

The standard physical assessment is done, focusing on:

- Appearance of the child—"sick" versus "not sick."
- Signs and symptoms of associated illnesses (viral, congenital, etc.).

Nursing Interventions

- Observe the infant in the ED for apnea spells (at rest and while crying).
- Have resuscitation equipment ready at bedside.
- Assist with diagnostic tests to rule out illnesses that may be causing apnea.
- Prepare the child and family for admission to the hospital.

Home Care and Prevention

- Provide instructions if the child is discharged home, including:

- Use of a home monitor and instructions on keeping a log of observations.
- Cardiopulmonary resuscitation skills.
- Follow-up with a home health nurse.
- Regular follow up as well as instructions on whom to call for assistance.

Hypoglycemia

Hypoglycemia is defined as a whole blood glucose concentration of less than 40 mg/dl in neonates regardless of age (Cornblath & Ichord, 1999; Karp, Scardino, & Butler, 1995).

Causes of hypoglycemia in the neonate can be classified as follows:

- Decreased glycogen storage:
  - Prematurity.
  - Small for gestational age.
- Hyperinsulinism:
  - Diabetic mother.
  - Insulin-secreting tumor.
- Other factors that increase glucose utilization:
  - Sepsis.
  - Asphyxia.
  - Cold stress.
- Metabolic causes:
  - Galactosemia.
  - Glycogen storage disease.

Pathophysiology

Pregnancy creates a "diabetic-like state" in all mothers from the effects of anti-insulin hormones, such as human placental lactogen, progesterone, and estrogen. Glucose crosses the placenta along concentration gradients via carrier-mediated diffusion. Only 40 to 50% of glucose volume delivered to the placenta gets to the fetus. Insulin and glucagon do not cross the placenta, but the fetus can produce significant amounts of insulin in response to hyperglycemia.

At birth, the maternal glucose source is lost. The neonate's stores of glycogen are usually depleted by 12 hours after birth, and the infant must perform gluconeogenesis to prevent hypoglycemia and to survive. The stress of birth, illness, and hypothermia increases the infant's glucose requirements beyond available stores. Illness and hypothermia can increase the metabolic rate and the glucose requirements.

Focused History

- Prematurity.
- Large or small for gestational age.
- Diabetic mother.
- Current and previous illnesses.
- Intake (oral or intravenous) and output.

Focused Assessment

The signs and symptoms of hypoglycemia can vary greatly. At the same glucose levels, some infants may be asymptomatic while others may exhibit the following signs and symptoms:

- Lethargy.
- Irritability/jitters.
- Apnea.
- Tachypnea.
- Cyanosis.
- Hypothermia.
- Hypotonia.
- Seizures.
- High-pitched cry.

Nursing Interventions

If an infant is suspected of being hypoglycemic, based on the history and signs and symptoms, obtain a blood glucose level immediately and initiate therapy as follows:

- Administer an intravenous bolus of 10% dextrose in water, 2 to 4 ml/kg. Concentrations greater than 10% should not be used unless diluted. If intravenous access cannot be obtained, formula can be administered via gavage (10U/kg). Glucagon, 0.1 mg/kg per dose, can also be given intramuscularly to mobilize hepatic glycogen stores. It is effective only if glycogen is still present.
- Initiate an intravenous infusion of glucose to supply 6 to 8 mg/kg/min of glucose.
- Give nothing by mouth, because of the risk of aspiration.
- Monitor glucose levels frequently.
- Treat underlying cause (e.g., sepsis or hypothermia).
- Reduce neonatal stress:
  - Use warming devices.
  - Cover the neonate's head to prevent heat loss.
  - Provide comforting measures such as swaddling and pacifiers.
  - Encourage the parents to hold the child.

Home Care and Prevention

Provide parental teaching to include recognition and prevention of hypoglycemia.

Hyperbilirubinemia

Hyperbilirubinemia is the result of accumulation of native or unconjugated bilirubin, or a mixture of both, in excess of its excretion. An excessive load can result from increased heme breakdown or from delayed excretion, which is caused by low levels of the enzyme (glucuronyl transferase) needed to conjugate bilirubin (Hinkes & Cloherty, 1998; Klein, 1995; Watson, 1999).

A normal newborn makes 6 to 10 mg/kg/day of bilirubin. Excessive accumulation of free bilirubin is neurotoxic, leading to kernicterus (acute bilirubin encephalopathy—deafness and mental retardation). Delayed excretion can be caused by low levels of conjugating enzymes, blocked bile ducts, or inability to pass stool, allowing reabsorption of bilirubin (enterohepatic reuptake).

In a healthy baby, bilirubin levels peak between 3 and 5 days after birth. Dehydration may result in elevated bilirubin levels.

Pathophysiology

Bilirubin is produced from the catabolism of heme (mostly from the breakdown of red blood cells). Native bilirubin (unconjugated) is water insoluble and has to be converted into the water-soluble form (conjugated bilirubin) by conjugation with glucuronic acid in the liver. Most unconjugated bilirubin is bound to albumin in the circulation in equilibrium with a small amount of free unconjugated bilirubin. Free unconjugated bilirubin is lipid soluble, rapidly crosses the blood-brain barrier, and is neurotoxic. Any condition that increases the breakdown of red blood cells or decreases the conjugating capacity of the liver, bilirubin-albumin binding, or bowel excretion can lead to hyperbilirubinemia.

Kernicterus (bilirubin encephalopathy) is a complication of high bilirubin levels, which may cause brain damage. The exact level of bilirubin that causes kernicterus is not known. However, it is desirable to keep blood bilirubin levels at less than 20 to 25 mg/dl.

Focused History

- Onset of jaundice.
- Blood type of baby and mother (if known).
- Other illnesses.
- Prematurity.
- Diabetes in mother.

Focused Assessment

- Skin color. (Bilirubin is visible as jaundice at a level of about 7 mg/dl, and yellow color progresses from head to toe.)
- Color of sclera.
- Pallor (as a sign of anemia).
- Hydration status.
- Neurologic status—tone; presence of high-pitched cry.
- Hepatosplenomegaly.
- Tachypnea.
- Vital signs.
- Color and frequency of stool.

Nursing Interventions

Treatment depends on the bilirubin level of the infant. The following nursing interventions might be performed:

- Obtain a stat bilirubin level and compare it to previous levels, if available. The upper limits of normal indirect bilirubin levels in full-term infants are as follows:
  - 13 mg/dl (bottle-fed).
  - 15 mg/dl (breast-fed).
- Obtain additional diagnostic studies to rule out other problems that might cause jaundice:
  - Septic workup.
  - Complete blood count.
  - Blood culture.
  - Toxoplasmosis, other, rubella, cytomegalovirus, herpes (TORCH) screen.
  - Clotting studies.
- Prepare for admission for phototherapy, arrangement for home phototherapy, or exchange transfusion. Exchange transfusion will require obtaining blood for a type and cross match for an exchange unit.

Home Care and Prevention (Burke, 1998)

- Place baby in a sunny area.
- Expose the baby's skin to sunlight.
- Keep the baby warm.
- Breast-feed more frequently to stimulate milk byproduction. (Increased intake by baby stimulates the intestine so that bilirubin can be excreted.)
- Report any changes to the physician or ED.
- Return to the infant's physician for follow-up.

Because of rapid discharge from the hospital after childbirth, mothers may have received limited education and support concerning newborn care, breast-feeding, and other information usually provided in the hospital. Also, many infants are being sent home with specialized care equipment, such as apnea, bradycardia, and pulse oximeter monitors. The ED nurse must be aware of the following:

- Home oxygen may be in use by many graduates of neonatal intensive care, especially those at high altitudes. The dose and usage may have to be reviewed with the family. A sufficient travel supply may have to be obtained as part of discharge planning.
- Monitors are usually prescribed for a specific reason, which can be elicited from the family. Continuation of their use may be necessary and may need to be reemphasized with the family.
- Immunizations may be due, and the ED nurse should be aware of the new immunization schedules (Chapter 5) so that the parent can be counseled concerning immunizations. It may be appropriate to provide these immunizations during the ED visit.
- Babies who were delivered at home may not have undergone mandated screening tests, such as those for phenylketonuria, hypothyroidism, galactosemia, and sickle cell anemia. Universal hearing screening may also have to be arranged.
- Mothers may need breast-feeding support. They can be referred to a local La Leche league or to a lactation specialist if one is available in the hospital.

Conclusion

Caring for the neonate in the ED requires that the nurse be aware of the many physiologic changes that take place from birth to 28 days. The neonate is not just a small child but an entirely different classification from the pediatric patient. Because neonates are discharged earlier after birth than they used to be and also because many babies are being born at home, the ED nurse must be aware of specific problems in this population, including thermoregulation, heart disease, and the increased risk for infection. Proper triage, assessment, and intervention are necessary to prevent complications of serious illnesses and congenital problems that have previously been undetected.

References

Behrman, R. E., & Shiono, P. H. (1997). Neonatal risk factors. In A. A. Fanaroff & R. J. Martin (Eds.), *Neonatal-perinatal medicine: Diseases of the fetus and infant* (6th ed., vol. 1, pp. 3-12). St. Louis: Mosby.

Burchett, S. K. (1998). Viral infections. In J. P. Cloherty & A. R. Stark (Eds.), *Manual of neonatal care* (4th ed., pp. 239-270). Philadelphia: Lippencott-Raven.

Burchfield, D. J. (1997). Acute distress in the neonatal and postnatal period. In R. M. Barkin (Ed.), *Pediatric emergency medicine* (2nd ed., pp. 205-222). St. Louis: Mosby.

Burke, S. S. (1998). Neonatal topics. In T. E. Soud & J. S. Rogers (Eds.), *Manual of pediatric emergency nursing* (pp. 660-685). St. Louis: Mosby.

Callow, L., Suddaby, E., & Slota, M. C. (1998). Cardiovascular system. In M. C. Slota (Ed.), *Core curriculum for pediatric critical care nursing* (pp. 144-273). Philadelphia: Saunders.

Carey, B. (1996). Evaluating and recording the neonatal history. In E. P. Tappero & M. E. Honeyfield (Eds.), *Physical assessment of the newborn* (pp. 9-19). Petaluma, CA: NICU.

Cleary, T., & Kohl, S. (1979). Overwhelming infection with group B beta-hemolytic *streptococcus* associated with circumcision. *Pediatrics, 64*(3), 301-303.

Cloherty, J. P., Scott, M. D., Feinberg, B. B., & Reke, J. T. (1998). Maternal conditions that affect the fetus. In J. P. Cloherty & A. R. Stark (Eds.), *Manual of neonatal care* (4th ed., pp. 11-30). Philadelphia: Lippincott-Raven.

Cornblath, M., & Ichord, R. (1999). Hypoglycemia in the neonate. *Seminars in Perinatology, 24*(2), 136-149.

Cornblath, M., & Schwartz, R. (1993). Hypoglycemia in the neonate. *Journal of Pediatric Endocrinology, 6*(2), 113-129.

Flaherty, L. (1996). Neonates and premature infants: Overview of differences and ED management. *Journal of Emergency Nursing, 22*(2), 120-124.

Goodwin, M. (1999). Apena of the newborn infant. In G. Avery, M. Fletcher, & M. McDonald (Eds.), *Neonatology: Pathophysiology and management of the newborn* (5th ed., pp. 151-163).

Greij, B. & McCracken, G. (1999). Acute infections. In G. Avery, M. Fletcher, & M. McDonald (Eds.), *Neonatology: Pathophysiology and management of the newborn* (5th ed., pp. 1189-1230). Philadelphia: Lippincott.

Guerina, N. G. (1998). Bacterial and fungal infections. In J. P. Cloherty & A. R. Stark (Eds.), *Manual of neonatal care* (4th ed., pp. 271-300). Philadelphia: Lippencott-Raven.

Hazinski, M. F. (1999). Children are different. In M. F. Hazinski (Ed.), *Manual of pediatric critical care* (pp. 1-13). St. Louis: Mosby.

Hinkes, M. T., & Cloherty, J. P. (1998). Neonatal hyperbilirubinemia. In J. P. Cloherty & A. R. Stark (Eds.), *Manual of neonatal care* (4th ed., pp. 175-209). Philadelphia: Lippincott-Raven.

Honeyfield, M. E. (1996). Principles of physical assessment. In E. P. Tappero & M. E. Honeyfield (Eds.), *Physical assessment of the newborn* (pp. 1-8). Petaluma, CA: NICU.

Karlsen, K. A. (2000). *Transporting newborns the S.T.A.B.L.E. way* (2nd ed.). Salt Lake City, UT: S.T.A.B.L.E. Transport Education Program.

Karp, T., Scardino, C., & Butler, L. (1995). Glucose metabolism in the neonate: The short and sweet of it. *Neonatal Network, 14*(8), 17-23.

Klein, A. (1995). Management of hyperbilirubinemia in the healthy full-term infant (online). Cedar Sinai Medical Center. Available: www.csmc.edu/neonatology/Syllabus/bili.klein.html.

Krebs, T. (1998). Cord care: Is it necessary? *Mother-Baby Journal, 3*(2), 5-12.

Lott, J. W. (1998). Assessment and management of cardiovascular dysfunction. In C. Kenner, J. Lott, & F. Flandermeyer (Eds.), *Comprehensive neonatal nursing* (2nd ed., pp. 306-355). Philadelphia: Saunders.

Medves, J. M., & O'Brien, B. A. C. (1997). Cleaning solutions and bacterial colonization in promoting healing and early separation of the umbilical cord in healthy newborns. *Canadian Journal of Public Health, 88*(6), 380-382.

Moore, K. L., & Persaud, T. V. N. (1993a). *The developing human* (5th ed., pp. 302-353). Toronto: Saunders.

Moore, K. L., & Persaud, T. V. N. (1993b). *The developing human* (5th ed.). Toronto: Saunders.

O'Toole, M. (Ed.). (1992). *Miller-Kane encyclopedia & dictionary of medicine, nursing, & allied health* (5th ed.). Philadelphia: Saunders.

Perlstein, P. (1997). Physical environment. In A. A. Fanaroff & R. J. Martin (Eds.), *Neonatal-perinatal medicine: Diseases of the fetus and infant* (6th ed., vol. 1, pp. 505-540). St. Louis: Mosby.

Redfearn, S. (1998). Cardiovascular system. In T. E. Soud & J. S. Rogers (Eds.), *Manual of pediatric emergency nursing* (pp. 233-265). St. Louis: Mosby.

Vargo, L. (1996). Cardiovascular assessment of the newborn. In E. P. Tappero & M. E. Honeyfield (Eds.), *Physical assessment of the newborn* (pp. 77-92). Petaluma, CA: NICU.

Watson, R. (1999). Gastrointestinal disorders. In J. Deacon & P. O'Neill (Eds.). *Core curriculum for neonatal intensive care nursing* (2nd ed., pp. 254-293). Philadelphia: W. B. Saunders.

Wiswell, T., Baumgart, S., Gannon, C., & Spitzer, A. (1995). No lumbar puncture in the evaluation for early neonatal sepsis: Will meningitis be missed? *Pediatrics, 95*(6), 803-806.

Wong, D. L. (1999). *Whaley & Wong's essentials of pediatric nursing* (6th ed.). St. Louis: Mosby—Year Book.

12

Common Chief Complaints

Donna Ojanen Thomas, RN, MSN
Treesa Soud, RN, BSN
Tracy Karp, RNC, MS, NNP

Introduction

Children present to the emergency department (ED) with a variety of vague, puzzling complaints. Some of these complaints represent a minor illness or a normal variant, while others represent a life-threatening condition. Whatever the cause, these symptoms often worry parents and frustrate ED staff because a cause for the symptom may not be readily apparent. Because young children cannot answer questions concerning history, signs, and symptoms they have been experiencing and cannot tell "where it hurts," the ED staff must rely on their assessment skills and the parents' impressions of what is wrong with the child.

The purpose of this chapter is to discuss common pediatric complaints seen in the ED, possible causes, nursing assessment, and care. Because many of the conditions represented by these complaints have been discussed elsewhere in this book, the reader will be referred to these chapters, and the information concerning nursing diagnosis, triage decisions, and interventions will not be repeated in all cases.

Fever

The generally accepted definition of normal body temperature used to be 37.0°C (98.6°F) for oral temperatures, 1.0° higher for rectal temperatures, and 1.0° lower for axillary temperatures. Recent work has indicated that the upper limit of normal body temperature is 37.7°C (99.9°F) in children (McCarthy, 1998). It was discovered that the baseline temperatures increase as children grow older, and one cannot rely on a single reading for every age group (Herzog & Coyne, 1993). Most of the current literature agrees that infants younger than 3 months are febrile if the rectal temperature is 38.0°C (100.4°F) or greater. Less consensus exists for children older than 3 months of age.

Fever is one of the most common symptoms in children that causes parents to seek outpatient treatment, often in the ED. The majority of children who present to the ED with fever are younger than 3 years of age. Two-thirds of all children will visit a physician for fever before the age of 2 years (Soman, 1985).

Fever has been studied throughout history. Even before the first thermometer was invented by Galileo in 1603, Hippocrates described fluctuating fevers found in malaria and typhoid fever (Stein, 1991). He used tactile observation to evaluate for the presence of fever. Later, Wunderlich studied 25,000 patients using a foot-long thermometer that had to be held in place under the axilla for 20 minutes. Wunderlich described the fever patterns of many diseases, including measles, pneumonia, scarlatina, and meningitis (Stein, 1991).

Fever in children is caused by a resetting of the thermoregulatory center in the hypothalamus by the action of cytokines released in response to various inciting agents (McCarthy, 1998). These agents are most often viral or bacterial pathogens. Once the thermoregulatory center is reset, it maintains a higher body temperature by mechanisms such as cutaneous vasoconstriction (heat conservation) or shivering (thermogenesis). The febrile response is less mature in young infants and they may have no fever or even hypothermia in the presence of infection.

The main causes of fever are viral illnesses. The degree of fever is related to the occurrence of bacteremia (McCarthy, 1998). Other causes of fever can include:

- Drug intoxications:
  - Atropine.
  - Scopolamine.
  - Belladonna.
  - Amphetamines.

- Bacterial infections:
  - Meningitis.
  - Sepsis.
  - Pneumonia.
- Collagen vascular diseases (Kawasaki disease) (Chapter 26).
- Organ rejection in transplant patients.
- Malignancies (leukemia or central nervous system tumors).
- Acute subdural hematomas.

Pediatric Considerations

Fever speeds up the basal metabolic rate, causing an increase in respiratory rate, oxygen consumption, cardiac output, and fluid and caloric requirements. The increased respiratory rate results in increased insensible water loss. This, coupled with the child's refusal to eat or drink, can contribute to dehydration. These symptoms are usually transient and treatable and will not harm a child who is not already compromised by an existing condition, such as cardiac disease.

Fever in itself is not harmful, despite what parents and even nurses seem to think. Parents often fear that the temperature will go "out of control" or that it will cause seizures or other serious conditions. In reality, temperatures rarely go higher than 41.1°C (106.0°F) because of a regulatory mechanism in the hypothalamus. The effects of fever may actually be helpful. Evidence suggests that fever increases the activity of white blood cells and the production of interferon, thus actually helping to fight infection. Fever may also enhance the effects of some antibiotics (Thomas, Riegal, Andreas, Murray, Gehrart, & Gocka, 1994).

Focused History

The following are important elements when obtaining a history in a febrile infant or child:

- Age of the child.
- Characteristics of the fever:
  - How was the fever measured?
  - When did it start?
  - What types of antipyretics or other treatments were given?
  - What was the child's response to the treatment?
- Underlying medical problems (such as immunocompromised status).
- Contact with any other infectious person.
- Current medications (especially antibiotics).
- Immunization status (Recent immunizations may cause fever).
- Birth history (Chapter 11).
- Caretaker's report of the child's well-being and activity level.

It is important to determine the method used by the parent to measure the temperature. Rectal measurements, with either a glass or an electronic thermometer, are quite accurate and generally preferred for children younger than 3 months of age. They are contraindicated in children with imperforate anus, those who are immunosuppressed, or in any child in whom a vagal response causing bradycardia could be harmful.

Tympanic thermometers work by measuring the magnitude of infrared radiation from the tympanic membrane and the surrounding ear canal. They are quick, easy to use, and well tolerated. Much of the literature suggests that they may not be as accurate in children younger than 3 months of age, and rectal temperatures are preferred in this age group (Stewart & Webster, 1992).

Axillary readings may not always be accurate because they also measure ambient temperature. Plastic strips placed on the forehead are popular and easy to use but may give falsely elevated readings (Betz, Hunsberger, & Wright, 1994).

Focused Assessment

Evaluating a child with fever may be difficult. Some of the effects of the fever may make the child look sicker than he or she is. Infants are hard to evaluate because the fever may be the only symptom present. An infant younger than the age of 3 months with a fever should be evaluated promptly because of the risk of serious infection without obvious symptoms.

The standard pediatric assessment is performed (Chapter 6). Other important considerations in the assessment include:

- Signs and symptoms of dehydration (Chapter 19).
- Rashes. A petechial or purpuric rash can indicate a serious bacterial infection requiring immediate attention (Chapter 22).
- Signs and symptoms of meningitis (Chapter 26).
- Signs of infection at operative sites or central lines, such as redness, draining, or swelling.

Several observation scales have been developed to help identify seriously ill children. One problem with these scales is that they are very hard to use for the young infant who does not localize signs of serious infection. Observation scales alone cannot be relied on to predict serious illnesses.

Nursing diagnoses and expected outcomes are listed below:

Nursing Diagnosis	*Expected Outcomes*
Hyperthermia	Temperature will be reduced by use of antipyretics, as appropriate.
Risk for infection	Child will be evaluated and serious infection will be ruled out or appropriately treated.
Fluid volume deficit (actual or potential)	Child will be hydrated with oral or intravenous fluids as necessary.

Triage Decisions

Emergent

The following children are at risk for serious illness associated with fever and should be categorized as emergent (Baraff et al., 1993):

- Toxic-appearing children (lethargy, poor perfusion, respiratory distress).
- Children younger than 28 days who have a temperature greater than 38.0°C (100.4°F).
- Children younger than 4 years who have a temperature greater than 41.0°C (105.8°F).

Urgent

- Children with preexisting conditions:
  - Ventroperitoneal shunts.
  - Congenital heart disease.
  - Asplenia.
  - Sickle cell disease.
  - Hematologic conditions.

Nonurgent

Fever in a child who is older than 3 months and is alert, oriented, and well hydrated, with no other signs or symptoms of illness.

Nursing Interventions

The main goal of treatment should be to treat the child, not the thermometer. The following interventions should also be considered:

- *Fever reduction measures:* The use of antipyretics and other physical measures are discussed in Table 12.1.

TABLE 12.1 Treatment of Fever

Antipyretics	*Symptomatic Care*
Acetaminophen (Tylenol, Tempra, etc.) *Dose:* Administer 15 mg/kg every 4 hours for temperatures higher than 38.3°C. Acetaminophen is available in liquids, in chewable tablets of varying strengths and flavors, and in adult tablets.	**Sponging** Sponging with tepid water is needed only for those children who are very uncomfortable (temperature greater than 40.0°C (104.0°F) and patients whose fever is caused by heat stroke (Betz et al., 1994). Do not allow the child to shiver, because shivering causes the temperature to rise even more as the body tries to conserve heat. Never use alcohol to sponge a child because skin absorption and inhalation can result in alcohol intoxication.
Ibuprofen (Pediaprofen, etc.) *Dose:* Administer 10 mg/kg every 6 hours. Liquid ibuprofen preparations are available and can be given to children 6 months or older. *Comment:* Use ibuprofen when acetaminophen is not effective in managing the fever. Ibuprofen's antipyretic effect lasts longer than that of acetaminophen. But because of the risk of renal impairment, do not give ibuprofen to children with sickle cell disease, cardiac problems, hypotension, or to those who are hypovolemic (Cassidy, 1993).	**Liquids** Offer liquids in any form the child will take (if not contraindicated by the child's condition). Popsicles, electrolyte solutions, or other liquids will help keep the child hydrated. Intravenous fluids may be necessary, depending on the child's condition. **Other methods** Application of cool compresses or ice packs to the forehead, axilla, and groin should be avoided in younger children to prevent rapid cooling and shivering.

TABLE 12.2 Laboratory Evaluation in Infants and Children with Fever

Patient Age and Characteristics	*Recommended Evaluation*
< 3 months	
	Full sepsis evaluation*
	Stool culture and chest roentgenogram by clinical indication
3 to 36 months	
Fever > 40.0°C (104°F)	Complete blood count (CBC), white blood cell (WBC)
Fever of any degree with no source found on examination	Blood culture Consider urine culture
Prolonged fever without source	
Initial evaluation	CBC, WBC, differential, platelet count, erythrocyte sedimentation rate, urinalysis
	Blood, urine, stool cultures
	Chest roentgenogram
	Consider lumbar puncture
	Antinuclear antibody, rheumatoid factor, C_3 complement
	Tuberculin skin test with anergy controls
Second-stage testing	Liver and kidney function studies
	Bone marrow aspiration
	Upper gastrointestinal contrast study with small-bowel follow-through

*A sepsis workup includes a CBC, WBC, urinalysis, lumbar puncture, and cultures of cerebrospinal fluid, blood, and urine (obtained by bladder catheterization).
From: McCarthy, 1998. Fever. *Pediatrics in Review, 19*(12), p. 406. Used with permission.

- *Laboratory evaluation:* Table 12.2 discusses laboratory evaluation in infants and children, based on age and characteristics.
- *Hospitalization:* Indicated for all children who appear toxic and for febrile infants younger than 28 days.
- *Outpatient management:* May be done based on laboratory tests, clinical signs and symptoms, and ability to provide follow-up care (patients can be reached by telephone).
- *Antibiotics:* Not routinely given on the basis of the fever alone, but based on the results of laboratory tests. The child may be instructed to return to the ED for intramuscular or intravenous antibiotics if he or she is discharged home.

Home Care

The following aspects of fever are important to discuss with family members (Nelson, 1998):

- Fever is a normal part of the body's response to infection.
- The fever will be present as long as the body is killing live microorganisms. Only when that task has been completed will the fever go away.
- Fever need not always be measured accurately at home. It is acceptable to feel a child's forehead and decide whether the fever is in the low, medium, or high category.
- Fever does not always have to be treated; it is not child abuse not to treat a child's fever.
- Acetaminophen and other fever-reducing medicines reduce fever for only a few hours; if the microorganisms are still present, the fever should come back.
- Antipyretic medicines are not without side effects; many a child has been seen in the ED with heme-positive emesis after receiving ibuprofen every 6 hours, usually on an empty stomach, for several days.
- High fever can cause a short, benign, febrile seizure in 3 to 5% of all children, but the seizure does not injure the brain. This event is difficult to prevent because febrile seizures usually occur during the first

few hours of a fever and because it has been shown that prophylactic administration of acetaminophen does not decrease seizure recurrence.

- How sick the child looks is most important, more important than any number on the thermometer.

When discussing fever with parents, do not use the term *fever control*. This term implies that fever is something that must be controlled or it might go out of control. However, ensure that parents are aware of the following:

- Children younger than 3 months of age with a fever have to be examined immediately because of the increased risk of serious infection.
- The child's physician should be contacted if the child at any age appears seriously ill or has a rectal temperature greater than 40.0°C (or 104.0°F).
- Aspirin or aspirin-containing products should never be given to a child, because of the risk of Reye's syndrome.

Abdominal Pain

Abdominal pain is a common complaint within the pediatric population, particularly among school-aged children and adolescents. The etiology of abdominal pain in children varies from serious, life-threatening emergencies to less serious disorders such as colic, constipation, or emotional disturbances. Certain conditions are more commonly associated with specific age groups. Table 12.3 lists the most common etiologies of abdominal pain, by age groups.

Respiratory illnesses are also associated with abdominal pain. Children with asthma exacerbation and associated muscle fatigue (from increased use of chest wall and abdominal muscles) may complain of abdominal pain. Pneumonia with muscular pain or diaphragmatic irritation resulting from coughing can also cause abdominal pain (Horton, Soud, Inman, & Standifer, 1998).

Unexplained pain in the lower abdomen is a common complaint among adolescent girls and creates a challenge. Although the cause is usually benign and self-limited, occasionally a serious underlying disorder exists (Cavanaugh, 1996). It is important to determine if the pain is gynecologic or nongynecologic in nature.

Recurrent abdominal pain with no known cause can also be related to a psychosocial problem, and a thorough history will help to identify stressors in school, family, or other personal circumstances.

The pathophysiology of abdominal pain depends on the underlying disorder or disease. The type and character of the pain provide important clues to the underlying pathology. Three neural pathways transmit visceral pain, somatic pain, and referred pain:

- *Visceral pain* emanates from the intra-abdominal organs with visceral peritoneum (Boenning & Klein, 1997). Visceral pain is characterized as deep or diffuse pain that is colicky or crampy and is often difficult to localize.
- *Somatic or parietal pain* emanates from the abdominal wall, base of the mesenteries, or the diaphragm (Boenning & Klein, 1997). It is characterized by sharp, localized pain that is often intense.
- *Referred pain* is pain that emanates from a site distant to the involved organ or area of pathosis. It may be sharp and localized or characterized as a distant ache.

TABLE 12.3 Most Common Etiologies of Abdominal Pain, by Age

Infancy	*Childhood*	*Adolescence*
Intussusception	Gastroenteritis	Ectopic pregnancy
Volvulus	Appendicitis	Pelvic inflammatory disease
Incarcerated hernia	Pancreatitis	Testicular torsion
Hirschsprung's disease	Henoch-Schonlein purpura	Inflammatory bowel disease
Necrotizing enterocolitis	Hemolytic-uremic syndrome	Biliary disease
Colic	Ulcers	
Perforation of the bowel	Constipation	
	Urinary tract infection	
	Functional causes of abdominal pain	

From: Boenning & Klein, 1997. Gastrointestinal disorders. In R. M. Barkin. *Pediatric emergency medicine, concepts in clinical practice* (2nd ed., p. 798). St. Louis: Mosby—Year Book.

Focused History

The history of the child with abdominal pain includes the following:

- Onset: When did the pain begin, and is it associated with anything in particular?
- Characteristics: sharp, dull, diffuse, localized, or colicky.
- Past medical history: underlying disorders, such as cystic fibrosis or sickle cell disease; previous abdominal surgery.
- Signs and symptoms associated with the pain: vomiting (bilious or not), diarrhea, constipation, fever, the presence of blood in the stool or emesis, abdominal distention, or the presence of a mass.
- Changes in feeding patterns or appetite.
- Changes in level of activity.
- Treatments attempted at home: enemas or the administration of an antiemetic, a cathartic, pain medication, or an antipyretic.
- Social history: The adolescent female should be interviewed separately to determine if any psychosocial stress is present. Also, determine if any new stressors (such as new school, divorce) exist.

Focused Assessment

The standard assessment is done (Chapter 6).

- Evaluate the infant's or child's appearance and level of activity.
- Evaluate the abdomen: symmetry, signs of abdominal distention, the presence of obvious masses, visible bowel loops, and the presence of peristaltic waves.
- Auscultate bowel sounds in all four quadrants. Ask the child to point to the most painful area of the abdomen prior to palpation.
- Palpate nonpainful areas prior to palpating the most painful area. Evaluate for pain to palpation and rebound tenderness.

Nursing diagnoses and triage decisions are discussed in Chapter 19.

Nursing Interventions

Specific diagnostic testing, treatment, and nursing interventions associated with abdominal pain are reviewed with each diagnostic category in Chapter 19.

In the adolescent female with unexplained lower abdominal pain, the following tests should be considered (Cavanaugh, 1996):

- Complete blood count.
- Sedimentation rate.
- Serum beta-human chorionic gonadotrophin.
- Urinalysis and urine culture.
- Flat plate of the abdomen.
- Sonogram of the abdomen and pelvis.
- Fresh stool for ova parasites, pH, reducing substances, and occult blood.
- Additional testing and referral to specialists. May be selected on an individual basis.

Home Care and Prevention

Instruct parents to follow up either in the ED or with the primary healthcare provider if the cause of the abdominal pain is not found.

- Explain any dietary restrictions or changes.
- Describe signs and symptoms that would require the family to return to the ED.
- Provide a referral to a child psychologist, if appropriate.

Limping

A *limp* is best described as a pathologic alteration of smooth, regular gait, in which weight bearing on the painful (or the weaker) limb is minimized (Teach, 1998). *Gait* requires an intact central nervous system, spinal cord, peripheral motor and sensory nerves, and skeletal muscles. It consists of two rhythmic phases:

- A weight-bearing phase (stance).
- A non-weight-bearing phase (swing).

Different types of gaits arise from different causes:

- Antalgic gait—a gait designed to minimize pain in the affected body part.
- Trendelenburg gait—a characteristic slump of the pelvis during the non-weight-bearing phase of gait on the side opposite a weak or painful hip. It does not necessarily indicate a painful condition.

A limp in a child is most often secondary to trauma (Mann, 1997). However, the causes could include benign as well as life-threatening conditions. Limp can be broadly divided into acute versus chronic conditions and painful versus painless conditions. The types of illness involved vary by age. For example, slipped capital femoral epiphysis is rare before adolescence, while toxic synovitis is most common in the school-aged child

TABLE 12.4 Etiologies of a Limp

Cause	*Examples*
Trauma	Soft-tissue injury
	Fracture
	Dislocation
	Sprain
	Foreign body
Infections	Osteomyelitis
	Septic arthritis
	Lyme disease
	Intervertebral diskitis
	Viral infections
Hip diseases	Transient synovitis
	Legg-Calvé-Perthes disease
	Slipped capital femoral epiphysis
Knee diseases	Osgood-Schlatter disease
	Painful patella syndrome
	Osteochondritis dissecans
Other causes	Henoch-Schönlein purpura
	Inflammatory bowel disease
	Serum sickness
	Acute rheumatic fever
	Systemic lupus erythematosus
	Sickle cell disease
	Neoplasms-osteogenic or Ewing's sarcoma

Modified from: Mann, 1997. Orthopedic emergencies. In E. Cranin & J. C. Gershel (Eds.), *Clinical manual of emergency pediatrics* (3rd ed., p. 511). New York: McGraw-Hill. Used with permission.

(Teach, 1998). Table 12.4 lists some etiologies of limp. These conditions are discussed in detail elsewhere in this book.

Focused History

The following history should be obtained:

- Recent trauma.
- Onset of limp (acute or chronic).
- Presence and location of pain.
- Onset and duration of symptoms.
- Recent illnesses.
- Associated symptoms (fever or rash).

Focused Assessment

The standard assessment is done (Chapter 6):

- Strength, reflexes, and sensation in extremities.
- Palpation of joints and muscle groups:
  - Range of motion in joints.
  - Size, strength, and sensation of both extremities.
- Signs and symptoms of inflammation (redness, warmth, and swelling).
- Evaluation of hips for pain. Several sources of hip or groin pain and limp originate in the lower spine, sacroiliac joints, pelvis, abdomen, and retroperitoneum (Teach, 1998):
- Iliopsoas abscess may present as limited hip flexion and extension.
- A torsion of the testis in a very young male may present as a refusal to walk because motion irritates the scrotal contents.

Triage decisions and nursing diagnoses are discussed in Chapter 21.

Nursing Interventions

Interventions specific to each condition are discussed in Chapter 21. Interventions for the child with a limp include the following:

- Radiographs to exclude fractures, avulsions, dislocations, and tumors.
- Diagnostic ultrasounds to detect joint effusions.
- Laboratory tests, including:
  - White blood cell count and evaluation of any aspirated synovial fluid.
  - Erythrocyte sedimentation rate to evaluate for inflammatory process.
  - Blood cultures.

Home Care and Prevention

- Instruct parents to follow up with the primary care provider or the ED, especially if:

- The child cannot walk.
- A high fever is present.

- Provide a referral to a specialist (such as an orthopedist or rheumatologist).
- Tell the parents whom to call for test results.

Complaint Specific to Infants: Crying

The crying infant creates stress for the caregiver and ED staff. The concerned parents are generally seeking an explanation for the crying, and this creates more stress for ED staff if the cause is not readily apparent.

Crying is a nonspecific response in infants and is also a necessary feature of normal psychomotor development in early infancy. It can be a means for an infant to express hunger, discomfort of some nature (often not readily apparent), or a desire to be held. However, it can also be indicative of a life-threatening illness. Crying begins as a response to a physiologic stress, such as hunger, discomfort, overstimulation or understimulation, or temperature change (Bolte, 1998). As the infant becomes conditioned to expect a response to his or her cry, it becomes a more purposeful tool for controlling the environment.

Crying levels increase from birth and peak at about 6 to 8 weeks. During peak times, the infant may cry for 2 to 3 hours per day. Crying episodes may also appear in clusters during the early afternoon and late evening (Maffei, 1997). A certain amount of inconsolable crying is normal in thriving infants in the first 12 weeks of life. Infants younger than 3 months old whose crying lasts longer than 3 hours per day, 3 days per week, and continues for more than 3 weeks, are said to have infantile colic (Wessel, 1954).

The causes of incessant crying in infants, especially those labeled as having colic, are obscure. However, when the crying is excessive, or uncharacteristic, the infant must be evaluated to rule out serious causes.

Conditions associated with abrupt onset of inconsolable crying in young infants are listed in Table 12.5.

Focused History

- Baseline feeding, sleeping, and crying patterns.
- Infectious symptoms (otitis media).
- Feeding intolerance (gastroesophageal reflux with esophagitis), change in infant formula.
- Vomiting, diarrhea, or signs of constipation.
- Recent immunizations (DTP reaction).
- Possibility of a drug reaction, including maternal drugs that may be transferred via breast milk.

TABLE 12.5 Conditions Associated with Abrupt Onset of Inconsolable Crying in Young Infants

Discomfort caused by identifiable illness

Head and neck

- Meningitis.*
- Skull fracture or subdural hematoma.*
- Glaucoma.
- Foreign body (especially eyelash) in eye.†
- Corneal abrasion.†
- Otitis media.†
- Caffey's disease (infantile cortical hyperostosis).
- Battered child syndrome.*
- Prenatal or perinatal cocaine exposure.

Gastrointestinal

- Excess air because of improper feeding or burping technique.
- Gastroenteritis.†
- Intussusception.*
- Anal fissure.†
- Milk intolerance.

Genitourinary

- Torsion of testis.
- Incarcerated hernia.*
- Urinary tract infection.

Integument

- Open diaper pin.
- Burn.
- Strangulated finger, toe, or penis (often because of an encircling hair).

Musculoskeletal

- Battered child syndrome.*
- Extremity fracture (following a fall).

Toxic and metabolic

- Drugs: aspirin, antihistamines, atropinics, adrenergics, or cocaine (including passive inhalation).*
- Metabolic acidosis, hypernatremia, hypocalcemia, or hypoglycemia.*
- Pertussis vaccine reactions.

- Colic—Recurrent paroxysmal attacks of crying†

*Life-threatening causes.
†Common causes.
From: Henretig, 1993. Crying and colic in early infancy. In G. R. Fleisher & S. Ludwig (Eds.), *Textbook of pediatric emergency medicine* (3rd ed., p. 144). Baltimore, MD: Williams & Wilkins. Used with permission.

- Past history (a suspicious history, including numerous ED visits, or a high-risk social situation raises the concern for abuse).
- History of fever.

Focused Assessment

The standard pediatric assessment is done (Chapter 6), focusing on the possible causes of crying (Table 12.5.) Nursing diagnoses are listed below.

Nursing Diagnoses	*Expected Outcomes*
Pain	Pain that may be causing discomfort will be alleviated by determining the cause and proper treatment.
Constipation	Constipation will be relieved. Parents will be instructed on how to prevent constipation in the future.
Risk for infection	Child will be evaluated to rule out serious infectious conditions.

Triage Decisions

Generally, a crying child should be categorized as urgent or emergent, if for no other reason than to remove the child and his or her distraught parents from the waiting room, but certainly to determine the cause of the crying. Table 12.6 lists "red flags" associated with intractable crying in infancy and early childhood.

Nursing Interventions

Nursing care will depend on the cause of the crying but will always include reassurance and support of the parents. Preparing the family for admission to the hospital may be necessary.

Parents may need to have some support for dealing with the crying as well. A home health nursing referral may be appropriate to assist the family with some parenting issues. An assessment of the family situation must be made to determine whether the parents are at risk for abusing their child.

Home Care and Prevention

If the child is discharged, the parents will need instructions on home care. If the reason for the crying has been labeled as colic, the following information should be given (Belmarich, 1997):

- Dispel common myths about colic, including:
  - Medications will help.
  - The infant is spoiled.
  - Colic is caused by parental inexperience and anxiety.

TABLE 12.6 Red Flags Associated with Intractable Crying in Infancy and Childhood

History
Fever in the infant younger than 12 weeks of age
Paradoxic irritability (infant does not want to be held)
Premature rupture of membranes, perinatal maternal fever or infection, or neonatal jaundice
Maternal drug use
Poor feeding or poor weight gain
Significant decrease in level of activity, cyanotic or apneic "spell," or seizure-like episode
Bilious or projectile vomiting
History not suggestive of classic infant colic syndrome
History suggestive of physical abuse (injury not consistent with reported history, inappropriate delay, or nonmaternal caregiver)
Antibiotic pretreatment (partially treated sepsis or meningitis)
History of recent head trauma
Lack of *Haemophilus* influenza type B immunization
Physical examination
Fever (rectal temperature > 38.0°C in the infant younger than 12 weeks of age)
Hypothermia
Heart rate greater than 230 beats per minute
Lethargy or poor eye contact
Paradoxic irritability
Pallor, mottling, poor perfusion, or weak pulse
Hypotonia, jitteriness, or poor feeding
Petechiae or ecchymosis
Meningismus or full fontanelle
Petechial hemorrhages or signs of basilar fracture or closed head injury
Tachypnea, retractions, nasal flaring, or cyanosis
Abnormal extremity movement (hip)
Abdominal tenderness or mass
Bloody stool (not just external streaks)
Bilious or projectile vomiting
Weight less than the fifth percentile for age

From: Bolte, 1998. In Aghababian, R. B., Allison, E. J., Braen, G. R., Fleisher, G. R., McCabe, J. B. (Eds.), *Emergency medicine: The core curriculum* (p. 628). Philadelphia: Lippincott-Raven. Used with permission.

- Explain measures that might help:
  - Increased holding and rocking of the baby.
  - More frequent feeding.
  - Use of a pacifier.
  - Environmental changes (stroller ride, infant swing, or car ride).
- Refer to family physician for follow-up care. Instruct parents to return to the ED if child has any new or unusual symptoms.
- Refer parents to outside support as necessary.

Other Common Infant Complaints

Other complaints specific to infants that are usually not serious, but are of concern to parents, are listed in Table 12.7, along with their common causes and ED nursing considerations.

Conclusion

A variety of nonspecific complaints may bring infants and young children to the ED. Many of these are self-limiting and benign, but some could represent serious conditions that need immediate attention. Fever is the most common complaint in the pediatric patient, resulting in many ED visits. The ED nurse has to focus on the parents' perceptions of the child's condition (remember, they know their child better than anyone else does), the history, and the assessment. An awareness of common causes of various common complaints will help the nurse to focus his or her assessment and provide proper interventions.

TABLE 12.7 Other Less Common Complaints in the Infant

Complaint	*Causes*	*Nursing Considerations*
Blood stools or hematemesis	Intestinal wall breakdown secondary to ischemia or hemorrhagic necrosis caused by emergent conditions, such as volvulus or Meckel's diverticulum (Chapter 19) or by formula intolerance.	A careful history and assessment will help to determine the cause. Generally these children should be seen urgently to rule out serious causes. Parents are usually very concerned to see blood.
	Viral gastroenteritis (rotavirus).	This is more common in older infants.
	Maternal blood, swallowed either at birth or from cracked nipples.	A history will help to determine this as a cause. The mother's nipples may also have to be evaluated for cracks and bleeding.
Bleeding	The causes of unusual bleeding may represent unique neonatal circumstances that, because of early discharge, were not discovered at birth, including: ■ Hemorrhagic disease of the newborn (HDN), which is a self-limiting disorder resulting from a deficiency of vitamin K-dependent clotting factors. ■ Hemophilia ■ Thrombocytopenia resulting from maternal antiplatelet antibodies.	This should be triaged emergently. Assessment should include birth history, trauma, illness, and medications. Look for bruising, cephalohematoma, enlarged liver, spleen, presence of petechiae, and jaundice. If the cause is a long-term condition, such as hemophilia (Chapter 25), the parents will need follow up and referral for counseling.
Common cold	Usually caused by a virus. Immunologically immature neonates are prone to frequent episodes of colds. Prematurity, congenital disorders, such as heart disease, and chronic illnesses increase the susceptibility of the neonate to colds.	A complete examination is necessary to rule out more serious conditions. There is no cure for the common cold, and antibiotics will not be helpful even though parents may want them. Supportive care with good follow up is the only treatment. Parents must be told to return if there is decreased intake, fever, or other symptoms. Cold symptoms usually resolve in about 2 weeks.

TABLE 12.7 (continued)

Complaint	*Causes*	*Nursing Considerations*
Circumcision problems	Problems include abnormal bleeding, infection, or meatal stenosis (late problems).	A small amount of bloody drainage may be observed when Plastibell falls off. Active bleeding, excessive swelling, and an odorous purulent discharge are abnormal. Treatment can include hygiene instructions to the parents, surgical consult, or complete septic workup.
Constipation	Can be caused by dietary changes, motility disorders, viral illnesses, and anal fissures. Congenital disorders may cause chronic constipation (Chapter 19).	Usually requires minimal interventions unless obstruction is suspected. Abdominal and rectal examinations are performed and a stool sample for occult blood is obtained. Digital rectal stimulation may be necessary to relieve impaction. Enemas are a last resort and are rarely used. A surgical or gastrointestinal consult may be necessary for chronic constipation.
Gynecomastia (enlarged breasts in the newborn with secretion of milky fluid)	Caused by influences of maternal estrogen from pregnancy or from maternal ingestion of birth control pills while breast-feeding.	This may persist for several weeks, but usually resolves in 2 weeks. If it does not resolve, further evaluation will be necessary. Mother may have to be instructed to stop using birth control pills.
Pseudomenses (a white, mucoid vaginal discharge or mild bleeding from the vagina)	Normal variant which may result from estrogen exposure; may occur with maternal birth control pill use.	This usually resolves in about 10 days.

References

Baraff, L. J., et al. (1993). Practice guidelines for the management of infants from 0-36 months of age with fever without source. *Pediatrics 92*(1), 1-12.

Belmarich, P. (1997). Gastrointestinal emergencies. In E. F. Crain & J. C. Gershel (Eds.), *Clinical manual of emergency pediatrics*, (pp. 191-253). New York: McGraw-Hill.

Betz, C. L., Hunsberger, M. M., & Wright, S. (1994). *Family centered nursing care of children* (2nd ed.). Philadelphia: Saunders.

Boenning, D. A., & Klein, B. L. (1997). Gastrointestinal disorders. In R. M. Barrkin, (Ed.), *Pediatric emergency medicine, concepts in clinical practice* (2nd ed.). St. Louis: Mosby—Year Book.

Bolte, R., (1998). Intractable crying in infancy and early childhood. In R. B. Aghababian, Allison, E. J., Braen, G. R., Fleisher, G. R., McCabe, J. B., & Moorehead, J. C., (Eds.). *Emergency medicine: The core curriculum* (pp. 622-630). Philadelphia: Lippincott-Raven.

Cassidy, J., (1993). Fever points. *Current Issues in Pediatric Medicine, 1*(1), 1.

Cavanaugh, R. M. (1996). Nongynecologic causes of unexplained lower abdominal pain in adolescent girls. *Clinical Pediatrics 35*(7) (pp. 337-341).

Henretig, F. M. (1993). Crying and colic in early infancy. In G. R. Fleisher, & S. Ludwig (Eds.), *Textbook of Pediatric Emergency Medicine* (3rd ed., pp. 144-146). Baltimore, MD: Williams & Wilkins.

Herzog, L., & Coyne, L. (1993). What is fever? Normal temperatures in infants less than three months old. *Clinical Pediatrics, 32*(3), 142.

Horton, M., Soud, T., Inman, C., & Standifer, P. (1998). Gastrointestinal system. In T. E. Soud & J. S. Rogers (Eds.), *Manual of pediatric emergency nursing* (pp. 332-363). St. Louis: Mosby.

Maffei, F. (1997). Special considerations in pediatric emergency care: The crying infant. In E. F. Crain & J. C. Gershel (Eds.), *Clinical manual of emergency pediatrics* (pp. 665-667). New York: McGraw-Hill.

Mann, R. (1997). Orthopedic emergencies: Limp. In E. F. Crain & J. C. Gershel (Eds.), *Clinical manual of emergency pediatrics* (pp. 510-515). New York: McGraw-Hill.

McCarthy, P. L. (1998). Fever. *Pediatrics in Review, 19*,(12), 401-407.

Nelson, D. (1998). Emergency treatment of fever phobia. *Journal of Emergency Nursing, 24*(1), 83-84.

Soman, M. (1985). Characteristics and management of febrile young children seen in a university family practice. *Journal of Family Practice, 21*, 117-122.

Stein, M. (1991). Historical perspective on fever and thermometry. *Clinical Pediatrics, Supplement.*

Stewart, J. V., & Webster, D. (1992). Re-evaluation of the tympanic thermometer in the emergency department. *Annals of emergency medicine 21*:2, 186–161.

Teach, S. J. (1998). Pediatric disorders: Limp. In R. B. Aghababian, Allison, E. J., Braen, G. R., Fleisher, G. R., & McCabe, J. B. (Eds.), *Emergency medicine: The core curriculum* (pp. 630-634). Philadelphia: Lippincott-Raven.

Thomas, V., Riegel, B., Andreas, J., Murray, P., Gehram, A., & Gocka, I. (1994). National survey of pediatric fever management practices among ED nurses. *Journal of Emergency Nursing, 20*(6), 505.

Wessel, M. A. (1954). Paroxysmal fussing in infancy, sometimes called "colic." *Pediatrics, 14*, 421–435.

13

Pain Assessment and Management

Pam Baker, RN, BSN, CEN, CCRN

Introduction

Until recently, the management of acute and chronic pain in infants, children, and adolescents presenting to the emergency department (ED) was neglected because of fallacies about the presence of pain, its physiologic consequences, and its alleviation or palliation (Table 13.1). Developmentally appropriate pain assessment scales, noninvasive cardiorespiratory monitoring technology, advanced pharmacologic agents, and nonpharmacologic modalities have changed emergency nursing approaches to the assessment, management, and evaluation of pain.

There are two pain-related etiologies: pain as a symptom of illness or injury and pain as the result of a procedure or treatment. Regardless of its etiology, pain must be ameliorated, controlled, or abated through pharmacologic and nonpharmacologic interventions. The acknowledgment of pain and the initiation of pain-relief measures promotes trust among children, their families, and emergency nurses. The purposes of this chapter are to differentiate pain experiences among infants, children, and adolescents and to outline pharmacologic and nonpharmacologic approaches to pain management.

Anatomy and Physiology of Pain

The perception of, interpretation of, and response to pain involves stimulus, receptors, pathways, and interpretive central nervous system structures. The pain response begins with a stimulus that activates a receptor site (nociceptor); this stimulus may result from:

- Stretching, tearing, cutting, or compression of skin or viscera.
- Release of chemicals at the injury site or hypoxic area, including bradykinin, serotonin, norepinephrine, leukokinins, histamine, potassium acids, acetylcholine, proteolytic enzymes, and prostaglandins (Willens, 1994).
- Interruption of blood flow, resulting in the release of substances such as lactic acid, bradykinin, and proteolytic enzymes.

Nociceptors

Nociceptors are located in the skin, periosteum, joint surfaces, arterial walls, subcutaneous tissues, muscles, viscera, and fascia. There are four classifications of nociceptors (Guyton, 2000):

1. *Mechanoreceptors* are stimulated by mechanical forces, such as shearing or stretching, resulting in the release of chemical mediators that stimulate chemoreceptors and intensify the pain response.
2. *Thermoreceptors* are stimulated by thermal stimuli. Their activation modulates the pain response (e.g., application of heat or cold to an area).
3. *Chemoreceptors* are stimulated by chemical mediators, which depolarize the nerve endings, decrease the receptor thresholds, and recruit surrounding cells to become nociceptors. The pain associated with inflammation arises because of stimulation of chemoreceptors.
4. *Polymodal nociceptors* are stimulated by mechanical, chemical, and thermal sensations.

TABLE 13.1 Facts and Fallacies about Children and Pain

Fallacy	*Fact*
Infants do not feel pain because they have an undeveloped nervous system, with poorly myelinated nerve fibers and immature cerebral functions.	Infants demonstrate behavioral, especially facial, and physiologic, including hormonal, indicators of pain. Neonates have the neural mechanisms to transmit noxious stimuli by 20 weeks' gestation. As early as the second trimester of pregnancy, the fetus has the anatomic and neurochemical abilities to experience discomfort (Anand & Hickey, 1987). It is proposed that infants have an anticipatory response to pain (McKenzie, 1997).
Children tolerate pain better than adults.	Children's tolerance for pain actually increases with age. Younger children tend to rate procedure-related pain higher than do older children.
Children cannot tell you where they hurt.	By 4 years of age, children can accurately point to the body area or mark the painful site on a drawing. Children as young as 3 years old can use pain scales.
Children always tell the truth about pain.	Children may not admit to having pain to avoid an injection or other unpleasant procedure; because of constant pain, they may not realize how much they are hurting. Children may believe that others know how they are feeling and may not ask for analgesia.
Children become accustomed to pain or painful procedures.	Children often demonstrate increased behavioral signs of discomfort with repeated painful procedures.
Behavioral manifestations reflect pain intensity.	Children's developmental level, coping abilities, and temperament, such as activity level and intensity of reaction to pain, influence pain behavior. Children with more active, resisting behaviors may rate pain lower than do children with passive, accepting behaviors.
Narcotics are more dangerous for children than they are for adults.	Narcotics (opioids) are no more dangerous for children than for adults. Addiction to opioids is extremely rare in children. Reports of respiratory depression are uncommon. By 3 to 6 months of age, healthy infants can metabolize opioids similar to other children.

Adapted from: Wong, 1999. Family-centered care of the child during illness and hospitalization. In Wong, D. L. (Ed.), *Whaley & Wong's nursing care of infants and children* (6th ed., pp. 1131–1209). St. Louis: Mosby—Year Book.

Prostaglandins further sensitize the nociceptors to the effects of other chemicals such as bradykinin and potassium. The release of potassium ions from the cell increases the nociceptor activity and facilitates transmission of the pain impulse (Emergency Nurses Association, 1995).

Nerve Fibers

Following nociceptor stimulation, the pain stimulus is transmitted to the spinal cord via A-delta or C peripheral afferent nerve fibers:

- A-delta fibers are fine, moderately myelinated fibers that rapidly conduct the pain stimulus. These fibers transmit the sharp, pricking sensations produced by mechanical stimuli. The pain is perceived as sharp and can be localized; its intensity is rapidly distinguished. Stimulation of these fibers produces the pain associated with acute conditions. The A fibers are stimulated only if the pain is above a certain threshold, preventing low levels of stimuli from causing pain. This threshold is different for everyone.
- C fibers are smaller and unmyelinated. These fibers are polymodal and produce pain that is described as dull, aching, or burning. C fibers are primarily found in the skin and deep tissues. Stimulation of the C fibers is responsible for the pain reported with chronic conditions.

Spinal Cord to Brain

The pain stimulus enters the spinal cord via the dorsal root. The fibers then bifurcate, synapse, and cross over to the opposite side of the cord. The synapse occurs between the first- and second-order neurons in specialized areas of the spinal cord gray matter (laminae). After the synapse, the stimulus from the A-delta fibers is transmitted via the cervicothalamic tract, terminating in the reticular formation, medulla, pons, and mesencephalon (Emergency Nurses Association, 1995). The stimulus from the C fibers is transmitted via the cervicothalamic tract, terminating in the reticular activating system, which is responsible for arousal and wakefulness. Termination of the C fiber stimulus in the reticular activating system explains why patients with chronic pain often are unable to sleep and arouse easier (Guyton, 2000). The stimulus from both sources is transmitted to the thalamus and then to the cerebral cortex for interpretation.

Gate Control Theory of Pain

The gate control theory of pain (Melzack & Wall, 1965) posits one explanation of pain perception and treatment effectiveness. According to this theory, a physiologic gate controlled by internal and external influences exists between the peripheral and central nervous systems. Pain stimuli can only be transmitted if the gate is open or partially open. The gate can be closed by competing stimuli or inhibitory impulses (Melzack & Wall, 1965). Stimulation of A-delta fibers by vibration, temperature changes, or touch can cause closure of the gate, a possible explanation for the effectiveness of massage, heat, cold, transcutaneous electrical nerve stimulation (TENS), and acupuncture in treating pain.

Short-Term and Long-Term Effects of Pain

The short-term, immediate effects of pain encompass physiologic, physical, and behavioral changes:

- Physiologic changes include stimulation of the autonomic nervous system, resulting in enhanced glucose breakdown, causing hyperglycemia. Additional hormonal changes include decreased insulin release and increases in plasma catecholamines, cortisol, glucagon, aldosterone, and other corticosteroids (Anand & McGrath, 1993). Eventually, the autonomic nervous system no longer maintains the hyperarousable state, and physiologic parameters return to previous levels.
- Physical changes include tachycardia, tachypnea, increased blood pressure, flushed skin, sweating, and dilated pupils.
- Behavioral changes include (Emergency Nurses Association, 1998):
  - Crying, grunting, or breath holding.
  - Facial grimacing; furrowing of the forehead; raised cheeks; lowered, drawn-together brows; broadened, bulging nose; or closing of the eyes.
  - Clinging to the caregiver or lack of movement.
  - Alteration in activity or behavior, such as decreased appetite, irritability, restlessness, aggressive behavior, or sleep problems.
  - Signs of muscle tension, clenched fists, guarding, or agitation.

The long-term effects of pain in the child include sleep disorders, withdrawal from friends and family, decreased ability to concentrate, and decreased activity levels (McGrath, 1993). These children experience learning problems and difficulty with social interactions.

The Experience of Pain

"Pain is an unpleasant sensory and emotional experience associated with actual or potential damage, or described in terms of such damage" (International Association for the Study of Pain, Subcommittee on Taxonomy, 1979). "Pain is whatever the experiencing person says it is and occurs whenever he says it does" (McCaffrey, 1979). These definitions illustrate the physical and psychological aspects of the pain experience. Both the response to and the interpretation of pain and its intensity are highly individualized; emergency nurses must recognize these individual responses and intervene accordingly.

Several factors affect children's pain experiences, including (Acute Pain Management Guideline Panel, 1992):

- The child's developmental, cognitive, and emotional levels (Table 13.2).
- The procedure to be completed.
- The duration of the procedure.
- The body areas involved.
- Previously implemented pharmacologic and nonpharmacologic therapies (Avner, 1997).

Emergency Nursing Care of Children in Pain

Emergency nurses must be astute to pain-related physical and behavioral cues. The presence of pain can be anticipated, such as prior to a procedure, or it can be suspected in an illness (otitis media) or injury (burn injury). Regardless of the pain's etiology (procedure, illness, or injury), the emergency nurse obtains a history and focused pain assessment, formulates nursing diagnoses, initiates pharmacologic and nonpharmacologic interventions, and evaluates their effectiveness.

Focused History

Preverbal children

- Parents' or caregivers' descriptions of the child's pain, including location, onset, and duration, as well as behavioral and activity changes.

TABLE 13.2 Developmental Considerations in Children's Pain

Age Group	*Characteristics*	*Nursing Interventions*
Infants	Easily comforted by caregiver and strangers. Ability to express pain is nonspecific.	Ask the caregiver to report changes in the infant's behavior.
Toddlers	Afraid of strangers and cling to caregivers when anxious. Able to use basic words to describe pain, such as "ouchie" or "boo-boo." May be able to localize pain.	Involving the caregiver in the child's care can reduce the toddler's and caregiver's anxiety.
Preschoolers and young school-aged children	More comfortable with certain adults other than caregivers (e.g., teachers). May view pain as a punishment and may blame someone for their pain. Are better able to describe and localize the pain. May believe the pain will magically disappear.	Include the child in the discussion of the need for the procedure and adequately prepare him or her for the procedure. Use concrete, simple terms that are appropriate for the developmental level.
Older school-aged children and young adolescents	Increased understanding of medical procedures and diagnoses. Strive to be independent but continue to depend on family support. Have limited experience with coping mechanisms, despite their mature understanding of pain. Changes in body image are very important. Late primary school children can conceive of physical pain and psychologic pain (e.g., someone dying). May view pain as a punishment (Wong, 1999).	To allow a child in this age group to maintain a sense of control over the situation, involve the child in his or her care and decisions related to that care (McKenzie, 1997). Explain procedures and health condition simply and honestly.
Adolescents	Able to explain the origin of their pain, can perceive several types of psychologic pain, and fear losing control during painful procedures (Wong,1999).	Encourage the adolescent to verbalize pain-relieving and coping strategies. Involve the adolescent in the selection of pain-relieving interventions.

- Previous coping strategies for pain, such as holding or rocking the child or distraction techniques.
- Home remedies or treatment (e.g., administration of acetaminophen or ibuprofen, application of ice or heat, administration of herbal products).
- Previous pain-related experiences (e.g., surgeries or fractures).

Verbal children

- Child's description of the pain, including location, radiation, severity, onset, quality, and duration.
- Parents' or caregivers' descriptions of the child's pain, including location, onset, and duration, as well as behavioral activity changes.
- Previous coping strategies for pain, such as thought-stopping or deep breathing.
- Home remedies or treatment (e.g., administration of acetaminophen or ibuprofen, or splinting).
- Previous pain-related experiences (e.g., surgeries or fractures).

Focused Assessment

After the child's underlying health condition is assessed, the pain assessment ensues:

- Observe the child's behavior and physical appearance for pain-related cues based on the child's age and developmental level (Wong, 1999):
  - Younger infants—Rigidity or thrashing of body, loud, inconsolable crying, and facial grimacing.
  - Older infants—Localized response to the area of pain; withdrawal of affected area; loud, inconsolable crying; facial grimacing; and resistance to or pushing away an applied stimulus (e.g., the nurse's hand or a bandage).
  - Young children—Loud crying or screaming, saying "ow," thrashing of arms or legs, pushing away an applied stimulus, and uncooperative behavior. For a painful procedure, these children may need measures for securing and positioning; they may cling to the caregiver or others, ask to have it "all done," and seek emotional support.
  - School-aged children—Clenched fists or teeth, body stiffness, closed eyes, and wrinkled forehead.

During a painful procedure, school-aged children may try verbal stalling ("Wait a minute.").

- Adolescents—State when and where it hurts. There may be decreased motor activity, increased motor tension, and body stiffness.

■ Elicit from the child the pain's location, radiation severity, onset, quality, and duration:

- Ask the verbal child to describe the pain: "Is it burning, or aching, or sharp?" "What do you think is causing it?"
- Ask the preverbal or frightened verbal child to point to the painful area: "Point to where you are hurting; show me where to put a bandage on mommy or daddy that shows me where you hurt."

■ Administer a self-report measurement. A self-report pain measurement tool allows the child to describe the location or intensity of pain. Drawings or dolls also can be used to identify the location of the pain. A number of pain rating scales are available to determine the intensity of a child's pain and the effectiveness of the interventions:

In children aged 5 years or younger (Wong, 1999):

- Oucher scale—This tool uses six pictures of a child's face, representing a range from "no hurt" to "biggest hurt ever." It also includes a vertical scale with numbers from 0 to 10 to use with older children. Ask the child to choose the face that best describes his or her pain.
- Poker chip tool—This tool uses four red poker chips placed in front of the child. Place the chips horizontally and tell the child that "these are pieces of hurt." Explain to the child that each chip represents a piece of hurt. Ask how many pieces of hurt the child has right now. Record the number of chips the child selected.
- Faces scale—This tool consists of six cartoon faces, ranging from a smiling face for "no pain" to a tearful face for "worst pain." Explain to the child that each face is for a person who feels happy because there is no hurt or sad because there is some or a lot of hurt. Ask the child to pick the face that best describes his or her pain.

In children older than 6 years of age (Wong, 1999):

- Numeric scale—This scale uses a straight line with end points that are labeled as "no pain" and "worst pain." Divisions with corresponding numbers from 0 to 10 are marked along the line. Ask the child to choose the number that best describes his or her pain.
- Visual analog scale—This scale uses a 10-cm horizontal line with end points marked "no pain" and "worst pain." Ask the child to place a mark on the line that best describes the amount of his or her pain. Measure the distance with a ruler from the "no pain" end and record the measurement as the pain score.
- Word-graphic rating scale—This scale uses descriptive words to categorize varying intensities of pain. Examples of the words along the scale may include "no pain," "little pain," "medium pain," "large pain," and "worst possible pain." Ask the child to mark on the line the words that best describe his or her pain. Measure the distance with a ruler from the "no pain" end to the mark and record the measurement as the pain score.

■ Evaluate physiologic parameters:

- Measure the child's blood pressure, heart rate, and respiratory rate; note tachycardia, tachypnea, or increased blood pressure.
- Assess the skin color, temperature, and moisture; note flushed skin color, warm skin temperature, and diaphoresis.

■ Consult with the caregivers regarding their impression of the child's condition and pain. Ask whether the child has responded to usual comforting measures or whether this episode is different. Validate the caregivers' reported signs and symptoms that indicate pain. Elicit their suggestions for pain relief interventions during this ED visit.

Nursing diagnoses and expected outcomes are listed below:

Nursing Diagnoses	***Expected Outcomes***
Acute pain or chronic pain	The child will experience relief of pain, as evidenced by:
	Diminishing or absent level of pain in child's self-report.
	Absence of physiologic indicators of pain, such as tachycardia, tachypnea, pallor, diaphoresis, and increased blood pressure.
	Absence of nonverbal cues of pain, such as crying, grimacing, inability to assume a position of comfort, or guarding.
	Ability to cooperate with care as appropriate.

Triage Decisions

Emergent

Severe pain related to a life-threatening health condition.

Urgent

Moderate pain from non-life-threatening health conditions that require rapid intervention to prevent suffering.

Nonurgent

Pain from health conditions where the child is stable and the pain can be alleviated with basic pharmacologic and nonpharmacologic interventions.

Nursing Interventions

Effective pain management integrates both pharmacologic and nonpharmacologic measures. Paramount to management of acute pain is the assurance of effective communication and promotion of positive interactions among the child, caregivers, and emergency team. In certain situations, the combination of therapeutic interventions, such as holding the child's hand, allowing the child to hold a doll or teddy bear, or distraction therapy, with effective communication may significantly decrease the child's pain and anxiety.

The selection of pharmacologic and nonpharmacologic pain management interventions, including the specific medication to be used, is individualized based on the child's underlying health condition and/or the procedure to be performed. The child who presents to the ED in pain should have that pain managed before a procedure is begun (Acute Pain Management Guideline Panel, 1992).

Pharmacologic Interventions

Analgesics and anesthetics are used to decrease or alleviate pain. Analgesics are used to decrease pain without causing a loss of consciousness. Analgesics are either nonnarcotic or narcotic. These agents alter the child's perception of the pain rather than affecting the painful stimulus. Anesthetics can be local, topical, regional, or general. Anesthetics alleviate pain by eliminating the presence of normal sensation.

Analgesics

Nonnarcotic analgesics

- Acetaminophen works centrally on nonopioid receptors in the brain to inhibit prostaglandin synthetase. It is generally well tolerated. There are relatively few side effects when given in therapeutic doses. Acetaminophen produces analgesic and antipyretic effects but lacks anti-inflammatory properties. It is available in liquid, pill, and suppository form (Selbst, 2000).
- Nonsteroidal anti-inflammatory drugs (NSAIDs) act on the peripheral nervous system to block the formation of prostaglandin. They possess analgesic, antipyretic, and anti-inflammatory properties. They are indicated for arthritic pain, viral syndromes, dysmenorrhea, and soft tissue injuries. The NSAIDs may cause gastrointestinal bleeding, nausea, vomiting, abdominal pain, renal and hepatic dysfunction, and sodium retention. Children who are sensitive to aspirin should not take NSAIDs, because there is a cross-reactivity. The NSAIDs are available in liquid or pill form (Selbst, 2000). Use with caution in children with dehydration and in infants younger than 6 months of age.
- Acetylsalicyclic acid (aspirin) is used to treat minor pain related to headache, arthritis, myalgia, arthralgia, or sunburn (Selbst, 2000). In high doses, aspirin produces anti-inflammatory effects. The side effects of aspirin include gastric irritation, which may cause nausea and vomiting; bleeding as a result of inhibition of platelet function; liver toxicity; and central nervous system problems. Aspirin has been linked to Reye's syndrome when administered during varicella or flu-like illnesses.

Narcotic analgesics

- Morphine sulfate is indicated for sickle cell crisis, burns, fractures, or other trauma. Its peak effect occurs within 20 minutes, and its duration is 3 to 4 hours. It may cause vasodilation, bronchospasm, and peripheral pooling because of a release of histamine. Therefore, it is not indicated for the child who is hypotensive (Selbst, 2000). Morphine potentiates respiratory depression when administered with benzodiazepines. Pruritis is a common side effect of morphine.
- Meperidine hydrochloride can be administered intramuscularly or intravenously. Its peak effect is quicker than that of morphine sulfate; its duration is 3 to 4 hours. Side effects include nervousness, tremors, disorientation, and seizures, especially in patients receiving monamine oxidase (MAO) inhibitors (Selbst, 2000).
- Fentanyl citrate is a synthetic opioid that can be administered intravenously, nasally, or orally (e.g., lollipops or sublingually). It is used to relieve pain during procedures. It causes less vasodilation and pruritus than does morphine sulfate. The onset of action is rapid, and the duration of action is 30 to 40 minutes. Fentanyl does not cause the release of histamine; therefore, it rarely causes hypotension. Respiratory depression, bradycardia, and chest and abdominal wall rigidity have been reported as potential side effects.

The side effects of opioid analgesics include hypotension, nausea and vomiting, urinary retention, constipation, confusion, dizziness, sedation, and respiratory depression. Opioids have the following effects in infants and children (Ragg, 1997):

- Neonates and small infants have decreased liver metabolism and decreased renal excretion of the medication but have increased penetration of the drug in the cerebrospinal fluid, thus increasing the risk of side effects.
- The binding of opioids to plasma is reduced in infants; as a result, more active drug is available to the tissues.
- The larger percentage of body water in infants may require higher loading doses of the water-soluble opioids.
- Neonates and infants may be more susceptible to apnea with rapid intravenous infusion of opioids because the drug is quickly delivered to the brain.
- Vomiting is less common following opioid injection in infants and small children.

Anesthetics

Local anesthetics

- Lidocaine hydrochloride is used for wound repair, foreign-body removal, lumbar puncture, and drainage of abscesses, or for nerve blocks. It is available with or without epinephrine. Lidocaine with epinephrine should never be used in areas with decreased blood supply, such as fingers, toes, nose, penis, and ears. Lidocaine is effective within several minutes and lasts approximately 1.5 to 2 hours (Selbst, 2000). There are no major side effects. To prevent pain with lidocaine hydrochloride:
  - Use lidocaine hydrochloride with bicarbonate. Buffering the lidocaine with 1 mEq of bicarbonate reduces the pain associated with the lidocaine injection. The solution consists of 1 mL of bicarbonate (1 mEq/L) mixed with 9 mL of lidocaine.
  - Rub the area prior to infiltration of the lidocaine may reduce the pain of infiltration. This action supports the gate control pain theory, which states that rubbing stimulates other nerve endings that may close the gate and block the transmission of the pain impulse (Selbst, 2000).
- EMLA is a topical lidocaine cream that can be used to anesthetize an area prior to intravenous line placement, venipuncture, lumbar puncture, and perirectal abscess or paronychia drainage (Selbst, 2000). The cream is placed on the skin and then covered with an occlusive dressing. The disadvantage is the need to apply the cream 45 to 60 minutes prior to the procedure. It may be advisable to have the triage nurse or primary nurse apply the cream as soon as possible if any of the aforementioned procedures are anticipated. Another disadvantage is that if the cream is applied to decrease pain during phlebotomy or intravenous cannulation, and the vein is not cannulated, the cream must be reapplied to another site, thus delaying the onset of treatment.
- Tetracaine hydrochloride, adrenaline, and cocaine hydrochloride (TAC) is a topical anesthetic prepared using 0.5% tetracaine, 1:2,000 adrenaline, and 11.8% cocaine. Because of the possible absorption and toxicity associated with TAC, it should never be applied near or on mucous membranes. The solution is applied as follows (Emergency Nurses Association, 1997):
  - The TAC solution is applied to a cotton ball while held in a gloved hand. The cotton ball is placed on the wound using a cotton-tipped applicator, or held in place with a gloved hand; a reliable parent can hold the TAC in place and comfort the child. An alternative is to place the remaining cotton over the wound and tape to apply pressure, ensuring that the TAC comes in contact with all of the wound's surfaces.
  - The TAC is left in place for 20 to 25 minutes. The wound ends should blanch. Supplemental infiltration with lidocaine may be required.
  - The TAC solution should not be used on ears, nose, fingers, toes, or penis, because of the epinephrine.
- Lidocaine hydrochloride, epinephrine, and tetracaine hydrochloride (LET) is a topical anesthetic made with lidocaine 4%, epinephrine 0.1%, and tetracaine 0.5%. Reportedly, LET is as effective as TAC and does not pose the risk associated with the absorption of cocaine in TAC (Shilling, Bank, Borchert, Klazko, & Uden, 1995). The LET solution is applied with the same technique used for applying TAC. With the addition of methylcellulose LET can be made into a gel and painted onto the wound. The LET solution should not be used on ears, nose, fingers, toes, or penis, because of the epinephrine.

Inhaled Anesthetics

Nitrous oxide is used for its analgesic, sedative, and amnestic properties. Nitrous oxide may be considered for use with painful treatments, such as orthopedic procedures, minor surgical procedures, dressing changes, venous cannulation, lumbar puncture, suturing, and dental procedures. The child must be awake and able to follow instructions. The gas is administered by a physician. Nitrous oxide is not used in children with an altered level of consciousness, respiratory distress, head injury, traumatic injury with a potential ruptured viscous abdominal distention, or history of eating within the previous two hours. Nitrous oxide may increase intracranial pressure and causes rapid expansion of air-filled spaces (e.g., pneumothorax).

The nitrous oxide is administered via a demand unit that mixes 50% nitrous oxide with 50% oxygen or via a constant flow device. Both systems must be equipped with an exhalation valve that empties into a scavenger unit to avoid staff exposure to the gas. Airway equipment, pulse oximeter, and cardiac monitor must be available at the bedside. The child must be observed continuously for respiratory or cardiac compromise. Once the procedure is completed, the child should be placed on 100% oxygen for several minutes.

Conscious Sedation

Conscious sedation is a medically controlled state of depressed consciousness that (1) allows protective reflexes to be maintained; (2) retains the patient's ability to maintain a patent airway independently and continuously; and (3) permits appropriate response by the patient to physical stimulation or verbal command (American Academy of Pediatrics, 1992, p. 1110).

Conscious sedation involves the use of a combination of medications, usually given intravenously, to induce sedation and analgesia. It is indicated for very painful procedures, such as closed reduction of a fracture, burn care, dental procedures, abscess drainage, and complex laceration repair (Cunningham & Crain, 1997). Because the child is sedated, the availability of naloxone hydrochloride and flumazenil is essential, as is the presence of equipment to stabilize the airway and to provide cardiorespiratory monitoring.

The combination of medications in conscious sedation provides analgesia, amnesia, altered pain perception, muscle relaxation, and euphoria. The medications of choice are an opioid analgesic and a benzodiazepine. The combination of medications is based on the age of the child, the degree of pain or anxiety, the probable duration of the procedure, and the physician's preference and experience with the medications (Cunningham & Crain, 1997).

Opioids are used in conscious sedation to provide analgesia by elevating the pain threshold and altering the child's mood. The side effects of all opioids include respiratory depression, sedation, and gastrointestinal effects. These effects, including the analgesic effect, can be reversed by naloxone hydrochloride. The opioids that may be used are as follows:

- Morphine sulfate is useful in longer procedures that may cause moderate to severe pain. Very careful monitoring of the young infant is needed when morphine is given because morphine is less protein-bound in newborns, resulting in higher "free" morphine levels. In these infants, the clearance of morphine is also slower (Cunningham & Crain, 1997).
- Fentanyl citrate is short acting; therefore, it is useful in brief procedures. It is often given in conjunction with midazolam hydrochloride. The child's oxygen saturation level is closely monitored, because respiratory depression may occur. Side effects include facial pruritus, chest wall rigidity, hypotension, bradycardia, nausea, and vomiting (Cunningham & Crain, 1993).
- Meperidine hydrochloride is useful for moderately to severely painful procedures. A higher incidence of nausea, vomiting, and dizziness is possible than occurs with other narcotics. It is not used for patients with head trauma and increased intracranial pressure or for patients taking MAO inhibitors (Cunningham & Crain, 1997).

The use of a benzodiazepine with the narcotic provides both analgesic and amnestic effects. The benzodiazepine is responsible for the amnestic and anxiolytic effects during conscious sedation. Midazolam hydrochloride is the most frequently used benzodiazepine. However, lorazepam or diazepam may also be ordered. A benzodiazepine is often used to calm the child during procedures requiring a local anesthetic (e.g., laceration repair). If the child develops respiratory depression from the benzodiazepine, flumazenil, a benzodiazepine antagonist, may be administered:

- Midazolam hydrochloride is a short-acting agent that causes sedation, amnesia, and anxiolysis. Its onset of action is 3 to 5 minutes, and it has a short half-life. Midazolam hydrochloride can be administered intravenously, nasally, or orally. The dose is repeated until the desired effect is obtained. When midazolam hydrochloride is used in conjunction with a narcotic, the benzodiazepine is administered first because it will potentiate the effects of the narcotic (Cunningham & Crain, 1997). The child's respiratory status should be monitored carefully because midazolam hydrochloride may cause respiratory depression.
- Lorazepam and diazepam both may cause respiratory depression. Diazepam may also cause headaches. Diazepam may be painful when administered intravenously.

Barbiturates may be administered as an alternative to benzodiazepines for sedation. Barbiturates depress the central and peripheral nervous systems and skeletal, cardiac, and smooth muscle. Because barbiturates do not cause analgesia, an analgesic should be administered in conjunction. Thiopental and pentobarbital sodium are the most commonly ordered barbiturates because they are short-acting.

Ketamine may be used for its sedative effects during short procedures. It must be used carefully, because it can produce marked sedation and an increase in oral and airway secretions. Therefore, atropine sulfate should be administered simultaneously to decrease the secretions. Ketamine can be administered intravenously, orally, intramuscularly, or rectally. It should not be used in children with cardiovascular disease, respiratory disease, head injury, or conditions with the potential for increased intracranial pressure (Cunningham & Crain, 1997). Some children may experience emergence reactions as a side effect of ketamine. This reaction includes visual hallucinations, anxiety, and unpleasant dreams. The use of a benzodiazepine with the ketamine may minimize or eliminate this reaction.

The child undergoing conscious sedation must be carefully and continuously monitored. One nurse should be present who is solely responsible for providing cardiorespiratory, oxygen saturation, and blood pressure monitoring throughout the procedure (Emergency Nurses Association, 1998). Each institution should have a protocol for conscious sedation that defines the monitoring parameters that must be followed. A bag-valve-mask device, oxygen, suction equipment, intubation equipment, and naloxone hydrochloride should be available.

The child's level of consciousness must be continuously evaluated and documented. Frequent assessment of pulse rate, respiratory rate, respiratory effort, blood pressure, and oxygen saturation must be completed and documented. Resuscitation equipment must be immediately accessible, and a physician must be present who can intubate and initiate pediatric advanced life-support protocols. After the procedure is completed, the child must be monitored until fully awake and reactive. The child must be discharged to a reliable adult who can observe the child.

Nonpharmacologic Interventions

There are a plethora of nonpharmacologic therapies to reduce procedural-, illness-, or injury-related pain. Nonpharmacologic interventions are used to enhance pharmacologic interventions. The success of nonpharmacologic therapies is often dependent on developing effective communication among the emergency team, the child, and the caregiver. Encouraging the caregiver to remain in the room during the child's care and to provide assistance with nonpharmacologic interventions will facilitate this process (Chapter 4). The caregiver should be educated on his or her role during the procedure (Chapter 4).

The nonpharmacologic intervention selected is based on the child's and caregiver's needs and preferences. A careful explanation of the procedure and the nonpharmacologic intervention is given. The availability of child-friendly and family-centered surroundings and rewards may help to alleviate the anxiety associated with pain (see Chapter 4).

- Apply heat, cold, or massage to the affected body area. These interventions may be effective based on the gate control theory of pain.
- Position the child as comfortably as possible. For example, elevating an injured extremity may be effective in decreasing pain, while the side-lying fetal position may be effective in decreasing lower back or abdominal pain.
- Use distraction techniques, such as reading, singing, having the child concentrate on a particular object, or counting. Toys for providing distraction are:
  - Bubbles. Have the child blow, count, and/or burst the bubbles.
  - Kaleidoscope or "magic wand." Have the child count the number of each confetti color or shape in the magic wand. Encourage the child to look through the kaleidoscope.
  - Music therapy. Play music that is familiar to the child. The adolescent may like to use headsets.
  - Games. Counting games, riddles, puppets, or a spongy ball to squeeze may be helpful.
  - Reading a story to the child. When read by the caregiver, familiar stories and books provide comfort to the child.
  - Videotapes. Allow the child to choose a videotape to watch.
- Use deep breathing and relaxation techniques by encouraging the child to take slow, deep breaths. Soap bubbles or party blowers can be used with the smaller child to facilitate deep breathing. Asking the child to blow out imaginary birthday candles or a penlight also promotes deep breathing.
- Initiate guided imagery, which can be facilitated easily by the caregiver. The child is asked to think of his or her favorite place or event; the caregiver then asks the child questions about the place or event. Ask the child and caregiver to develop a story as they discuss the situation.
- Consider using hypnosis, an effective technique that may be difficult to initiate in the ED. Self-hypnosis can be encouraged in children who practice it for chronic pain; hypnosis can be initiated by an emergency team member who is proficient in its use.
- Encourage biofeedback in children who are able to cooperate or who are experienced in its use.
- Facilitate progressive relaxation by encouraging the child to tighten and relax different muscles (Bernardo & Conway, 1998).

Evaluation of the Effectiveness of Pharmacologic and Nonpharmacologic Interventions

The effectiveness of initiated pain management techniques is continuously evaluated throughout the ED visit:

- Ask the verbal child if pain is present; if present, ask about its quality and severity; ask the preverbal child to point to the pain or to nod or shake the head if pain is present or absent.
- Readminister the same pain assessment tool.
- Ascertain the caregivers' impression of how the child is feeling and whether the pain is decreased or alleviated.
- Observe the child's behavior and note any changes.
- Observe the child's physiologic response, including changes in vital signs, respiratory effort, and oxygen saturation.

If the evaluation demonstrates that pain is not alleviated, the treatment protocol is altered to include:

- Administration of another dose of the same medication.
- Administration of a different medication.
- Administration of the same medication but adding another medication to potentiate the effects.
- Initiation of other nonpharmacologic interventions.

Prevention of Pain

Procedure-related pain can be reduced or prevented through the combination of pharmacologic and nonpharmacologic therapies. Chronic pain may be ameliorated by teaching the child and caregiver selected therapeutic methods (e.g., distraction therapy, biofeedback, or hypnosis) that can be initiated at home and practiced in the ED as needed. Referrals to pain clinics can be initiated. Illness or injury-related pain should be recognized and treated; after the underlying pathology is corrected, the pain should subside with appropriate management. In one study of children discharged from an ED with analgesics, 96% of the parents believed their child's pain was well controlled (Chan, Russell, & Robak, 1998).

Conclusion

The management of pain in the ED requires an integrated approach of pharmacologic and nonpharmacologic therapies. Policies and procedures should be in place for expediting the initiation of pain-relieving measures. Early and continued assessment of pain in the child is essential to providing appropriate care. This assessment presents many challenges, particularly in the preverbal child. The caregiver is an essential link in the assessment, intervention, and evaluation process. The caregiver can identify the specific signs that indicate the child is in pain and can be involved in the treatment process to alleviate the pain. Emergency nurses are the child's advocate in pain management.

References

Acute Pain Management Guideline Panel. (1992, February). *Acute pain management: Operative or medical procedures and trauma.* Clinical practice guideline (AHCPR Publication No. 92-0032). Rockville, MD: Agency for Health Care Policy and Research, Public Health Service, U.S. Department of Health and Human Services.

American Academy of Pediatrics. (1992). Guidelines for monitoring and management of pediatric patients during and after sedation for diagnostic and therapeutic procedures. *Pediatrics, 89*(6), 1110-1115.

Anand, K., & Hickey, M. (1987). Pain and its effects on the human neonate and fetus. *New England Journal of Medicine, 31*(7), 1321-1329.

Anand, K., & McGrath, P. (Eds.). (1993). *Neonatal pain and distress.* Amsterdam: Elsevier.

Avner, J. R. (1997). Pain management techniques. In F. M. Henretig & C. King (Eds.), *Textbook of pediatric emergency procedures* (pp. 437-444). Baltimore, MD: Williams & Wilkins.

Bernardo, L. M., & Conway, A. E. (1998). Pain assessment and management. In T. Soud & J. Rogers (Eds.), *Manual of pediatric emergency nursing* (pp. 686-711). St. Louis: Mosby—Year Book.

Chan, L., Russell, T., & Robak, N. (1998). Parental perception of the adequacy of pain control in their child after discharge from the emergency department. *Pediatric Emergency Care, 14*(4), 251-3.

Cunningham, S. J., & Crain, E. F. (1997). Conscious sedation. In F. M. Henretig & C. King (Eds.), *Textbook of pediatric emergency procedures* (pp. 445-454). Baltimore, MD: Williams & Wilkins.

Emergency Nurses Association. (1998). *Emergency nursing pediatric course: Instructor manual.* Park Ridge, IL: Author.

Emergency Nurses Association. (1995). *Course in advanced trauma nursing: A conceptual approach* (pp. 253-278). Park Ridge, IL: Author.

Emergency Nurses Association. (1997). *Orientation to emergency nursing: Diversity in practice.* Park Ridge, IL: Author.

Emergency Nurses Association. (1998). Conscious sedation. Des Plaines. IL: Author.

Guyton, A. C. (2000). Somatic sensations. II. Pain, headache, and thermal sensations. In A. C. Guyton (Ed.), *Textbook of medical physiology* (9th ed., pp. 552-563). Philadelphia: Saunders.

International Association for the Study of Pain, Subcommittee on Taxonomy. (1979). *Pain terms: a list with definitions and notes on usage, 6*(3), 249-252.

McCaffrey, M. (1979). Misconceptions that hamper assessment. In M. McCaffrey (Ed.), *Nursing the patient in pain* (2nd ed., p. 14). Philadelphia: Lippincott.

McGrath, P. A. (1993). Psychological aspects of pain perception. In N. L. Schechter, C. B. Berde, & M. Yaster (Eds.), *Pain in infants, children, and adolescents* (pp. 39-63). Baltimore, MD: Williams & Wilkins.

McKenzie, I. (1997). Developmental physiology and psychology. In I. McKenzie, P. B. Gaukroger, P. Ragg, & T. Brown (Eds.), *Manual of acute pain management in children* (pp. 7-11). New York: Churchill Livingstone.

Melzack, R., & Wall, P. (1965). Pain mechanism: A new theory. *Science, 150*, 971-979.

Ragg, P. (1997). Opioids in children. In I. McKenzie, P. B. Gaukroger, P. Ragg, & T. Brown (Eds.), *Manual of acute pain management in children* (pp. 25-38). New York: Churchill Livingstone.

Selbst, S. M. (2000). Sedation and analgesia. In G. R. Fleisher & S. Ludwig (Eds.), *Textbook of pediatric emergency medicine* (4th ed., pp. 59-82). Baltimore, MD: Williams & Wilkins.

Shilling, C. G., Bank, D. E., Borchert, B. A., Klazko, M. D., & Uden, D. L. (1995). Tetracaine, epinephrine (adrenaline), and cocaine (TAC) versus lidocaine, epinephrine, and tetracaine (LET) for anesthesia of lacerations in children. *Annals of Emergency Medicine, 25*(2), 203-208.

Willens, J. (1994). Pain management in the trauma victim. In V. D. Cardona, P. D. Hurn, P. J. B. Mason, A. M. Scanlon, & S. W. Veise-Berry (Eds.), *Trauma nursing: From resuscitation through rehabilitation* (2nd ed., pp. 325-362). Philadelphia: Saunders.

Wong, D. L. (1999). Family-centered care of the child during illness and hospitalization. In D. L. Wong (Ed.), *Whaley & Wong's nursing care of infants and children* (6th ed., pp. 1131-1209). St. Louis: Mosby—Year Book.

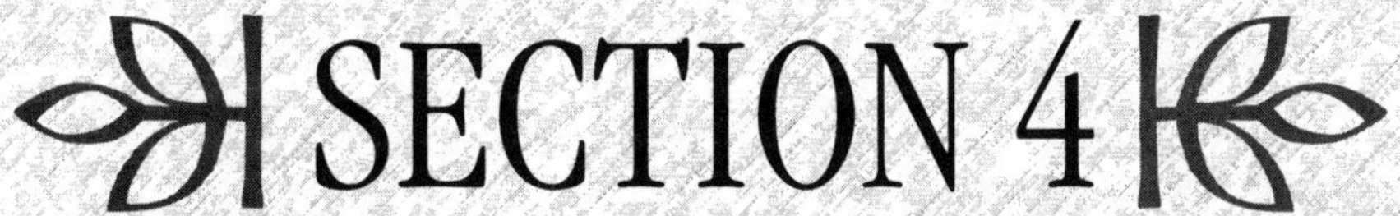

Resuscitation

14

Neonatal Resuscitation

Sarah A. Martin, RN, MS, PCCNP, CPNP, CCRN
Tracy Karp, RN, NNP
David C. LaCovey, NREMT-P

Introduction

Although the optimal setting for neonatal resuscitation is in the delivery room with trained personnel and neonatal-specific equipment, the emergency department (ED) may have to be transformed into a delivery room to attend to an unanticipated birth. Unanticipated births occur in about one in every 300 births (Brunette & Sterner, 1989); about one in 160 births occurs at home or enroute to the hospital. ED staff need to be prepared and have the necessary equipment to resuscitate an infant born unexpectedly. Chances for successful outcomes for the neonate requiring resuscitation are increased with advanced preparation of personnel and necessary equipment.

An educational program offered by the American Heart Association provides in-depth knowledge in neonatal resuscitation: Neonatal Resuscitation Program (Kattwinkel, 2000). Emergency nurses can attend this course to obtain this specialized knowledge. The purposes of this chapter are to describe the factors leading to neonatal resuscitation and to outline the process of neonatal resuscitation.

Etiology of Unanticipated Birth

The trigger for normal labor is unknown, and the length of labor is dependent on the mother's parity. For the average primigravida, about 11 hours are required for cervical dilation and about 1.1 hours are needed for delivery. For the average multigravida, about 7 hours are required for cervical dilation and about 0.4 hours are needed for delivery.

The following conditions can initiate labor:

- Obstetric:
  - Trauma.
  - Vaginal bleeding.
  - Infection.
  - Drug use (cocaine or amphetamines).
- Fetal distress:
  - Placental insufficiency.
  - Presentation abnormalities (breech, transverse lie, shoulder dystocia).
  - Anemia.
  - Asphyxia neonatorium.

The need for resuscitation of the neonate is rare. However, as many as 80% of neonates weighing less than 1,500 g require some resuscitative intervention (Alesanbrini, 2000). Conditions associated with neonatal resuscitation are outlined in Table 14.1.

Birth is a time of significant physiologic transition, as the cardiac and pulmonary circulation of the fetus transforms to neonatal circulation. The restrictive nature of the birth canal compresses the infant's thorax during a vaginal delivery and expels fluid from the lungs. The birth process reduces airway resistance in the lungs and allows the neonate to take the first breath. Gas exchange is transferred from the maternal-placental unit to ventilation and perfusion in the neonate's pulmonary system. With this transition, there is a decrease in pulmonary artery pressure and an increase in systolic blood pressure. The blood no longer flows from the pulmonary artery through the ductus arteriosus to the aorta; it is redirected into the neonate's pulmonary artery and into the lungs.

Focused History

- Maternal health history:
  - Prenatal care. Lack of prenatal care may result in a high-risk delivery.
  - Parity.
  - Number of live births.

TABLE 14.1 Selected Conditions Associated with Increased Risk for Neonatal Resuscitation

Antepartum Maternal Factors	*Intrapartum Maternal or Fetal Factors*
> 35 years or < 16 years	Breech or other abnormal presentation
Diabetes	Infection
Bleeding in second or third trimester	Prolonged labor
Chronic illness	Prolonged rupture of membranes
Drug therapy (e.g., magnesium, adrenergic blocking agents, and lithium)	Prolapsed cord
Substance abuse	Maternal narcotic administration with 4 hours of delivery
Previous fetal or neonatal death	Operative delivery
No prenatal care	Meconium-stained amniotic fluid
Pregnancy-induced or chronic hypertension	Emergency cesarean section
Anemia/isoimmunization	Fetal bradycardia
Infection	Abruptio placenta
Multifetal gestation	Placenta previa
Postterm gestation	
Premature rupture of membranes	
Oligohydramnios/polyhydramnios	
Diminished fetal activity	

Adapted from: American Heart Association, 2000, *Guidelines 2000 for cardiopulmonary resuscitation and emergency cardiovascular care* (p. 346), Dallas, TX: Author.

   - Previous pregnancy complications, such as gestational diabetes and hypertension. Both are associated with an increase in perinatal morbidity.
   - Previous health history.
- Current labor history:
   - Number of babies anticipated.
   - Date of the last menstrual period, needed to estimate the gestational age to determine whether the unborn neonate is premature (less than 37 weeks gestation).
   - Color of the amniotic fluid. Meconium-stained fluid suggests potential risk of meconium aspiration and the need for specialized respiratory care.
   - Time that membranes ruptured. Prolonged rupture of membranes can be associated with infectious complications.
   - Duration of labor and contraction status.
   - Presence of unusual vaginal bleeding.
   - Maternal drug or alcohol use, to anticipate possible narcotic withdrawal.
   - Fetal activity.

Nursing Assessment and Interventions for the Mother

- Measure the mother's heart rate, respiratory rate, and blood pressure.
- Initiate measures to support airway, breathing, and circulation, as needed.
- Assess the mother's contraction status and cervical dilation.
- Attach a fetal heart monitor to measure the fetal heart rate and tolerance to contractions.
- Provide reassurance to the mother. Contact other family members or support persons at the mother's request.
- Administer analgesics as needed.
- Assist with the infant's delivery.
- Prepare for the delivery of the placenta.
- Perform fundal massage.
- Observe and record the amount of bleeding.
- Prepare for transfer and/or transport to a hospital with maternity capabilities, as needed (Chapter 10).

TABLE 14.2 Nursing Diagnoses and Expected Outcomes

Nursing Diagnoses	*Expected Outcomes*
Ineffective airway clearance related to prematurity or meconium aspiration.	The neonate will maintain a patent airway, with or without airway adjuncts, suctioning, and positioning.
Ineffective thermoregulation, related to environmental temperature, skin wet with amniotic fluid, and large body surface area.	The neonate will maintain normothermia through the use of external heat sources.
Altered tissue perfusion (cardiopulmonary, cerebral, renal, gastrointestinal, and peripheral) related to cardiopulmonary instability or arrest.	The neonate will be well perfused, as evidenced by normotension, capillary refill < 3 seconds, strong peripheral pulses, adequate urinary output, and quiet, alert wakefulness.

Nursing Assessment and Interventions for the Neonate

- Prepare to perform the four categories of neonatal resuscitation (American Heart Association, 2000):
  - Rapid assessment and initial steps in stabilization.
  - Ventilation, including bag-mask or bag-tube.
  - Chest compressions.
  - Administration of medications or fluids.
- Perform a rapid assessment and initial steps in stabilization:
  - Place the neonate supine with the head in a neutral position for optimal airway patency.
  - Dry and place the infant in a radiant warmer; avoid hyperthermia.
  - In the neonate *without* meconium present, suction the neonate's mouth and then the nose.
  - In the neonate *with* meconium present (American Heart Association, 2000), suction meconium from the hypopharnyx immediately upon delivery of the head. Perform direct tracheal suctioning to remove meconium from the airway if the infant has absentce of depressed respirations, heart rate < 100, or poor muscle tone.

FIGURE 14.1 Algorithm for resuscitation of the newly born infant

1. Evaluate the adequacy of respiratory effort:
   - Auscultate breath sounds for:
     - Rate.
     - Presence and equality.
     - Adventitious breath sounds.
   - Inspect the chest for:
     - Equal movement.
     - Use of accessory muscles.
   - Observe for signs of respiratory distress or insufficiency (Chapter 16):
     - Respiratory insufficiency may yield an inadequate heart rate; thus the heart rate should be evaluated immediately following the initial respiratory assessment.
   - Stimulate (by drying, warming, or suctioning) the neonate to promote spontaneous respiratory effort.
   - Initiate positive-pressure ventilation with 100% forced inspiratory oxygen if there is inadequate respiratory effort or heart rate is less than 100 beats per minute. Continue positive-pressure ventilation if there is:
     - Apnea or gasping respirations.
     - Heart rate of less than 100 beats per minute.
     - Persistent central cyanosis.
2. Assess the circulatory status:
   - Palpate the base of the umbilical cord for pulsations:
     - Rate.
     - Quality.
   - Palpate the brachial and/or femoral arteries for:
     - Rate.
     - Quality.
     - Comparison with the umbilical cord.
   - Auscultate the heart for rate (American Heart Association, 2000):
     - If the apical rate is > 100 beats per minute (bpm), continue ongoing assessment of respiratory effort.
     - If the heart rate is < 60 bpm despite adequate positive pressure ventilation for 30 seconds, initiate chest compressions.
     - Use the two-thumb technique to compress the sternum one-third the depth of the anterior/posterior chest diameter.
     - Compress at 3 compressions to 1 ventilation with 90 compressions and 30 breaths to achieve 120 events per minute.

- Administer resuscitation medication (epinephrine) if the heart rate remains at < 60 bpm despite 30 seconds of adequate ventilation and compression (Table 14.3).
- Murmurs (Chapter 17).
- Evaluate peripheral perfusion:
  - Palpate pulses in all four extremities for rate, quality, equality.
  - Measure capillary refill.
  - Measure skin temperature by touching the skin: Temperature is assessed because hypothermia is poorly tolerated by the stressed neonate.
  - Inspect skin color.
- Calculate an Apgar score (Table 14.4):
  - The Apgar score is a universal statistical assessment tool utilized at all births.

TABLE 14.3 Commonly Used Resuscitation Medications

Medication	*Dose/Route*	*Indication for Use*	*Action*	*Side Effects*	*Nursing Implications*
Epinephrine (Adrenaline®)	E.T., I.V., U.V.: 0.01–0.03 mg/kg (1:10,000) every 3 to 5 minutes	Cardiac arrest. Symptomatic bradycardia unresponsive to oxygen administration, ventilation, and chest compressions. Hypotension not related to volume depletion.	Alpha-adrenergic effect (vasoconstriction) increases systemic vascular resistance and increases systolic and diastolic BP. Beta-adrenergic action increases myocardial contractility, increases heart rate, relaxes smooth muscle in the skeletal muscle vascular bed and in the bronchi.	Tachycardia, hypertension, increased myocardial oxygen consumption, cardiac arrhythmias, decreased renal and splanchnic blood flow.	Incompatible with alkaline solutions. Tissue irritant; extravasation may be treated with phentolamine. Dilute with 3–5 ml of normal saline prior to E.T. administration.
Sodium bicarbonate ($NaHCO_3$) 4.2%	I.V., U.V.: 1–2 mEq/kg of a 0.5 mEq/ml solution as a single dose, may repeat with 0.5 mEq/kg	Used for documented metabolic acidosis.	Elevates the plasma pH.	Edema, cerebral hemorrhage (especially with rapid injection of the hyperosmotic $NaHCO_3$), hypernatremia, hypocalcemia.	Administer over 2 minutes. Tissue necrosis can occur with extravasation. Do not mix $NaHCO_3$ with calcium salts, catecholamine, and atropine.
Naloxone (Narcan®)	I.V., U.V., I.M., E.T.: Birth to 5 years or ≤ 20 kg: 0.1 mg/kg. May be administered every 2 to 3 minutes.	Reverse the effects of narcotic overdose.	Pure opiate antagonist that reverses the effect of narcotics.	Rare and related to the abrupt reversal of narcotic. Hypertension, hypotension, tachycardia, ventricular arrhythmias, cardiac arrest, nausea, vomiting, and increased sweating.	Dilute with 3 to 5 cc of saline prior to endotracheal administration.
Dextrose	I.V., U.V.: $D_{10}W$ 5–10 ml/kg	Hypoglycemia; hypothermia.	Glucose provides a significant energy source during episodes of ischemia.	Hyperglycemia.	Hypertonic glucose ($D_{25}W$ or $D_{50}W$) is hyperosmolar and may sclerose peripheral veins. The concentration of glucose administered to neonates should not exceed $D_{10}W$.
Normal saline solution or Ringer's lactate	I.V., U.V.: 10 ml/kg repeat if needed	Hypovolemia. Failure to respond to resuscitation measures. (Suspect shock or blood loss.)	Expands the intravascular volume.	Intracranial hemorrhage.	Administer slower over 5–10 minutes.

I.V. = intravenous; E.T. = endotracheal; I.M. = intramuscular; U.V. = umbilical vein.
From: American Heart Association, 2000; Taketomo, Holding, & Kraus, 2000

TABLE 14.4
Apgar Score

Sign/Score	***0***	***1***	***2***
Heart rate	Absent	<100	>100
Respirations	Absent	Slow, irregular	Good, crying
Muscle tone	Limp	Some flexion	Active motion
Reflex irritability	No response	Grimace	Cough or sneeze
Color	Blue or pale	Pink body with blue extremities	Completely pink

From: Apgar, 1953. A proposal for a new method of evaluation of the newborn infant. *Anesthesia Analogues, 32*, 260–267.

- An Apgar score is never used to determine the need for resuscitation.
- Establish intravenous access, with the umbilical vein as (UV) the preferred route. Considerations during UV cannulation are (American Heart Association, 2000):
  - The depth of catheter placement should not exceed 5–6 cm; this action avoids cannulation of the portal vein.
  - The UV catheter should be flushed with normal saline solution prior to insertion; this action avoids the introduction of air into the central circulation.
- Obtain serial laboratory tests, such as:
  - Arterial blood gases.
  - Electrolytes.
  - Glucose. Prepare to administer intravenous glucose as needed.
  - Complete blood count.
- Measure urinary output amounts.
- Monitor intravenous fluid amount.
- Perform a rapid general assessment to identify any obvious congenital anomalies:
  - Inspect the neonate's general appearance, particularly for any dysmorphic features.
  - Observe for any missing body appendages.
  - Note any midline defects, such as encephalocele, oomphalocele/gastroschisis, myelomeningocele, or facial or cleft palates.
  - Observe for an anal opening.
  - Observe the infant's movement of all extremities; note any bruising or swelling.
- Provide post-resuscitation care:
  - Perform continuous cardiorespiratory and oxygen saturation monitoring.
  - Continue supplemental oxygen and mechanical ventilation.
  - Secure venous access sites.
  - Perform serial neurologic examinations.
  - Provide gastric decompression with the insertion of a nasogastric tube.
  - Maintain normothermia with the application of external heat sources.
- Provide the mother and other family members with frequent updates of the infant's condition.
- Prepare for transfer or transport to the newborn nursery or neonatal intensive care unit (Chapter 10). Ensure that the neonate is STABLE:
  - Blood *S*ugar is normal.
  - *T*emperature is normal.
  - *A*irway and breathing are adequate.
  - *B*lood pressure is normal.
  - Appropriate *L*aboratory tests are obtained to rule out infection, including complete blood count and blood cultures. Antibiotics (ampicillin and gentamicin) should be started for any neonate needing resuscitation.
  - *E*motional support is provided for the family.
- Ensure that any congenital anomalies are appropriately protected.
- Provide support (clergy, social work) if the neonate dies in the emergency department (Chapter 28).

Prevention

Prevention of neonatal resuscitation begins with adequate prenatal care. The reduction of maternal risk factors associated with increased perinatal morbidity should be initiated early in pregnancy.

References

Alessanbrini, E. (2000). Neonatal resuscitation. In G. R. Fleisher, & S. Ludwig (Eds.), *Textbook of pediatric emergency medicine* (4th ed., pp. 33-46).

American Heart Association. (2000). *Guidelines 2000 for cardiopulmonary resuscitation and emergency cardiovascular care* (pp. 343-357). Dallas, TX: Author.

Apgar (1953). A proposal for a new method of evaluation of the newborn infant. *Anesthesia Analogues, 32,* 260-267.

Brunette, D., & Sterner, S. (1989). Prehospital and ED delivery: A review of eight years' experience. *Annals of Emergency Medicine, 18*(10), 116-118.

Kattwinkel, J. (2000). *Textbook of neonatal resuscitation*. Elk Grove, IL: American Academy of Pediatrics and American Heart Association.

Taketomo, C., Hodding, J., & Kraus, D. (2000). *Pediatric dosage handbook* (7th ed.). Cleveland, OH: Lexi-comp.

15

Pediatric Resuscitation

Sarah A. Martin, RN, MS, PCCNP, CPNP, CCRN
David C. LaCovey, NREMT-P

Introduction

Cardiopulmonary arrest is rarely a sudden event in the pediatric population. Unlike adults, in children the usual etiologic factor of cardiopulmonary arrest is respiratory failure. Therefore, it is of the utmost importance that emergency nurses recognize the child in respiratory distress and intervene accordingly. Early recognition and intervention may prevent cardiac and respiratory failure, thus minimizing subsequent multiple-organ system dysfunction and associated morbidity and mortality. Despite prompt emergency interventions, survival outcomes for the pediatric victim of cardiac arrest are poor; mortality is as high as 91% (Zaritsky, Nadkarni, Getson, & Kuehl, 1987). In a study of 100 children in respiratory and/or cardiac arrest admitted to a children's hospital emergency department (ED), only 15% were successfully resuscitated and eventually discharged (Schindler, Bohn, Cox, McCrindle, Jarvis, Edmonds, & Barker, 1996). No children who required two doses of epinephrine or more than 20 minutes of resuscitation survived (Schindler et al., 1996).

The successful resuscitation of infants and children requires knowledge of the etiology, assessment, interventions, and outcomes of the need for advanced life support. The purpose of this chapter is to outline the nursing assessment and interventions for pediatric resuscitation. In-depth knowledge can be obtained by attending a standardized course on pediatric advanced life support (Pediatric Advanced Life Support Course or Advanced Pediatric Life Support Course).

Etiology

Cardiopulmonary arrest occurs most commonly in infants (younger than 1 year of age) and in adolescents. In most instances, the cause of cardiac arrest is respiratory failure. The etiologies of arrest in the infant and child are diverse (Table 15.1). Studies estimate that 43 to 80% of cardiac arrests in infants and young children, are secondary to respiratory compromise; however, after 1 year of age, trauma is the leading cause of death (Scott & Wiebe, 1996). Children with congenital heart disease may present with cardiac arrest unrelated to respiratory failure.

Focused History

Events leading to the cardiopulmonary arrest

- Trauma related.
- Suspected child maltreatment (Chapter 46).
- Illness related:
  - Symptoms.
  - Length of illness.
  - Current treatment.

Length of time the child had no cardiac or respiratory function

Initiation of cardiopulmonary resuscitation (CPR)

- When CPR was initiated.
- Who initiated CPR.
- Length of time CPR was administered prior to ED arrival.
- Child's response to CPR (pulses regained or pulses absent).

TABLE 15.1 Etiologies of Cardiac and Respiratory Arrest in Infants and Children

Etiology	*Younger than 1 Year*	*1 to 12 years*	*Adolescence*
Respiratory	Pneumonia Bronchiolitis Upper airway obstruction (e.g., foreign body, croup, epiglottitis) Sudden infant death syndrome (SIDS) Apparent life-threatening event (ALTE)	Bronchopulmonary dysplasia Asthma Upper airway obstruction (e.g., foreign body) Bronchiolitis	Asthma
Cardiac disease	Congenital heart disease Dysrhythmias Cardiomyopathy	Congenital heart disease Dysrhythmias Cardiomyopathy	Congenital heart disease Dysrhythmias
Central nervous system	Seizures Meningitis Hydrocephalus	Seizures Coma	
Infectious disease	Sepsis Pneumonia Meningitis	Meningitis Pneumonia Sepsis	
Trauma	Child maltreatment Burns/smoke inhalation	Drowning Child maltreatment Burns/smoke inhalation Intracranial hemorrhage (subdural hematoma, epidural hematoma, intraventricular hemorrhage)	Pedestrian, motor vehicle, or bike crashes Homicide Falls Homicide Pedestrian, bike, and motor vehicle crashes
Congenital anomalies	Chromosomal abnormalities Inborn errors of metabolism		

Initiation of advanced life-support measures

- Airway maintenance with endotracheal intubation.
- Defibrillation.
- Initiation of an intravenous or intraosseous infusion.
- Administration of endotracheal, intravenous, or intraosseous medications.

Previous health history

- Any prodromal signs and symptoms that the child exhibited.
- Chronic health conditions (e.g., congenital heart disease, bronchopulmonary dysplasia, sickle cell disease, asplenia, central nervous system condition, epilepsy, or asthma).
- Allergies.
- Current over-the-counter and prescribed medication regimens.
- Immunization status.
- Medications prescribed for other persons in the home (e.g., suspected poisoning, Chapter 44).

Table 15.2 outlines the results of the focused history.

Nursing Assessment and Interventions

1. Initiate basic life support maneuvers (Table 15.3).
2. Assess the airway for patency; presence of secretions or foreign bodies (chewing gum, teeth, or small objects).
3. Assess respiratory effort. Inspect the chest for:
   - Work of breathing:
     - Accessory muscle use and retractions.
     - Head bobbing.
     - Nasal flaring.
     - Grunting.
   - Chest expansion and symmetry.
   - Color:

TABLE 15.2 Nursing Diagnoses and Expected Outcomes

Nursing Diagnoses	*Expected Outcomes*
Ineffective airway clearance related to respiratory failure or arrest, and altered level of consciousness.	The child will have a patent airway, as evidenced by: • Insertion and maintenance of an airway adjunct. • Equal chest expansion. • Equal breath sounds in all lobes. • Adequate oxygen saturation.
Decreased cardiac output related to cardiopulmonary insufficiency and/or cardiac arrest.	The child will have adequate cardiac output, as evidenced by: • Normotension. • Heart rate normal for age. • Capillary refill < 3 seconds. • Warm and dry skin.
Ineffective family coping related to the child's respiratory and/or cardiac failure/arrest.	Parents will begin to demonstrate effective coping as evidenced by: • Verbalization of an accurate understanding of their child's condition. • Recognition of the need to accept support from others.

TABLE 15.3 Basic Life Support for the Infant, Child, and Adolescent

Maneuver	*Infant (<1 year)*	*Child (1–8 years)*	*Adolescent (>8 years)*
Airway	Head tilt—chin lift (jaw thrust if trauma present)	Head tilt—chin lift (jaw thrust if trauma present)	Head tilt—chin lift (jaw thrust if trauma present)
Breathing	*Initial*: 2 effective breaths at 1 to 1-½ seconds/breath *Subsequent*: 20 effective breaths/minute	*Initial*: 2 effective breaths at 1 to 1-½ seconds/breath *Subsequent*: 20 effective breaths/minute	*Initial*: 2 effective breaths at 2 seconds/breath *Subsequent*: 12 effective breaths/minute
Circulation:			
Pulse check	Brachial artery	Carotid artery	Carotid artery
Compression area Compression width	Lower 1/2 of sternum 2 fingers	Lower 1/2 of sternum Heel of 1 hand	Lower 1/2 of sternum Both hands (heel of 1 hand, with other hand on top)
Depth	Approximately 1/3 to 1/2 the depth of the chest	Approximately 1/3 to 1/2 the depth of the chest	Approximately 1-½ to 2 inches for normal-sized older child
Rate of compressions	At least 100/minute	Approximately 100/minute	Approximately 100/minute
Compression-ventilation ratio	5:1	5:1	15:2
Foreign-body airway obstruction	Back blows/chest thrusts	Abdominal thrusts/ back blows/chest thrusts	Abdominal thrusts/back blows/ chest thrusts

Adapted from: American Heart Association, 2001, p. 117.

- Central cyanosis is a sign of respiratory failure and reflects hypoxemia.
- Peripheral cyanosis reflects poor peripheral perfusion and compensatory vasoconstriction secondary to shock or hypothermia.

■ Signs of surface trauma (e.g., bruising or open wounds).

4. Auscultate the chest for:
   - Respiratory rate (bradypnea or apnea).
   - Quality of breath sounds/presence of adventitious sounds.
   - Equality of breath sounds.
5. Measure oxygen saturation.

6. Assess cardiac function. Auscultate the heart for:
   - Rate:
     - As a compensatory response to a decreased cardiac output, children may initially increase their heart rate.
     - A decreased heart rate is generally an ominous sign and may occur in the presence of significant hypoxemia.
   - Quality and murmurs.
   - Rhythm.
7. Measure blood pressure.
8. Assess systemic perfusion
   - Inspect the skin for:
     - Color.
     - Temperature.
   - Palpate peripheral pulses for:
     - Quality.
     - Equality.
     - Rate.
   - Assess capillary refill.
   - Measure urinary output.
9. Assess neurologic status
   - Assess level of consciousness with the Glasgow coma scale or AVPU method (alert, responds to verbal stimuli, responds to painful stimuli, unresponsive).
   - Inspect pupils for:
     - Equality.
     - Response to light.
     - Size.
10. Expose the patient:
    - Measure the core temperature:
      - Hypothermia may be present and may affect the efficacy of administered medications.
11. Initiate Pediatric Advanced Life Support Measures (for patients not responsive to basic life support maneuvers):
    - Prepare for tracheal intubation.
    - Provide ventilatory assistance:
      - Oxygenate the patient with 100% forced inspiratory oxygen using bag-valve-mask ventilation.
      - Prepare for mechanical ventilation (Chapter 16).
    - Continue chest compressions.
    - Secure venous access.
      - Attempt peripheral venous access.
      - If peripheral venous access is not attained within three attempts or 90 seconds, attempt intraosseous access.
      - Secure central venous access if attempts at peripheral venous and intraosseous access are unsuccessful and a practitioner skilled in the procedure is present.
    - Administer resuscitative medications (Table 15.4).
    - Obtain blood for laboratory testing, such as:
      - Arterial blood gases.
      - Electrolytes.
      - Glucose.
      - Complete blood count.
      - Toxicology testing (in suspected poisoning).
12. Offer parents frequent updates on their child's condition:
    - The unexpected cardiac or respiratory arrest is a time of crisis (Chapter 28).
    - Consider having the family present during resuscitation (Emergency Nurses Association, 1996; American Heart Association, 2000).
    - Consult pastoral care staff and social services to assist with crisis intervention.
13. Perform post-resuscitation care:
    - Continue frequent assessment of cardiopulmonary function.
    - Administer humidified oxygen at the highest possible concentration unless objective assessment by blood gas or noninvasive monitoring reflects adequate arterial saturation.
    - Obtain serial neurologic evaluation.
    - Insert a nasogastric tube for gastric decompression.
    - Insert an in-dwelling bladder catheter for bladder decompression.
    - Maintain normothermia with warming lights, warm blankets, or warm intravenous fluids; avoid hyperthermia.
    - Prepare for transfer or transport to a pediatric intensive care unit (Chapter 10).

Prevention

The prevention of pediatric cardiopulmonary arrest is early recognition of respiratory distress. The initiation of measures to relieve respiratory distress prevents further cardiopulmonary compromise. Other general preventive measures include anticipatory guidance (Chapter 4), injury and illness reduction (Chapter 5), and poison prevention (Chapter 44).

TABLE 15.4 Commonly Used Resuscitation Medications

Medication	*Dose/Route*	*Indication for Use*	*Action*	*Side Effects*	*Nursing Implications*
Epinephrine (Adrenaline®)	I.V., I.O.: Initial dose 0.01 mg/kg (1:10,000) Second and subsequent doses may be considered: I.V., I.O.: 0.01–0.1 mg/kg Initial and subsequent doses E.T.: 0.1 mg/kg (1:1,000)	• Cardiac arrest • Symptomatic bradycardia unresponsive to oxygen administration and ventilation • Hypotension not related to volume depletion	Alpha-adrenergic effect (vasoconstriction) increases systemic vascular resistance and increases systolic and diastolic BP. Beta-adrenergic action increases myocardial contractility, increases heart rate, relaxes smooth muscle in the skeletal muscle vascular bed, and in the bronchi.	Tachycardia, hypertension, increased myocardial oxygen consumption, cardiac dysrhythmias, anxiety, headache, weakness, tremor, decreased renal and splanchnic blood flow.	Incompatible with alkaline solutions. Tissue irritant; extravasation may be treated with phentolamine.
Atropine	I.V., E.T., I.O.: 0.02 mg/kg May be administered through the E.T. tube at 2 to 3 times the I.V. dose.	• Symptomatic bradycardia • Prevent or treat vagally mediated bradycardia	Parasympatholytic drug that accelerates sinus or atrial pacemakers and atrioventricular conduction.	Tachycardia, palpitations, fatigue, headache, restlessness, impaired GI motility, and blurred vision.	Dose must be sufficient to produce vagolytic effects. Minimum dose in a child is 0.1 mg and a maximum dose of 0.5 mg in a child and 1.0 mg for an adolescent.
Sodium Bicarbonate	I.V.: 1 mEq/kg as a single dose	• Used for documented metabolic acidosis	Elevates the plasma pH.	Edema, cerebral hemorrhage (especially with rapid injection), hypernatremia, gastric distension.	Tissue necrosis can occur with extravasation. Do not mix $NaHCO_3$ with calcium salts, catecholamines, and atropine.
Dextrose	Child $D_{25}W$ 2–4 ml/kg I.V./I.O.	• Hypoglycemia	Glucose provides a significant energy source during episodes of stress.	Hyperglycemia	Hypertonic glucose ($D_{25}W$ or $D_{50}W$) is hyperosmolar and may sclerose peripheral veins. The concentration of glucose administered to neonates should not exceed $D_{10}W$.
Calcium chloride 10%	20 mg/kg I.V., I.O. may repeat 1 minute as necessary	• Emergency treatment of hypocalcemic tetany. • Treatment of hypermagnesemia. • Cardiac disturbances related to hyperkalemia, hypocalcemia, or calcium channel blocking agent toxicity.	Mediates nerve and muscle performance via action potential excitation threshold regulation.	Vasodilation, hypotension, bradycardia, cardiac arrhythmias, ventricular fibrillation, lethargy, coma, erythema, tissue necrosis, muscle weakness	

(continued)

TABLE 15.4 Commonly Used Resuscitation Medications (continued)

Medication	*Dose/Route*	*Indication for Use*	*Action*	*Side Effects*	*Nursing Implications*
Adenosine (Adenocard)	I.V.: 0.1 mg/kg (up to 6 mg) 0.2 mg/kg for second dose	• Treatment of supraventricular tachycardia	Causes a temporary block of AV node conduction.	Transient, due to its short half life	Administer at the injection site closest to the patient using the 2-syringe technique, (administer the medication, then a 5 cc flush of normal saline solution). Provide continuous cardiorespiratory monitoring during administration.
Amiodarone	I.V., I.O.: 5 mg/kg, up to a maximum of 15 mg/kg/day	• Ventricular tachycardia • Ventricular ectopy	Causes vasodilation and AV nodal suppression.	Prolonged Q-T interval. Slows conduction to ventricles.	Administer over 20–60 minutes. Do not administer simultaneously with Procanamide.
Lidocaine	I.V., I.O., E.T.: 1 mg/kg	• Ventricular tachycardia • Ventricular fibrillation • Ventricular ectopy	Decreases automaticity. Suppresses ventricular dysrhythmias.		Follow initial administration with a lidocaine infusion. The infusion rate should be 20–50 mcg/kg/min. Start the infusion within 15 minutes of the initial bolus dose.
Procainamide	I.V.: 15 mg/kg over 30–60 minutes	• Atrial fibrillation • Atrial flutter • Supraventricular tachycardia	Sodium channel blocker	Myocardial and circular depression; seizures; muscle twitching; drowsiness; disorientation; hypotension.	Do not administer simultaneously with Amiodarone. Stop administration with hypotension or if the QRS complex widens to > 50% of baseline.

From: American Heart Association, 2000; American Heart Association, 2001; Takemoto, Hodding, & Kraus, 2000.
I.V. = intravenous; E.T. = endotracheal; I.O. = intraosseous.

References

American Heart Association. (2000). *Guidelines 2000 for cardiopulmonary resuscitation and emergency cardiovascular care* (pp. 253–290; 291–342) Dallas, TX: Author.

American Heart Association (2001). Pediatric advanced life support. *Instructor's Manual.* Dallas, TX: Author.

Emergency Nurses' Association. (1996). Family presence at the bedside during invasive procedures and/or resuscitation. Park Ridge, IL: Author.

Schindler, M., Bohn, D., Cox, P., McCrindle, B., Jarvis, A., Edmonds, J., & Barker, G. (1996). Outcome of out-of-hospital cardiac or respiratory arrest in children. *New England Journal of Medicine, 335*(20), 1473–1479.

Scott, S., & Wiebe, R. (1996). Introduction. In G. Strange, W. Ahrens, S. Lelyveld, & R. Schafermeyer (Eds.), *Pediatric emergency medicine: A comprehensive study guide* (pp. 1–3). New York: McGraw-Hill Companies, Inc.

Taketomo, C., Hodding, J., & Kraus, D. (2000). *Pediatric dosage handbook* (7th ed.). Cleveland, OH: Lexi-comp.

Zaritsky, A., Nadkarni, V., Getson, P., & Kuehl, K. (1987). CPR in children. *Annals of Emergency Medicine, 16*(10), 1107–1111.

SECTION 5

Specific Emergencies

16

Respiratory Emergencies

Jacqueline Jardine, RN, C

Introduction

Respiratory disease accounts for almost 10% of pediatric ED visits. Approximately 20% of all pediatric hospital admissions are due to respiratory illness (Baker & Ruddy, 2000). The anatomy and immaturity of the respiratory system make children more prone to complications and significant morbidity. Presenting symptoms and illnesses range in severity from minor to life-threatening.

Emergency nurses must know the implications of these symptoms to recognize the need for immediate intervention. Accurate assessment is the first step in reducing the risk of progression of respiratory distress to respiratory failure and cardiac arrest. The purpose of this chapter is to review common respiratory conditions in the pediatric patient as well as the signs and symptoms and nursing interventions for these conditions.

Respiratory function depends on the following:

- Adequate oxygenation to maintain perfusion.
- Effective elimination of carbon dioxide.

Gas exchange occurs between the lung capillaries and the walls of the alveoli. The pressure gradient of the gases between alveolar air and pulmonary blood causes oxygen to diffuse from the alveoli to the blood, and carbon dioxide to diffuse from the blood to the alveoli (Wong, 1999; Ashwill & Droske, 1997). Ventilation occurs through inspiration and expiration, as intrathoracic pressures change and air moves into and out of the lungs. *Respiratory distress* occurs when the work of breathing or respiratory rate increases to maintain the respiratory function needed to meet the body's requirements (Strange, 1998). *Respiratory failure* occurs when there is an inability to maintain either the normal delivery of oxygen to the tissues or the normal removal of carbon dioxide from the tissues (Howard & Goldstein, 1999).

Disease processes that cause illness that lead to respiratory distress or failure include (Chameides & Hazinski, 1997):

- Decreased lung compliance and/or increased airway resistance, resulting in increased work of breathing and increased oxygen demand.
- Direct interference with exchange of oxygen or carbon dioxide.
- Mismatch of ventilation and perfusion, causing shunting of pulmonary blood through the lung so that hypoxemia and (to a lesser extent) hypercarbia occur.

Embryologic Development of the Respiratory System

The development of the respiratory system begins as early as the 16th week of gestation. The following briefly describes the development of the lungs, upper airway, and the pulmonary circulation (Webster, Grant, Slota, & Killian, 1998).

Lungs

The lungs develop in three different stages:

- *Glandular stage:* This stage lasts from conception to the 16th week of development. The lungs begin as buds on the embryonic gut 28 days after conception. These divide until about the 16th week. By the fourth week of gestation, a long bud branches from the primitive esophagus to form airways and alveolar spaces. The larynx develops during weeks 7 to 10.
- *Canalicular stage*: This stage lasts from the 16th to the 24th week of gestation. Vascularization of the lung occurs. The first capillaries can be identified in the middle of this phase. Alveolar ducts develop on the terminal bronchioles. Airways are lined with large cuboidal cells filled with glycogen. At about 18 weeks, some of the epithelial cells become alveolar epithelial type II cells, which synthesize pulmonary surfactant.
- *Alveolar stage*: This stage is from the 24th week to birth. Alveolar ducts surrounded by capillaries appear at 26 weeks. Alveoli and alveolar capillaries appear at 30 weeks.

Upper Airway

- *Nose*: The nasal cavities begin as widely separated pits on the face at 4 weeks. At birth, the maxillary sinuses are the largest sinuses. The ethmoidal cells are present and increase in size throughout life. The frontal and sphenoidal sinuses do not begin to invade the frontal and sphenoid bones until several years after birth.
- *Pharynx*: The oropharyngeal membrane between the foregut and the stomodeum begins to disintegrate to establish continuity between the oral cavity and the pharynx.
- *Larynx*: During the fourth week of embryologic life, the laryngotracheal groove begins as a ridge on the ventral portion of the pharynx. Vocal cords begin to appear in the eighth week.
- *Trachea*: The trachea begins to develop in the 24-day-old embryo. At 26 to 28 days, a series of asymmetric branchings of the primitive lung bud initiate the development of the bronchial tree.

Pulmonary Circulation

Development of the pulmonary circulation closely follows development of the airway and alveoli:

- *Preacinar arteries* develop in utero and branch along the airways.
- *Muscular arteries* end at the level of the terminal bronchiole in the fetus and newborn but gradually extend to the alveolar level during childhood.

Pediatric Considerations

Infants and young children have anatomic and physiologic characteristics that predispose them to respiratory distress (Webster et al., 1998):

- Infants are obligatory nose breathers until the age of 6 months, because the elongated epiglottis, positioned high in the pharynx, almost meets the soft palate. However, they are still able to mouth breathe, because blocked nares do not lead to complete upper airway obstruction. By the sixth month, growth and descent of the larynx reduces the amount of obstruction. Nasal breathing doubles the resistance to airflow and proportionately increases the work of breathing.
- The child's epiglottis is longer and more flaccid than that of an adult. The more anterior and cephalad epiglottis in a newborn may make intubation more difficult.
- A small upper airway makes infants more susceptible to obstruction from edema, foreign bodies, or congenital anomalies. In the infant and small child, the narrowest portion of the airway is the cricoid cartilage ring. This is the only point within the larynx at which the walls are completely enclosed in cartilage. Swelling from trauma or infection can lead to additional narrowing in this area, producing large increases in airway resistance.
- Smaller lower airways predispose the infant to mucus plugs and ventilation-perfusion mismatch.
- Infants have a limited alveolar space and therefore a smaller area for gas exchange (Wong, 1999).
- Infants have a more compliant chest wall and poorly developed intercostal muscles. Lungs are not well supported; if the airway is obstructed, active inspiration may result in paradoxic chest movement with sternal and intercostal retractions (Chameides & Hazinski, 1997).
- The tidal volume of infants and toddlers is largely dependent on the movement of the diaphragm; high intrathoracic pressure or abdominal distention compromises respiration because the intercostal muscles are unable to lift the chest wall (Chameides & Hazinski, 1997).

Focused History

The following history should be obtained for all children who present to the emergency department (ED) with a respiratory complaint or signs and symptoms of respiratory distress:

- Past medical history, including preexisting medical conditions that may contribute to the respiratory distress (cardiac disease, chronic conditions such as cystic fibrosis, and bronchopulmonary dysplasia).
- Immunization status.
- Onset of symptoms.
- Associated symptoms.
- Medications that the child is taking (including over-the-counter medications).

Other history depends on the signs and symptoms. These are discussed later in more detail, for each individual disease or condition.

Focused Assessment

Physical Assessment

The standard assessment, focusing on the signs and symptoms of respiratory distress (Chapter 6) is done for all children presenting with a respiratory complaint. The initial recognition of respiratory distress is more important than determining the cause. When the assessment is performed:

- The child should be allowed to remain with the caregiver and maintain a position in which he or she is most comfortable and able to breathe with the least amount of effort. Often, the child in moderate-to-severe distress will sit upright with the head, neck, and jaw extended.
- The child should be approached as gently as possible; anxiety increases the need for oxygen. Observing the child without touching (the "across-the-room assessment") can reveal many signs and symptoms of distress.
- The assessment should begin with the least intrusive procedures.
- Physical assessment of the child in respiratory distress includes
  - Airway patency.
  - Respiratory rate. Normal respiratory rates in children are (Rogers, 1998):

    Infants = 30–60 breaths per minute

    Toddlers = 24–40

    Preschoolers = 22–34

    School-age children = 18–30

    Adolescents = 12–16
- Work of breathing: location and depth of retractions, nasal flaring, grunting, and use of accessory muscles.
- Presence of inspiratory or expiratory wheezes or inspiratory stridor.
- Quality of breath sounds: diminished or absent.
- Changes in skin color: pallor, mottling, or cyanosis.
- Changes in mental status: confusion or inability to recognize caregiver.
- Restlessness or fatigue.

Psychosocial Assessment

Respiratory distress causes anxiety to both the child and the caregiver. The goal of the ED nurse is to reduce that anxiety by providing a calm environment, individualizing interventions, and considering the child's needs. These needs may include:

- Allowing the parent to remain with the child as much as possible.
- Providing information about the illness and the child's condition. Often the parent has to be told what the findings are and what they mean. For example, "Your child is breathing very noisily, but I can hear good air movement and her color is good. We will continue to observe her."
- Providing privacy.
- Allowing the child to make choices when possible.
- Providing age-appropriate toys and distraction.

Nursing Diagnoses	***Expected Outcomes***
Ineffective breathing pattern	The breathing pattern will improve. The respiratory rate will be normal for age. Signs and symptoms will be decreased or absent. Color will be normal.
Ineffective airway clearance	The airway will be clear after appropriate interventions, and the child will be able to maintain an open airway with or without assistance.
Potential fluid volume deficit	The child will be well hydrated after intravenous or oral fluid intake.

Triage Decisions

Emergent

Any of the following symptoms:

- Cyanosis or pallor.
- Marked retractions with inspiratory stridor.
- Lethargy or restlessness.

- Signs of dehydration and inability to take oral fluids.
- Any signs of respiratory failure or shock.
- Fever, sore throat, and drooling, with or without other symptoms.
- Apnea spells.

Urgent

- Mild retractions and stridor.
- Alert and able to take oral fluids.
- History of asthma or other preexisting condition.

Nonurgent

- Normal color and breath sounds.
- No retractions.
- Occasional cough.
- No signs of dehydration.

Nursing Interventions

The following interventions are generally performed for the child in respiratory distress. Additional interventions are included under specific conditions:

1. Provide supplemental oxygen:
   - Administer by a method best tolerated by the child and that will deliver the highest concentration.
   - Allow the child to maintain a position of comfort.
   - Ensure that pediatric emergency airway equipment is available.
2. Maintain normal temperature to minimize oxygen and fluid requirements.
3. Encourage oral fluids and provide intravenous fluids as ordered.
4. Be ready to assist with intubation:
   - Rapid-sequence induction may be performed.
   - Rapid-sequence induction may be used to induce anesthesia and neuromuscular blockade in fully or partially conscious children before intubation and is indicated for children requiring emergency intubation in the ED (Soud, 1998). Table 16.1 lists the steps in rapid-sequence induction.
5. Prepare for mechanical ventilation if the intubated child will be in the ED for extended periods of time:
   - Appendix A at the end of this chapter discusses the use of mechanical ventilation.
   - Generally, if a patient is being mechanically ventilated in the ED, it is desirable to have a respiratory therapist present.
6. Monitor vital signs.
7. Monitor pulse oximetry:
   - Pulse oximetry measures oxygen saturation but does not measure effectiveness of ventilation.
   - Failure to detect a pulse signal may be a mechanical error or an indication that the child is in a low-perfusion state and requires urgent treatment (Chameides & Hazinski, 1997).
   - Use data in conjunction with assessment and appearance of the child. Do not rely on the monitor to be the only reflection of the child's condition.
8. Perform frequent reassessments.
9. Keep parents informed of the progress in the child's condition, assessment findings, and reason for interventions.
10. Prepare the child and parents for admission to the hospital.

Selected Respiratory Emergencies

Croup (Laryngotracheobronchitis)

Croup is a viral infection that causes inflammation of the upper respiratory tract, initially in the pharynx, spreading down to the larynx and occasionally further along the respiratory tract (Fleisher, 2000). Croup is usually seen in the late fall and winter and is caused predominantly by the parainfluenza virus. Other viral agents include rhinovirus, influenza A, and respiratory syncytial virus. Children between the ages of 6 months and 3 years are primarily affected (Fleisher, 2000).

Pathophysiology

The infection causes endothelial damage, mucus production, loss of ciliary function, and edema along the upper respiratory tract (Fleisher, 2000). The characteristic stridor occurs as the child inspires air through a small, edematous airway.

History

- Gradual onset of symptoms; may be over 1 to 2 days.
- Cold symptoms.
- Cough, worse at night; generally described as a barking, seal-like cough.

TABLE 16.1 Steps in Rapid-Sequence Induction

Step	*Comments*
1. Preoxygenate. The child should already be on cardiac and oximetry monitors, and have an intravenous line.	Preoxygenate with 100% oxygen for 2 to 5 minutes (by nonrebreather mask or bag-valve-mask).
2. Premedicate.	Medications for premedication may include: ■ Atropine—Used to prevent bradycardia due to vagal response during procedure. ■ Lidocaine—Used to prevent increased ICP response to intubation and suppress cough reflex.
3. Administer sedatives.	Sedatives include: ■ Thiopental—Depresses the CNS; does not provide analgesia. Used in children with head injury because it reduces cerebral blood flow and oxygen consumption. ■ Ketamine—Produces analgesia, amnesia, and dissociation from the environment with protection of respiratory drive. Drug of choice for children with asthma, respiratory failure, or shock. ■ Diazepam—Produces sedation but no analgesia. Can cause respiratory depression. ■ Midazolam—Same as diazepam, but is faster acting and has shorter duration.
4. Administer muscle relaxant.	Muscle relaxants include: ■ Succinylcholine ■ Vecuronium ■ Rocuronium
5. Monitor child throughout procedure.	Observe for bradycardia, which most always indicates hypoxia. Observe skin color, perfusion, and capillary refill. If signs of hypoxia occur, the procedure should be stopped and the patient should be hypoventilated.
6. Secure tube and confirm placement.	The child should be restrained to prevent him or her from pulling tube. Tube placement is confirmed by auscultation, chest X-ray, or improvement in the child's condition.

Data from: Soud, 1998.

- Low-grade fever (temperature less than 38.5°C).
- Hoarse voice.

Focused Assessment

The airway assessment described earlier in this chapter is performed. Assessment findings depend on the severity of the illness and may include:

- Tachypnea and tachycardia.
- Inspiratory stridor.
- Expiratory wheezing.
- Suprasternal and subcostal retractions, indicating increased work of breathing.
- Cough.
- Signs and symptoms of dehydration because of an inability to take oral fluids.
- Low-grade fever.

Although presenting symptoms may be minor, children with croup are at risk for upper airway obstruction and respiratory failure.

Nursing Interventions

- Administer oxygen as tolerated by the child and if the oxygen saturation is less than 90 to 95%.
- Perform frequent reassessment, including vital signs, location and degree of retractions, frequency and type of cough, breath sounds, and behavior, to detect any deterioration in the child's condition.
- Monitor oxygen saturation.
- Encourage fluids.
- Administer medications as ordered.
    - Racemic epinephrine, administered by nebulizer, may be prescribed for moderate-to-severe croup:
    - The dose is 0.25 ml, diluted with 3-5 ml of normal saline (Fleisher, 2000).
    - Symptoms may be relieved for up to 2 hours following the aerosol treatment.
    - Children are commonly observed in the ED for 2 to 3 hours because of the rebound effect of racemic epinephrine, which may cause the condition to worsen.
- The efficacy of steroid therapy is still being questioned:
    - Intramuscular dexamethasone, 0.6 mg/kg may be ordered (Fleisher, 2000).
    - Oral steroids may be given if the child can tolerate oral intake.

Home Care and Prevention

- Provide clear oral and written instructions to the parents.
- Review the signs of increasing distress and when to return to the hospital.
- Provide discharge instructions that include measures that may help if the child develops symptoms at home:
    - Use a vaporizer to provide a cool mist.
    - Sit with the child in a bathroom filled with steam.
    - Take the child out into the cool night air or sit by an open window.
    - Encourage the child to drink cool fluids.
    - Manage fever—antipyretics.
- In severe cases, the child may require admission to the hospital.

Epiglottitis (Supraglottitis)

Epiglottitis is a life-threatening bacterial infection causing inflammation and swelling of the epiglottis and surrounding tissue. The incidence of epiglottitis has decreased greatly since the introduction of the *Haemophilus influenzae* type b (Hib) vaccines (Ball & Bindler, 1999). Recent studies show a 95% decrease in the incidence of invasive Hib disease since 1988; it now occurs primarily in undervaccinated children or in infants too young to have completed the primary series of vaccination (American Academy of Pediatrics, 1997). Other causative organisms include *Streptococcus pneumoniae* and staphylococcus (Ball & Bindler, 1999).

Pathophysiology

Infection of the epiglottis occurs when organisms pass through the mucosal barrier, resulting in bacteremia. The infection causes inflammation and edema of the epiglottis and rapidly spreads to the entire supraglottic area, resulting in increased secretions and a narrowed upper airway.

History

The history is often key to differentiating croup and epiglottitis:

- Sudden onset of symptoms; may be within 2 to 4 hours of presenting to the ED.
- High fever.
- Severe sore throat or difficulty swallowing.
- Drooling (not always present).
- Absence of cough or minimal cough. (Severe sore throat makes coughing painful and the child will resist coughing.)

Assessment

Children with epiglottitis often look sick and anxious. However, symptoms of respiratory distress may be absent, and a well-appearing child with minimal symptoms may progress to complete airway obstruction in less than 4 hours. Adolescents may present only with complaints of fever, sore throat, and difficulty swallowing. The assessment should be limited to determining the degree of respiratory distress. Interventions to support the airway must be started. Avoid upsetting the child, because this may lead to laryngospasm and subsequent airway obstruction. The following areas should be assessed:

- Respiratory rate, nasal flaring, the location and depth of retractions, and the presence of stridor.

- Skin color, for pallor or cyanosis.
- Drooling or inability to swallow.

Nursing Interventions

Interventions are directed at maintaining a patent airway. If possible, allow the child to remain with the caregiver:

- Administer oxygen as tolerated by the child.
- Prepare equipment for bag-valve-mask ventilation and intubation:
  - Direct visualization of the epiglottis and intubation will usually take place in the operating room, but the ED should be prepared to intubate.
- An X-ray may be ordered if the airway is stable and there is a question about the diagnosis:
  - Radiographic anteroposterior and lateral views of the neck will show the degree of airway narrowing. This assists in determining the immediate management of the patient but is rarely needed.
  - In most cases of severe respiratory distress X-rays should not be performed prior to intubation. The RN and MD should accompany the patient to radiology, equipped with emergency airway equipment.
- After the airway is secure, begin an intravenous infusion and antibiotics (usually ampicillin and a cephalosporin to cover *hemophilus influenzae* and *staphylococcus aureous*).
- Explain all procedures and treatments to the child and caregiver.
- Prepare for admission procedures and/or transfer to the operating room.

Home Care and Prevention

Children with epiglottitis will be admitted to the hospital. Because the Hib vaccine appears to be helping to reduce the incidence of epiglottitis, question caregivers about the immunization status of all children presenting to the ED. Educate parents on the need to keep immunizations current. It is hoped that the incidence of epiglottitis resulting from Hib disease will be eradicated in children younger than 5 years (American Academy of Pediatrics, 1997).

Bronchiolitis

Bronchiolitis is an inflammatory disease of the bronchioles caused by a viral infection. Bronchiolitis occurs primarily in children younger than 2 years of age and the infection is most severe in infants under 6 months (Ball & Bindler, 1999). It is seen mainly in the winter and spring. Pathogens include influenza virus, parainfluenza virus, adenovirus, and rarely *Mycoplasma pneumoniae* (Fleisher, 2000; Wong, 1999). The most common pathogen is the respiratory synctial virus (RSV). Respiratory synctial virus is responsible for at least 50% of the children admitted with bronchiolitis and is considered the most important pathogen in infancy and early childhood (Wong, 1999). Outbreaks of illness caused by RSV are commonly seen during the winter months. Infants, especially those with a history of prematurity, congenital heart disease, or bronchopulmonary dysplasia, are very susceptible to this virus and are at high risk for complications, including respiratory failure.

Pathophysiology

The infection causes inflammation and necrosis of the epithelial cells lining the bronchioles and bronchi. Sloughing of these cells results in a narrowing of the lumen. Edema and increased mucus production further obstruct the narrowed airways and result in tachypnea and wheezing. Hyperinflation and atelectasis may occur distal to the obstruction.

History

Symptoms of respiratory distress may occur over a few days but can occur over hours. Tachypnea is often the first sign and may be accompanied by audible wheezing. Apnea may be the initial symptom in high-risk infants. Other historical findings include:

- Cold for 1 to 2 days.
- Low-grade fever, runny nose, and decreased appetite.
- Cough, sometimes with vomiting.
- Difficulty breathing.
- Apnea spells, described by parents.

Assessment

The appearance of the child with bronchiolitis will depend on the stage of the illness and the degree of respiratory distress. The rate and work of breathing are observed before any intrusive procedures are performed. Assessment findings include:

- Respiratory rate: Often 50 to 80 breaths per minute or higher. Respirations may be shallow.
- Retractions: Signs of respiratory fatigue include a reduction in respiratory rate and a concurrent increase in retractions.
- Wheezing and a prolonged expiratory phase. Breath sounds may be unequal because of the irregular pattern of obstruction.
- Tachycardia.
- Signs of dehydration because of the inability to take oral fluids secondary to increased work of breathing.

Skin turgor, fontanelles, urinary output, and the presence or absence of tears should be evaluated.

- Neurologic status: The child may be alert or appear restless or fatigued. Apnea spells may indicate the need for intubation.
- Low-grade fever.

Nursing Interventions

- Ensure the availability of equipment to provide respiratory support.
- Allow the caregiver to stay with and hold the infant or child.
- Monitor respiratory rate, heart rate, and oxygen saturation.
- Assess the child frequently. Document and report changes in work of breathing, breath sounds, or neurologic and hydration status.
- Administer oxygen.
- Suction the child (nasopharyngeal) frequently to remove secretions. This often alleviates respiratory distress and improves oxygen saturation levels.
- Give oral fluids. Administer intravenous fluids as ordered.
- Administer medications as ordered:
  - Currently controversy exists about the efficacy of albuterol in treating bronchiolitis, even though it is widely used (Lugo, Salyer, & Dean, 1998).
  - A bronchodilator, delivered via nebulizer, is the initial treatment.
  - Albuterol, 0.1 to 0.3 cc of a 0.5% solution may be repeated every 20 minutes (Fleisher, 2000).
  - Tremors, tachycardia, and vomiting are possible side effects of albuterol.
- Keep the caregiver informed about procedures and any changes in the child's condition.

Home Care and Prevention

Discharge instructions should include:

- Signs that may indicate that the child should be returned to the hospital.
- Information on medications.
- Instructions to keep infant at home and away from crowds.
- Instructions for home use of oxygen, if prescribed.

Infusions of high-dose immunoglobulin, containing high titers of respiratory syncytial virus-neutralizing antibody, have been given prophylactically to prevent RSV in high risk children (Wong, 1999).

Asthma

Asthma is defined as a chronic inflammatory disorder of the airways in which many cells or cell elements play a role (Expert Panel on the Management of Asthma, 1997). The life-threatening potential of this illness is not always realized by patients, parents, or healthcare professionals (Kulick & Ruddy, 2000)

Asthma is the most common chronic disease of childhood, affecting more than 5 million children younger than 21 years, accounting for 5 to 12% of annual ED visits (Henderson, 2000). Despite many changes in therapy, there has been an increase in the number of hospitalizations and asthma-related deaths since the 1960s (Kulick & Ruddy, 2000). The reason is not fully understood, and research into the etiology and treatment of asthma continues.

The airway of the asthmatic child is more reactive and sensitive than is the unaffected airway. Some degree of inflammation of the airway is always present. The degree of airway reactivity determines the severity of chronic asthma. When the child is exposed to certain triggers, the airway becomes hyperresponsive, resulting in bronchospasm, increased inflammation, and mucus production. These triggers may include:

- Allergens.
- Upper respiratory tract infection.
- Exercise.
- Weather.
- Environmental irritants, such as cigarette smoke and pollution.
- Emotional stress.

Pathophysiology

When an asthmatic individual is exposed to a trigger, histamine and other mediators are released, causing an inflammatory response in the bronchial wall, swelling, bronchospasm, and increased production of mucous. Air trapping occurs, resulting in hyperinflation of the chest, making it a less efficient muscle of inspiration and forcing the use of accessory muscles (Connors, 1996). Ventilation-perfusion abnormalities result in a decrease in arterial oxygen saturation (Kulick & Ruddy, 2000). Metabolic changes also take place as the increased work of breathing increases the oxygen and energy requirements. Young children are more susceptible to status asthmaticus because of the differences in their respiratory anatomy and physiology (Kulick & Ruddy, 2000).

History

- Tightness in the chest, shortness of breath, coughing, and wheezing.
- Fatigue, inability to exercise, or chest pain with exercise.
- Allergy or cold symptoms, runny nose, itchy eyes, or sneezing.
- Family history.
- Number and severity of previous episodes.
- Previous hospitalizations and intubations.
- Previous steroid use.
- Current medications and those given before arrival at the ED.
- Recent upper respiratory tract infection or known exposure to other triggers.
- Duration of current symptoms.

Assessment

The child should be quickly assessed for the degree of respiratory distress. The following signs and symptoms may be apparent during the assessment:

- Tachypnea. A decrease in respiratory rate may not be a sign of improvement but may signal fatigue and impending respiratory failure.
- Wheezing on expiration (may progress to inspiratory and expiratory wheezing) with a prolonged expiratory phase. Absence of wheezing may indicate a severe obstruction with little airflow.
- Unequal breath sounds that may vary from loud and coarse to quiet and high pitched.
- Inability to speak, which has been correlated with hypoxia and a decreased peak flow rate (Connors, 1996).
- Pallor or cyanosis.
- Deteriorating mental status and increased tachycardia, which indicate increasing hypoxemia.
- Other signs and symptoms of respiratory distress, including nasal flaring, intercostal retractions, and the use of accessory muscles.

Nursing Interventions

In addition to the standard interventions performed for the child in respiratory distress, the following should be done as appropriate:

- Obtain a baseline peak expiratory flow rate (PEFR) using a peak flow meter:
  - This measures the speed at which air is forced out of the lungs.
  - Children older than 4-5 years of age can usually perform this test and children with chronic asthma often use it at home.
  - It is helpful to compare the child's PEFR to the predicted rate for age or the child's normal rate.
  - Normal PEFR varies based on sex and height as well as characteristics of each meter model. A rate of less than 80% of predicted or personal best is considered abnormal; a rate of less than 50% indicates moderate to severe obstruction (Kulick & Ruddy, 2000).
  - The PEFR also measures the efficacy of medication when the initial measurement is compared to the rate following treatment.
- Administer medications as ordered:
  - A beta-adrenergic bronchodilator is delivered by nebulizer or metered-dose inhaler (MDI) and may be combined with an anticholinergic.
  - Oral systemic steroids suppress and reverse airway inflammation and are recommended for moderate to severe exacerbations or for patients who fail to respond promptly and completely to an inhaled B_2-antagonist (Expert Panel on the Management of Asthma, 1997).
  - Table 16.2 lists medications for asthma management and recommended dosages.
- Monitor the child for tremors, tachycardia, and vomiting, possible side effects of the medication.

Home Care and Prevention

Asthma is disruptive for the child and family as well as potentially life-threatening. The goal of allowing children to lead active, healthy lives can be accomplished by educating not only the child and family, but also teachers, friends, and anyone else involved in the child's care. Ensure that they are well informed about possible triggers and how they may be avoided, and that they are able to recognize early warning signs and provide the necessary intervention. Discharge instructions should include recognition of early warning signs, information on medications to be administered at home, and possible asthma triggers. The importance of good follow-up and compliance in taking medications, both bronchodilator and anti-inflammatory, must be emphasized.

Pneumonia

Pneumonia is an inflammation of the lung tissue, usually caused by a viral or bacterial infection. Approximately 1 in 50 children in the United States has pneumonia annually (Fleisher, 2000). The organism causing pneumonia varies according to age and may be bacterial or viral in

TABLE 16.2 Recommended Drug Dosages for Asthma Exacerbations

Medication	***Dosage***	***Comments***
Inhaled short-acting B_2 agonists		
• Albuterol nebulizer solution (5 mg/ml)	0.15 mg/kg (minimum dose 2.50 mg) every 20 minutes for three doses, then 0.15 to 0.30 mg/kg, (up to 10.00 mg) every 1 to 4 hours, as needed; or 0.50 mg/kg/hour by continuous nebulization	For optimal delivery, dilute aerosols to minimum of 4 ml at oxygen flow of 6 to 8 L/min.
• Metered-dose inhaler (MDI) (90 mg/puff)	Four to eight puffs every 20 minutes for three doses, then every 1 to 4 hours as needed	The use of an MDI with a spacer/holding chamber is as effective as nebulized therapy if the child is able to coordinate the inhalation maneuver.
Systemic (injected) B_2 antagonists		
• Epinephrine 1:1,000 (1 mg/ml)	0.01 mg/kg (up to 0.30 to 0.50 mg) every 20 minutes for three doses, subcutaneously	Systemic therapy has no proven advantage over aerosol.
• Terbutaline (1 mg/ml)	0.01 mg/kg every 20 minutes for three doses, then every 2 to 6 hours, as needed, subcutaneously	Systemic therapy has no proven advantage over aerosol.
Anticholinergics		
• Ipratropium bromide (Atrovent) nebulizer solution (0.25 mg/ml)	0.25 mg every 20 minutes for three doses, then every 2 to 4 hours	May mix in same nebulizer with albuterol. Should not be used as first-line therapy; should be added to B_2 antagonist therapy.
Anticholinergics		
• Ipratropium bromide (Atrovent) nebulizer solution (18 mg/puff)	Four to eight puffs, as needed	Dose delivered from MDI is low and has not been studied in asthma exacerbations.
Corticosteroids		
• Prednisone • Methylprednisolone • Prednisolone	1.00 mg/kg every 6 hours for 48 hours, then 1.00 to 2.00 mg/kg/day (maximum = 60.00 mg/day) in two divided doses, until PEFR is 70% of predicted or personal best	

Adapted from: Expert Panel on the Management of Asthma, 1997. *Expert panel report 2: Guidelines for the diagnosis and management of asthma* (Publication No. 97-4051A, pp. 44–45). Bethesda, MD: National Institutes of Health, National Heart, Lung and Blood Institute.

origin. The majority of cases are viral. Causal agents include RSV, parainfluenza virus, adenovirus, rhinovirus, measles, rubella, varicella, and enteroviruses. By age group, the most common bacterial agents are:

- Newborn: Predominantly group B streptococci, the majority caused by aspiration of the organism during delivery.
- Under 3 years: *Streptococcus pneumoniae*, *Staphyloccus aureus*, and *Haemophilus influenzae*.
- Over 3 years: *Mycoplasma pneumoniae*, *Streptococcus pneumoniae*.

Children with chronic and acute conditions are at increased risk to develop pneumonia (Ashwill & Droske, 1997).

Pathophysiology

Infection causes an inflammation in the lung tissue, leading to exudation of fluid and fibrin deposits. Accumulation of this exudate causes the lobar consolidation visible on an X-ray.

History

The history is influenced by the causative agent (viral or bacterial):

- Viral pneumonia:
  - Development over several days.
  - Upper respiratory tract infection for several days.

    - Cough.
    - Low-grade fever.
- Bacterial pneumonia:
    - Abrupt onset.
    - Contact with other children who are sick.
    - High fever with chills.
    - Increased respiratory rate.
    - Wet-sounding cough.
    - Tired, less active, decreased appetite.
    - Chest or abdominal pain.

Assessment

The overall appearance may be of a child who looks sick and is lethargic, especially those children with a bacterial infection. Assessment findings may include:

- Tachypnea; grunting respirations.
- Decreased breath sounds; diffuse wheezing.
- Retractions.
- Circumoral pallor or cyanosis.
- Cough.
- Fever; hot and dry skin.
- Chest or abdominal pain.

Nursing Interventions

In addition to interventions for the child in respiratory distress, the following should be done:

- Provide fever management.
- Encourage oral fluids.
- Administer medications as ordered. Oral, intravenous, or intramuscular antibiotics may be given, depending on the suspected organism.
- Prepare the child for a chest X-ray.

Home Care and Prevention

- Educate the caregiver about the importance of continuing antibiotic therapy and of returning for recheck if requested.
- Discuss signs and symptoms of respiratory distress that require the family to return to the ED.
- Consider immunization with Pneumovax (to prevent pneumococcal pneumonia) in children with preexisting conditions, such as cardiac or respiratory disease.

Foreign-Body Aspiration

An aspirated foreign body may cause complete or partial obstruction of the upper or lower airway. Diagnosis is complicated by the similarity of the presenting symptoms to those of other respiratory illnesses.

Aspiration of a foreign body occurs most commonly in children younger than 4 years of age (Ball & Bindler, 1999). Sixty-five percent occur in children younger than 2 years old (Schunk, 2000). Part of a child's normal development is to experiment and explore. This includes placing objects in the mouth. Factors contributing to the risk of aspiration include the child's being given food and toys that are, by shape and size, inappropriate for the child's age. Ingestion of objects, especially coins, which lodge in the esophagus, may also cause respiratory distress (Schunk, 2000).

Pathophysiology

The effect of the aspirated body depends on the size, shape, and composition of the object, where it becomes lodged, and the local tissue reaction to the foreign body (Schunk, 2000). Aspiration that causes an immediate and complete obstruction of the airway is a life-threatening event. This is more likely to occur if the foreign body is lodged in the upper airway. If the foreign body lodges in the bronchi, the symptoms may develop over several days. Symptoms result when air is trapped, leading to emphysema or atelectasis, pneumonia, or tissue erosion.

Focused History

The history may include:

- Coughing or a choking spell.
- Wheezing or episodes of stridor.
- Recurrent respiratory tract infections.
- A history of an ingestion.

Assessment

Findings will depend on the location and degree of obstruction. In addition to the standard respiratory assessment, the following should be evaluated:

- Breath sounds: wheezing or decreased or unequal air movement.
- Other signs and symptoms of respiratory distress, including color, mental status, and retractions.

Nursing Interventions

- Acute obstruction:
    - Initiate measures to relieve the airway obstruction in accordance with American Heart Association guidelines (Chapter 15).

  - If a laryngoscopy, bronchoscopy, cricothyroidotomy, or tracheotomy is required, prepare for transfer to the operating room. Have tracheotomy tray and Magill forceps immediately available in the ED.
- Chronic obstruction:
  - Establish an IV line and administer antibiotics as prescribed. A complete blood count and blood culture may be ordered.
  - Obtain a chest X-ray.

Home Care and Prevention

- Provide education regarding age-appropriate foods and toys.
- Encourage caretakers to attend cardiopulmonary resuscitation classes.

Other Respiratory Conditions

There are several preexisting conditions that may contribute to or cause respiratory distress in children. These include structural defects, such as kyphoscoliosis, tracheomalacia, and congenital defects, as well as cardiopulmonary conditions such as heart disease, cystic fibrosis (CF), and bronchopulmonary dysplasia (BPD). The most important aspect of caring for a child with a preexisting condition is to determine what the child's normal respiratory status is. The caregiver knows the child better than anyone and should be asked, "How do you think your child looks today?". Cystic fibrosis and bronchopulmonary dysplasia will be discussed here because they may be more commonly encountered in the ED. Other cardiac conditions are discussed in Chapter 17.

Cystic Fibrosis

Cystic fibrosis is an autosomal-recessive inherited disorder of the exocrine glands and mucosal surfaces caused by a variety of mutations of the CF gene. It is a generalized disorder that affects multiple body organs, including the lungs, bowels, sweat and salivary glands, pancreas, liver, and male reproductive tract (Rogers, 1998).

Patients with CF have, among other interrelated abnormalities, an increase in viscosity of mucus secretions and an increased susceptibility to chronic colonization of the respiratory tract by certain bacteria, especially *Pseudomonas aeruginosa*.

These children may be brought to the ED for complaints related to respiratory infections. The goal should be to recognize and treat these infections promptly to prevent further complications. The child is treated as any other child with respiratory distress, but it is extremely important to involve the caregiver because he or she will be familiar with usual treatment and the child's baseline condition. Prior records will have to be obtained and the child's physician should be consulted. Chest physiotherapy may be needed in the ED as well.

Bronchopulmonary Dysplasia

Bronchopulmonary dysplasia is an acquired, chronic cardiopulmonary disease characterized by respiratory distress, oxygen dependence, and abnormal chest X-rays that persist beyond 1 month of age (Rogers, 1998). Factors contributing to the development include oxygen toxicity, positive-pressure ventilation, pulmonary inflammation, and nutritional deficiencies; premature infants are at highest risk for development of BPD because of the immaturity of their lungs. Signs and symptoms include tachypnea, shallow breathing, dyspnea, retractions, cough, and wheezing. Infants with BPD often have feeding difficulties and are irritable.

Infants with BPD may present to the ED with viral respiratory infections, such as RSV. Again, it is important to ask the parent's perception of the child's condition and how it compares to the baseline. The infant with BPD with signs of respiratory distress must be treated emergently. Treatment includes administration of oxygen therapy, diuretics, and bronchodilators.

The incidence of BPD in infants older than 30 weeks has decreased in recent years, mostly because of the advent of therapy such as surfactant, high-frequency jet ventilation, and steroid administration. However, the overall incidence has increased because of the improved survival rates of extremely premature neonates.

Conclusion

Children with respiratory problems are at risk for progression to severe respiratory distress and respiratory failure. If cardiopulmonary arrest occurs, the chance for survival is poor. Children present to the ED with symptoms ranging from mild to severe distress. Rapid observation of the child's general appearance, accurate assessment of signs and symptoms, effective intervention, and frequent reassessment are vital to the successful management of respiratory emergencies. Caregivers are a very important resource in determining the severity of illness in children with chronic respiratory conditions.

References

American Academy of Pediatrics. (1997). *Haemophilus influenzae* infections. In G. Peter (Ed.), *1997 red book: Report of the Committee on Infectious Diseases* (24th ed. pp. 220-231.). Elk Grove Village, IL: American Academy of Pediatrics.

Ashwill, J., & Droske, S. (1997). The child with an acute respiratory disorder. In J. Ashwill & S. Droske (Eds.), *Nursing care of children. Principles & practice* (1st ed., pp. 810-859). Philadelphia: W. B. Saunders Company.

Baker, M. D., & Ruddy, R. (2000). Pulmonary emergencies. In G. Fleisher & S. Ludwig (Eds.), *Textbook of pediatric emergency medicine* (4th ed., pp. 1067-1086). Philadelphia: Lippincott Williams & Wilkins.

Ball, J., and Bindler, R. (1999). Alterations in respiratory function. In J. Ball & R. Bindler (Eds.), *Pediatric nursing caring for children* (2nd ed., pp. 407-463). Stamford, CT: Appleton & Lange.

Chameides, L., & Hazinski, M. F. (Eds.). (1997). *Textbook of pediatric advanced life support* (pp. 2-1B2-3, 4-1B4-5). Dallas: American Heart Association.

Connors, K. (1996). Asthma. In G. Strange, W. Ahreus, S. Lelyveld, & R. Schatermeyer (Eds.), *Pediatric emergency medicine, A comprehensive study guide.* (pp. 165-172). New York: McGraw Hill.

Expert Panel on the Management of Asthma. (1997). *Expert panel report 2: Guidelines for the diagnosis and management of asthma* (Publication No. 97-4051A). Bethesda, MD: National Institutes of Health, National Heart, Lung and Blood Institute.

Fleisher, G. (2000). Infectious disease emergencies. In G. Fleisher & S. Ludwig (Eds.), *Textbook of pediatric emergency medicine* (4th ed., pp. 725-793). Philadelphia: Lippincott Williams & Wilkins.

Henderson, D. (2000). Cooling with asthma: The National Institutes of Health asthma guidelines. *Journal of Emergency Nursing, 26*(1), 70-75.

Howard, C., & Goldstein, L. (1999). Respiratory failure and the need for ventilatory support. In C. Scanlon, R. Wilkins, & J. Stoller (Eds.), *Egan's fundamentals of respiratory care* (7th ed., pp. 819-831). St. Louis: Mosby.

Kulick, R., & Ruddy, R. (2000). Allergic emergencies. In G. Fleisher & S. Ludwig (Eds.), *Textbook of pediatric emergency medicine* (4th ed., pp. 999-1015). Philadelphia: Lippincott Williams & Wilkins.

Lugo, R. A., Salyer, J. W., & Dean J. M. (1998). Albuterol in acute bronchiolitis-continued therapy despite poor response? *Pharmacotherapy, 18*(1), 198-202.

Rogers, J. (1998). Respiratory system. In T. E. Soud & J. S. Rogers (Eds.), *Manual of pediatric emergency nursing* (pp. 193-232). St. Louis: Mosby.

Schunk, J. E. (2000). Foreign body ingestion/aspiration. In G. Fleisher & S. Ludwig (Eds.), *Textbook of pediatric emergency medicine* (4th ed., pp. 267-273). Philadelphia: Lippincott Williams & Wilkins.

Soud, T. (1998). Respiratory failure and shock. In T. E. Soud & J. S. Rogers (Eds.), *Manual of pediatric emergency care* (pp. 107-127). St. Louis: Mosby.

Strange, G. (1998). Respiratory distress. In G. Strange (Ed.), *American College of Emergency Physicians and American Academy of Pediatrics: The Emergency Medicine Course* (3rd ed., pp. 3-16). Pains Texas & Elk Grove Village, IL.

Webster, W. F., Grant, M. J., Slota, M. C., & Kilian, K. M. (1998). Pulmonary system. In M. C. Slota (Ed.), *Core curriculum for pediatric critical care nursing* (pp. 33-43). Philadelphia: Saunders.

Wong, D. (1999). The child with respiratory dysfunction. In D. Wong (Ed.), *Nursing care of infants and children* (6th ed., pp. 1456-1532). St. Louis: Mosby.

A

Overview of Pediatric Ventilator Care

Robin Long, RN, MSN, PNP

Indications for Mechanically Assisted Ventilation

Respiratory failure occurs when children are unable to achieve an adequate oxygen-carbon dioxide exchange on their own. Mechanically assisted ventilation in children can be necessary for several reasons:

- The inability to initiate breathing, as in disorders of the central nervous system.
- The inability to process brain-diaphragm signals via the phrenic nerve, as in the case of diaphragmatic or chest wall disorders.
- The inability to establish respirations because of diseases of the airway or acute trauma.

Frequently a child will be placed on a ventilator in the ED because a bed is not readily available in the intensive care unit, and the child needs artificial ventilation. The ideal situation is to have a respiratory therapist present to assist in the care of this patient because ED nurses may not be familiar with ventilator care. This discussion includes basic information about ventilators and their care.

If mechanical ventilation is indicated, it will be delivered by either an endotracheal tube or a tracheostomy. It is essential that the airway be maintained for a child who is mechanically ventilated. Emergencies that require immediate intervention are accidental extubation or decannulation, a difficult tracheostomy tube reinsertion, a mucus plug in the endotracheal tube, or water entering the artificial airway from the ventilator tubing. Appropriate measures have to be taken immediately to resecure the airway and to ventilate the child.

Methods

Artificial ventilation may be delivered to a child through two different methods:

1. *Negative-pressure ventilation (NPV).* Negative-pressure ventilation affects ventilation by application of negative pressure around the thorax for the inspiratory phase of respiration. This creates a pressure gradient inside the thoracic cavity, causing air to flow into the lungs. The application of negative pressure to the thorax produces a more physiologic method of ventilation than does positive-pressure ventilation (PPV). The popularity of NPVs has decreased since the introduction of PPV. Some patients still are candidates for NPV. They must have a compliant chest wall and no upper airway obstruction to assure adequate ventilation. The patient's medical condition must be stable for a period of time before the patient is sealed in the device.

2. *Positive-pressure ventilation (PPV).* Positive-pressure ventilation is achieved by applying pressure greater than atmospheric pressure to the airways to promote inspiration; expiration is passive. There are two types of positive-pressure ventilation: pressure or volume. The two types differ in the manner by which inspiration is stopped: pressure or volume. The pressure-limited ventilators are usually simpler and less expensive than the volume-limited types. The volume-limited devices are more widely used because of the constant tidal volumes they are able to deliver. If small volumes are needed, a pressure-limited ventilator may be used. A volume-limited ventilator can be set to function as a pressure-limited ventilator by setting the relief valve for maximum pressure at the desired ventilating pressure.

   Ventilators are designed to deliver oxygen mixtures through stabilized pressure and/or volume. Pressure-preset ventilators deliver a set pressure at a predetermined rate, but their amount of tidal volume varies with each breath. Volume-preset ventilators deliver a preset air volume at a predetermined rate, but the amount of pressure varies with each breath. Volume-preset ventilators are typically more portable than are pressure-preset devices.

Settings

Many settings on a ventilator must be preset before the child is connected to the ventilator:

- Intermittent mandatory ventilation (IMV), or breath rate per minute.
- Tidal volume (TV) or volume of air delivered per breath.
- Peak inspiratory pressure (PIP).
- Positive end-expiratory pressure (PEEP).
- Percentage of oxygen (FIO_2).
- Humidification temperature and alarms.

Each ventilator has a high-pressure alarm and a low-pressure alarm. Ventilator settings must be checked frequently. Ventilator alarms must be on at all times, and all ED nurses need to know how to respond to the alarms.

Troubleshooting

Many problems may arise with ventilators. While troubleshooting the ventilator, the nurse should always double-check the settings and look for leaks, obstructions, and resets as well as other common problems. The following problems can occur:

- *Leaks.* Effective positive-pressure ventilation depends on maintenance of an airtight connection between the ventilator and the patient's lungs. A leak can result in failure to ventilate the lungs adequately. If the patient does not seem to be getting enough volume to breathe, there may be a leak in the system. The nurse should always check to make sure that none of the tubing has been disconnected from either the ventilator or the patient.
- *Obstructions.* Failure to ventilate also can result from plugs, kinks, and other obstructions. Tubing can be kinked or crimped behind a moved bed or other equipment. Patient circuits may be incorrectly assembled, creating inappropriate ventilation.
- *Resets.* When a problem in the system arises, the nurse should always recheck the ventilator settings. Dials are sometimes accidentally moved and reset, or the settings may be changed by another team member. If a problem arises, the nurse should always consider the possibility that the settings have been adjusted without his or her knowledge.
- *Obstruction of the right mainstem bronchus.* When an endotracheal tube is displaced and slips too far down the trachea, the tube enters the right mainstem bronchus and occludes the left mainstem bronchus. As a result, the right lung is overventilated and the bronchus to the left lung is completely obstructed. The treatment is to pull the endotracheal tube back and reposition it.
- *Decreased venous return.* Positive-pressure ventilation impedes venous return. This may reduce cardiac output and lower blood pressure, especially during the inspiratory phase. The body attempts to compensate for these developments by retaining fluid and expanding blood volume. If hypotension becomes serious, it may be necessary to augment the intravascular volume rapidly with intravenous fluids or blood.

A respiratory therapist or an intensive care nurse should be contacted for any problem. Ideally, if a patient is held in the ED on a ventilator, a respiratory therapist or nurse familiar with ventilators should be present.

17

Cardiovascular Emergencies

Sarah A. Martin, RN, MS, PCCNP, CPNP, CCRN
Michelle R. Morfin, RN, MS, PCCNP, CCRN

Introduction

Cardiovascular emergencies in children arise from congenital or acquired heart conditions. Although most congenital cardiac lesions are diagnosed during the antenatal period or early in infancy, cardiac lesions may be detected during emergency department (ED) treatment. Children with congenital heart disease (CHD) may present to the ED with congestive heart failure (CHF) or sequelae of their condition, prompting rapid intervention. Children with acquired cardiac disease (e.g., dysrhythmias, endocarditis, myocarditis, and pericarditis) are more likely to be diagnosed in the ED; however, the priorities of cardiopulmonary support remain the same for either group. Furthermore, children with heart transplants may present to the ED with signs of heart failure or organ rejection. The purpose of this chapter is to compare and contrast selected congenital and acquired cardiac conditions and to describe the emergency nursing care of children with cardiovascular emergencies.

Embryologic Development of the Cardiovascular System

Cardiac embryologic development occurs between the third through tenth week of gestation. The origin of cardiac tissue is the mesoderm (Smith et al., 1996). A crescent of mesoderm is formed from a pair of endothelial tubes. These endothelial tubes grow, fuse, and establish a single, straight cardiac tube at approximately 20 days gestation. Cellular development around the cardiac tube results in the formation of a distinct myocardium and endocardium. The contractile activity of the heart with the forward flow of blood is initiated at 22 days gestation (Smith et al., 1996). The regulation of heart rate, vascular tone, and cardiac output through sympathetic innervation and circulating catecholamines is present in the fetus as early as 24 to 26 days gestation.

At 25 days gestation, continued growth of the cardiac tube in the confined chest wall causes twisting or looping of the heart. Normally, the bulboventricular mass (as it is now referred to) loops to the right (D-dextro looped), and becomes the right ventricle. If the bulboventricular mass loops to the left (L-levo looped), the right ventricle forms on the left side, resulting in ventricular inversion. Growth of the proximal bulboventricular mass results in the right ventricular mass, while the growth of the midportion results in the ventricular outflow tracts. Growth of the distal portion results in the truncus arteriosus, which eventually divides and becomes the pulmonary artery and aortic root.

Septation of the ventricles occurs after looping. The primitive ventricles are connected through an interventricular foramen, which is the only means by which the right ventricle has access to the circulating blood flow necessary for growth. As the ventricles enlarge, the muscular septum arises from the ventricular floor and grows toward the atrioventricular canal, or endocardial cushion, which is the central portion of endocardial tissue that gives rise to the tricuspid and mitral valves. Until the sixth week of gestation, a communication persists between the ventricles; this is eventually closed by tissue from growth of the muscular septum, endocardial cushion, and conal truncal tissue.

Atrial septation occurs much in the same way ventricular septation does, except that the atrial septum is multilayered. The septum primum forms first and grows toward the endocardial cushion. A communication persists through the ostium primum. As the septum primum joins the atrioventricular canal, small perforations in the septum primum join, to give rise to the septum secundum. The foramen ovale is a flap-like valve that is left open between the growth of the septa primum and secundum, which allows for right-to-left blood flow throughout the remainder of gestational life. As atrial septation occurs, the common pulmonary vein is being formed from the posterior atrial wall. The conal-truncal tissue gives rise to the truncus arteriosus, the common pathway for blood flow exiting the fetal heart. It is ultimately separated into a pulmonary artery and aorta under the influence of blood flow and conal-truncal separation around the 34th day gestation. As the truncus arteriosus grows, it spirals so that the pulmonary artery arises from the right ventricle and the aorta arises from the left ventricle. Interruptions in any of these processes can result in a ventricular septal defect (VSD), transposition of the great vessels (TGV), persistent truncus arteriosus, or unequal-sized great arteries (Srivastava & Baldwin, 2001; Mahony, 2001).

Pediatric Considerations

The unique anatomy and physiology of the child contribute to altered physiologic responses to disease states and therapeutic modalities. An immature sympathetic nervous system contributes to a decreased response to sympathetic output and increased sensitivity to parasympathetic output (i.e., vagal input). Thus, there is an inability to alter vascular tone to environmental and external stressors. In newborns and infants, immaturity of the cardiac conduction system and autonomic innervation as well as numerous metabolic and functional alterations in the developing conduction system contribute to cardiac dysrhythmias.

Cardiac output per kilogram of body weight is higher in the child than in the adult (Table 17.1). The stroke volume is fixed; therefore, cardiac output is altered through heart-rate variability. The higher the heart rate, the lower the stroke volume, because there is less filling time. The response of children to the exogenous administration of catecholamines is under investigation; therefore, correct dosing of vasoactive drugs is determined at the bedside with titration to patient response.

Etiology

The etiology of cardiovascular conditions arises from congenital or acquired processes, as described in this chapter.

Focused History

Family history

- Congenital heart defects.
- Valvular heart disease and/or murmurs.
- Cardiovascular surgery.

Patient history

- Heart defects:
  - Type of defect.
  - Repair completed or scheduled.
  - Current medications.
- Heart disease.
- Cardiovascular surgery.

Symptoms of the presenting illness

- Fever (presence and duration).
- Fatigue.
- Chest pain.
- Dyspnea.
- Cyanosis.
- Exercise intolerance.
- Edema.

Focused Assessment

Physical Assessment

1. Assess the respiratory system.
   - Auscultate the chest for:
     - Adventitious sounds.
     - Respiratory rate. In the child with impending cardiac failure, the respiratory rate may be slow, fast, or labored.

TABLE 17.1 Cardiac Parameters in the Pediatric Population

Parameter	*Definition*	*Normal Values*
Cardiac output is the volume of blood ejected from the heart in 1 minute.	Heart rate times stroke volume	*Infant:* 200 ml/kg/min *Child:* 150 ml/kg/min *Adult:* 100 ml/kg/min
Cardiac index	Cardiac output / Body surface area	2.8 to 4.2 L/min/m^2
Stroke volume	(Cardiac output (ml/min))/Heart rate	60 to 90 ml/beat

From: Hazinski (1999). Cardiovascular disorders. In M. Hazinski (Ed.), *Manual of pediatric critical care* (pp. 84–288). St. Louis: Mosby—Year Book.

TABLE 17.2 Pathologic Cardiac Murmurs

Murmur Assessment	*Associated Cardiac Lesions*
Short, loud, midsystolic murmur	Stenotic lesions (e.g., aortic stenosis)
Holosystolic murmurs (lasting throughout systole)	Mitral or tricuspid regurgitation
	Ventricular septal defects
Diastolic murmurs	Aortic or pulmonary valve dysfunction
	Mitral valve/Tricuspid valve stenosis
Continuous machinery murmur	Patent ductus arteriosus

2. Assess the cardiovascular system.
   - Auscultate for:
     - Rate. Broad categories for the evaluation of heart rate are (American Heart Association, 2000): bradyarrhythmias; tachyarrhythmias; pulseless electrical activity; ventricular fibrillation.
     - Rhythm.
     - Clarity. Faint or muffled heart tones may be indicative of tamponade or pericardial effusion.
     - Benign murmurs (Toepper, 1996):

       Low-grade (I/VI to III/VI).

       Short in two words duration.

       Occur early in systole.
     - Pathologic murmurs (Toepper, 1996) (see Table 17.2):

       Louder.

       Longer.

       Timing in the cardiac cycle and location suggests their representative pathology.

       Rubs may be indicative of pericardial effusions.
3. Evaluate cardiac rhythm by initiating cardiorespiratory monitoring.
4. Measure the blood pressure.
   - Blood pressure for the child with suspected congenital cardiac disease should be obtained in both the upper, especially right arm (preductal), and lower extremities for comparison.
5. Assess peripheral perfusion.
   - Palpate peripheral pulses for:
     - Equality.
     - Quality. Although pulse quality is a subjective assessment finding, pulse intensity is often ranked on a 0 to 4+ scale (Chapter 6).
   - Measure core and skin temperature.
     - An elevated core body temperature in the presence of peripherally cool, mottled skin temperature reflects a compensatory vasoconstriction with a resultant shunting of blood flow centrally to preserve vital organ perfusion.
     - Diaphoresis reflects sympathetic response to intrinsic catecholamine release.
   - Inspect the skin, nailbeds, and oral mucosa for:
     - Color.
     - Lesions.
     - Clubbing (results from long-standing cyanotic heart disease).
     - Turgor.
   - Measure capillary refill.
     - Prolonged capillary refill (greater than 3 seconds) reflects compensated cardiac output.
6. Assess level of consciousness with the Alert, Responds to Verbal Stimuli, Responds to Painful Stimuli, Unresponsive (AVPU) scale, or Glasgow coma scale (GCS) methods (Chapter 6).
   - With a significant decrease in cardiac output, cerebral perfusion can become impaired, resulting in irritability, agitation, or lethargy.
   - Seizures may be indicative of embolic events, especially in children with unrepaired septal defects.

Psychosocial Assessment

- Assess the child's previous experience with healthcare providers.
- Assess the parent's knowledge of their child's condition; assess their coping strategies.

See Table 17.3 for a nurse's assessment.

Triage Decisions

Categorize the following patients as requiring emergent, urgent, or nonurgent care.

Emergent

- Infant or child with evidence of cardiac decompensation or hemodynamic compromise, as evidenced by hypotension, profound bradycardia or tachycardia, decreased peripheral perfusion, faint heart sounds, dyspnea with grunting respirations, or signs and symptoms of severe congestive heart failure.

TABLE 17.3 Nursing Diagnoses and Expected Outcomes

Nursing Diagnoses	*Expected Outcomes*
Decreased cardiac output related to myocardial dysfunction	The child will have adequate cardiac output, as evidenced by: ▪ Normal sinus rhythm. ▪ Control of symptomatic dysrhythmias with pharmacologic or electrical intervention. ▪ Hemodynamic stability.
Impaired tissue perfusion related to decreased cardiac output	The child will have adequate tissue perfusion, as evidenced by: ▪ Capillary refill time < 2 seconds. ▪ Warm, dry skin. ▪ Pink mucous membranes.
Fluid volume deficit related to inadequate intravascular volume	The child will be hemodynamically stable, as evidenced by: ▪ Adequate cardiac output. ▪ Level of consciousness appropriate for age and development. ▪ Adequate urinary output.
Altered family process related to the diagnosis of cardiovascular dysfunction	The family will demonstrate appropriate coping strategies, as evidenced by: ▪ Verbalizing an appropriate understanding of their child's health condition. ▪ Accepting support from staff and other family members.

- Infant or child with suspected or confirmed dysrhythmia with signs of compromised cardiac output.
- Tachypneic child with poor perfusion and pulmonary congestion/edema.
- Child who has evidence of embolic events with fever and pain.

Urgent

- Infant or child with tachycardia, systolic murmur, irregular rhythm, precordial chest pain, pericardial friction rub, low-grade fever, mild signs and symptoms of CHF, and possible dysrhythmia without compromised cardiac output.
- Acutely ill child who is febrile, has a new murmur or a change in murmur, and exhibits pallor and weight loss.

Nonurgent

- Child with adequate cardiovascular perfusion.
- Child with neurologic status appropriate for age and level of development.
- Child with a low-grade fever with fatigue and change in activity level.

Nursing Interventions

1. Assess and maintain airway, breathing, and circulation.
   - Initiate maneuvers to maintain airway patency, such as positioning and suctioning and insertion of an airway adjunct.
   - Prepare for endotracheal intubation in the child who cannot maintain airway patency.
   - Administer 100% oxygen through a nonrebreather mask; initiate assisted ventilation in the child who is not maintaining adequate respiratory effort.
   - Initiate cardiorespiratory monitoring; measure continuous oxygen saturation:
     - Analyze the ECG rhythm on the cardiac monitor.
     - Obtain a 12-lead electrocardiogram (ECG), if indicated.
   - Obtain blood pressure in the upper and lower extremities.
2. Obtain venous access and initiate an intravenous infusion at the ordered rate.
   - Obtain blood for laboratory studies, such as:
     - Complete blood count.
     - Electrolytes.

- Administer medications, as needed.

3. Prepare for diagnostic studies, as needed:
   - Chest radiograph.
   - Echocardiogram.
4. Reassess the child's neurologic and cardiovascular status.
5. Insert an indwelling bladder catheter to measure urinary output.
   - Urinary output less than 1 ml/kg/hour can reflect inadequate renal perfusion.
6. Inform the family frequently about the child's condition; provide emotional support to the child and family.
7. Prepare for transfer and transport to a tertiary care facility, as indicated (Chapter 10).

Congenital Heart Disease

Etiology

The incidence of congenital heart disease in the general population is 1% (Park, 1996). Maternal infection (e.g., rubella), medication usage, excessive smoking or alcohol intake, maternal age over 40 years, insulin-dependent diabetes, and genetics may contribute to the development of CHD. Many infants born to high-risk mothers are diagnosed as CHD *in utero* due to advances in fetal echocardiography.

Early hospital discharges coupled with physiologic changes in circulation may mask symptoms of cardiac defects in the first few days of life. With the closure of the patent ductus arteriosus (PDA) within the first 7 days of life, ductal-dependent lesions may become apparent, as the infant develops shock-like signs and symptoms. Often, CHD is associated with other congenital anomalies or syndromes. Abnormal development of the heart may be coupled with abnormal development of other structures that develop simultaneously during gestation such as tracheal esophageal fistula, renal agenesis, and diaphragmatic hernias (O'Brien, Baker, & Boisvert, 2000).

Table 17.4 summarizes common cardiac lesions and their incidence, pathophysiology, assessment findings, and interventions.

Prevention

Early and thorough prenatal care may prevent the development of cardiac defects, although their true etiology remains unknown. Minimizing identified maternal risk factors also may lessen the incidence of congenital heart disease.

Selected Cardiovascular Emergencies

Congestive Heart Failure

Congestive heart failure is a clinical syndrome manifested by inadequate cardiac output to meet ongoing metabolic demands. The most common causes of CHF in the pediatric population are congenital and acquired heart disease. For the child with congenital heart disease, the most common cause of heart failure is the sequelae of lesions with left-to-right shunting (Table 17.5). These lesions result in increased pulmonary blood flow and decreased systemic flow, yielding impaired cardiac performance as the heart is unable to keep up with the body's metabolic demands. The transplanted heart also may fail; Table 17.6 highlights significant clinical features of and interventions for children with heart transplants.

Etiology

Volume and/or pressure overload lesions are the most common etiologies of CHF. Volume overload lesions are the most common cause of CHF in the first 6 months of life and include (Park, 1996):

- Ventricular septal defects.
- Patent ductus arteriosus.
- Truncus arteriosus.
- Endocardial cushion defects.

Pressure overload lesions include:

- Critical aortic stenosis.
- Coarctation of the aorta.
- Pulmonary stenosis.

Acquired heart disease is the second most common etiology of CHF in children. The age of onset for acquired heart disease is nonspecific. Acquired heart diseases include:

- Myocarditis.
  - Myocarditis is more common in children greater than 1 year of age, although fulminant cases have occurred in the newborn period.
- Dilated cardiomyopathy.
  - Dilated cardiomyopathy can occur at any age.
- Endocardial fibroelastosis.
  - Ninety percent of endocardial fibroelastosis cases in the first 8 months of life (Park, 1996).
- Valvular heart disease.
- Acute rheumatic fever.
- Endocarditis.

TABLE 17.4 Common Cardiac Lesions

Lesion/Incidence	*Description of Lesion*	*Pathophysiology*	*Assessment*	*Intervention*
Lesions with increased pulmonary blood flow				
Atrial septal defect (ASD)/5–10%	Abnormal opening between the atria. Three types: primum—opening at the lower end of the septum; secundum—opening near the center of the septum; sinus venosus—opening near the junction of the superior vena cava and the right atrium.	As left atrial pressures are higher than right atrial pressures, there is increased oxygenated blood flow to the right atrium. There is an increase in right atrial and right ventricular blood flow. Over decades, there is increased pulmonary blood flow with the possible sequela of pulmonary hypertension.	Patients are usually asymptomatic. Grade II/VI or III/VI systolic ejection murmur at the upper-left sternal border. In large, untreated defects CHF and pulmonary hypertension can occur. Atrial arrhythmias may occur with long-standing defect because of right atrial enlargement.	Surgical correction with the opening sutured or closed with a patch Device closure by an interventional cardiologist
Ventricular septal defect (VSD)/20–25%	Abnormal opening between the right and left ventricles. May be classified as membranous or muscular. Defects vary in size.	Blood flows through the defect to the pulmonary artery. Increased pulmonary blood flow may eventually result in pulmonary hypertension. Right ventricular and atrial enlargement may result from an increased workload.	Patients with small VSDs may be asymptomatic. Grade II/VI to V/VI systolic murmur may be audible at the left lower sternal border. CHF may be present.	Palliative surgery: Pulmonary artery banding may be performed in the infant to decrease pulmonary blood flow. The defect may be closed with sutures or a patch. Device closure by an interventional cardiologist
Patent ductus arteriosus (PDA)/5–10% (excluding premature infants)	Persistent patency of a normal fetal structure in which there is a connection between the pulmonary artery and the aorta.	There is a left-to-right shunt. The length and width of the ductus and the pulmonary vascular resistance (PVR) determine the magnitude of the shunt. Congestive heart failure (CHF) may develop if the ductus is large.	Grade I/VI to IV/VI continuous machinery murmur. Signs and symptoms of congestive heart failure may occur.	Subacute bacterial endocarditis prophylaxis when indicated. Treatment of congestive heart failure. Thoracotomy may be performed and the ductus tied off and/or ligated (cut). Device closure by an interventional cardiologist
Lesions with decreased pulmonary blood flow				
Transposition of the great vessels (TGV)/5% (D-transposition)	Aorta and pulmonary artery arise from the morphologically wrong ventricle so that the aorta arises from the right ventricle and the pulmonary artery arises from the left ventricle.	There is complete separation of pulmonary and systemic circulations, whereby hypoxemic blood circulates only to the body and hyperoxemic blood circulates solely to the lungs. Defects such as a PDA, ASD, or VSD are necessary to allow the mixing of unoxygenated and oxygenated blood that is crucial to survival. Blood flow pattern: body to right atrium to right ventricle to aorta to body; lungs to left atrium to left ventricle to pulmonary artery to lungs.	Cyanosis is usually present from birth. Signs and symptoms of CHF with dyspnea and poor feeding. May be tachypneic but without retractions.	Immediate management: hyperoxia test to confirm presence of CHD. Blood gas analysis, prostaglanden E1 (CPGE1) (Table 17.9) infusion, oxygen administration for severe hypoxia, administration of digoxin and diuretics followed by urgent balloon atrial septostomy (Wernovsky, 2001). Long-term: complete corrective surgery (arterial switch procedure), done in the neonatal period.
Obstructive defects				
Aortic stenosis (AS)	Narrowing at the valvular, subvalvular, or supravalvular level of the aortic valve.	If the stenosis is severe, left ventricular hypertrophy may develop. With critical AS, CHF and shock may develop in infants.	With mild-to-moderate AS, children may be asymptomatic.	Aortic valve commissurotomy, valvuloplasty, valve replacement, excision of membrane subvalvular AS, or widening of the area with a patch for discrete

TABLE 17.4 (continued)

Lesion/Incidence	*Description of Lesion*	*Pathophysiology*	*Assessment*	*Intervention*
Obstructive defects				
Aortic stenosis (AS) (continued)				supravalvular AS. Infants with critical AS are either operated on in an urgent manner or transferred to the cardiac catheterization laboratory for balloon valvotomy. Children with a peak systolic pressure gradient of 50 to 80 mm Hg may be electively operated on (Park, 1997). Children with mechanical valve replacements will receive Coumadin therapy.
Coarctation of the aorta	Narrowing or kinking of the aorta.	With severe lesions, infants are symptomatic and show signs of CHF. Ductal dependent coarctations lie just beyond the left subclavian artery; systemic circulation depends upon ductal flow. As the ductus closes, systemic circulation is blocked by the coarctation, resulting in shock.	The infant may be symptomatic or asymptomatic, depending on the defect's location and severity. The infant may exhibit signs and symptoms of CHF. The hallmark sign of this defect is discrepant blood pressures in the upper and lower extremities (blood pressure higher in the upper extremities).	Medical management includes aggressive treatment of CHF; PGE1infusion (Table 17.9) for ductal-dependent coarctation. The need for surgery is urgent in the presence of CHF (Park, 1997). Surgery should be performed as soon as the defect is diagnosed or for a gradient = 20 min.
Tetralogy of Fallot/10%	Composed of four lesions: VSD, pulmonary stenosis (PS), right ventricular hypertrophy (RVH), and overriding aorta.	The VSD allows for communication between the ventricles. Pulmonary stenosis is a constricted area of the pulmonary artery or valve that decreases blood flow to the lungs with a resultant right ventricular outflow tract obstruction. The RVH results from the increased PVR as a result of pulmonary stenosis and an overriding aorta.	Symptoms of cyanotic heart disease include cyanosis, clubbing, dyspnea on exertion, and hypoxic spells. "Tet" spells are caused by an acute increase in PVR, or a decrease in oxygen availability versus demand, and are characterized by hypercyanosis (DeBoer, 1996).	Tet spell: knee-to-chest positioning, oxygen administration, Morphine sulfate, 0.1–0.2 mg/kg/dose, and/or Propranolol (Inderal) 0.15–0.25 mg/kg/dose. May require a higher propanolol dose at 1–2 mg/kg/dose over 6 hours. Elective repair is usually completed at any time after 3 to 4 months of age (Park, 1997). Arrhythmias may develop later, including ventricular tachycardia.
Ductal-dependent lesions/systemic flow—dependent lesions				
Hypoplastic left-heart syndrome/< 1%; 9% of CHD in newborns	Critical mitral and aortic stenosis with underdevelopment of the left-sided cardiac structures: left atrium and ventricle, aorta, aortic valve, and mitral valve. Usually accompanied by a small patent foramen ovale and large PDA. Usually no VSD.	During fetal life, PVR is greater than systemic vascular resistance (SVR). After birth, SVR rises dramatically, and the ductus arteriosus closes, resulting in markedly decreased cardiac output, shock, hypoxia, and metabolic acidosis. Survival depends on size of the ASD, presence of a PDA, and timing of diagnosis; 75% are diagnosed in the first week of life (Freedom, Black & Benson, 2001).	Birth weight is normal. Ten percent have associated extracardiac anomaly (Freedom, Black, & Benson, 2001). Tachypnea, dyspnea, crackles, weak peripheral pulses, peripheral vasoconstriction, and hepatomegaly. Usually no significant murmur. May not be severely cyanotic.	Immediate care includes: Intravenous PGE1 infusion (Table 17.9) to maintain ductal patency and intubation to control ventilation, manipulate PVR, and decrease metabolic acidosis. Urgent balloon atrial septostomy (Park, 1996). Long-term options: no surgical intervention with certain death in 1 month, Norwood procedure followed by staged surgical repair, or cardiac transplant.

TABLE 17.4 (continued)

Lesion/Incidence	*Description of Lesion*	*Pathophysiology*	*Assessment*	*Intervention*
Cyanotic lesions with high pulmonary blood flow				
Truncus arteriosus/< 1% (Mair, Edwards, Julsrud, Seward, & Danielson, 2001)	Single arterial blood vessel arising from base of the heart gives rise to coronaries, pulmonary artery, and aorta. Single, semilunar valve (truncal valve) most often dysplastic and incompetent (regurgitant). Most have a VSD.	There is complete mixing of systemic and pulmonary venous blood within the heart. Both ventricles are subjected to increased pressure and flow. Incompetent truncal valve contributes to ventricular overload. Preferential blood flow to lungs because PVR is less than SVR after birth, which leads to pulmonary hypertension.	There is cyanosis with signs and symptoms of CHF: tachypnea, dyspnea, and poor feeding. With a large VSD, no murmur may be heard. May hear systolic/diastolic murmur, depending on truncal valve morphology (Mair et al., 2001). May have bounding peripheral pulses with wide pulse pressure. Congestive heart failure will start when PVR begins to fall (around 4 to 6 weeks of life).	Medical management to relieve CHF. Surgical intervention before 3 months of life to prevent irreversible PHTN (ideally completely correct defect at 4 to 6 weeks of life) (Mair et al., 2001). Type of surgery depends on coronary and truncal valve anatomy.

TABLE 17.5 Causes of Congestive Heart Failure According to Age and Congenital Heart Disease

Age	*Congenital Heart Disease*
Birth	Hypoplastic left-heart syndrome
	Tricuspid regurgitation/Ebstein's anomaly
Week 1	Transposition of the great arteries
	Hypoplastic left-heart syndrome
	Total anomalous pulmonary venous return
	Critical aortic stenosis
	Critical pulmonic stenosis
Weeks 1 to 4	Coarctation of the aorta associated with other anomalies
	Critical aortic stenosis
	Large left-to-right shunt lesions in premature infants (e.g., ventricular septal defect and patent ductus arteriosus)
Weeks 4 to 6*	Some left-to-right shunt lesions (e.g., endocardial cushion defect)
Weeks 6 to 16	Large ventricular septal defect
	Large patent ductus arteriosus
All ages	Post-cardiac-repair status

Adapted from: Park (1996). *Pediatric Cardiology for Practitioners* (3rd ed., p. 402). St. Louis: Mosby—Year Book.

*Large left-to-right shunting lesions, such as the ventricular septal defect and patent ductus arteriosus, do not cause CHF until the pulmonary vascular resistance falls at 4 to 6 weeks to allow for excessive left-to-right shunting.

Other etiologies of CHF include:

- Dysrhythmias.
  - Supraventricular tachycardia.
  - Complete heart block.
- Pulmonary diseases.
  - Bronchopulmonary dysplasia.
  - Cystic fibrosis.
  - Primary pulmonary hypertension.
  - Cor pulmonale from obstructive pulmonary disease.
- Muscular dystrophy (in adolescents).
- Metabolic derangements.
  - Anemia.
  - Acidosis.
  - Hypoglycemia.

Congestive heart failure is the result of a number of pathologic phenomena of cardiac performance and resultant compensatory mechanisms. The endpoint of CHF is the inability of the heart to pump an adequate amount of blood to meet the metabolic needs of the body. Heart failure in children is generally characterized by four hemodynamic states (O'Brien et al., 2000):

- Volume overload.
  - Usually related to congenital heart lesions with increased pulmonary blood flow from left-to-right shunting.
  - Associated with findings of right ventricular hypertrophy.
- Pressure overload.

TABLE 17.6 Considerations for the Child with a Heart Transplant

Indications	*Physiologic Considerations*	*Sign of Rejection*	*Concerning Symptoms*	*Emergency Treatment*
Select complex congenital heart defects (e.g., hypoplastic left-heart syndrome, single ventricle disease, post Fontan procedure); cardiomyopathy; cardiac tumors	Denervated myocaridum results in a loss of autonomic control of heart rate. Electrocardiogram may demonstrate two P waves: the donor and the recipient SA nodes are present.	*Infants:* Irritability, lethargy, poor feeding, and tachycardia. *Children:* Decreased exercise tolerance, marked fatigue, elevated temperature, signs of congestive heart failure. A gallop or pericardial friction rub may be present. Dysrhythmias occur. Cardiomegaly on chest radiograph.	Any evidence of atherosclerosis; any signs of infection or rejection; exposure to varicella	Obtain a 12-lead electrocardiogram if rejection is suspected. Contact the transplant center. Provide care as previously outlined. For varicella exposure: administer V-ZIG. Review the patient's complete medication list; for example, is the child on *Pneumocystis carinii* prophylaxis? Obtain axillary or tympanic temperature measurement, because some transplant centers recommend avoiding rectal temperature measurement in immunosuppressed children. Obtain blood cultures, complete blood count, and chest radiograph for children presenting with fevers.

    - Results in impaired systolic myocardial performance.
    - Decreased systemic perfusion and increased afterload from obstructive congenital heart lesions.
- High cardiac output demands.
    - In high-output failure, myocardial systolic function is preserved, and diastolic dysfunction is present.
    - Conditions that lead to high-output failure include sepsis and severe anemia, in which there is a normal volume status but cardiac output is inadequate for tissue metabolic needs.
- Decreased myocardial contractility from:
    - Acquired heart disease (e.g., cardiomyopathy, pericarditis).
    - Acidosis.
    - Ventricular dilation: overstretching of cardiac myofibrils.

In failure states, there is decreased cardiac output with a compensatory ventricular dilation, hypertrophy, and neurohormonal stimulation. Ventricular dilation and hypertrophy occur in response to the demand for increased cardiac output.

- Dilation of the cardiac muscle increases the stretch of the fibers, initially increasing the force of contraction. Over time, dilation causes a decreased contractile force.
- Hypertrophy of the cardiac muscle results in greater tension and increased pressure in the ventricle, with a resultant compensatory increased systolic ejection force.
- Dilation and hypertrophy can have potentially negative effects over time, because there is decreased muscle compliance as a higher filling pressure is required to produce the same stroke volume.

Neurohormonal stimulation includes the renin-angiotensin system and sympathetic-adrenergic discharge.

- Stimulation of the renin-angiotensin and aldosterone system promotes reabsorption of salt and water, with a resultant increase in circulating blood volume to increase preload.

- Baroreceptors stimulate the sympathetic nervous system, releasing catecholamines, when there is a decrease in cardiac output.
- Catecholamines increase the force and rate of myocardial contraction and cause peripheral vasoconstriction.
- Atrial naturetic hormone, produced directly by the right atrial myocytes, is an endogenous diuretic released in response to changes in right atrial pressures.

Focused History

Maternal history (factors associated with an increased incidence of CHD)

- Infection.
- Illnesses.
- Medication usage.
- Maternal CHD.

Patient history

- Failure to thrive or inappropriate growth and development in infants with CHF.
  - There is an increased compensatory sympathetic discharge as a result of increased stress on the child's physiologic state.
- Feeding history (infant).
  - Protracted feeding time.
  - Diaphoresis or tachypnea during feeding.
  - Falling asleep quickly after or during feeding.
- Energy level and exercise tolerance (older child).
  - Shortness of breath.
  - Puffy eyelids/exercise intolerance.
  - Swollen feet.

Focused Assessment

Physical Assessment

Specific cardiovascular assessment parameters are evaluated.

1. Assess the respiratory system.
   - Auscultate the chest for:
     - Adventitious sounds. Pulmonary congestion is evidenced by tachypnea, dyspnea, orthopnea (older children), wheezing, crackles, and cough, which may reflect left- or right-sided heart failure.
     - Respiratory rate.
2. Assess the cardiovascular system.
   - Auscultate the heart for:
     - Rate. Tachycardia, loud murmurs, and gallop rhythm are auscultated in the child with impaired cardiac performance.
   - Palpate peripheral pulses for:
     - Equality.
     - Rate.
     - Quality. Weak pulses may be detected.
     - Rhythm.
3. Inspect the skin for:
   - Capillary refill (delayed).
   - Color (mottling).
   - Temperature (diaphoresis).
   - Edema:
     - Periorbital edema (infants).
     - Peripheral edema (children).
     - Neck vein distension (older children).
     - Hepatomegaly > 2 cm below the right costal margin (infants).
4. Assess the neurologic system.
   - Assess the child's level of consciousness with the GCS or AVPU (Chapter 6).
5. Obtain other assessment parameters:
   - Measure urinary output (oliguria).
   - Plot height and weight on a growth chart to determine growth failure.

Psychosocial Assessment

- Assess the parents' knowledge of the child's condition.
- Assess the family's support systems.
- Assess the child's understanding of the current health condition.

Nursing Interventions

1. Place the patient in a position of comfort.
2. Administer supplemental oxygen therapy as needed.
3. Initiate cardiorespiratory and oxygen saturation monitoring.
4. Obtain venous access and initiate an intravenous infusion:
   - Administer medications as needed to relieve pulmonary and systemic venous congestion, improve myocardial performance, and, if possible, reverse the underlying disease process through:
     - Diuretic therapy. Treats relative volume overload by decreasing the workload of the heart and reducing pulmonary and systemic congestion.

- Inotropic agents. Digoxin (Lanoxin®), the most commonly administered inotropic agent for treatment of CHF, delays atrioventricular conduction, decreases the heart rate, and subsequently increases cardiac filling and output.
- Afterload-reducing agents. Counteract the compensatory response of increased sympathetic tone in the presence of decreased cardiac output. With afterload reduction, the stroke volume is augmented without a change in the cardiac contractile state.

- Obtain blood specimens for:
  - Arterial or venous blood gas.
  - Complete blood count with differential.
  - Electrolytes.

5. Obtain accurate measurements of intake and output.
6. Weigh the child or estimate the child's weight.
7. Prepare for diagnostic procedures:
   - Obtain a 12-lead ECG.
   - Obtain anteroposterior and lateral chest radiographs.
8. Prepare for transfer and transport to a tertiary care facility, as needed (Chapter 10).

Home Care and Prevention

Early diagnosis of cardiac conditions and close medical follow-up help to prevent occurrences of CHF. Monitoring of the child's health allows for adjustments in medication doses to assist in management of CHF. Palliative or corrective cardiovascular surgery may be indicated to prevent or treat CHF. Parents should be taught how to administer medications at home and should be taught the signs of impending CHF, such as activity intolerance and poor feeding.

Dysrhythmias

Dysrhythmias are a relatively infrequent finding in the pediatric patient; however, early recognition of abnormal cardiac rates and rhythms in children is essential to prompt intervention. Common pediatric dysrhythmias include sinus tachycardia, sinus bradycardia, supraventricular tachycardia (SVT), and premature ventricular contractions (PVCs). Regardless of the underlying etiology, treatment of pediatric dysrhythmias is always guided by the principle that rhythm disturbances in children are usually more benign and are generally better tolerated than are their counterparts in adults (Toepper, 1996).

Etiology

Rhythm disturbances occur for different reasons in children than they do in adults. Certain forms of CHD may predispose a child to dysrhythmias, but dysrhythmias often occur in the absence of any such disease. Hypovolemia, electrolyte disturbances, and hypoxia are the most common causes of pediatric dysrhythmias in patients without underlying heart disease (Toepper, 1996). Drug exposures and toxicities must also be considered. Table 17.7 outlines common pediatric dysrhythmias and their characteristics. Because SVT and sinus tachycardia are difficult to differentiate, their specific characteristics are highlighted in Table 17.8.

Dysrhythmias can be precipitated or can occur idiopathically. They are generally well tolerated in children for some time; however, eventually, dysrhythmias can compromise cardiac output if left untreated. This is especially true if the dysrhythmia is a compensatory mechanism for an abnormal state (e.g., tachycardia for hypovolemic states). Such compensatory mechanisms can stress the myocardium and should be evaluated fully before being deemed benign. In some instances, a dysrhythmia is a symptom of an underlying disease process that needs further medical evaluation (e.g., cardiomyopathy, myocarditis, hyperthyroidism, or cardiac tumors). Toxicities can cause a variety of rhythm disturbances by virtue of the drug's chemical composition, exerting effects on the myocardium as well as the conduction system (Chapter 44).

Focused History

Patient history

- Repaired or unrepaired CHD.
- History of Wolff-Parkinson-White syndrome.
- Signs and symptoms of cardiopulmonary distress:
  - Tachypnea.
  - Diaphoresis.
  - Dyspnea.
  - Palpitations or chest pain (older child). Elicit from the older child a description of what the child's chest feels like (e.g., pounding, fluttering, skipping, racing, or jumping).
- Precipitating events (activity, fever, or anxiety).
- Possible ingestions of medications or other poisons.
- Previous experience with similar symptoms.
- Previous consultation with a pediatric cardiologist.

Family history

- Abnormal heart rhythms.
- Mitral valve prolapse.
- Wolff-Parkinson-White syndrome.

TABLE 17.7 Common Pediatric Dysrhythmias

Rhythm	*ECG Characteristics*	*Causes*
Sinus tachycardia	Regular rhythm Normal P, QRS, T sequence	Fever, anemia, congestive heart failure, anxiety, hypovolemia (resulting from dehydration or fluid loss), and circulatory shock
Sinus bradycardia	P-waves usually observed QRS usually normal	Vagal stimulation, increased intracranial pressure, hypothermia, hypoxia, sedation, hyperkalemia, and digitalis toxicity
Premature ventricular contractions	Widened QRS complexes fall early in cardiac cycle	Acquired heart disease, drug toxicities, electrolyte imbalances, increased intracranial pressure, ingestion of toxic substances, acidosis
Supraventricular tachycardia	Regular rhythm P waves may not be observed QRS usually very narrow	Reentry mechanism involving either an accessory pathway (e.g., Wolff-Parkinson-White syndrome) or the atrioventricular node. Idiopathic supraventricular tachycardia without underlying heart disease is found more commonly in infants than in older children. Congenital heart lesions are more prone to supraventricular tachycardia (e.g., Ebstein's anomaly, single ventricle disease, and L-TGA).

TABLE 17.8 Supraventricular Tachycardia versus Sinus Tachycardia

	Sinus Tachycardia	*Supraventricular Tachycardia*
Rate	Heart rate greater than normal for age, usually < 220 beats/minute.	Heart rate > 230 beats/minute.
History	Fever; volume loss as a result of hemorrhage; vomiting; diarrhea; pain; sepsis; shock.	Usually paroxysmal onset with nonspecific findings: irritability, lethargy, and poor feeding.
Electrocardiogram findings	Rate is greater than normal for age. Rhythm is regular. P-wave axis is normal. P-QRS-T wave sequence. QRS duration is normal.	Rhythm is usually regular, but may have beat-to-beat variability. P-waves may not be identifiable. QRS duration is normal (< 0.08 second) in most children (> 90%). With persistent tachycardia, ST- and T-wave changes consistent with myocardial ischemia may be present.

- Other conduction disturbances (e.g., long Q-T syndrome).

Focused Assessment

Physical Assessment

1. Assess the respiratory system.
   - Auscultate the chest for:
     - Respiratory rate.
     - Rhythm.
     - Adventitious sounds.
   - Inspect the chest for:
     - Accessory muscle use.
2. Evaluate the cardiovascular system.
   - Auscultate the heart for:
     - Rate.
     - Rhythm.

  - Clarity.
  - Murmurs.
- Evaluate cardiac rhythm by initiating cardiorespiratory monitoring.
- Measure the blood pressure.
- Assess peripheral perfusion:
  - Palpate peripheral pulses for equality; quality; regularity.
  - Measure core and skin temperatures.

Nursing Interventions

1. Maintain airway patency.
2. Administer supplemental oxygen, if indicated.
3. Initiate cardiorespiratory and oxygen saturation monitoring.
   - Increase the volume of the QRS to detect dysrhythmias and to determine rhythm regularity.
4. Obtain venous access and initiate an intravenous infusion.
   - Obtain blood for laboratory studies:
     - Arterial blood gas.
     - Complete blood count with differential.
     - Electrolytes.
     - Toxicology screening, in cases of suspected poisoning.
5. Obtain diagnostic tests:
   - Twelve-lead ECG.
   - Chest radiograph.
6. Initiate dysrhythmia-specific interventions:
   - Bradycardia.
     - Provide supplemental oxygenation.
     - Initiate oxygen saturation monitoring.
     - Initiate chest compressions, if needed.
     - Initiate external cardiac pacing in unstable patients.
   - Sinus tachycardia.
     - Determine and treat the underlying cause. Pharmacologic therapy is inappropriate for sinus tachycardia that is symptomatic of an underlying condition such as fever, hypovolemia, pain, or anxiety.
   - Supraventricular tachycardia.
     - Perform synchronized cardioversion in children with cardiovascular compromise.
     - Attempt vagal maneuvers in children without cardiovascular compromise (Schamberger, 1996). Infants tend to respond well to an ice bag (for up to 10 seconds) to the forehead, face, or cheeks. Children tend to respond better to coughing and breath holding (Valsalva maneuver) on command, if able to cooperate.
     - Administer adenosine (Adenocard®) in children with cardiovascular compromise: Administration causes temporary atrioventricular node conduction block, interrupting the reentry circuit mechanism. Adenosine has negative chronotropic and inotropic effects. Administer 0.1 mg/kg via rapid intravenous bolus and rapid 5-cc normal saline flush. The two-syringe technique must be used because of the short half-life of the drug (<1.5 seconds), where two-needled or needleless devices on the syringes are given at the intravenous port proximal to the patient (i.e., t-connector) (American Heart Association, 2000).
     - Administer digoxin. In cases where SVT may precipitate or result in CHF, digitalization may be helpful in providing inotropic support and in preventing recurrence in older children (Park, 1996). In the absence of CHF, infants may benefit from digitalization to prevent recurrence of SVT once converted to normal sinus rhythm.
     - Consider overdrive esophageal pacing. Overdrive esophageal pacing has proven to be effective in some patients, especially once pharmacologic management is initiated. This is usually performed by a pediatric cardiologist.
   - Premature ventricular contractions.
     - Determine and eliminate the etiology if known (e.g., electrolyte disturbance or hypoxemia).
     - Benign PVCs (patient asymptomatic). No therapy is indicated.
     - Unifocal PVCs. May be benign, even if they occur as bigeminy.
     - Multifocal PVCs. May signify greater pathology.
     - Initiate lidocaine therapy for symptomatic PVCs or PVCs with increasing frequency (e.g., couplets or triplets).
7. Provide the family with frequent updates on their child's condition; provide psychosocial support as needed.
8. Prepare for transfer and transport to a tertiary care facility, as needed (Chapter 10).

Home Care and Prevention

Close medical follow-up of children predisposed to cardiac dysrhythmias should be assured. The therapeutic benefit of prescribed pharmacologic agents on hospital discharge should be evaluated and monitored. Parents should be encouraged to practice home safety measures with medication and poison storage. Parents and older children can be taught to recognize signs of and predisposing factors for dysrhythmia and to initiate measures to prevent or ameliorate their effects.

Acquired Heart Disease

Recognition of acquired heart disease in infants and children is often difficult because patients may have vague presenting signs and symptoms. The spectrum of presentation ranges from fever, tachypnea, congestion, and respiratory distress, to fulminant CHF and cardiovascular compromise, with shock and life-threatening dysrhythmias. Prompt recognition of infants and children in the ED who present with acquired heart disease is essential not only to save the lives of these patients, but also to protect them from the potential sequelae of untreated acquired heart disease.

Endocarditis

Etiology

Infective endocarditis, excluding postoperative endocarditis in pediatric patients, accounts for approximately 0.5 to 1.0 per 1,000 hospital admissions annually (Park, 1996). Although endocarditis can affect children of all ages, it is most commonly seen in children older than 10 years of age and is rarely seen in infants (Dajani & Taubert, 2001). Patients at risk for endocarditis include those with structural heart defects and bacteremia. All children with CHD are at risk for acquiring infective endocarditis, especially those with turbulent, high-flow lesions, including tetralogy of Fallot, ventricular septal defect, and patent ductus arteriosus (Park, 1996). Other patients at risk include those with mitral and aortic valve abnormalities and those undergoing congenital heart surgery with prosthetic shunts, baffles, homografts, or conduits.

In the emergency department, endocarditis in a patient with undiagnosed CHD may present with vague symptomatology that may be overlooked and result in a delay in diagnosis and treatment. Any delay in treatment can result in damage to the heart structure itself. Infective endocarditis is a microbial infection of the endothelium, or the inner lining of the heart, which may include the semilunar or atrioventricular valves. Prosthetic valves are also frequently involved. The most common causative bacteria are Gram-positive cocci (80%); *Streptococcus viridans* and *Staphylococcus aureus* are the most common (Dajani & Taubert, 2001). Fungi can also be responsible for infective endocarditis with a greater virility and poorer prognostic clinical course.

For endocarditis to occur, bacteria must enter the bloodstream via a secondary event (e.g., a dental procedure). Turbulent blood flow from the CHD slowly erodes the endothelial lining in the area of the defect. Platelets and fibrin are deposited in the endothelium as a normal protective mechanism, allowing thrombus formation. Bacteria already in the bloodstream become entrapped in the fibrin network of the thrombus, bacterial multiplication occurs, and vegetative growth ensues, including invasion of the valves and possibly the conduction system. Destruction of the vegetation by phagocytosis cannot occur because of the encasement of bacterial colonies in the fibrin network. These vegetative lesions are very friable and may break off, causing embolic events. Finally, valve closure is impaired because of vegetative growth, causing regurgitation and CHF.

Focused History

Patient history

- Underlying cardiac disease.
- Prior surgeries or procedures (e.g., cardiac catheterization).
- History of recent illness or exposures.
- Recent dental cleanings or procedures or complaints of toothache.
- Lack of prophylactic antibiotics prior to dental procedures.
- Presence of any prosthetic devices, such as pacemakers, central lines, cardiac graft, or artificial valve.
- Signs and symptoms the child has experienced:
  - Fatigue.
  - Anorexia.
  - Fever.

Focused Assessment

Physical Assessment

1. Assess the respiratory system.
   - Auscultate the chest for:
     - Respiratory rate.
     - Equality of breath sounds.
     - Adventitious sounds.
2. Assess the cardiovascular system.
   - Auscultate the heart for:
     - Rate.
     - Rhythm.
     - Clarity.
     - Murmurs. Extracardiac sounds may be auscultated.
   - Inspect the skin for:
     - Color. Pale skin may result from decreased perfusion. Petechiae in the extremities, nailbeds, and mucous membranes may be evidence of embolic events.

- Temperature. Cool extremities may indicate poor peripheral perfusion.
- Measure capillary refill.
  - Delayed capillary refill (> 3 seconds) may indicate early shock.

3. Assess the neurologic system.
   - Measure the child's level of consciousness with the GCS or AVPU method.
4. Assess the abdomen.
   - Palpate the abdomen for organ enlargement resulting from right-sided heart failure:
     - Hepatomegaly.
     - Splenomegaly.
     - Lymphadenopathy.
5. Assess the oral cavity for:
   - Caries.
   - Lesions.
   - Gingival disease.

Nursing Interventions

1. Maintain airway patency.
2. Administer supplemental oxygen, as needed.
3. Initiate cardiorespiratory and oxygen saturation monitoring.
4. Obtain venous access and initiate intravenous therapy.
   - Obtain blood for laboratory studies:
     - Complete blood count with differential.
     - Blood cultures.
     - Erythrocyte sedimentation rate.
   - Obtain urine for urinalysis.
5. Administer medications as ordered:
   - Antibiotics.
   - Antipyretics.
   - Intravenous hydration.
6. Provide anticipatory guidance for child and family for lengthy treatment regimen (2 to 6 weeks) and possible surgical intervention.

Home Care and Prevention

Children with CHD who present to the ED for treatment require antibiotic prophylaxis prior to invasive procedures such as (Mott, 1994):

- Dental procedures with probable bleeding.
- Biopsies.
- Wound debridement.
- Incision and drainage of an infected site.
- Bronchoscopy.
- Urethral catheterization with a suspected urinary tract infection.

The recommended pediatric prophylaxsis dose should not exceed the adult dose (American Heart Association, 1997). The recommendation for standard general prophylaxis is amoxicillin, 2.0 g for an adult and 50 mg/kg for a child, administered orally 1 hour before a procedure (American Heart Association, 1997). Parents should be taught about requirements for antibiotic prophylaxis so that they can inform the ED staff of this need. Children should be taught to practice good dental hygiene to prevent dental caries.

Myocarditis and Pericarditis

Myocarditis is an inflammation of the myocardium, or the heart muscle. Often there is an associated myocellular necrosis (Towbin, 2001). Presentation can range from mild symptoms that go undiagnosed to severe decompensation and sudden death in children. Myocarditis is more common in children greater than 1 year of age.

Pericarditis is an inflammation of the pericardium, or the outer lining of the heart. Although similar in etiology to myocarditis, pericarditis follows a more benign clinical course, usually with fewer long-term sequelae. Table 17.9 compares the etiology, ECG findings, and assessment findings for myocarditis and pericarditis.

Focused History

- Recent upper respiratory tract infection.
- Signs of cardiac decompensation.

Focused Assessment

Physical Assessment

1. Assess the respiratory system.
   - Auscultate the chest for:
     - Respiratory rate.
     - Equality of breath sounds.
     - Adventitious sounds.
2. Assess the cardiovascular system.
   - Auscultate the heart for:
     - Rate.
     - Rhythm.
     - Clarity.
     - Murmurs. Extracardiac sounds, such as a pleural friction rub, may be auscultated.

TABLE 17.9 Myocarditis versus Pericarditis

	Myocarditis	*Pericarditis*
Etiology	■ Viral pathogens: ■ Coxsackie B virus (50%) ■ Echovirus (Suddaby, 1996) ■ Human immunodeficiency virus ■ Enterovirus ■ Bacterial pathogens: ■ *Haemophilus influenzae* ■ Fungal pathogens ■ Collagen-vascular disease ■ Toxic myocarditis following drug or exotoxin exposure ■ Acute rheumatic fever ■ Lyme disease	■ Viral pathogens similar to those involved in myocarditis ■ Bacterial pathogens: ■ Staphylococcus aureus, Streptococcus pneumoniae, streptococci, Haemophilus influenzae, and Tuberculosis mycobacterium can result in purulent pericarditis ■ Post-pericardiotomy syndrome ■ Acute rheumatic fever ■ Rheumatoidal diseases ■ Oncologic disease treatment (e.g., chemotherapy, radiation) ■ Uremia associated with renal failure
Electrocardiogram findings	Low QRS voltage ST-segment and T-wave abnormalities Prolonged QT interval Dysrhythmias	ST-segment elevation
History	Sudden onset is common in younger children (Baker, 1994). May have history of recent upper respiratory tract infection, flu-like symptoms, or vague complaints, such as malaise and lethargy.	Predominant presenting complaint is precordial chest pain (80%) exacerbated by breathing, coughing, or exercise and alleviated by sitting upright (Park, 1996).
Physical examination findings	Signs and symptoms of CHF: tachypnea, gallop, tachycardia, poor feeding, diaphoresis at rest, and hepatomegaly Loud systolic murmur Active precordium	Precordial pain may radiate to shoulder or neck. Respiratory distress is uncommon in the absence of tamponade. Pericardial friction rub is loudest while the patient leans forward. Cardiac tamponade: Distant heart tones, tachycardia, quiet precordium, pulsus paradoxus, hypotension, hepatomegaly, and peripheral vasoconstriction. Purulent pericarditis is associated with high fever (>38.5°C).
Pathophysiology	Can result from a cell-mediated immunologic process as well as viral infection (Suddaby, 1996). Myocardial inflammation interferes with normal structural and cellular function of the myocardium, which becomes soft, flabby, and pale with scarring on gross anatomic exam (Park, 1996).	Two factors contribute to development: 1. Speed of fluid accumulation. 2. Competence of the myocardium. ■ Several compensatory mechanisms are initiated as inflammation/effusion/tamponade develops: ■ Systemic and pulmonary vasoconstriction to improve diastolic filling.

TABLE 17.9 (continued)

	Myocarditis	*Pericarditis*
Pathophysiology (continued)	Viral invasion is followed by leukocyte and antigen-antibody complex infiltration. Immune response with subsequent cytokine byproduction leads to inflammation. Autoimmune response and viral persistence can complicate recovery. Microvascular spasm and reperfusion injury occur secondary to vascular endothelial damage. Over time, the edematous, necrotic muscle area is reabsorbed and replaced with scar tissue. Some patients will develop chronic myocarditis with cardiomegaly, severe congestive heart failure, ventricular dysfunction, and valvular regurgitation (Towbin, 2001).	▪ Increased systemic vascular resistance to increase blood pressure. ▪ Tachycardia to increase cardiac output. ■ Cardiac tamponade is a rare but serious complication (Toepper, 1996). Tamponade results from excessive pericardial effusion, which is rarely associated with viral disease. ■ For ductal-dependent lesions, administer Prostaglandin E1 (PGE1) infusion to maintain ductal patency: ▪ Dose: 0.05–0.1 mcg/µg/kg/min. ▪ Side effects: apnea, hypotension, fever, flushing, seizurelike activity, and jitteriness.

- Inspect the skin for:
  - Color. Pale skin may indicate decreased perfusion.
  - Temperature. Cool extremities may indicate poor peripheral perfusion.
- Measure capillary refill.
  - Delayed capillary refill (> 3 seconds) may indicate early shock.

3. Assess the neurologic system.
   - Measure the child's level of consciousness with the GCS or AVPU method.
4. Assess the abdomen.
   - Palpate the abdomen for organ enlargement resulting from right-sided heart failure:
     - Hepatomegaly.
     - Splenomegaly.
     - Lymphadenopathy.

Nursing Interventions

1. Maintain airway patency.
2. Administer supplemental oxygen, as needed.
3. Initiate cardiorespiratory and oxygen saturation monitoring.
4. Place the child in a position of comfort or in a semi-Fowler's position.
5. Obtain venous access and initiate intravenous therapy.
   - Obtain specimens for myocarditis laboratory testing:
     - Complete blood count with differential.
     - Electrolytes.
     - Blood culture.
     - Stool culture.
     - Throat viral culture.
   - Obtain specimens for pericarditis laboratory testing:
     - Blood culture.
     - Electrolytes.
     - Viral culture.
6. Prepare for a possible pericardiocentesis for both therapeutic and diagnostic value in symptomatic patients (Rheuban, 2001).
   - Send a sample of pericardial fluid for culture.
   - Prepare for intravascular volume replacement following pericardiocentesis (pericarditis).
7. Prepare the child and parents for procedures and offer emotional support and information.
8. Monitor vital signs and cardiovascular and respiratory status closely.
9. Administer medications, as prescribed:
   - Antipyretics.
   - Analgesics.
   - Diuretics.
   - Inotropic agents.
   - Corticosteroids.
   - Nonsteroidal anti-inflammatory drugs.
   - Intravenous gamma globulin.

10. Prepare for transfer and transport to a tertiary care facility, as needed.

Home Care and Prevention

Although prevention of myocarditis is difficult, aggressive initial treatment may prevent chronicity. Routine primary pediatric care should be provided to detect illness and prevent complications. Thorough postcardiothoracic surgical care and follow-up are imperative.

Prompt recognition of hemodynamic compromise and subtle signs and symptoms of CHF will prevent further decompensation.

Conclusion

Infants and children may present for ED treatment related to acquired or congenital heart disease. Children with chronic cardiac problems are faced with numerous issues related to their normal growth and development. The child with a heart or a heart-lung transplant has unique needs related to an immunocompromised state as well as infection and rejection. Astute emergency nursing assessments, coupled with emotional support and timely interventions, lend themselves to improved outcomes for these patients and families.

References

American Heart Association (2000). *Guidelines 2000 for cardiopulmonary resuscitation and emergency cardiovascular care.* Dallas, TX: American Heart Association (pp. 291-342).

American Heart Association. (1997). Recommendations by the American Heart Association by the Committee on Rheumatic Fever, Endocarditis, and Kawasaki Disease. *Circulation, 96*, 358-366.

Baker, A. (1994). Acquired heart disease in infants and children. *Critical Care Nursing Clinics of North America, 6*, 175-186.

Dajani, A. S., & Taubert, K. A. (2001). Infective endocarditis. In H. D. Allen, E. B. Clark, H. P. Gutgesell, & D. J. Driscoll (Eds.), *Moss and Adams' heart disease in infants, children, and adolescents: Including the fetus and young adult* (6th ed., vol. 2, pp. 1297-1310). Philadelphia: Lippincott Williams & Wilkins.

DeBoer, S. (1996). The case of the blue baby: ED management of tetralogy of Fallot. *Journal of Emergency Nursing, 22*, 73-76.

Freedom, R. M., Black, M. D., & Benson, L. N. (2001). Hypoplastic left heart syndrome. In H. D. Allen, E. B. Clark, H. P. Gutgesell, & D. J. Driscoll (Eds.), *Moss and Adams' heart disease in infants, children, and adolescents: Including the fetus and young adult* (6th ed., vol. 2, pp. 1011-1026). Philadelphia: Lippincott Williams & Wilkins.

Hazinsky, M. (1999). Cardiovascular disorders. In M. Hazinski (Ed.), *Manual of pediatric critical care* (pp. 84-288). St. Louis: Mosby—Year Book.

Mahony, L. (2001). Development of myocardial structure and function. In H. D. Allen, E. B. Clark, H. P. Gutgesell, & D. J. Driscoll (Eds.), *Moss and Adams' heart disease in infants, children, and adolescents: Including the fetus and young adult* (6th ed., vol. 1, pp. 24-40). Philadelphia: Lippincott Williams & Wilkins.

Mair, D. D., Edwards, W. D., Julsrud, P. R., Seward, J. B., & Danielson, G. K. (2001). Truncus arteriosus. In H. D. Allen, E. B. Clark, H. P. Gutgesell, & D. J. Driscoll (Eds.), *Moss and Adams' heart disease in infants, children, and adolescents: Including the fetus and young adult* (6th ed., vol. 2, pp. 910-923). Philadelphia: Lippincott Williams & Wilkins.

Mott, S. (1994). Cardiac emergencies. In S. J. Kelley (Ed.), *Pediatric emergency nursing* (pp. 199-227). Norwalk, CT: Appleton & Lange.

O'Brien, P., Baker, A. L., & Boisvert, J. T. (2000). The child with cardiovascular dysfunction. In L. D. Wong (Ed.), *Whaley and Wong's nursing care of infants and children* (6th ed., pp. 1583-1647). St. Louis: Mosby—Year Book.

Park, M. K. (1996). *Pediatric cardiology for practitioners* (3rd ed.). St. Louis: Mosby—Year Book.

Park, M. K. (1997). *The pediatric cardiology handbook* (2nd ed.). St. Louis: Mosby—Year Book.

Rheuban, K. S. (2001). Pericardial diseases. In H. D. Allen, E. B. Clark, H. P. Gutgesell, & D. J. Driscoll (Eds.), *Moss and Adams' heart disease in infants, children, and adolescents: Including the fetus and young adult* (6th ed., vol. 2, pp. 1287-1296). Philadelphia: Lippincott Williams & Wilkins.

Schamberger, M. S. (1996). Cardiac emergencies in children. *Pediatric Annals, 25*(6), 339-344.

Smith J. B., Ley, S. J., Curley, M. A. Q., Elixson, M. E., & Dodds, K. M. (1996). Tissue perfusion. In M. A. Q. Curley, J. B. Smith, & P. A. Maloney-Harmon (Eds.), *Critical care nursing of infants and children* (pp. 155-245). Philadelphia: Saunders.

Srivastava, D. & Baldwin, H. S. (2001). Molecular determinants of cardiac development. In H. D. Allen, E. B. Clark, H. P. Gutgesell, and D. J. Driscoll (Eds.), *Moss and Adams' heart disease in infants, children, and adolescents: Including the fetus and young adult* (6th ed., vol. 1, pp. 3-23). Philadelphia: Lippincott Williams & Wilkins.

Suddaby, E. C. (1996). Viral myocarditis in children. *Critical Care Nurse, 16*, 73-82.

Towbin, J. A. (2001). Myocarditis. In H. D. Allen, E. B. Clark, H. P. Gutgesell, & D. J. Driscoll (Eds.), *Moss and Adams' heart disease in infants, children, and adolescents: Including the fetus and young adult* (6th ed., vol. 2, pp. 1197-1215). Philadelphia: Lippincott Williams & Wilkins.

Toepper, W. C. (1996). Dysrhythmias. In J. Kircher & M. Navrozov (Eds.), *Pediatric emergency medicine: A comprehensive study guide* (pp. 203-207). New York: McGraw Hill.

Wernovsky, G. (2001). Transposition of the great arteries. In H. D. Allen, E. B. Clark, H. P. Gutgesell, & D. J. Driscoll (Eds.), *Moss and Adams' heart disease in infants, children, and adolescents: Including the fetus and young adult* (6th ed., vol. 2, pp. 1027-1086). Philadelphia: Lippincott Williams & Wilkins.

18

Neurologic Emergencies

Nancy Eckle, RN, MSN

Introduction

Neurologic emergencies are relatively common in the pediatric population. Neurologic dysfunction may result from either a direct insult to the nervous system or as a secondary effect from a systemic process. Evaluation of the neurologic status of the pediatric patient is a vital component in the emergency nurse's assessment of illness and injury.

When evaluating neurologic function, emergency nurses must be aware of the infant's and child's corresponding developmental stages and milestones as well as age-appropriate levels of neurologic functioning. The purpose of this chapter is to describe common neurologic emergencies and to outline emergency nursing interventions for their recognition and treatment.

Embryologic Development of the Neurologic System

Neurologic (central nervous system [CNS]) malformations cause 75% of fetal deaths and 40% of deaths during infancy; 90% of central nervous system malformations are defects in neural tube closure (Farley Hardin-Mooney, 1998). Because many of these neonates receive early surgical intervention, children with congenital neurologic malformations are likely to receive emergency department (ED) treatment, whether related or unrelated to their neurologic condition. Therefore, it is important to understand the embryologic development of the nervous system.

The embryologic development of the nervous system is a complex process. Derived from the ectoderm of the embryo, the neural groove develops in the midline of the embryo. The neural groove is bordered by neural folds, which close in the fourth week of embryonic life to form the hollow neural tube (Williams, Warwick, Dyson, & Bannister, 1989; Gilman & Newman, 1996). The neural tube and surrounding tissues are composed of several different types of cells. Through continued cellular differentiation and cellular migration, the structures of the *central* and *peripheral* nervous systems develop (Gilman & Newman, 1996; Williams et al., 1989).

The *central nervous system* comprises the brain and spinal cord, which arise from the neural tube. Before closure of the neural tube is completed, the development of the brain begins. At the rostral end of the neural tube, three vesicles emerge. These vesicles further differentiate to ultimately form the cerebral hemispheres, cerebellum, pons, medulla and internal structure of the brain (Gilman & Newman, 1996; Sarnat, 1996; Williams et al., 1989).

The *peripheral nervous system* originates from a ridge of ectodermal cells along the neural folds. As the neural tube closes, the neural crests are formed. The neural crest cells migrate through the embryo and differentiate to form the peripheral nervous system, chromaffin cells (found in the adrenal medulla and carotid bodies), and other nonneural structures (Gilman & Newman, 1996; Sarnat, 1996).

The embryonic growth of the nervous system includes the differentiation of neuroepithelial cells, which results in the formation of mature neurons. Cellular migration and differentiation also result in the development of the glial cells, dendrites, axonal pathways, membrane excitability, neurotransmitters, and myelination (Sarnat, 1996).

Neurologic disorders may arise from alterations in the structural development of the spinal cord, brain, or bony structures; chromosomal abnormalities; enzyme deficiencies; inborn errors of metabolism, or hypoxic ischemic injury to the CNS. Table 18.1 compares developmental errors and their outcomes.

TABLE 18.1 Neurologic Developmental Errors and Their Descriptions

Developmental Error	*Description*
Defective closure at the cranial end of the neural tube	
• Posterior defects (more common)	*Anencephaly*—Soft, bony part of the skull and part of the brain are missing.
	Encephalocele—Herniation of brain and meninges into a saclike structure through a skull defect.
	Occipital meningocele—Meninges and spinal fluid in a sac through a vertebral defect that does not involve the spinal cord; occurs in the cervical, thoracic, and lumbar spine.
• Anterior midline defects	*Cyclopia*—Single midline orbit and eye.
Defective closure of the caudal end of the neural tube	*Myelomeningocele* (spina bifida cystica)—Herniation of a sac with meninges, spinal fluid, and a segment of the spinal cord and nerves through an opening in a vertebrae. Eighty percent are located in the lumbar and lumbar sacral regions (a final area that closes). The level of the myelomeningocele indicates the level of neurologic involvement; higher levels are associated with extensive levels of neurologic involvement. For example, a thoracic-level lesion involves flaccid paralysis of the lower extremities, abdominal muscle weakness, and absence of bowel and bladder control; and a sacral-level lesion involves normal neurologic function of the lower extremities and bowel and bladder control.
	Two associated conditions are:
	Arnold-Chiari II malformation—The possible herniation of the cerebellum, cerebral tonsils, brain stem, and fourth ventricle through the foramen magnum; this can be life-threatening.
	Tethered cord—The spinal cord is trapped (tethered) from scar tissues as the child grows, causing scoliosis, altered gait, loss of muscle strength, changes in bowel and bladder function, and back pain.
Failure of the posterior laminae to fuse/malformation of the axial skeleton	*Spina bifida occulta*—Abnormal hair growth along the spine; midline dimple cutaneous angioma; lipoma or dermoid cyst. Most (80%) are located in the lumbar-sacral regions.
Malformations of the axial skeleton	*Craniosynostosis*—Premature closure of the cranial sutures during the first 18 to 20 months of life, causing abnormal skull expansion and growth.
	Microcephaly—Cranial size is below average for the infant's age and other characteristics.
	Congenital hydrocephalus—Increased volume of cerebro spinal fluid because of blockage within the ventricles, overproduction of cerebro spinal fluid (CSF), or a reduced reabsorption of CSF.

From: Chandrasoma & Taylor, 1995; Farley et al., 1998.

Pediatric Considerations

Neurologic development is sequential, and, over time, neurologic responses change to become those seen in adults. Developmental milestones in motor function (Table 18.2), reflexes (Table 18.3), and head growth (Table 18.4) are highlighted.

Etiology

Neurologic conditions arise from a variety of causes, including alterations in:

- Cerebral blood flow.
- Intracranial pressure (ICP).
- Level of consciousness.
- Motor function.
- Sensory function.

They also may be precipitated by:

- Metabolic disturbances (e.g., diabetic ketoacidosis or hypoglycemia).
- Infection.

TABLE 18.2 Major Motor Milestones during the First 24 Months of Life

Age	*Motor Development*
Newborn/young infant	The newborn has clenched fists (Berg, 1996a; Swaiman, 1999a). The young infant's normal posture is flexion of the upper and lower extremities with somewhat jerky but vigorous movements.
3 to 4 months	The extremities are more supple and movements become smoother. Hands are open, and the infant will grasp for objects (Berg, 1996a; Swaiman, 1999b).
6 months	The infant should grasp object with one hand, roll from prone to supine, and sit with support (Berg, 1996a; Swaiman, 1999b).
8 months	The infant should be able to roll supine to prone and transfer objects between hands (Berg, 1996a; Swaiman, 1999b).
10 months	The infant sits well, stands while holding on, and grasps and picks up smaller objects; finger-thumb opposition is present (Berg, 1996a; Swaiman, 1999b).
12 months	The infant stands while holding on and walks with support.
24 months	The toddler gains independent walking skills and the ability to climb and descend stairs (Berg, 1996a; Swaiman, 1999b).

TABLE 18.3 Primitive Reflexes

Reflex	*Age*	*Description*
Moro reflex (startle reflex)	Present until 6 months of age	A sudden release of support that allows the infant's head to drop (in relation to the body) to a pillow or the examiner's hand will elicit the reflex. The infant will open his or her hands, extend and abduct the upper extremity, and then flex the arms, as in an embrace (Berg, 1996a; Swaiman, 1999b).
Tonic neck reflex	Present until 6–7 months of age	Turning the infant's head to one side results in extension of the arm and leg of the side the head is rotated toward and flexion of the arm on the opposite side (Berg, 1996a; Swaiman, 1999b).
Palmar reflex (grasping reflex)	Present until 6–8 months of age, but less evident by 2–3 months of age	Placement of the examiner's finger in the infant's palm results in the infant's grasping the finger. The infant's grasp will tighten with attempts to remove the finger (Berg, 1996a; Brucker, 1996; Swaiman, 1999b).
Babinski's reflex	Present until about 2 years of age	Stroking the sole of the infant's foot from the heel to the toes will elicit the response, fanning of the toes and flexion of the great toe (Brucker, 1996).

- Toxic exposures.
- Alcohol or substance abuse.
- Hypoxia or anoxia.
- Intracranial hemorrhage or central venous thrombosis.
- Shock.
- Direct and secondary trauma to the central and peripheral nervous system.
- Stroke.
- Seizures.

Focused History

- Onset of the patient's present illness:
  - Sequence and development of neurologic symptoms suggestive of ICP.

TABLE 18.4 Cranial Development

Characteristic of Cranial Development	*Implications*
The head accounts for one-fourth of the infant's total body height (compared with one-eighth of the adult's total body height).	The infant's head represents a larger body surface area from which to lose heat. The head presents a larger area for injury to be sustained.
The infant's skull bones are separated by suture lines that form two fontanelles (anterior and posterior) and allow room for expansion with increased intracranial pressure. The adult skull is fixed and cannot expand.	The posterior fontanelle typically closes by 8 weeks of age. The anterior fontanelle closes by 18 months of age. The softer skull affords less protection from injury. Open fontanelles allow for brain expansion with increased intracranial pressure, thus delaying brain stem herniation.
The infant's head is the fastest-growing body part.	Head circumference should be measured regularly through the first 5 years of life to detect increased or decreased growth.

From: Farley et al., 1998.

  - Changes in level of consciousness, activity level, mentation, communication, sensation, vision, and/or motor abilities. Consciousness is a state of full awareness; alterations in the level of consciousness encompass a range of conditions described by a variety of terms. Definitions of the familiar terms (such as *confusion*, *lethargy*, and *obtunded*) are often obscure and vary among parents and healthcare providers.
- Child's behaviors:
  - In infants, changes in social behaviors and interaction should be evaluated, including (Ashwal, 1999) changes in feeding, sleeping, and waking patterns; response to comforting; delays in developmental milestone attainment or regression.
- Symptoms:
  - Headache: location, quality, and duration; changes in vision or visual disturbances.
  - Vomiting.
  - Fever.
- Medications (over-the-counter and prescribed):
  - Dose.
  - Time of last dose.
  - Compliance with dosing regimen.
- Past health history:
  - Past history of congenital or chronic illness or condition and course of treatment.
  - Presence of a persistent neurologic deficit and normal baseline neurologic function, including usual level of activity, usual and current interactions with others and the environment, baseline cognitive level, usual movement patterns, and muscle tone.
- Recent falls or injury:
  - Time of occurrence.
  - Mechanism of injury.
  - Changes in behavior since injury.
- Seizures:
  - Onset, duration, and description of seizure activity.
  - Postictal state.
- Immunization status.
- Developmental milestones achieved (Chapter 4).

Focused Assessment

Physical Assessment

1. Assess the neurologic system (primary assessment):
   - Assess the level of consciousness: A rapid method for evaluating the child's level of consciousness is the AVPU system (Dolan, 1997):

     A = Alert.

     V = Responds to verbal commands.

     P = Responds only to pain.

     U = Unresponsive.
   - Assess the pupillary size and response:
     - Pupils should be equal in size.
     - Pupils should be round.
     - Pupils should react to light.
     - Reactions should be equal and brisk.
2. Perform a detailed neurologic assessment (secondary assessment):
   - Inspect the head for shape and symmetry.
     - Examine the fontanelles: The anterior fontanelle should be examined when the infant is quiet and positioned at a 45-degree angle.
     - The anterior fontanelle may appear sunken in infants who are dehydrated.

- The anterior fontanelle may be bulging in an infant with increased intracranial pressure.
- Measure the infant's head circumference and compare it to the age-defined diameter:
  - An enlarged head may be indicative of hydrocephalus.
  - A small head may be indicative of microcephaly.
- Palpate the head for:
  - Overriding sutures.
  - Hematomas.
  - Step offs.
  - Bruits over the skull.
- Observe the face and head for:
  - Bruises (indicative of child abuse, Chapter 4).
  - Lacerations.
  - Other signs of trauma.
- Assess the level of consciousness:
  - Use an objective scale to describe the level of consciousness to facilitate trending of the patient's responses and improve communication among healthcare providers. The scale must be used in conjunction with a prudent neurologic assessment.
  - Measure the level of consciousness with the Glasgow coma scale (GCS) (Table 18.5).

3. Assess orientation and mentation:
   - The GCS verbal response is used to evaluate mentation and orientation.
   - In children, orientation is evaluated through age-appropriate questions.
   - In infants or preverbal children, orientation is evaluated through observation of their:

TABLE 18.5 Glasgow Coma Scale

Parameter	*Description*	*Score*	
Eye opening	Observe eye-opening activity in relation to stimulus required to elicit the response (Dolan, 1997; Hector, 1986).	*> 2 Years old* 4 Spontaneously 3 To verbal stimuli 2 To pain 1 No response	*< 2 Years old* 4 Spontaneously 3 To speech 2 To pain 1 No response
Best verbal response	Observe the response to questions. In preverbal children, spontaneous vocalization and vocal responses to pain are observed to score this parameter (Dolan, 1997; Hector, 1986).	*> 2 Years old* 5 Oriented/uses appropriate words and phrases 4 Confused 3 Inappropriate words/screams/cries 2 Nonspecific sounds 1 No response	*< 2 Years old* 5 Coos, babbles 4 Irritable, cries 3 Cries to pain 2 Moans to pain 1 No response
Best motor response	Observe the response to verbal commands or painful stimuli. In children younger than 2 years of age, this parameter is scored by observing for spontaneous movements, response to touch, or response to painful stimulus (Dolan, 1997; Hector, 1986).	*> 2 Years old* 6 Obeys command 5 Localizes pain 4 Withdraws to pain 3 Flexion response to pain 2 Extension response to pain 1 No response	*< 2 Years old* 6 Normal spontaneous movement 5 Withdraws to touch 4 Withdraws to pain 3 Abnormal flexion 2 Abnormal extension 1 No response

- Social behaviors.
- Interaction with the environment.
- Recognition of parents and/or familiar objects.

■ Evaluate the cranial nerves. A gross evaluation of cranial nerve function can be completed relatively quickly. However, the child's condition and developmental level may preclude evaluation of all cranial nerves. Basic cranial nerve evaluation involves eye movement and function (cranial nerves II, III, IV, and VI) (Hector, 1986):

- Equal rise of eyelids.
- Equality of pupil size; reactivity to light and accommodation.
- Infants younger than 3 months of age should blink at bright light.
- Infants older than 3 months of age should follow a dangling object, moving the head to follow the object (Ashwal, 1999).
- Evaluation of extraocular movements through the six fields of gaze, visual acuity, visual tracking, and color identification in the conscious child. Complete evaluation of all extraocular movements may not be possible in children younger than 2 to 3 years of age.
- The position of eyes at rest and the presence of abnormal spontaneous eye movement are noted in the unconscious child or child with an altered level of consciousness (Dolan, 1997). Note the presence of eye deviation, dysconjugate gaze, nystagmus, doll's eyes.

■ Evaluate the remaining cranial nerves and reflex responses (Table 18.6).

■ Evaluate motor function; compare to the major motor milestones attained up to age 24 months: GCS motor response, symmetry of movement, posture.

■ Evaluate muscle tone:

- Muscle tone is the muscle tension or resistance of the muscle to passive movement (Berg, 1996a; Brucker, 1996). Abnormalities in muscle tone are related to the location of the neurologic lesion. In the infant, extension and/or scissoring of the legs when lifted vertically denotes increased muscle tone and corticospinal disorder (Berg, 1996a). Table 18.7 highlights the types of abnormal muscle tone.
- Muscle tone and power are assessed in upper and lower extremities.
- Child: Ask the child to execute movements such as pushing against the examiner's hands with his or her hands and then feet, grasping the examiner's hands and fingers, and moving extremities against resistance.

■ Evaluate muscle power:

- Muscle power is graded based on the movement with gravity and resistance. Normal power is the ability to move or contract the muscle against gravity and maximal resistance (Berg, 1996a; Brucker, 1996):

  5 = Normal power and strength.

  4 = Movement against gravity and variable resistance.

  3 = Movement against gravity.

  2 = Movement with gravity eliminated.

  1 = Muscular contraction without movement.

  0 = No muscular contraction.

- Infant: Pull the infant to a sitting position and evaluate the infant's strength and control of the body (Brucker, 1996). Observe the infant's strength, such as withdrawal from touch, to assess motor power.

■ Evaluate mobility.

■ Evaluate reflexes:

- Tendon reflexes are elicited in the upper and lower extremities. If the child is unable to relax the extremity being examined, the reflex may not be elicited.
- Reflexes (including the primitive reflexes) should be evaluated in terms of strength and symmetry. Continued presence of primitive reflexes beyond the expected age of cessation may indicate neurologic dysfunction. Asymmetric reflex responses may indicate injury.
- *Clonus* is a rhythmic contraction and relaxation of the muscle when the wrist, ankle, or great toe is flexed. Clonus may be present with motor neuron lesion, cerebral cortex injury, or in metabolic disease (Brucker, 1996).

■ Evaluate cerebellar function:

- The cerebellum regulates motor function, coordination of movement and balance, and maintains muscle tone. Observe the child's gait (crawling or walking), balance while standing and/or sitting, performance of repetitive motions.
- Disturbances of balance and/or involuntary movements are indicative of neurologic dysfunction.

Psychosocial Assessment

■ Assess the family's understanding of the child's underlying neurologic-related health condition, as needed.

■ Assess the child's and family's understanding of the child's current neurologic-related health condition.

■ Assess the child's and family's usual coping strategies.

TABLE 18.6 Cranial Nerve and Reflex Responses

Cranial Nerve and Reflex	*Responses*
Cranial nerves IX and X	Ability to swallow Ability to cough Presence of the gag reflex Clarity of speech
Cranial nerves V, VII (corneal reflex)	Ability to blink
Cranial nerves III, VI, VIII (oculocephalic and oculo-vestibular responses)	Only tested for severe brain stem dysfunction *Doll's eyes* Absence of doll's eyes (abnormal): • Eyes move in the same direction as the head is turned Presence of doll's eyes (normal): • Eyes move in the opposite direction as the head is turned *Ice water caloric test* Nystagmus (normal response) No eye movement or asymmetric eye movement (abnormal response).
Cranial nerves V and VII (facial movement and expression)	Facial symmetry with movement; in infants, facial symmetry during crying and sucking Ability to raise eyebrows, smile, clench teeth, chew Presence of tears with crying Presence and strength of suck reflex
Cranial nerves XI and XII (motor and muscular function)	Ability to shrug shoulders Ability to turn head and move upper extremities Ability to stick out the tongue In infants, midline tongue position when crying
Cranial nerve VIII (hearing)	Response to verbal commands and ability to answer questions Ability to repeat words Ability of the infant < 3 months to stop spontaneous movements or sucking in response to voice or sound and then resume the activity Ability of the infant > 3 months to quiet to the sound of voice or sound, turn head or eyes toward sound, and vocalize in response to sounds or voice

From: Brucker, 1996; Emergency Nurses Association, 1995; Hazinski, Headrick, & Bruce, 1999.

Nursing Diagnoses	*Expected Outcomes*
Altered tissue and cerebral tissue perfusion	The patient will demonstrate adequate tissue and cerebral perfusion. The patient's ICP will be within normal limits (5–15 mm Hg). The patient will demonstrate age and developmentally appropriate neurologic function. The patient will demonstrate vital signs within normal limits for developmental age.
High-risk for injury	The patient will be free of injury or secondary complications.
Knowledge deficit related to disease	The patient and family will verbalize an understanding of the patient's medications and process and therapeutic regimen treatment regimen.

TABLE 18.7 Types of Muscle Tone Abnormality

Type of Abnormality	*Characteristics*
Hypertonia or spasticity	Persistent increased muscle tension. With passive stretch of the muscle, there is increased muscle tone or resistance to the movement, which then suddenly gives way or relaxes (Berg, 1996b; Brucker, 1996).
Hypotonia	Decreased muscle tension and decreased resistance to passive movement. Infants may also exhibit a weak cry, weak suck, and decreased spontaneous movements. In the hypotonic infant, movement of the infant's arm across the chest and neck will result in the elbow crossing the midline (positive scarf sign) (Berg,1996b).
Abnormal posture or asymmetry of function or strength	Indicative of significant neurologic dysfunction. *Decorticate rigidity:* Flexion of elbows, wrist, and fingers, and extension of legs and ankles, indicating ischemia or damage to the cerebral hemispheres (Hazinski et al., 1999). *Decerebrate posturing:* Extension of arms and legs with rigidity, indicating diffuse cerebral injury or ischemia or damage to brain stem structures (Hazinski, 1999). *Flaccidity:* Absence of muscle tone.

Triage Decisions

Emergent (Murphy, 1997; Thomas, 1991)

- Current seizure activity.
- Inability to maintain a spontaneous patent airway.
- Respiratory distress or hypoventilation.
- Compromised perfusion.
- Seizure longer than 15 minutes.
- Multiple seizures.
- Decreased level of consciousness and GCS score less than 12.
- Difficult to arouse following a first-time seizure or febrile seizure.
- Prehospital pharmacologic intervention for seizure control.
- Incapacitating headache in the child with a cerebrospinal fluid (CSF) shunt.
- Incapacitating headache with slurred speech, facial asymmetry, and extreme hypertension.

Urgent (Murphy, 1997; Thomas, 1991)

- Awake and alert after first-time seizure or febrile seizure.
- Seizure after head trauma.
- Focal seizure.
- Inconsolability or irritability.
- History of toxic substance ingestion.
- Atypical seizure in the patient with known seizure disorder.
- Signs of meningeal irritation (e.g., nuchal rigidity).
- History of seizure disorder and noncompliance with medication regimen.
- Inconsolability or irritability, vision changes or photophobia, frequent vomiting, abdominal pain and tenderness, fever, signs of meningeal irritation, and severe headache in the child with a CSF shunt.
- Severe headache in the presence of frequent vomiting, signs of meningeal irritation, focal motor or sensory weakness, and hypertension.

Nonurgent

- None.

Nursing Interventions

- Assess and maintain airway, breathing, and circulation:
  - Initiate maneuvers to maintain airway patency, such as positioning and suctioning and insertion of an airway adjunct.
  - Prepare for endotracheal intubation for the child who cannot maintain airway patency.
  - Administer 100% oxygen through a nonrebreather mask; initiate assisted ventilation in the child who is not maintaining adequate respiratory effort and/or if the GCS score is less than 9.
  - Initiate cardiorespiratory monitoring; measure continuous oxygen saturation.
- Initiate spinal immobilization if trauma is suspected.
- Obtain venous access and initiate an intravenous infusion at maintenance rate:
  - Obtain blood for laboratory studies: serum medication levels (e.g., valproic acid), toxicology screen, glucose and electrolytes.

- Administer analgesics for pain control, as needed (Chapter 13). Closely monitor patients receiving narcotic analgesics that may alter the level of consciousness.
- Monitor neurologic status:
  - Observe for changes in level of consciousness.
  - Observe for seizures.
- Protect from injury.
- Provide psychosocial support to the patient and family.
- Prevent complications.
- Prepare for transfer and transport to a tertiary care facility (Chapter 10) or prepare for hospitalization, as needed.

Home Care and Prevention

Patients and families may need time to understand the home care process involved with a neurologic disorder that suddenly presents in their child. Learning about seizures, headaches, or other neurologic conditions helps patients and parents to feel a sense of control. It is important to teach the older child and parents the importance of diligence with prescribed medications to prevent future seizures or other neurologic problems. Finally, older children and families require knowledge of first aid and cardiopulmonary resuscitation and how to access their local emergency medical services agency.

Emergency nurses may want to learn more about specific neurologic conditions to prepare teaching materials for parents and other caregivers. Several helpful organizations are:

- Spina Bifida Association of America (202/944-3285) www.sbaa.org.
- United Cerebral Palsy Association, Inc. (800/827-5827) www.ucpa.org.
- Epilepsy Foundation of America (800/EFA-1000) www.epilepsyfoundation.org.

Selected Neurologic Emergencies

Seizures

Etiology

Seizures are among the more common events that trigger an ED visit. A *seizure* occurs when there is a sudden, abnormal, excessive cerebral electrical discharge. The rate and progression of the electrical discharge, the child's age, and the specific area of the brain involved influence the clinical presentation, which may vary (Fuchs et al., 1997; Holmes, 1996). The incidence of seizures during childhood is high. *Febrile seizure* is the most common seizure occurring in childhood; the typical age of onset is between 3 months and 5 years of age (Fuchs et al., 1997). In the United States, 2 to 4% of children will experience a febrile seizure before the age of 5 years (Holmes, 1996). Febrile seizures are categorized as simple and complex (Table 18.9).

Seizures are caused by a number of factors that interrupt normal brain function (Table 18.10).

Epilepsy is defined as recurrent unprovoked seizures (Holmes, 1996). The average incidence of epilepsy in childhood ranges from 46 to 86 per 100,000 children; the incidence is higher in children younger than 9 years of age (Holmes, 1996). Seizures brought on by acute events such as fever, infection of the central nervous system, or following head trauma are not considered epilepsy. Epileptic seizures are classified into two general categories, partial and generalized (Table 18.11).

Nonepileptic paroxysmal events, such as breath-holding spells, may be mistaken for seizures because the child exhibits twitching or clonic-tonic movements at the end of the episode. Differentiation between these

TABLE 18.9 Comparison of Simple and Complex Febrile Seizures

Simple Febrile Seizures	*Complex Febrile Seizures*
Associated with a febrile illness with no CNS infection (Holmes, 1996).	Associated with a febrile illness with no CNS infection with additional characteristics (Holmes, 1996).
Have generalized clonic-tonic or tonic motor activity.	Have prolonged generalized seizure activity.
Last less than 10 to 15 minutes.	Last greater than 15 minutes.
Have no focal onset.	Have focal characteristics.
Usually occur in the first 24 hours of the febrile illness.	Have recurrent seizure with the same illness; more than one seizure in 24 hours.

TABLE 18.10 Etiologies of Seizure

- Acute seizures (Chiang, 2000)
  - Infection (meningitis, encephalitis, brain abscess, shigellosis)
  - Trauma
  - Intracranial bleeding
  - Toxic exposures
  - Metabolic disturbances, including electrolyte imbalances and hypoglycemia
  - Anoxia
  - Brain tumors
  - Fever
- Recurrent seizures or seizure disorders
  - Idiopathic
  - Injury to the CNS caused by trauma, anoxia, hemorrhage, toxin exposure, or infectious disease
  - Congenital disorders
  - Degenerative disorders

episodes and seizures may be difficult and require electroencephalographic evaluation. Syncope is also considered a nonepileptic paroxysmal event (Chiang, 2000).

Status epilepticus is a medical emergency. Generalized seizure activity results in increased tissue oxygen demand arising from muscle contractions, increased cerebral metabolic requirements, increased cerebral blood flow, and potentially increased intracranial pressure. Brain damage may occur if insufficient oxygen is delivered to the brain to meet metabolic needs (Brucker, 1996; Holmes, 1996; Chiang, 2000). Characteristics of status epilepticus are:

- Continuous generalized seizure lasting longer than 30 minutes.
- Recurrent seizures that occur without full recovery of consciousness between seizures.
- Risk for respiratory depression and hypoxia.

Focused History

- History of patient's present illness:
  - Onset of the present illness.
  - Events prior to seizure onset: changes in expression, repetitive gestures, facial expression, or crying; any potential ingestion of toxic substance; recent trauma.
  - Description of body movements or seizure activity.
  - Duration of movements or seizure; number of seizures.
  - Level of awareness during seizure.
  - Color change during seizure; presence of respiratory compromise.
  - Postictal behaviors.
  - Associated symptoms (such as fever, vomiting, headache, stiff neck, and back pain).
  - Dietary intake and output.
  - Parent's or caretaker's impressions. If the child has a known seizure disorder, ask whether this seizure was typical of the child's usual seizure activity.
  - Current medications (dose, time of last dose, and compliance with dosing regimen).
- Past health history:
  - Neurologic, metabolic, or bleeding disorders.
  - Previous seizures, febrile seizures, and last seizure episode.
  - Family history of febrile seizures, seizure disorder, or epilepsy.
  - History of CSF shunt device (ventriculoperitoneal shunt), last revision date.
  - Presence of a persistent neurologic deficit.

Focused Assessment

Physical Assessment

1. Assess the respiratory system:
   - Auscultate the chest for:
     - Respiratory rate.
     - Respiratory effort. Respiratory rate, depth, and effort may be decreased during a seizure and in the postictal phase. Increased secretions and an altered level of consciousness increase the patient's risk for aspiration and respiratory compromise.
2. Assess the cardiovascular system:
   - Auscultate the heart for:
     - Rate. *Tachycardia* is typically present during a seizure and may be related to fever, dehydration, or shock and sepsis. *Bradycardia* may be present in patients with elevated ICP or in those who are experiencing airway obstruction, respiratory depression, hypoventilation, or apnea.
     - Measure blood pressure, including pulse pressure:
       - Alterations in blood pressure (hypotension or hypertension) may arise from a variety of causes. It is critical to evaluate blood pressure readings in relation to the child's age to determine the presence of hypertension, hypotension, and abnormal pulse pressures. Rising

TABLE 18.11 Categories of Epileptic Seizures

Category of Seizure	*Description*
Partial seizures Simple partial seizures (Fenichel, 1997a; Fuchs et al., 1997; Holmes, 1996).	Motor, sensory, autonomic, or psychic manifestation without a loss of consciousness. Focal motor activity. Somatosensory symptoms (headache, pins-and-needles sensation, metallic taste). Autonomic symptoms (flushing, sweating, salivation). Typically last less than 1 minute without postictal symptoms (Holmes, 1996).
Complex partial seizures (Fenichel, 1997a; Fuchs et al., 1997; Holmes, 1996).	Arise from any region of the brain (temporal, frontal, parietal, occipital). Rare in children younger than 10 years of age. Involve an impairment of consciousness. Repetitive automatic behavior—purposeful but inappropriate motor movement, such as facial grimacing, fumbling movements, or running. Last 30 seconds to several minutes. Postictal symptoms may include lethargy, confusion, fear, sadness.
Generalized seizures Absence (Fenichel, 1997a)	Brief lapse of awareness without loss of consciousness (5 to 15 seconds). Staring. Minor motor movement: blinking or nystagmus. Changes in muscle tone.
Tonic-clonic (Fenichel, 1997a; Fuchs et al., 1997; Holmes,1996).	Loss of consciousness. Stained muscle contraction and rigidity of extremities and trunk (tonic); alternates with rhythmic jerking and flexor spasm of the muscles (clonic). May experience aura. Incontinence of urine and/or stool. Postictal state may last hours; deep postictal sleep is typical.
Myoclonic (Fenichel, 1997a; Fuchs et al., 1997; Holmes,1996)	Brief, sudden muscle contraction may be generalized or limited to individual muscle groups; face, trunk, or extremities may be involved. Drooping of the head may occur. Patient may fall to the ground. Contraction may be subtle, resembling tremors. May occur as a component of absence seizure or start of generalized tonic-clonic seizure. Usually no loss of consciousness.
Atonic (Fuchs et al., 1997; Holmes,1996)	Sudden loss of muscle tone. Begin without warning. Patient will fall to the ground if standing. Consciousness impaired. Associated with myoclonic jerks Rare.
Tonic (Holmes, 1996)	Brief; usually less than 60 seconds. Tonic contraction of muscles; sudden increase extensor muscle tone consciousness impaired. Contraction of respiratory and abdominal muscles may result in periods of apnea or high-pitched cry. Occur more frequently at night. Patient typically will fall to the ground if standing. Postictal state may include confusion, lethargy, and headache.

systolic readings and widening pulse pressures are associated with increased ICP and/or early septic shock.

- Measure skin and core temperature:
  - Body temperature may be elevated following a prolonged seizure.
  - The presence or absence of fever is dependent on the etiology of the seizure (e.g., CNS infection or febrile seizure).

3. Assess the neurologic status:
   - Assess the child's level of consciousness, orientation, mentation.

- Calculate the GCS score.
- Evaluate the cranial nerves for:
  - Pupil reaction.
  - Extraocular eye movement.
  - Blinking.
  - Gag reflex.
  - Facial symmetry.
- Evaluate eye position and movement:
  - Deviation may be present.
  - Nystagmus may be present.
- Evaluate motor function:
  - Spontaneous motor response and/or response to stimulus.
  - Posture and muscle tone.
  - Muscle power.
  - Reflexes.
- Observe the child's balance while sitting or standing:
  - Ataxia may be present.
- Describe seizure activity if present or reoccurs:
  - Focal versus generalized motor activity.
  - Progression of motor activity.
  - Type of motor activity (clonic-tonic, clonic, myoclonic, etc.).
  - Duration of seizure: spontaneous resolution; resolution with medication administration.
  - Incontinence of urine and/or stool.
- Assess for signs of meningeal irritation:
  - Nuchal rigidity (neck pain and stiffness).
  - Kernig's sign (inability to completely extend leg when patient lies on back with thigh flexed to 90 degrees).
  - Brudzinski's sign (flexion of the hip and knee in response to forward flexion of the neck).
  - Opisthotonos (severe arching of the neck and back caused by extensor muscle spasm).
  - Photophobia (increased sensitivity to light).
- Assess the head for:
  - Injury or surface trauma.
  - Bulging anterior fontanelle in infants with open anterior fontanelle.

4. Assess the integumentary system:
   - Inspect the skin for:
     - Presence of petechial or purpuric rash. Such rashes may indicate sepsis or meningitis.
     - Surface trauma. Suspicious bruises and bruises in varying stages of healing may be indicative of child maltreatment (Chapter 46).

Psychosocial Assessment

- Assess the family's coping strategies: Observing their child having a seizure, especially a first-time seizure, can be very distressing to the parents.
- Assess and observe the child's and family's interaction patterns: A lack of concern about the seriousness of the child's condition or unhealthy family interaction patterns may indicate child maltreatment or neglect and warrant further investigation (Chapter 46).

Nursing Interventions

1. Assess and maintain airway, breathing, and circulation:
   - Initiate measures to protect the airway:
     - Suction the oropharynx, as needed, to remove secretions.
     - Initiate the jaw thrust—chin lift maneuver to maintain the airway, as needed.
     - Prepare for endotracheal intubation if prolonged airway patency is needed.
     - Initiate spinal immobilization if trauma is suspected.
     - Prepare to turn or turn the patient in a side-lying position if vomiting occurs.
     - Loosen restrictive clothing.
   - Assure adequate breathing and ventilation:
     - Administer 100% oxygen via nonrebreather mask during active seizure, deep postictal state, or respiratory distress.
     - Initiate bag-valve-mask ventilation with 100% oxygen for hypoventilation and apnea.
   - Initiate cardiorespiratory and oxygen saturation monitoring.
2. Obtain venous access and initiate intravenous infusion at a maintenance rate:
   - Obtain blood for laboratory studies:
     - Electrolytes.
     - Glucose.
     - Calcium.
     - Magnesium.
     - Toxicology screen.
     - Complete blood count.
     - Anticonvulsant levels, if the child routinely takes an anticonvulsant medication.

- Consider prothrombin time and partial thromboplastin time in the neonate or infant.
- Administer medications, as prescribed:
  - Pharmacologic intervention should be initiated as soon as possible for seizures lasting 5 minutes or longer to stop the seizure because of the risk of brain injury (Holmes, 1996; Gorelich, 2000; Chiang, 2000) (Table 18.12).
  - Treat documented hypoglycemia. Administer 10% dextrose, intravenously (neonates). Administer 25% dextrose, intravenously (infants and older).
  - Administer additional medications as prescribed:
    - Antibiotics for a CNS infection.
    - Calcium chloride for hypocalcemia.
    - Normal or hypertonic saline for hyponatremia.
    - Gastric decontamination and/or specific antidote for a toxin.
    - Osmotic diuretic for increased intracranial pressure.

3. Monitor the neurologic status:
   - Observe duration and characteristics of seizure activity and signs of improvement.
4. Reassess the child's cardiopulmonary and neurologic status.
5. Prepare for and assist with diagnostic procedures:
   - Neuroimaging (CT scan, MRI): focal seizure, suspected intracranial bleed, suspected intracranial lesion, or signs of increased intracranial pressure.
   - Lumbar puncture and CSF analysis: suspected CNS infection.
6. Inform the family frequently about their child's condition; provide psychosocial and emotional support to the patient and family.
7. Protect the patient from injury:
   - Put side rails up; pad rails as needed.
   - Place the patient in a side-lying position after the seizure to protect from aspiration of secretions and/or emesis.
8. Prepare for transfer and transport to a tertiary care facility (Chapter 10) hospital admission, or discharge to home.

Home Care and Prevention

The patient and family should be educated about the child's disease process and subsequent plan of care, including follow-up with the child's primary care physician. Although additional teaching and follow-up will be necessary, basic instructions on seizure management and appropriate first-aid measures can be taught on ED discharge (Ball, 1998):

- Seizure prevention:
  - Supervise the child's baths and swimming; ensure that someone is at home when an adolescent is bathing or swimming.
  - Purchase and have the child wear a safety helmet when bicycling, tree-climbing, skateboarding, snowboarding, skiing, rollerblading, or doing other activities that place the child at risk for a head injury.
  - Keep bathroom and bedroom doors unlocked to allow quick access in case of an emergency.
  - Obtain a medical identification bracelet for the child who may be eventually or potentially diagnosed with a seizure disorder.
  - Administer antiseizure and antipyretic medications as prescribed.
- First aid for a seizure:
  - Remain calm and remain with the child.
  - Protect the child from injury by removing dangerous objects and placing the child on the floor in a side-lying position.

TABLE 18-12 Medications for Acute Seizures

Medications for Acute Seizures	*Medications Used following Benzodiazepam Administration*
Lorazepam, I.V.: Lorazepam is the drug of first choice because of rapid onset and duration.	Phenytoin, I.V., at a rate no greater than 1 mg/kg/min (maximum 50 mg/min).
Diazepam, I.V.: or rectally if there is no I.V. access.	Fosphenytoin. Fosphenytoin dosage is expressed in phenytoin sodium Eqs (PE). Fosphenytoin may be given I.V. at a rate no greater than 150 mg.
Midazolam, I.M., if no I.V. access.	Phenobarbital, I.V., at a rate no greater than 1 mg/kg/min.
Consider Pyridoxine (neonatal seizure).	

I.V. = Intravenously; I.M. = Intramuscularly.

- Place a folded jacket, blanket, or towel under the child's head to prevent injury if the child is lying on a hard surface, such as an uncarpeted floor.
- Avoid placing fingers, any objects, fluids, or food in the child's mouth during or after the seizure.
- Talk calmly to the child after the seizure; explain what happened; reassure the child.

■ Contact emergency medical services when:
- The child's seizure continues for more than 5 minutes.
- The child develops respiratory distress.
- The seizure activity continues without a postictal phase.

Cerebral Spinal Fluid Shunt Dysfunction

Etiology

The placement of a CSF shunt is the current treatment of choice for hydrocephalus. Hydrocephalus may be acquired (e.g., posttrauma or brain tumor) or congenital. In both types of hydrocephalus, excess CSF accumulates in the ventricular system because of (Brucker, 1996; Ashwal, 1999):

- Excessive production of CSF.
- Obstruction of CSF flow in either the ventricles or subarachnoid space.
- Abnormal absorption of CSF.

The most common type of CSF shunt is the ventriculoperitoneal shunt. The proximal end of the ventriculoperitoneal shunt is placed in the lateral ventricle, and the distal end terminates in the peritoneal cavity. CSF shunts may also terminate in the jugular vein (ventriculojugular shunt) or the right atrium (ventriculoatrial shunt). The shunt device drains excess CSF from the ventricles via a pressure gradient. A one-way value in the shunt tubing prevents retrograde flow of CSF.

Shunt function can be impaired by (Bragg, Edwards-Beckett, Eckle, Principe, & Terry, 1994a):

- Obstruction.
- Infection:

  Most shunt infections occur within 2 months of surgery (Steele, 2000).

  Signs of meningeal irritation (e.g., nuchal rigidity) have been reported in only 33% of patients (Steele, 2000).

  Signs suggestive of shunt infection may include (Steele, 2000):
  - Fever (42% of patients).
  - Irritability.
  - Swelling.
  - Erythema.
  - Tenderness around the shunt.
  - Ventriculoperitoneal shunt—Abdominal pain with guarding and rebound tenderness due to pus drainage into the peritoneal cavity.
  - Signs of increased ICP.
- Catheter migration.
- Disruption of shunt integrity.

Signs and symptoms of shunt dysfunction are related to increasing intracranial pressure. When the shunt device is not functional, excess CSF accumulates, and intracranial pressure increases. Initial symptoms may be vague or intermittent; symptoms of shunt malfunction are listed in Table 18.13.

Focused History

- Onset of the patient's present illness and development of neurologic symptoms.
- Associated symptoms:
  - Morning headache with vomiting.

TABLE 18.13 Signs of Shunt Malfunction

Initial Symptoms	*Additional Symptoms*
Vomiting	Vision changes
Decreased activity	Seizures
Nausea	Tense or bulging anterior fontanelle (in infants)
Headache	Gait or balance abnormalities
Irritability/behavior change	Altered mental status
"Sunset" eyes (downward gaze)	Fever (if infection is present)
	Increased head circumference

From: Bragg et al., 1994b; Steele, 2000.

- Signs of increased intracranial pressure (e.g., vomiting, headache, and changes in level of consciousness or activity).
- Dietary intake and output:
  - Changes from normal feeding habits; anorexia.
  - Last bowel movement; problems with constipation (Bragg, Edwards-Beckett, Eckle, Principe & Terry, 1994b).
- Parent or caretaker's impressions:
  - Changes in school performance or achieved developmental milestones.
- Current medications (dose, time of last dose, and compliance with dosing regimen).
- Shunt-related history:
  - Type of shunt.
  - Reason for shunt placement.
  - Previous or last episode of shunt dysfunction.
  - Date of last shunt revision.
- History of seizure disorder.
- History of spina bifida or myelomeningocele.
- Presence of a persistent neurologic deficit. Determine baseline function.

Focused Assessment

Physical Assessment

- Assess the respiratory system:
  - Auscultate the chest for respiratory rate. Tachypnea often is present.
  - Ausculate the respiratory pattern. Changes in respiratory pattern and apnea may develop if ICP remains high or continues to increase.
- Assess the cardiovascular system:
  - Auscultate the heart for rate. Tachycardia may be present in young children. Bradycardia may be present in adolescents.
  - Measure the blood pressure and pulse pressure. Blood pressure fluctuations are seen initially and then rising systolic blood pressure and widening pulse pressure as ICP increases. Young children may exhibit the triad of wide pulse pressure, increased systolic blood pressure, and tachycardia. Adolescents may exhibit the more classic triad of wide pulse pressure, rising systolic blood pressure, and bradycardia (Holmes, 1996).
  - Assess core and skin temperature. Fever may be present with CNS or shunt infection.
- Assess the neurologic system:
  - Assess level of consciousness with AVPU or GCS. Alterations in level of consciousness may be subtle initially, including irritability, lethargy, or decreased eye contact.
  - Evaluate the cranial nerves. Sluggish pupil response may be noted. Palsies of cranial nerves IV and VI may also be present, affecting the patient's eye movements and tracking of objects. Upward eye movement may be difficult. Papilledema may be present and result in blurred vision and headache (Steele, 2000; Brucker, 1996; Hazinski et al., 1999).
  - Evaluate motor function. Increased tone of lower extremities and positive Babinski's reflex may be present in child who is walking (Steele, 2000; Hazinski et al., 1999). Patients with myelomeningocele may have a baseline alteration in lower extremity motor function or paralysis.
  - Assess balance. Uncoordinated movement, inability to sit unassisted, ataxia, or abnormal gait may be present.
  - Inspect the head. Infants may have an increased head circumference and tense, bulging anterior fontanelle; widened or separated sutures; dilated scalp veins; downturned or "sunset eyes." (Brucker, 1996; Hazinski et al., 1999)
- Assess for other neurologic-related findings:
  - Incontinence.
  - High-pitched cry.

Psychosocial Assessment

- Assess the child's and family's understanding of the child's underlying health condition.
- Assess the child's and family's prior experience with the healthcare system.
- Assess the child's and family's coping strategies:
  - Children with ongoing health conditions develop a repertoire of coping skills for hospitalizations and procedures. Early evaluation of these skills helps the emergency nurse to plan approaches to care and treatment.

Nursing Interventions

1. Assess and maintain airway, breathing, and circulation:
   - Assure adequate breathing and ventilation:
     - Administer 100% oxygen via nonrebreather mask, as needed.
     - Initiate bag-valve-mask ventilation with 100% oxygen for hypoventilation and apnea.
   - Initiate cardiorespiratory and oxygen saturation monitoring, as needed.

- Assess patient for signs of shock/septic shock when shunt or CNS infection is suspected.

2. Obtain venous access and initiate intravenous infusion at prescribed rates:
   - Obtain blood for laboratory studies:
     - Electrolytes.
     - Glucose.
     - Complete blood count.
     - Cultures as indicated.
   - Administer medications, as prescribed:
   - Administer antipyretics to decrease fever and maintain normothermia to decrease metabolic demand. Acetaminophen may administered rectally if the patient is vomiting or shunt malfunction is suspected.
     - Administer nonnarcotic analgesics for headache.
     - Administer antibiotics for suspected infection as prescribed for preoperative care.
     - Administer other medications as indicated to treat increased ICP.
3. Monitor neurologic status for signs of increased ICP.
4. Reassess cardiopulmonary and neurologic status.
5. Position the patient to promote venous outflow:
   - Place the patient in a position of comfort.
   - Elevate the head of the bed 30 degrees.
   - Maintain the head and neck in midline.
6. Prepare for and assist with diagnostic procedures:
   - Computerized tomographic scan to evaluate shunt function.
   - Shunt-series radiographs to assess shunt continuity.
   - Lumbar puncture and CSF analysis if meningitis is suspected.
   - Shunt tap to evaluate for shunt infection.
   - Bladder catheterization or assisting the child to void to obtain a urine culture and urine specimen.
7. Inform the family frequently about their child's condition; provide psychosocial and emotional support to the patient and family.
8. Prepare for transfer and transport to a tertiary care center (Chapter 10), hospitalization and possible surgical procedure, or discharge to home.

Home Care and Prevention

Children who have CSF shunts and their families are taught to assess the shunt's integrity on a regularly scheduled basis by inspecting the shunt and observing the child's behavior (Ball, 1998). In general, parents are taught to (Ball, 1998):

- Inspect the child's head for CSF, an indication of shunt leakage.
- Palpate and observe the shunt, which is generally looped subcutaneously behind an ear. The shunt should feel and look round and full, not flat.
- Observe the shunt for redness, edema, or tenderness.
- Observe the child for fever or irritability, early indications of shunt infection.
- Observe for signs of shunt blockage:
  - Fatigue.
  - Stiff neck.
  - Nausea.
  - Seizures.
  - Visual disturbances.
  - Fever.
  - Vomiting.

Children and parents know that during a "growth spurt" the shunt may have to be revised. The child is taught to avoid contact sports, but other activities are generally not limited. Emergency nurses should incorporate the family's knowledge into the plan of care during ED treatment and should help to clear up any misconceptions on discharge. Regular follow-up with the child's primary care physician should be encouraged.

Headaches

Etiology

Headaches are common complaints in children and adolescents, occurring in approximately 10% of children aged 5 to 15 years (Ball, 1998). Headaches tend to be more common in females than in males (Ball, 1998). Approximately 12% of adolescents miss at least one day of school each month for headache-related complaints (Ball, 1998). Headaches in children and adolescents are often mild and of minimal consequence. Although a commonly associated symptom of the febrile response in systemic illnesses, headache can be a symptom of life-threatening conditions. A child presenting with a complaint of headache must be carefully evaluated for signs and symptoms associated with emergent conditions.

Headache pain generally results from vascular or meningeal irritation. Common causes of headache in children include (King, 2000; Goerlich, 2000):

- Febrile illness.
- Sinus and dental infections.
- Trauma.
- Migraine.

These causes of headache affect the pain-sensitive structures of the intracranial vascular structures and cranium. Pain-sensitive intracranial vascular structures include:

- The venous sinuses.
- Portions of the large cerebral arteries.
- The dura mater at the base of the skull.

The pain sensitive structures of the cranium include:

- The sinus cavities.
- The teeth.
- The muscles of the head and neck.
- The scalp.
- The orbits.

Headache pain results from inflammation, traction on intracranial structures, muscle contraction, or vasodilation that affects the pain-sensitive structures (King, 2000). Severity and associated characteristics are important factors in identifying the etiology of headaches. Table 18.14 compares headaches and their causes and assessment findings.

Focused History

Patient history

- Headache-specific history:
  - Quality of pain: throbbing; pressure; squeezing.
  - Location of pain: unilateral or bilateral; frontal, temporal, occipital, or above or behind the eye.
  - Duration of pain: episodic or constant.
  - Precipitating events.
- Headache-relief measures and their success.
  - Position change exacerbates pain (may be present with traction headache).
  - Pain awakens from sleep (may be present with traction headache or increased ICP).
  - Relieved by sleep (may get some relief with sleep during migraines).
- Associated symptoms:
  - Rhinitis.
  - Fever.
  - Nausea.
  - Vomiting.
  - Sore throat.
  - Stiff neck.
  - Visual changes.
  - Toothache.
- Changes in dietary intake and output.
- Parent's or caretaker's impressions.
- Current medications:
  - Over-the-counter and prescribed.
  - Dose, time of last dose, and dosing regimen.
- Recent head trauma.
- Recent emotional stress.
- Past medical history:
  - Blood and bleeding disorders. Children with blood and bleeding disorders are at greater risk for bleeding from relatively minor head trauma (e.g., hemophilia). Children with sickle cell disease are at higher risk for cerebral infarction and intracranial hemorrhage.
  - Previous similar headache episodes; history of migraine.
  - History of neurologic, metabolic, renal, cardiac, or blood disorders.
  - History of hypertension.
  - Use of birth control pills.
  - Allergies.
  - Previous sinus infections or dental problems.

Family health history

- Family history of migraine or headaches.

Focused Assessment

Physical Assessment

Assess the respiratory system

- Auscultate the chest for respiratory rate.

Assess the cardiovascular system

- Auscultate the heart for rate.
- Measure the blood pressure:
  - Headache and hypertension may be present in children with renal disease.
  - Children with congenital heart disease (e.g., coarctation of the aorta) may also present with an associated hypertension (Chapter 17).
- Measure core and skin temperature:
  - Fever may be present, with flushed cheeks and pale skin.

Assess the neurologic system

- Assess level of consciousness with the GCS or the AVPU method:

TABLE 18.14 Description, Causes, and Assessment Findings of Different Headache Types

Headache Type	*Description*	*Possible Causes*	*Associated Symptoms, Characteristics, and Clinical Findings*
Inflammatory	Infections cause inflammation of pain-sensitive intracranial or extracranial structures and lead to meningeal irritation and increased ICP.	Meningitis Encephalitis Intracranial abscess	Neck stiffness Fever Vomiting Altered level of consciousness
	Infection and inflammation of a sinus causes headache as a primary symptom.	Sinusitis	Rhinitis, nasal congestion, morning cough Facial pain (maxillary) Occipital pain (sphenoid) Frontal pain (frontal sinus in older children) Fever
	Dental infections can cause headaches.	Abscesses	Localized symptoms of tooth pain and sensitivity Fever
Vascular	Increased intracranial vasodilation or arterial dilation cause vascular headaches. Migraine is the most common recurrent headache in children.	Fever related to a viral or systemic illness	Pain in frontal and/or bitemporal area Throbbing Often unilateral pain, but may become generalized Aura may be present (pain begins as the aura wanes) Visual disturbances Transient motor deficits Nausea Vomiting Abdominal pain Photophobia
	Headaches may occur prior to a seizure, in the postictal phase, or may be the only manifestation of the seizure.	Varying causes of seizures	No specific characteristics
	Hypoxia associated with decreased cerebral perfusion results in arterial dilation.	Congestive heart failure Hypertension Vasoocclusive event, such as sickle cell disease or severe anemia	Throbbing quality Frontal bitemporal headache
Traction	Traction headaches are caused by conditions that shift intracranial structures and place traction on, or cause stretching of, the pain-sensitive dura and/or blood vessels at the base of the brain.	Intracranial hemorrhage Intracranial hematoma Cerebral edema Hydrocephalus Tumors Brain abscess	Symptoms of increased ICP. Focal neurologic deficits Drowsiness Vomiting Diplopia Headaches associated with increased ICP; morning headaches with generalized pain, nausea, and vomiting; the child may be awakened from sleep Signs of brain abscess: fever, altered level of consciousness, focal motor weakness, and/or other neurologic deficits
Tension/muscle contraction	Tension headaches are caused by a sustained contraction of the head and neck muscles. These are more common in adolescents than in younger children.	Tension Fatigue	Feeling of tightness or pressure in the back of head and neck; occasionally generalized

ICP = Intracranial pressure.
From: King, 2000; Fenichel, 1997b; Hockaday, 1996.

    - Alterations in level of consciousness may be associated with life-threatening infection of the CNS, increased ICP, intracranial mass, or intracranial hemorrhage.
- Evaluate cranial nerves, including an ocular examination:
    - Transient difficulties with speech may be present during migraines.
    - Intracranial tumor and/or increased ICP may cause altered cranial nerve function.
    - Visual acuity disturbances and papilledema may be present.
- Evaluate motor function:
    - Transient motor deficits may be present with migraine; however, a complete evaluation is needed to rule out other causes, such as brain lesion or increased ICP.
- Assess balance:
    - Ataxia while sitting or standing may be evident.
- Assess for signs of meningeal irritation:
    - Nuchal rigidity.
    - Kernig's sign.
    - Brudzinski's sign.
    - Photophobia.
- Assess for sinus pain by:
    - Palpating the sinuses.
    - Observing for edema over the sinuses.
- Listen for bruits over skull and neck.
    - Assess the pain with an age-appropriate pain scale and assessment techniques (Chapter 13).

Psychosocial Assessment

- Assess the child's previous experience with headaches.
- Assess the child's and the family's coping strategies.
- Assess the child's previous pain experience and strategies to cope with pain.

Nursing Interventions

1. Assess and maintain airway, breathing, and circulation.
2. Reassess the child's neurologic status.
3. Apply pain-relief measures:
    - Darken the room if the child is photophobic.
    - Apply a cool compress for a vascular headache.
    - Administer analgesic medications, as prescribed:
        - Mild analgesics, such as acetaminophen, coupled with rest and/or sleep, will relieve the pain of most headaches.
        - Other medications may be administered for more severe headaches or migraine headaches not responsive to acetaminophen.
    - Administer medications to treat an underlying condition (e.g., hypertension or sinusitis) that is causing the headache.
    - Administer antipyretic therapy for fever; maintain normothermia to decrease metabolic demand.
4. Employ nonpharmacologic interventions to relieve pain (Chapter 13):
    - Guided imagery.
    - Hypnosis.
5. Allow the child to rest and/or sleep.
6. Reassess the child's cardiovascular and neurologic status to detect improvement or worsening of condition.
7. Reassess for pain using the same age-appropriate pain scale and assessment techniques (Chapter 13).
8. Prepare for and assist with diagnostic procedures:
    - Neuroimaging: computerized tomography scan or magnetic resonance imaging for suspected intracranial lesion, intracranial bleeding, or abscess.
    - Lumbar puncture and CSF analysis if CNS infection is suspected (meningitis or encephalitis).
    - Laboratory studies, as indicated, dependent on the patient's presenting symptoms and examination.
9. Inform the family frequently of the child's condition; provide psychosocial and emotional support to the patient and family.
10. Prepare for transfer and transport to a tertiary care facility (Chapter 10), hospitalization, or discharge to home.

Home Care and Prevention

Headaches can be devastating to the child and family. The patient and family will need education concerning procedures, medications, and pain-relief measures. Home care measures are taught according to the type of headache diagnosed in the patient. Selected home care measures include (Ball, 1998):

- Having the child lie in a dark, quiet room.
- Alternating the placement of hot and cold packs on the child's forehead.
- Administering over-the-counter or prescribed analgesics or anti-inflammatories.
- Teaching the child special relaxation techniques and recognition of specific triggers that bring on the headache.

Conclusion

Neurologic emergencies pose a unique situation for emergency nurses because of the neurologic differences among infants, children, and adolescents. These emergencies can range from life-threatening to urgent conditions. Recognition of signs of increased intracranial pressure and rapid initiation of measures to prevent complications are the foundation for the emergency nursing care of children with neurologic conditions.

References

Ashwal, S. (1999). Congenital structural defects. In K. F. Swaiman & S. Ashwal (Eds.), *Pediatric neurology: Principles & practice* (3rd ed., pp. 234-300). St. Louis: Mosby—Year Book.

Ball, J. (Ed.). (1998). Neurologic section. In J. Ball (Ed.), *Mosby's pediatric patient teaching guides* (pp. I1-I12). St. Louis: Mosby—Year Book.

Berg, B. O. (1996a). The clinical evaluation. In B. O. Berg (Ed.), *Principles of child neurology* (pp. 5-22). New York: McGraw-Hill.

Berg, B. O. (1996b). Hypotonia. In B. O. Berg (Ed.), *Principles of child neurology* (pp. 1451-1458). New York: McGraw-Hill.

Bragg, C. L., Edwards-Beckett, J., Eckle, N., Principe, K., & Terry, D. (1994a). Shunt dysfunction and constipation: Could there be a link? *Journal of Neuroscience Nursing, 26*(2), 91-94.

Bragg, C. L., Edwards-Beckett, J., Eckle, N., Principe, K., & Terry, D. (1994b). Ventriculoperitoneal shunt dysfunction and constipation: A chart review. *Journal of Neuroscience Nursing, 26*(5), 265-269.

Brucker, J. M. (1996). Neurologic disorders. In J. M. Brucker & K. D. Wallin (Eds.), *Manual of pediatric nursing* (pp. 251-297). Boston: Little, Brown.

Chandrasoma, P. & Taylor, C. R. (1995). *Concise pathology* (2nd ed., pp. 902-916). Norwalk, CT: Appleton & Lange. RB37C456 1995

Chiang, V. W. (2000). Seizures. In G. R. Fleisher & S. Ludwig (Eds.), *Textbook of pediatric emergency medicine* (4th ed., pp. 573-579). Philadelphia: Lippincott Williams & Wilkins.

Dolan, M. (1997). Head trauma. In R. M. Barkin (Ed.), *Pediatric emergency medicine: Concepts and clinical practice* (2nd ed., pp. 236-251). St. Louis: Mosby—Year Book.

Emergency Nurses Association. (1995). *Course in advanced trauma nursing: A conceptual approach* (pp. 287-331). Park Ridge, IL: Author.

Farley, J., Hardin-Mooney, K. (1998). Alterations of neurologic function in children. In K. McCance & S. Huether (Eds.), *Pathophysiology: The biologic basis for disease in adults and children* (3rd ed., pp. 591-624). St. Louis: Mosby—Year Book.

Fenichel, G. M. (1997a). *Clinical pediatric neurology: A signs and symptoms approach* (3rd ed., pp. 1-46). Philadelphia: Saunders.

Fenichel, G. M. (1997b). *Clinical pediatric neurology: A signs and symptoms approach* (3rd ed., pp. 77-90). Philadelphia: Saunders.

Fuchs, S. M., Barkin, R., Bhende, M., Gonzalez del Rey, J., Holtzman, D., Isaacman, D., Karasic, R., & Paul, R. (1997). Neurologic disorders. In R. M. Barkin (Ed.), *Pediatric emergency medicine: Concepts and clinical practice* (2nd ed., pp. 972-1024). St. Louis: Mosby—Year Book.

Gilman, S., & Newman, S. W. (1996). *Essentials of clinical neuroanatomy and neurophysiology* (9th ed., pp. 3-16). Philadelphia: Davis.

Gorelich, M. H. (2000). Neurologic emergencies. In G. R. Fleisher & S. Ludwig (Eds.), *Textbook of pediatric emergency medicine* (4th ed., pp. 701-723). Philadelphia: Lippincott Williams & Wilkins.

Hazinski, M. F., Headrick, C., & Bruce, D. (1999). Neurologic disorders. In M. F. Hazinski (Ed.), *Manual of pediatric critical care* (pp. 371-445). St. Louis: Mosby—Year Book.

Hector, J. E. (1986). Neurologic evaluation and support in the child with an acute brain insult. *Pediatric Annals, 15*(1):16-22.

Hockaday, J. M. (1996). Migraine in childhood. In B. O. Berg (Ed.), *Principles of child neurology* (pp. 693-706). New York: McGraw-Hill.

Holmes, G. L. (1996). Epilepsy and other seizure disorders. In B. O. Berg (Ed.), *Principles of child neurology* (pp. 223-284). New York: McGraw-Hill.

King, C. (2000). Headache. In G. R. Fleisher & S. Ludwig (Eds.), *Textbook of pediatric emergency medicine* (4th ed., pp. 459-465). Philadelphia: Lippincott Williams & Wilkins.

Murphy, K. A. (1997). *Pediatric triage guidelines* (pp. 62-79). St. Louis: Mosby.

Sarnat, H. B. (1996). Neuroembryology. In B. O. Berg (Ed.), *Principles of child neurology* (pp. 602-627). New York: McGraw-Hill.

Steele, D. W. (2000). Neurosurgical emergencies, non-traumatic. In G. R. Fleisher & S. Ludwig (Eds.), *Textbook of pediatric emergency medicine* (4th ed., pp. 1621-1629). Philadelphia: Lippincott Williams & Wilkins.

Swaiman, K. F. (1999a). Neurologic examination of the term and preterm infant. In K. F. Swaiman & S. Ashwal (Eds.), *Pediatric neurology: Principals and practice* (3rd ed., pp. 39-53). St. Louis: Mosby-Yearbook.

Swaiman, K. F. (1999b). Neurology examination after the newborn period until 2 years of age. In K. F. Swaiman & S. Ashwal (Eds.). *Pediatric Neurology: Principals and Practice* (3rd ed., pp. 27-38).

Thomas, D. O. (1991). Seizures. In D. O. Thomas (Ed.), *Quick reference to pediatric emergency nursing* (pp. 153-159). Gaithersburg, MD: Aspen Publications.

Williams, P. L., Warwick, R., Dyson, M., & Bannister, L. H. (1989). Embryology. In P. L. Williams, R. Warwick, M. Dyson, & L. H. Bannister (Eds.), *Gray's anatomy* (37th ed., pp. 177-201). New York: Churchill Livingstone.

19

Gastrointestinal Emergencies

Treesa Soud, RN, BSN

Introduction

Gastrointestinal (GI) complaints are common among the pediatric population; the most common complaints are diarrhea, vomiting, and abdominal pain (Chapter 12). For most infants and children, these symptoms represent a relatively minor illness (such as gastroenteritis) that can be easily treated. These symptoms may also be indicative of a life-threatening illness such as appendicitis, volvulus, or intussusception. The purposes of this chapter are to review common gastrointestinal complaints of the infant and child, to describe signs and symptoms of serious gastrointestinal illnesses, and to discuss nursing care and management of the child with a gastrointestinal complaint.

Embryologic Development of the Gastrointestinal System

The formation of the gastrointestinal system is dependent on embryologic folding by the fourth week of gestation. Development of the gut is nearly complete by the 20th week of gestation, and functional maturity occurs by the 33rd to 34th week of gestation, providing nutrition to support fetal growth. (Martin & Derengowski, 1997). By week 34, coordinated sucking and swallowing and nutritive sucking occur in preparation for extrauterine tasks. Birth heralds a neonatal phase of gastrointestinal adaptation to the demands of enteral nutrition. Gastrointestinal development is concluded by weaning from milk to a solid diet (Weaver, 1996).

Some congenital anomalies occur early in the development of the fetus. These conditions can result in life-threatening emergencies if they are not detected and treated. The etiology and treatment of some of these conditions are discussed later in this chapter.

Pediatric Considerations

- The abdominal wall is less muscular in the infant and toddler, making the abdominal organs easier to palpate. In the infant, the liver can be palpated 1 to 2 cm below the right costal margin (Martin & Derengowski, 1997).
- The contour of the abdomen is protuberant in young children because abdominal muscles are immature.
- Gastric motility is decreased and somewhat irregular in comparison to that of the adult. Gastric emptying is more frequent.
- Gastroesophageal reflux is common during the first 6 months of life because of inappropriate relaxation of the lower esophageal sphincter.
- The neonatal liver is immature but develops during the first year of life. Toxic substances are inefficiently detoxified.
- Caloric requirements per kilogram of weight are higher in children than in adults. The basal metabolic rate is highest during the first two years of life. The basal metabolic rate increases 12% with each centigrade of temperature greater than 37°C.
- Losses from vomiting and diarrhea as a result of gastrointestinal infections or disease can cause dehydration and shock in the neonate and child, because the percentage of extracellular fluid volume is higher than that of an adult.

Focused History

The history includes information related to the chief complaint and the symptoms. The following information should be obtained:

- Events surrounding the illness.
- Associated symptoms.
- Changes in feeding or elimination patterns.
- Character and location of pain associated with the illness: sharp, dull, diffuse, localized, or colicky. (Chapter 12 for more information on abdominal pain as a chief complaint.)
- Changes in the child's activity level.
- Significant medical history, such as cystic fibrosis, sickle cell disease, or previous abdominal surgery.
- Family history of gastrointestinal problems or congenital conditions.

Focused Assessment

Physical Assessment

The physical examination includes the standard pediatric assessment; special attention is paid to the following when the abdomen is examined:

- Observe the abdomen for symmetry, abdominal distention, obvious masses, visible bowel loops, and peristaltic waves.
- Inspect the umbilicus of young infants for hernias, ulceration, discharge, or granulation tissue.
- Auscultate the abdomen for bowel sounds in all four quadrants:
    - Bowel sounds are normally heard every 10 to 13 seconds.
    - Auscultate breath sounds to rule out the possibility of pneumonia or reactive airway disease because abdominal pain may be a presenting symptom in young children with respiratory disorders (Horton, Soud, Inman, & Standifer, 1998).
- Palpate the abdomen:
    - First ask the child to point to the most painful area of the abdomen; palpate nonpainful areas before palpating the most painful area.
    - Evaluate pain to palpation and rebound tenderness.
    - Table 19.1 describes abdominal physical findings and their meaning.
- Percussion:
    - Percussion is not routinely done but can be performed by lightly tapping the abdomen to emit a sound.

TABLE 19.1 Abdominal Physical Findings and Their Meaning

Physical Finding	*Meaning*
Abdominal distention	Peritonitis; intestinal obstruction; ileus with gastroenteritis
Visible bowel loops	Intestinal obstruction; intussusception
Asymmetry	Appendiceal abscess; tumor
Point tenderness	Appendicitis; cholecystitis
Guarding	Peritonitis; appendicitis; abscess
Rigidity	Cholecystitis
Rebound	Infarcted bowel
Palpable mass	Tumor or cyst; intussusception; chronic constipation
Gas palpable in cecum	Not appendicitis
High-pitched bowel sounds	Intestinal obstruction
No bowel sounds	Peritonitis; infarcted bowel; perforated appendix or bowel
Rectal examination—tenderness or bogginess on right	Appendicitis

From: Schnaufer & Mahboubi, 1993. Abdominal emergencies. In G. R. Fleisher, & S. Ludwig (Eds.), *Textbook of pediatric emergency medicine* (3rd ed., p. 1308). Baltimore: Williams & Wilkins. Used with permission.

- Percussion is used to determine the presence of tympany and to detect free fluid, hepatic and splenic borders, a distended bladder, or other masses (Horton et al., 1998).
- Rectal examination:
    - Prepare the child for a rectal examination, which is usually performed by the physician.
    - Tell the child what will happen and instruct him/her to take deep breaths throughout the examination.

Psychosocial Assessment

The abdominal assessment can be difficult to perform in the young child because pain and fear can cause the child to cry throughout the examination. The result is abdominal wall rigidity and no overt clues to the intensity or location of the pain. Additionally, young children cannot verbalize their fears or describe the location or characteristics of their pain. Approaching the child in a calm manner and using distraction, such as talking about the child's favorite activity or cartoon character, may assist in gaining cooperation.

Communicating the need for therapeutic intervention is important for both the child and family. Each intervention should be described to the child in age-appropriate terminology. Fear and pain can overwhelm the child. A consistent, caring nurse can help to allay anxiety. Parents should be allowed to remain with the child as much as possible.

The emergent nature of an illness means the parents have had little time to prepare. Anxiety and guilt are common and normal reactions. The parents should be allowed to express their concerns, and their questions should be answered honestly. They should be kept informed regarding the plan of care and offered frequent updates.

Table 19.2 outlines the nursing diagnoses and expected outcomes.

Triage Decisions

Emergent

- Toxic-appearing; exhibits signs or symptoms of shock.
- Altered level of consciousness.
- Underlying illness or pathology (e.g., sickle cell disease or diabetes) that may predispose to rapid deterioration.
- Severe abdominal pain, distention, and/or fever (may be unable to walk or may walk bent over because of the pain).
- Signs of hemorrhage, shock, or abdominal obstruction.
- Bilious vomiting; vomiting coupled with acute-onset abdominal pain and/or abdominal distention.
- Abdominal mass; discoloration or swelling over the mass.
- Signs and symptoms of respiratory distress; drooling, fever, or refusal of food and liquids; evidence of esophageal perforation (e.g., bloody sputum); or ingestion of a button battery.

Urgent

- Well-appearing infant or child with signs and symptoms of moderate dehydration.
- Well-appearing child with diffuse abdominal pain.
- Infant or child with a history of moderate to severe rectal bleeding but no signs of volume loss or shock.
- Any infant with a history of significant vomiting and weight loss.
- Well-appearing infant or child with a firm, discrete abdominal mass and irritability, abdominal pain, or vomiting.

Nonurgent

- Well-appearing child with signs and symptoms of mild dehydration.

TABLE 19.2 Nursing Diagnoses and Expected Outcomes

Nursing Diagnoses	*Expected Outcomes*
Potential for fluid volume deficit related to intestinal losses or decreased fluid intake and vomiting.	Intestinal losses will decrease, as evidenced by decreased frequency of stooling, decreased emesis, and increased fluid intake (intravenous or oral).
Potential for altered nutrition (less than body requirements) related to intestinal losses and inadequate intake to meet the body's demands.	Nutrition status will be corrected by prescribed fluids and diet to replace losses.
Pain related to abdominal cramping and diarrhea or other pathology.	Pain will be relieved by correction of the problem, pharmacologic or surgical intervention, or other nonpharmacologic interventions.

- Well-appearing infant or child with a history of chronic constipation and no other symptoms.
- Well-appearing child with none of the above-mentioned signs or symptoms.

Nursing Interventions

Specific diagnostic testing, treatment, and nursing interventions associated with abdominal pain are reviewed with each diagnostic category within this chapter. As with all ED patients, stabilization of the airway, breathing, and circulation has priority. The following interventions may be anticipated for the child with an abdominal complaint:

- Allow the child to have nothing by mouth (NPO) after arrival in the ED.
- Initiate intravenous fluids to replace losses and correct shock.
- Insert a nasogastric tube to decompress the stomach.
- Administer antibiotics and other medications (such as pain medications), as ordered.
- Obtain laboratory work and X-rays, as ordered.
- Prepare the child for surgery and/or admission to the hospital.
- Provide the family with support and information.

Specific Gastrointestinal Medical Emergencies

Gastroenteritis

Gastroenteritis, or acute, infectious diarrhea, is one of the most common complaints encountered within the pediatric population. Within the first five years of life, an estimated 20 to 35 million episodes of diarrhea will occur annually in children in the United States (Behrman, Kliegman, & Jenson, 2000).

Gastroenteritis may be caused by a bacterial, viral, or parasitic invasion that produces inflammation of the gastrointestinal tract:

- *Viral* etiologies account for approximately 80% of all infectious diarrheas. These include:
  - Rotavirus (the most common etiology).
  - Norwalk virus.
  - Adenovirus.
  - Coxsackie virus.
  - Echovirus; astrovirus.
  - Caliciviruses.
- *Bacterial* etiologies account for 10 to 15% of cases of gastroenteritis in the pediatric population. These include:
  - *Campylobacter* (the most common etiology).
  - *Escherichia coli*.
  - *Salmonella*.
  - *Shigella*.
  - *Yersinia enterocolitica*.
- *Parasites* that can produce diarrhea include:
  - *Giardia lamblia* (the most common etiology).
  - *Cryptosporidium*.

Pathophysiology

When the gastrointestinal tract is invaded by a viral agent, destruction of the mucosal cells of the villi begins. Injury to the intestinal epithelial cells decreases the surface area available for absorption and impairs water and electrolyte transport. Bacterial invasion of the gastrointestinal tract also produces direct damage to the villi and can produce toxins stimulating an inflammatory response. The formation of mucosal ulcerations, which erode the blood vessels, will lead to bleeding.

Focused History

- Onset of the diarrhea.
- Frequency of stooling.
- Consistency and color of the stool.
- Presence or absence of blood or mucus in the stool.
- Fluid intake and urinary output.
- Weight loss.
- Associated findings, such as the presence of fever, vomiting, abdominal pain, rash, runny nose, or cough.

Focused Assessment

The standard assessment is performed, beginning with an evaluation of the child's overall appearance and age-appropriate activity level:

- Assess the airway for patency.
- Evaluate breathing for rate and rhythm. Tachypnea or deep breathing may indicate fever and/or metabolic acidosis associated with tissue hypoxia from fluid losses.
- Evaluate the circulatory status for signs of decreased peripheral perfusion, which may indicate dehydration or shock:
  - Assess the skin color.
  - Assess the strength of peripheral pulses.
  - Assess skin turgor.
  - Evaluate capillary refill.
  - Examine the condition of the fontanelle in infants.

TABLE 19.3 Dehydration: Clinical Findings that Correlate with Weight Loss

Symptom	*Mild*	*Moderate*	*Severe*
Weight loss (infants and young children)	3-5%	5-10%	10-15%
Weight loss (children > 10 years)	3-5%	5-7%	7-9%
Eyes	Normal	Sunken	Sunken; no tearing
Mucous membranes of the mouth	Moist to sticky	Dry	Dry to parched
Skin color	Normal	Normal to pale	Pale, mottled
Skin turgor	Normal	Decreased	Tenting
Anterior fontanelle (infants)	Normal	Sunken	Sunken
Pulse	Normal	Rapid	Rapid
Blood pressure	Normal	Normal to low	Low
Urinary output	Normal	Decreased	Decreased to absent
Mental status	Normal	Normal to lethargic	Lethargic to coma

From: Soud & Rogers, 1998. *Manual of pediatric emergency nursing.* (p. 316). St. Louis: Mosby—Year Book. Used with permission.

- Inspect mucus membranes for moistness and the eyes for the presence of tearing and/or a sunken appearance.

- Clinical findings, correlated with weight loss, are then used to determine the degree of dehydration. These findings are described in Table 19.3.

Nursing Interventions

Initially the airway and breathing are stabilized, as required by the child's condition. If dehydration is present, the method of rehydration will depend on the child's clinical presentation and the degree of dehydration.

Severe Dehydration

- Obtain immediate venous access and administer a 20 ml/kg bolus of normal saline or lactated Ringer's solution. Take the following approach to parenteral fluid therapy:
  - Initially restore or maintain perfusion by administering a 20 ml/kg bolus of normal saline, 5% dextrose in normal saline, or lactated Ringer's.
  - Use normal saline or lactated Ringer's solution for subsequent bolus therapy, as necessary, to maintain or restore perfusion.
  - Calculate fluid and electrolyte deficits in milliliters, based on the child's weight loss and the suspected degree of dehydration. Each kg of weight loss is equal to 1,000 mL of fluid loss.
  - Calculate daily maintenance fluid requirements (Table 19.4).
  - Replace abnormal ongoing losses, such as vomiting and diarrhea, milliliter for milliliter.
  - Calculate other sources of abnormal losses, such as fever, which increases the metabolic rate by 10 to 12% per degree Centigrade greater than 37°C.
  - Treat for isotonic (equal proportions of sodium and water have been lost through vomiting and diarrhea) dehydration. Fluid therapy begins with the administration of one-half of the fluid deficit and one-third of the maintenance requirements, given over the first 8 hours of treatment, using 5% dextrose in half normal saline. Because potassium losses are common, even if serum potassium levels remain normal, add 20 mEq/L of potassium to the solution once renal function has been established (when the child voids). Replace the remaining fluids (half of the deficit and two-thirds of the maintenance) over the next 16 hours of therapy.
- During fluid therapy, record all intake and output; monitor perfusion and neurologic status.
- The child with moderate-to-severe dehydration usually requires hospitalization.

Mild to Moderate Dehydration

- Treat with parenteral fluid therapy or oral fluid (enteral) therapy.

TABLE 19.4 Calculations for Maintenance Fluid

1–10 kg	100 ml/kg/day
11–20 kg	1000 + (50 ml/kg for each kg > 10 kg)
> 20 kg	1500 + (20 ml/kg for each kg > 20 kg)
Example 1: 6-month-old weighing 8 kg	
8 kg	100 ml × 8 kg = 800 ml
	800 ml ÷ 24 hr = 33.3 ml/hr
Example 2: 12-year-old weighing 44 kg	
20 kg	1500 ml
+ 24 kg	+ 1480 ml (24 kg × 20 ml)
44 kg	2980 ml ÷ 24 hr = 124 ml/hr

- Replace fluid losses with an oral rehydration solution (ORS), such as Pedialyte or Rehydralyte, if the child is able to tolerate oral fluid:
  - Use a formula that estimates fluid losses to determine oral replacement therapy, or allow the child to drink an ORS as desired (drinking no greater than 200 ml/kg in 24 hours) (Sacchetti, Brilli, & Barkin, 1997).
  - Vomiting alone is not a contraindication to the administration of an ORS; offer children with a history of vomiting frequent, small amounts of the solution rather than large amounts.
  - Infants require early reintroduction of normal nutrients into their diet. Allow infants who are breast-feeding to continue to do so and use the ORS to replace ongoing losses.
  - The treatment of formula-fed infants is more controversial. Some physicians recommend using a lactose-free formula instead of lactose-containing formulas during the acute phase of diarrhea. Others recommend the sole administration of an ORS for a brief (6- to 12-hour) period with rapid progression back to formula feeding, supplemented with the ORS.

Diagnostic Testing

Infants and children with gastroenteritis and mild dehydration rarely require specific diagnostic testing unless a coexisting illness is suspected (e.g., in the presence of fever and a toxic appearance).

- A stool culture or other specific testing (e.g., for rotavirus or parasites) may be ordered, depending on the suspected underlying etiology. Stool may also be evaluated for the presence of blood. If blood is present, a stool culture is performed.
- Children with moderate to severe dehydration may require testing, such as:
  - Serum electrolytes to assist in determining the severity, type (isotonic, hypertonic, or hypotonic), and degree of dehydration. Serum sodium and potassium values do not always reflect total body stores. Potassium stores are usually depleted in the dehydrated child. In the presence of metabolic acidosis (which occurs with moderate to severe dehydration), intracellular potassium is exchanged for the circulating hydrogen ion, resulting in normal serum potassium level.
  - Blood glucose. The blood glucose level may be low because of decreased intake and increased losses.
  - Hematocrit and hemoglobin. In a dehydrated child, the hematocrit will be higher than normal because of hemoconcentration.
  - Blood urea nitrogen, creatinine, and a urinalysis. The blood urea nitrogen will be elevated. (It may not be elevated if the child has had decreased protein intake.) The creatinine level will be higher than normal. (Normal values in children are much lower than those in adults.) Urinary specific gravity will be elevated.

Home Care and Prevention

If the infant or child is to be discharged home, the following instructions must be given:

- Explain signs and symptoms of dehydration and shock:
  - Decreased or absent urination.
  - Dry mucous membranes.
  - Sunken fontanelle (in infants).
  - Sunken eyes.
  - Lack of tears.
  - Excessive sleepiness or lethargy.
- Provide instructions for use of ORS:

- Give the infant a full-strength ORS and then progress to breast-feeding or a nonlactose formula.
- For older children with both vomiting and diarrhea, give an ORS or sports drink for at least 24 hours.
- For children of any age, wait at least 2 hours following emesis before offering small, frequent amounts of liquid (10 to 15 ml every 15 to 20 minutes). Many physicians recommend early introduction of bland foods, such as rice cereal. With the initiation of formula or solid foods, the diarrhea may recur but should resolve quickly.

- Provide information on the need for adequate hand washing and proper disposal of diapers to prevent the spread of infection to other family members.
- Explain that the diapered child must remain out of day care until the diarrhea has subsided.

Specific Gastrointestinal Surgical Emergencies

Appendicitis

Appendicitis is the most common acute surgical condition of the abdomen during childhood. It is caused by inflammation of the appendix, initiated by an obstruction of the appendiceal lumen. Appendicitis is rarely seen in children younger than 2 years of age but becomes more common as children approach the teenage years. Until puberty, boys and girls are equally affected; after the age of 15 years, twice as many boys are affected as girls (Strahlman, 1997).

Pathophysiology

Appendicitis is caused by an obstruction of the appendiceal lumen, which can result from a fecalith (hard lump of feces) or from edema of the lymphoid tissue caused by a viral or bacterial infection. Other causes include parasites (e.g., pinworms), carcinoid tumors, and foreign-body obstruction. Appendicitis is rare in children younger than 2 years of age because of a lack of lymphatic tissue in infants and because the appendiceal lumen is funnel-shaped and not easily obstructed (Friedman & Sheynkin, 1995).

When the lumen of the appendix is obstructed, the accumulation of mucoid material causes an increase in intraluminal pressure. Aerobic and anaerobic bacteria within the appendix begin to proliferate. As intraluminal pressure rises, infection and edema impede blood flow, causing ischemia and necrosis. With continued pressure, ischemia and infarction can cause the appendix to become gangrenous. The gangrenous appendix may perforate, releasing bacteria into the abdominal cavity. Young children with appendicitis are more susceptible to early perforation of the appendix because the wall of the appendix is very thin. In this age group, diffuse peritonitis results, because the immature omentum is incapable of "walling off" the infection.

Focused History

The presentation of appendicitis is highly variable in the child, and classic findings are not always present. A high index of suspicion is maintained for any child with a history of abdominal pain. The history should include the onset, location, and character of the abdominal pain:

- Early signs of appendicitis:
  - Diffuse periumbilical or midabdominal pain.
  - Abdominal pain with coughing and walking.
- Progressive appendicitis:
  - Anorexia, nausea, and vomiting.
  - Low-grade fever.
  - Normal bowel habits, constipation, or diarrhea.
  - Pain localized to the right lower quadrant.
- Perforated appendix:
  - Increasing fever.
  - Rapid, shallow respirations.
  - Diffuse abdominal pain.
  - Irritability or lethargy.

Focused Assessment

The standard pediatric assessment is done. The child's initial clinical appearance depends on the degree of progression of the disease. Early in the course of the illness, the child may complain of diffuse abdominal pain. As the illness progresses, the child may walk bent forward while splinting the abdomen, may refuse to jump during the examination, or may refuse to walk. An additional finding may be refusal or inability to get onto the examination table without assistance. Children with appendicitis prefer to lie very still in bed with the head of the bed elevated and the knees flexed. Assessment findings include:

- An altered respiratory pattern, such as rapid, shallow respirations or grunting, both of which can indicate pneumonia or shock, or may be the result of severe abdominal pain. Auscultation of the lung fields and a chest X-ray is required to rule out the presence of pneumonia.
- Tachycardia. The child's skin may be flushed or excessively pale.
- Continuous but poorly defined or localized abdominal pain (early):
  - The pain characteristically localizes in the right lower quadrant of the abdomen at McBurney's point (two-thirds the distance from the pubis to

the anterosuperior iliac spine) with progression of the disease.

- Because the location of the appendix can vary, pain may localize in other areas, such as the pelvis, in the right upper quadrant under the gallbladder, over the bladder, or in a retrocecal site (Rowe, 1995).

- Hypoactive or hyperactive bowel sounds, making auscultation of the abdomen of little benefit in determining the presence of appendicitis.
- Rebound tenderness in older children, if peritoneal irritation is present.
- Localized right vault tenderness, a mass (abscess), or a retrocecal appendix, as revealed by a rectal examination, performed by the emergency care practitioner (Rowe, 1995).
- Signs and symptoms of perforation:
  - Diffuse abdominal tenderness (younger children).
  - Immediate relief of pain.
  - Signs and symptoms of toxicity, such as pale skin and marked tachypnea and tachycardia.
  - A rigid and extremely tender abdomen.
  - Markedly decreased or absent bowel sounds.

Nursing Interventions

1. Assess and stabilize the airway, breathing, and circulation as required.
2. Place child NPO.
3. Give a 20 ml/kg bolus of Ringer's lactate solution or normal saline solution if the child is hypovolemic.
4. Monitor for signs of progression of the illness:
   - Obtain vital signs frequently.
   - Monitor intake and output.
   - Observe peripheral perfusion for signs of toxicity or shock.
   - Assess the intensity, location, and character of the abdominal pain to evaluate the progression of the illness:
     - Severe pain requires the administration of an analgesic.
     - A complete surgical evaluation should be performed before an analgesic is given.
5. Administer broad-spectrum antibiotics if appendicitis is suspected.
6. Prepare the child for surgery.
7. Insert a nasogastric tube if a perforated appendix is suspected.
8. Perform diagnostic testing:
   - Complete blood count and differential:
     - Early in the course of illness, the white blood cell count is usually between 10,000 and 15,000/mm^3.
     - The differential may reveal increasing numbers of bands and polymorphonuclear leukocytes.
     - With perforation of the appendix, the white blood cell count markedly increases.
   - Urinalysis:
     - An excessive number of white blood cells in the urine may indicate the presence of a urinary tract infection or may indicate that the inflamed appendix lies over a ureter or adjacent to the bladder.
   - Abdominal X-rays:
     - The appearance is usually normal early in the course of the illness.
     - As the illness progresses, the abdominal X-ray often reveals diminished air in the gastrointestinal tract, the result of anorexia and/or vomiting; however, this finding is not diagnostic.
     - A diagnostic finding (when identified) is the presence of a calcified fecalith in the right lower quadrant.
     - Radiographic findings that may indicate a perforated appendix include the presence of free air in the abdomen or evidence of peritonitis.
   - Serum electrolyte levels, to determine the degree of dehydration and identify fluid shifts.
   - Ultrasound, to determine the diameter of the appendiceal lumen and to observe for an abdominal mass or free fluid within the abdominal cavity.
   - Chest X-ray, to rule out pulmonary problems, such as right lower lobe pneumonia, as a cause of the abdominal pain.
   - Barium enema, occasionally ordered to determine the patency of the appendix.

Home Care and Prevention

If signs and symptoms are nonspecific for appendicitis, the parents may be instructed to return with the child in a specified amount of time, usually 6 to 8 hours, for reevaluation. The parents must be given specific information about signs and symptoms that require immediate return to the ED, and they must understand the importance of follow-up. The child should be placed NPO or should be put on a clear liquid diet until the return visit takes place.

Meckel's Diverticulum

Meckel's diverticulum is a congenital anomaly in which there is an outpouching (evagination) of the small intestine. It occurs early in gestation when the vitelline duct, which is located at the umbilicus, fails to close completely. Although Meckel's diverticulum may be an isolated abnormality, it frequently occurs in association with other congenital disorders, such as Down syndrome and cardiac defects (Rowe, 1995).

Meckel's diverticulum affects approximately 2% of the population and is usually painless (Rowe, 1995). Symptoms related to the anomaly occur in 4 to 35% of affected individuals (Rowe, 1995). Typically, symptomatic patients are young children; about 45% are younger than 2 years of age (Klein, 1997a). Males have a higher overall incidence of Meckel's diverticulum; however, among symptomatic patients, there is a relatively equal distribution between the sexes (Rowe, 1995).

Pathophysiology

Early during embryonic development, the vitelline (omphalomesenteric) duct connects the gut to the yolk sac at the umbilicus. After about 7 weeks of gestation, this duct regresses and eventually is completely reabsorbed. In some children, a fibrous cord or band of tissue may persist between the umbilicus and the bowel, serving as a lead point for later complications. In some cases, the vitelline duct fails to obliterate, leading to several types of deformities, such as a vitelline duct cyst, a patent vitelline duct (allowing passage of gas or bilious drainage), or prolapse of the proximal and distal bowel through a patent duct (Rowe, 1995).

Meckel's diverticulum is the most common of the vitelline duct disorders and is represented by an outpouching of the gut that contains all layers of the intestinal wall and may also contain ectopic tissues, such as ectopic gastric mucosa or ectopic pancreatic tissue (Rowe, 1995).

In symptomatic infants and children the most common complications include:

- Bloody stools, which can be caused by ulceration and hemorrhage of ectopic gastric mucosa within the diverticulum.
- Intestinal obstruction, which can be caused by volvulus around or herniation through a still attached fibrous band of tissue, prolapse of the bowel through the duct, or ileocolic intussusception in which the diverticulum acts as a lead point (Klein, 1997a; Rowe, 1995).
- Inflammation, which can occur when peptic ulceration or obstruction leads to diverticulitis or with perforation that causes diffuse peritonitis or a localized abscess (Klein, 1997a).

Focused History

The initial history for the infant or child with Meckel's diverticulum can vary significantly, depending on the severity of the disorder:

- A history of vomiting, abdominal distention, and abdominal pain may be associated with intestinal obstruction.
- The history associated with rectal bleeding may reveal intermittent bouts of significant bleeding. During these bouts, stools are characteristically brick red or currant jelly in appearance.

Focused Assessment

- Assess general appearance.
- Assess airway and breathing.
- Assess circulatory status for signs and symptoms of shock (weak or absent peripheral pulses, delayed capillary refill, hypotension, and altered mental status) that may be the result of significant rectal bleeding, intestinal obstruction, or sepsis.
- Perform an abdominal assessment:
  - Auscultate for bowel sounds.
  - Palpate for the presence of abdominal pain, tenderness, or distention, which can represent an obstruction or perforation. These findings can easily be misinterpreted as appendicitis. If intussusception is present (discussed later in this chapter), a palpable mass may be present.
- Evaluate the stool for the presence of overt and occult blood:
  - Tarry stools may be seen if the bleeding is minor.

Nursing Interventions

1. Place on supplemental oxygen and give fluid bolus if signs of shock are present (Chapter 17).
2. Prepare the child for surgery once the presumptive diagnosis of Meckel's diverticulum is made.
3. Evaluate the child frequently while awaiting surgery:
   - Monitor vital signs.
   - Evaluate for signs of shock.
   - Record approximate blood losses from the stools (Wong, 1997).
   - Communicate the expected treatment to the family. When possible, the parents should be allowed to remain with the child.
4. Perform diagnostic testing:
   - Diagnostic testing is based on the child's presenting symptoms and the suspected underlying etiology; for example, a history of rectal bleeding requires the evaluation of the stool for occult blood.
   - Other diagnostic testing that may be ordered, depending on symptomatology, includes:
     - Complete blood count.

- Blood urea nitrogen.
- Electrolytes.
- Blood glucose.
- Blood type and crossmatch if significant blood loss is suspected.
- Abdominal X-rays to rule out an intestinal obstruction or a perforation.

Pyloric Stenosis

Pyloric stenosis is an obstruction at the pyloric sphincter resulting from a hypertrophied pyloric muscle. The condition, which is usually manifested in the second to fifth week of life, is one of the most common disorders to require surgery during infancy. Although many theories have been suggested regarding the cause of pyloric stenosis, the etiology remains unknown.

The overall incidence of pyloric stenosis is approximately 1 in 250 births. The disorder affects white infants more commonly than it does African-American or Asian infants (Klein, 1997b). There is a 5:1 male-to-female incidence of pyloric stenosis. The first-born male is at highest risk (Schnaufer & Mahboubi, 2000; Jedd, Melton, Griffin, 1988). Children of parents who had the condition are more likely to develop pyloric stenosis; the children of mothers who had the disease are significantly more likely to develop the condition (Schnaufer & Mahboubi, 2000). Siblings of children with hypertrophic pyloric stenosis are also more likely to be affected than is the general population.

Pathophysiology

During the first few weeks of life, the pylorus appears to function normally. Within several weeks, however, hypertrophy and hyperplasia of the circular pyloric muscle develop, partially obstructing the pyloric channel. With continued irritation and inflammation of the mucosa, a complete obstruction can occur. Constant peristaltic movements against the obstructed lumen can produce marked gastric dilation and hypertrophied musculature (Horton et al., 1998). Blood-streaked emesis may result from the persistent vomiting, which can produce a mucosal tear or gastritis.

Metabolic derangements and dehydration result from the continued vomiting. With prolonged vomiting, shock can occur. Losses of hydrogen ion and chloride with gastric contents can lead to metabolic alkalosis. Compensatory mechanisms cause sodium to move into the cells and potassium to move out of the cells and be excreted in the urine. The results are hypokalemia, hypochloremia, and occasionally hyponatremia.

Focused History

The typical history is that of an infant who eats well in the first few weeks of life. Within a 2- to 5-week period, the following symptoms occur:

- The infant vomits after some feedings. Following vomiting, the infant eats vigorously but may vomit again.
- As the obstruction progresses, the infant vomits with every feeding and the vomiting becomes projectile or "forceful."
- The vomitus in infants with pyloric stenosis typically includes formula or breast milk from the last feeding and does not contain bile.
- The vomitus may have a brownish discoloration or bloody streaks, caused by gastritis or mucosal tears resulting from prolonged vomiting.
- There may be a positive family history of pyloric stenosis.

Focused Assessment

The standard assessment is done. If the vomiting has been excessive and prolonged, the infant will show signs of growth retardation and nutritional deprivation, such as weight loss and loss of subcutaneous tissue. Other findings include:

- Signs of dehydration (e.g., sunken eyes, absence of tears, dry mucous membranes of the mouth, tenting skin, and decreased urination).
- Gastric peristaltic waves from left to right following feeding.
- Diminished or absent bowel sounds.
- An enlarged pylorus, or "olive," palpated in the upper abdominal quadrant, to the right of the midline:
    - To facilitate palpation of the olive, gentle elevation of the infant's lower extremities while the infant is sucking may be required.
    - Occasionally, gastric emptying with a nasogastric tube is necessary to allow palpation of the olive.

Nursing Interventions

1. Assess airway and breathing and stabilize, as required by the infant's condition.
2. Assess circulatory status.
3. Obtain intravenous access to replace fluids and electrolytes to correct dehydration and metabolic abnormalities.
4. Treat severe dehydration by restoring circulating volume with one or more boluses of 20 ml/kg of normal saline or lactated Ringer's solution:

- Follow the same replacement therapy protocol described in the section on gastroenteritis.
- Higher doses of potassium chloride, up to 30 to 40 mEq/L, may be ordered.
- Administer potassium only after renal function has been established (when the infant voids).
- Place infants receiving high doses of potassium chloride on a cardiac monitor and place intravenous fluid on a pump.
- Assess the infusion-site frequently for signs of infiltration.

5. Insert a nasogastric tube.
6. Maintain NPO status.
7. Prepare for admission to the hospital:
   - Give parents information regarding the plan of care, including the anticipated time of surgery and the reason for delaying immediate surgery:
     - Definitive treatment for pyloric stenosis is surgical intervention after fluid and electrolyte imbalances have been corrected.
     - Because this correction can take from 24 to 36 hours, the infant generally does not go directly to the operating room from the ED but instead is admitted to a general surgical unit for stabilization.
8. Perform diagnostic testing:
   - Definitive diagnosis of pyloric stenosis is most often made by palpation of an olive coupled with classic clinical findings.
   - In the cases where an olive may not be palpable, the following testing may be performed:
     - Ultrasonography.
     - Upper gastrointestinal series. Confirmatory findings include a positive "string sign," which represents the narrowed pyloric opening.
     - Serum electrolytes. The most common diagnosis findings associated with pyloric stenosis include hypochloremia and hypokalemia, which produce metabolic alkalosis.

Malrotation with Volvulus

Malrotation of the bowel is a congenital condition resulting from an abnormal rotation of the intestine during embryonic development. This anomaly can result in torsion (malrotation) of the intestines and obstruction of the blood supply to the bowel. Although malrotation with volvulous usually occurs *in utero* or early neonatal life, the disorder can go unrecognized until childhood (Schnaufer & Mahboubi, 2000).

Pathophysiology

With abnormal fetal development of the bowel, varying degrees of volvulus can occur at the points of abnormal fixation. Volvulus, or twisting of the small intestine, may produce a partial or complete obstruction of the intestine. In addition, twisting of the mesentery, which contains the blood supply to the intestines, can compromise arterial and venous blood flow and produce bowel ischemia and necrosis within 1 to 2 hours. Without emergent surgical intervention, necrosis of the bowel can lead to perforation and peritonitis, which may ultimately produce septic shock.

Focused History

Prodromal symptoms vary, depending on the degree of intestinal obstruction:

- Several days or weeks of feeding problems, vomiting, and weight loss.
- Sudden onset of abdominal pain coupled with bilious vomiting.

Focused Assessment

The standard assessment is done. Signs and symptoms vary, depending on the degree of obstruction and the length of time elapsed prior to arrival in the ED. The infant with a history of acute-onset abdominal pain and vomiting may initially appear well hydrated and may be actively crying. These infants can rapidly become ill, appearing with grunting respirations, an altered mental status, signs of dehydration, and/or signs of shock.

The most remarkable findings in the infant or child with volvulus are:

- The presence of severe, constant abdominal pain.
- Bilious emesis.
- Abdominal distention:
  - Distention may be mild or absent, depending on the location of the obstruction.
  - Palpation of the abdomen will reveal diffuse tenderness; however, this finding may be difficult to identify in the small, already crying infant.
- Rectal bleeding:
  - This signals bowel ischemia and probable necrosis, which can also be associated with bloody emesis.

Nursing Interventions

Assess and stabilize the airway and breathing, as dictated by the infant's clinical condition. In addition, perform the following interventions to prepare the child for surgery and to monitor the child's condition while in the ED:

1. Monitor pulse oximetry and heart rate.

2. Obtain intravenous access to correct fluid deficits:
   - Fluid replacement therapy is described in the section on gastroenteritis.
   - Treatment for shock is reviewed in Chapter 17.
   - Because of the need for rapid surgical intervention, fluid stabilization may not be completed prior to surgery.
3. Insert a nasogastric or orogastric tube to decompress the gastrointestinal tract.
4. Administer broad-spectrum antibiotics.
5. Obtain blood for typing and cross matching.
6. Continuously monitor vital signs, respiratory status, circulatory status, neurologic status, and intake and output, because infants with volvulus can rapidly decompensate.
7. The nurse or physician should accompany the infant or child for all diagnostic testing.

Intussusception

Intussusception is a bowel obstruction caused by the telescoping of one section of bowel into the more distal segment. The majority of children with intussusception are between the ages of 3 months and 5 years. The highest incidence is in infants between the ages of 5 and 9 months (Rowe, 1995). Intussusception occurs more frequently in males than in females.

In most cases, intussusception occurs in otherwise healthy infants and children, and there is no known etiology. There is higher incidence of cases in the spring and winter corresponding to the peak incidence of viral illnesses (both gastrointestinal and respiratory). Other cases have been associated with constipation, parasites, or the ingestion of a foreign body. Pathologic conditions, such as Meckel's diverticulum or a gastrointestinal tumor or cyst, can precipitate an intussusception. Children with cystic fibrosis and children with Henoch-Schönlein purpura are also more prone to the development of intussusception.

Pathophysiology

Intussusception results when one portion of the intestine telescopes into the distal portion. This causes a complete or partial bowel obstruction involving constriction of the mesentery and venous stasis. When blood flow to the intestines is compromised, the bowel becomes edematous, further impairing blood flow. Increased production of mucus from cellular damage mixed with bloody fluid leaking from the engorged bowel, forms the classic currant-jelly stool (Horton et al., 1998). If the intussusception is untreated, arterial blood flow will cease and bowel necrosis will result. Eventually, perforation and peritonitis may occur.

Focused History

Classic history:

- Otherwise healthy infant or child who suddenly cries with colicky, abdominal pain:
  - The parent may say the pain seemed to go away and the infant went to sleep or was comfortable, only to later cry out with the same symptoms.
  - The parents may relate a history of lethargy between episodes as the episodic pain progresses.

Atypical findings:

- Lethargy and poor feeding.
- Vomiting.

Focused Assessment

The standard pediatric assessment is done. Physical findings can reveal classic findings or may be nonspecific. The following assessment findings may be present:

- Irritability.
- Pale skin.
- Lethargy.
- A toxic-appearing, shock-like state that may mimic a postictal state or sepsis.
- A soft abdomen (early in the illness) and sometimes a sausage-shaped mass, usually in the right upper quadrant.
- A distended and rigid abdomen as the obstruction progresses.
- Blood in the stool:
  - The classic current-jelly stool is often a late finding of intussusception.

Nursing Interventions

1. Assess and stabilize the airway, breathing, and circulation as required by the infant's or child's condition.
2. Obtain venous access to address fluid and electrolyte needs.
3. Anticipate a barium or air enema if perforation is not suspected.
4. Prepare for surgical intervention if perforation has occurred:
   - Obtain laboratory specimens.
   - Administer broad-spectrum antibiotics.
   - Insert a nasogastric tube to relieve gastric distention and prevent emesis.
5. Continuously monitor the child for signs and symptoms of sepsis:
   - Monitor vital signs.

- Monitor circulatory status, including skin color and peripheral pulses.
- Monitor neurologic status.

6. Administer an intravenous dose of morphine, 0.1 mg/kg, or another appropriate analgesic for pain management as necessary.
7. Perform diagnostic testing:
   - The degree of diagnostic testing depends on the initial presentation, but usually consists of:
     - Complete blood count, white blood cell count, and differential.
     - Serum electrolytes.
     - Blood urea nitrogen.
     - Blood type and cross match (if perforation is suspected).
     - Plain film abdominal X-rays. Findings are often inconclusive and depend on the location, severity, and duration of the symptoms.
     - Ultrasonography. A highly reliable method of identifying intussusception, it is particularly useful in children with an atypical presentation or in whom perforation is suspected.
     - Air enema. The definitive diagnosis and treatment for most cases of intussusception (unless perforation is suspected) is an air enema, which both identifies the presence of the obstruction and in many cases reduces the intussusception (Swischuk, 1994). This procedure is contraindicated if a perforation is suspected. When reduction with an enema is unsuccessful, emergent surgical intervention is required.

Incarcerated Hernias

Hernias are the result of a congenital anomaly that allows an organ, such as the small bowel, cecum, ovary, fallopian tubes, or appendix, to protrude through an opening in the musculature. In infants and young children, these openings generally occur in the inguinal or umbilical areas, but they can also occur in the scrotal and femoral areas.

Umbilical hernias are the most commonly seen hernias in infants. A higher percentage of umbilical hernias occur in African-American infants younger than 6 weeks of age and in low-birth-weight infants. Most umbilical hernias close by 3 years of age and require no intervention.

Inguinal hernias occur in approximately 3 to 5% of all live births and are more prevalent in preterm infants (Rowe, 1995). Boys have a significantly higher percentage of inguinal hernias than do girls.

Pathophysiology

When an organ such as the bowel or an ovary protrudes through a muscular opening, the organ can become incarcerated or trapped. Progressive edema can lead to venous obstruction and decreased arterial blood supply, resulting in necrosis and gangrene. If the obstruction is in the bowel, perforation can occur.

Umbilical hernias rarely become incarcerated; inguinal hernias are more prone to incarceration. Inguinal hernias, which occur in the groin or scrotal area, are more likely to become incarcerated in the first year of life. They are most commonly seen on the right side, and incarceration is most prevalent in girls. In girls, however, the incarceration usually involves the ovary rather than the intestines (Schnaufer & Mahboubi, 2000). In boys, pressure on the spermatic cord from the incarceration can cause the testicle to infarct.

Focused History

- A bulge in the umbilical area, groin, or scrotal area.
- A bulge that tends to worsen with crying or straining.

If the hernia is incarcerated, the following history may also be present:

- Uncontrolled crying and irritability.
- Abdominal pain.
- Vomiting.

Focused Assessment

The standard assessment is performed. Findings include:

- A crying, irritable infant.
- A firm, discrete mass felt in the abdomen or groin.

Additional findings depend on the location and degree of obstruction, and the duration of the incarceration. These symptoms may include:

- Local tenderness and swelling over the mass.
- Abdominal distention.
- Erythematous or discolored skin over the mass.

Nursing Interventions

1. Continuously evaluate the infant or child or with an incarcerated hernia to monitor for changes in circulatory status and level of consciousness.
2. Treatment for an incarcerated hernia in a stable infant with no signs of toxicity or peritonitis is manual reduction of the hernia:
   - Place the infant in the Trendelenburg position.
   - Apply a cold pack to the area.
   - Administer sedatives as necessary to facilitate manual reduction.

- When sedation is used, monitor the heart rate and pulse oximetry according to hospital sedation policy.
- Prepare for admission to the hospital for observation and possible elective surgical repair if manual reduction is successful.
- When the infant is quiet and the abdomen is relaxed, apply gentle manual pressure to the mass.
- Elective hernia repair is usually performed within the next few days.

3. When manual reduction is unsuccessful, emergent surgical reduction is required:
   - Maintain NPO status.
   - Record color, consistency, and frequency of emesis.
   - Observe the child for signs of intestinal obstruction (e.g., vomiting or abdominal distention).
   - Prepare for emergency surgical intervention.
4. Perform diagnostic testing:
   - The diagnosis of an incarcerated hernia is based on clinical findings.
     - Diagnostic testing may include abdominal X-ray; ultrasound and/or color-flow Doppler to verify blood flow to the organ.

Hirschsprung's Disease (Congenital Aganglionic Megacolon)

Hirschsprung's disease is a disorder of the large intestine that causes inadequate motility of the affected part of the intestine. The result is a functional obstruction of the large intestine and interference with the normal mechanism of defecation. Hirschprung's disease is a congenital disorder, and evidence suggests that the affected population has a genetic predisposition to the disease.

Hirschprung's disease accounts for one-fourth to one-third of all intestinal obstructions in neonates. The disease is most prevalent in males, and the incidence of Hirschsprung's disease is higher in children with Down syndrome.

Pathophysiology

Hirschprung's disease is caused by the absence of ganglionic cells in the colon. The affected segment may involve a very small portion of the bowel or the entire colon. The obstruction is most commonly located in the rectum and the portion of the large intestine proximal to the rectum. The result of the obstruction is spasm, abnormal motility, and enlargement of the colon proximal to the aganglionic segment. The aganglionic section will be narrow and nonfunctional. Intestinal obstruction or chronic constipation will result. Erosion and eventual ulceration of the colon above the aganglionic section of bowel can lead to acute enterocolitis, perforation, and peritonitis.

Focused History

Neonates and infants

- Failure to pass meconium within the first 24 to 48 hours following birth.
- Constipation alternating with diarrhea, if the condition is not diagnosed in the first 48 hours after birth.

Older children

- Chronic constipation, abdominal distention, and bloating or gas.
- Frequent use of enemas, suppositories, or rectal stimulation to assist the child with defecation.
- Vomiting uncommon.

Infants or children

- Acute enterocolitis
  - Fever.
  - Explosive diarrhea.
  - Abdominal tenderness.
  - Vomiting.

Focused Assessment

The standard assessment is done. Table 19.5 lists the clinical manifestations of children with Hirschsprung's disease. Most children who present to the ED with undiagnosed Hirschprung's disease appear to be well, although some may appear poorly nourished and anemic. On rare occasions, an infant or child will have a toxic appearance as a result of acute enterocolitis and peritonitis. Other assessment findings may include:

- Abdominal distention and visible peristalsis.
- A palpable fecal mass.
- Ribbon-like and foul-smelling stools.
- A narrow rectum with little or no feces.

Nursing Interventions

The infant or child with signs of peritonitis or sepsis requires emergent management:

- Maintain the airway, breathing, and circulation.
- Stabilize fluid and electrolyte levels.
- Perform a full sepsis workup.
- Administer broad-spectrum antibiotics.

TABLE 19.5 Clinical Manifestations of Hirschprung's Disease

Newborn Period
Failure to pass meconium within 24 to 48 hours after birth
Reluctance to ingest fluids
Bile-stained vomitus
Abdominal distention
Infancy
Failure to thrive
Constipation
Abdominal distention
Episodes of diarrhea and vomiting
Ominous signs (often signify the presence of enterocolitis):
▪ Explosive, watery diarrhea
▪ Fever
▪ Severe prostration
Childhood*
Constipation
Ribbon-like, foul-smelling stools
Abdominal distention
Visible peristalsis
Easily palpable fecal masses
Child usually poorly nourished and anemic

*Symptoms are more chronic.
From: Wong, 1997. *Whaley and Wong's essentials of pediatric nursing* (5th ed., p. 817) St. Louis: Mosby—Year Book. Used with permission.

Most infants and children suspected to have Hirschprung's disease are stable and require only supportive nursing care while awaiting diagnostic testing:

- Obtain vital signs, weight, and abdominal circumference.
- Administer single or multiple enemas, as ordered, to relieve abdominal distention and empty the bowel.
- Prepare for admission to a surgical floor and/or surgery:
  - The urgency of treatment depends on the child's age and clinical presentation.
  - Usually the infant or child will require a temporary colostomy to treat or to prevent enterocolitis and to allow the proximal bowel to resume normal size and tonicity.
  - Definitive repair can then be performed electively.
  - In newborns, definitive repair is sometimes delayed until the infant is between 6 and 12 months of age.
- Perform diagnostic testing:
  - Abdominal X-ray: The abdominal X-ray will reveal large, dilated loops of intestine and the absence of gas.
  - Barium enema: The barium enema will identify the dilated bowel proximal to the narrowed aganglionic section of bowel. Confirmation of the diagnosis is made with suction rectal biopsy.
  - Anorectal manometric examination.

Gastrointestinal Foreign Body

Ingestion of foreign bodies is common in young children, particularly in infants, toddlers, and preschoolers. Increasing mobility, natural curiosity, and an affinity for mouthing objects, coupled with decreased supervision, make children in these age groups particularly prone to ingestions. The foreign bodies most commonly ingested by children are:

- Coins.
- Buttons.
- Marbles.
- Small toy parts.
- Screws and tacks.
- Button batteries.
- Chicken or fish bones.
- Straight pins.

Pathophysiology

The majority of foreign bodies ingested by infants and children pass to the stomach and through the GI tract without incident. In some children, however, ingested foreign bodies become lodged in one of these physiologically narrow areas in the esophagus: the cricopharyngeal muscle; the aortic arch; or the gastroesophageal junction (Swischuk, 1994). The cricopharyngeal area is the most common site of lodged foreign bodies in children. The gastroesophageal junction is the least common site (Swischuk, 1994).

The danger from a foreign-body ingestion is that an irregular or pointed object may puncture or tear the esophagus; the object may compress the trachea and cause respiratory distress; or the object may become lodged in a portion of the esophagus. A lodged object, particularly one that is undetected, can lead to tissue erosion and eventual perforation. Ingestion of button batteries is of particular concern because a button battery lodged in the esophagus can rapidly produce liquefaction necrosis and electrochemical burns (Sheikh, 1993).

Focused History

Medical care is not sought for the majority of children with gastrointestinal foreign-body ingestions because the ingestion was not observed and the child exhibited no symptoms. Parents who do bring their child to the ED usually observed the ingestion or suspect an ingestion and report the following history:

- Observation of the infant or child mouthing an object that disappeared.
- Observation of the child coughing and gagging after playing with a small object.

The following history would be suggestive of an ingested object when the parents did not observe the incident:

- Coughing and gagging.
- Increased salivation.
- Refusal to eat or drink.
- Pain or discomfort with feeding.
- Vomiting.

Focused Assessment

The majority of children who have ingested a foreign body appear to be well and have no overt signs and symptoms of an ingestion. Assessment findings may include:

- Coughing, gagging, and/or salivation.
- Signs and symptoms of respiratory distress, including tachypnea and retractions (if the object is compressing the trachea).

Nursing Interventions

Treatment depends on the type of foreign body ingested and its location. Because the majority of foreign bodies pass through the gastrointestinal tract without incident, most children are sent home and the parents are told to observe for the presence of the object in the stool. Objects lodged in the esophagus may be treated in one of several ways:

- They may be removed by endoscopy.
- They may be watched for up to 12 hours (if they are located in the lower third of the esophagus and are smooth and round).
- They may be removed with the indwelling urinary catheter method (if smooth and round):
  - Insert an indwelling urinary catheter into the esophagus below the object.
  - Inflate the catheter and remove the object.
  - This procedure is done using fluoroscopy.
- Button batteries lodged anywhere in the esophagus are removed emergently by endoscopy because esophageal burns can occur within hours of the ingestion.

The child with signs and symptoms of respiratory distress requires the following nursing interventions:

- Prepare for airway support as preparations are made for a portable X-ray and emergent removal of the foreign body.
- Provide supplemental oxygen.
- Allow the child to maintain a position of comfort.
- Prepare for surgical intervention if the child has signs or symptoms of esophageal perforation.
- Accompany the unstable child for all diagnostic testing and/or to the operating room.
- Prepare the child for esophagoscopy or balloon catheter removal if the object is lodged in the esophagus:
  - Administer sedation as ordered.
  - Accompany the child to the radiology department.
  - Prepare for ventilatory support.
- Perform diagnostic testing:
  - Anteroposterior and lateral X-rays include the neck, chest, and abdomen.
  - The use of a metal detector is an alternative to X-ray evaluation in the child who ingested a metal object such as a coin (Biehler, Tuggle, & Stacy, 1993).
  - Computerized tomographic scan or barium swallow may be necessary if the object is radiolucent and is suspected to be lodged in the esophagus.

Home Care and Prevention

When children are discharged following removal of an esophageal foreign body, parents are given the following instructions:

- Provide a clear liquid diet for 12 to 24 hours and then progress to a regular diet.
- Seek immediate care if the child begins to have severe abdominal pain, bloody stools, bloody emesis or repeated emesis, or develops a fever, whether the object was removed or not.
- Prevent future episodes of ingestion:
  - Lock cabinets.
  - Remove small objects from the child's environment.

In addition, parents should be given information concerning cardiopulmonary resuscitation classes.

Conclusion

Abdominal complaints are common and most are benign. The life-threatening emergencies that affect the gastrointestinal tract are commonly surgical emergencies that can result in shock and sepsis; however, medical conditions, such as gastroenteritis, can cause dehydration, electrolyte imbalances, and shock. Nurses must understand the pathology behind these conditions and accurately assess and treat children who present to the ED with complications resulting from these conditions.

References

Behrman, R. E., Kliegman, R. M., & Jenson, H. B. (2000). *Nelson's textbook of pediatrics* (16th ed., pp. 765-768). Philadelphia: Saunders.

Biehler, J. L., Tuggle, D., & Stacy, T. (1993). Use of the transmitter-receiver metal detector in the evaluation of pediatric coin ingestions. *Pediatric Emergency Care, 9*, 208-210.

Friedman, S. C., & Sheynkin, Y. R. (1995). Acute scrotal symptoms because of perforated appendix in children: Case report and review of literature. *Pediatric Emergency Care, 11*, 181-182.

Jedd, M. B., Melton, L. J., & Griffin, M. (1988). Factors associated with infantile hypertrophic pyloric stenosis. *American Journal of Diseases of Children, 142*, p. 334.

Klein, B. L. (1997a). Meckel's diverticulum. In R. M. Barkin. (Eds.), *Pediatric emergency medicine, concepts in clinical practice* (2nd ed., pp. 854-856) St. Louis: Mosby—Year Book.

Klein, B. L. (1997b). Pyloric stenosis, infantile hypertrophic. In R. M. Barkin, (Ed.), *Pediatric emergency medicine, concepts in clinical practice* (2nd ed., pp. 856-857). St. Louis: Mosby—Year Book.

Martin, S., & Derengowski, S. (1997). In M. C. Slota (Ed.), *Core curriculum for pediatric critical care nursing* (pp. 424-460). Philadelphia: Saunders.

Rowe, M. I. (1995). *Essentials of pediatric surgery*. St. Louis: Mosby—Year Book.

Sacchetti, A., Brilli, R. J., & Barkin, R. M. (1997). Fluid and electrolyte balance. In R. M. Barkin (Eds.), *Pediatric emergency medicine, concepts in clinical practice* (2nd ed., pp. 166-169). St. Louis: Mosby—Year Book.

Schnaufer, L., & Mahboubi, S. (2000). Abdominal emergencies. In G. R. Fleisher & S. Ludwig (Eds.), *Textbook of pediatric emergency medicine* (3rd ed., pp. 1513-1538). Philadelphia: Lippincott, Williams & Wilkins.

Sheikh, A. (1993). Button battery ingestions in children, *Pediatric Emergency Care, 9*(4), 224-229.

Soud, T. E., Inman, C., Horton, M. S., & Standifer, P. (1998). Gastrointestinal disorders. In T. E. Soud & J. S. Rogers (Eds.), *Manual of pediatric emergency nursing*. (pp. 332-363). St. Louis: Mosby—Year Book.

Soud, T., & Rogers, J. S. (1998). *Manual of pediatric emergency nursing*. St. Louis: Mosby—Year Book.

Strahlman, R. S. (1997). Appendicitis. In R. A. Hoekelman, (Ed.), *Primary pediatric care* (3rd ed., pp. 1187-1189). St. Louis: Mosby—Year Book.

Swischuk, L. E. (1994). *Emergency imaging of the acutely ill or injured child* (3rd ed.). Baltimore: Williams & Wilkins.

Weaver, L. T. (1996). Anatomy and embryology. In W. A. Walker, P. R. Durie, R. J. Hamilton, J. A. Walker Smith, & J. B. Watkins (Eds.), *Pediatric gastrointestinal disease* (2nd ed., pp. 9-17). St. Louis: Mosby.

Wong, D. L. (1997). *Whaley and Wong's essentials of pediatric nursing* (5th ed.). St. Louis: Mosby—Year Book.

20

Genitourinary Emergencies

Christine Nelson, RNC, MS, PNP

Introduction

The genitourinary (GU) system includes organs of the urinary system and the reproductive system. The urinary system maintains the optimal environment for metabolism by excreting waste products from the body and consists of the kidneys, ureters, bladder, and urethra. The reproductive system supplies hormones, as well as eggs and sperm, for sexual growth and fertility. The male reproductive system consists of the scrotum, testicles, and penis, and the female reproductive system consists of the vagina, labia minora and majora, ovaries, and uterus. Because the urologic and reproductive systems are in close anatomic proximity, they are discussed together.

GU conditions range from common, simply treated illnesses to emergent health conditions. Children may present to the emergency department (ED) with congenital GU conditions or acquired conditions that are diagnosed in the ED. Children with kidney transplants also may require ED treatment. Emergency nurses must be able to recognize the presence of these conditions and initiate appropriate treatment measures. The purpose of this chapter is to discuss common congenital and acquired GU conditions and to outline emergency nursing treatment of GU concerns.

Embryologic Development of the Genitourinary System

Urinary System

The urinary system separates from the rectum at about 6 weeks of gestational age. Protein codes on the Y chromosome initiate development of male genitalia at 7 to 8 weeks' gestation. The embryonic kidneys develop as three distinct, sequentially replaced organs; the collecting ducts form by the fifth fetal month (Gilman & Mooney, 1998). Errors in the development of the collecting ducts may result in polycystic kidneys (Gilman & Mooney, 1998). Fetal urine is produced by 10 to 11 weeks' gestation. In utero, the placenta functions as the major filtering system. As the kidneys mature *in utero,* the cloaca becomes the urogenital sinus and differentiates into the vesicourethral canal, forming the bladder and upper urethra; the urogenital sinus becomes the main part of the urethra (Gilman & Mooney, 1998).

Embryologic variations in urinary system development can lead to structural abnormalities, ranging from minor, surgically correctable conditions to those that are incompatible with life. Structural abnormalities of the urinary system cause approximately 45% of the cases of renal failure in children (Gilman & Mooney, 1998). Table 20.1 outlines common urinary system abnormalities.

Genitalia

For a brief period of development, the embryo has a common genital structure prior to differentiating into male or female structures. Slight abnormalities during the development of the reproductive structures can cause significant malformations. For example, a hermaphrodite is an individual who has gonads and internal and external reproductive structures of both genders. Genital abnormalities may result from congenital or acquired conditions. Table 20.2 describes common male and female genital abnormalities.

Male development

The inner portion of the medulla joins with the mesonephric duct; further differentiation forms the seminiferous tubules, efferent ductules, epididymis, and ductus differens. The genital tubercle elongates and forms the penis. The urethral folds fuse, leaving an opening in the distal end. The labioscrotal swellings form the scrotum.

Female development

The outer portion of the undifferentiated gonads undergoes greater development for later reproduction purposes. The gonads differentiate to form ovaries. The müllerian

TABLE 20.1 Common Urinary System Abnormalities

Condition	*Description*
Ectopic kidneys	Failure of the kidneys to ascend from the pelvis to the abdomen. Kidney function is usually normal.
Horseshoe kidney	Fusion of the kidneys as they ascend, creating a single, U-shaped kidney. While these children are usually asymptomatic, they may have hematuria following trauma to the pelvic region, a midline abdominal mass, or ureteropelvic junction obstruction.
Renal aplasia	Failure of the uterine duct to differentiate into kidney-forming tissues *in utero*, resulting in the absence of one or both kidneys.
Hypoplastic or dysplastic kidneys	Development of small, normal kidneys. This may affect one or both kidneys. Bilateral hypoplastic kidneys are a common cause of pediatric renal failure.
Renal dysplasia	Abnormal differentiation of renal tissues. This can be associated with obstruction of the urinary collection system.
Renal agenesis	Failure of one or both of the kidneys to grow. This condition can be hereditary or random. Unilateral renal agenesis occurs in 1 of 1,000 live births, usually in males. Usually the left kidney is absent. The remaining kidney compensates in size, and the child usually leads a healthy life.
Duplication of the urinary collection system	Duplication arising from embryologic maldevelopment. It is usually more common in females and can be familial. The duplication can be bilateral. Vesicoureteral reflux or ureteral obstruction may be present.
Vesicoureteral reflux	Impaired valvular function at the ureterovesical junction that leads to the reflux of bladder urine into the ureter or kidneys. In the presence of a urinary tract infection, such reflux of infected urine can lead to pyelonephritis, renal scarring, and chronic renal damage.
Prune-belly syndrome	Absence of abdominal musculature as well as renal and urinary tract abnormalities and cryptochordism. Males are affected more frequently and severely than are females. Other congenital malformations may be present.

From: Ellis, 1997; Gilman & Mooney, 1998.

ducts between the ovaries form the uterus and vagina. There is less elongation of the genital tubercle as it forms the clitoris. The urethral folds, which do not fuse as they do in males, form the labia that surround the vagina.

Pediatric Considerations

Although all of the kidneys' nephrons are present at birth, they are not fully developed. The tubules and glomeruli are variable in size, accounting for the limited ability of the newborn to conserve sodium and excrete sodium loads. This variability resolves around 12 to 14 months of age.

Renal blood flow and the glomerular filtration rate are low at birth and gradually increase as the child develops. This is an important consideration when drugs excreted by the renal system are prescribed and when fluid requirements are calculated.

The total extracellular fluid volume is significantly greater in infants than adults. Infants are less able to concentrate urine, making it much more diluted than it is in adults (Barber, 2000). Mature renal function is usually reached at 1 to 2 years of age (Barkin & Rosen, 1999).

The infant's bladder is a cylindrical abdominal organ with a 15- to 20-ml urine capacity; the bladder descends into the pelvis over time (Pye & Soud, 1998). As bladder volume increases, the ability to retain urine improves; with the maturation of the neurogenic pathways by 2 to 3 years of age, bladder sphincter control occurs, and the child learns voluntary bladder control (Pye & Soud, 1998).

Etiology

The etiology of GU health conditions arises from congenital or acquired processes as described in this chapter.

Focused History

- Patient history:
    - Activity level. A decrease in activity or performance of developmentally appropriate skills may be related to renal disease.
    - Onset and duration of symptoms.

TABLE 20.2 Selected Genital Abnormalities

Finding	*Description*	*Implication*
Hypospadius	Urethral opening on the ventral (underside) of penis	Urinary stream aims downward.
Chordee	Ventral bowing of the penis caused by tight band of fibrous tissue	May make catheterization difficult.
Microphallus	Abnormal smallness of the penis	May make catheterization difficult.
Crypto-orchidism	Absence of one or both testes from the scrotal sac	Should be referred to a specialist if finding persists after 6 months of age.
Hydrocele	Collection of serous fluid in the scrotal sac; scrotal size may increase with activity and decrease with rest	Referral for management is necessary if the problem persists after 1 year of age or if there is discomfort.
Labial adhesions	Fusion of tissue between the labia minora that covers vaginal opening.	Treatment in prepubescent females is necessary only if urinary or vaginal drainage is impaired. May make catheterization difficult.

  - Interventions that relieve or worsen the symptoms.
  - Fever.
  - Abdominal or back pain.
  - Recent injuries or illness.
  - Urination patterns: changes in the urine force or stream; dribbling enuresis; incontinence.
  - Change in urine color or hematuria.
  - Urine odor.
  - Urinary frequency and volume.
  - Dysuria or urgency.
  - Sexual history (if applicable).
  - Congenital or acquired genitourinary conditions.
- Family history:
  - Renal disease.
  - Renal abnormalities.
  - Hypertension.
  - Congenital defects.

Focused Assessment

Physical Assessment

1. Assess the cardiovascular system:
   - Measure blood pressure:
     - Hypertension in infants without aortic coarctation can result from a renovascular disorder, such as renal venous thrombosis, arterial thrombosis, or renal artery stenosis (Ellis, 1997).
     - Hypertension in children may be associated with renal disorders (Ellis, 1997), such as nephritis and chronic renal failure.
   - Observe the skin for color, turgor, and markings:
     - Generalized edema may be present in renal failure.
     - Pallor may be a sign of renal dysfunction.
     - Poor skin turgor may be associated with dehydration.
     - Café au lait spots, neurofibromas, and other skin lesions may suggest renal disorders (Ellis, 1997).
2. Assess the abdomen:
   - Observe the size and shape of the abdomen:
     - Ascites, distention, rigidity, or tenderness may be associated with renal problems.
   - Auscultate the great vessels:
     - Bruits auscultated over great vessels may indicate arteriopathy.
     - Bruits noted in the epigastric area may indicate renovascular disease.
   - Palpate the abdomen:
     - Palpate the bladder for distention. A distended bladder may be palpable above the symphysis pubis. Persistent bladder distention may indicate a blockage or other emptying abnormality. An enlarged bladder or gynecologic lesion may be palpated as a midline mass in the pelvis (Bellinger, 1997).

- Palpate the kidneys (rarely palpable except in neonates or very thin children). Enlarged kidneys may be palpated as upper abdominal or flank masses (Bellinger, 1997), indicating a tumor or hydronephrosis.
- Percuss the back for costovertebral angle tenderness:
  - Fist percussion at the costovertebral angle may elicit tenderness as the kidneys are jarred, indicating possible infection or injury.

3. Assess the genitalia:
   - Inspect the external genitalia for abnormalities:
     - Note abnormalities in appearance, open or closed wounds, visible foreign bodies, discharge or bleeding, rashes, lesions, and scars.
   - Inspect the external male genitalia for (Bellinger, 1997):
     - Scrotal size and character.
     - Location and size of the testes.
     - Swelling or nodules.
     - Penis size. The foreskin is examined for adhesions to the glans, and the meatus is noted for its size and location (Bellinger, 1997).
   - Inspect the female external genitalia for (Bellinger, 1997):
     - Size and location of the clitoris, urethral meatus, vaginal introitus, and hymenal ring.
4. Assess the child's height and weight for age and overall appearance; plot height and weight on a growth chart:
   - Frequent or chronic urinary tract infections or chronic renal disease are associated with failure to thrive.
   - Congenital scoliosis, facial or external ear deformities, and multiple congenital anomalies may be associated with urologic conditions (Bellinger, 1997).

Psychosocial Assessment

- Assess the child's understanding of sexual function; determine the significance of this understanding.
- Assess the child's terminology for urination.
- Assess the family's understanding of their child's preexisting GU condition:
  - Assess the family's understanding of their child's sexual activity.
- Assess the child's prior experience with healthcare professionals and with a GU examination or treatment:
  - Injuries and illnesses of the genitourinary system can be difficult for a young patient concerned about modesty, body image, and body integrity.
  - Children, especially those of school age, find it difficult to have their genitalia examined by a stranger after so much emphasis is placed on stranger avoidance. There is also anxiety because very little can be visualized, as the majority of the genitourinary system is not easily assessed.

Triage Decisions

Emergent

- Fever > 38.2°C (100.8°F) in infants 3 months of age or younger.
- Signs of sepsis and shock (suspected renal failure, post-neonatal male circumcision, post-female circumcision, vaginal bleeding).
- Altered level of consciousness.
- Signs of renal failure.
- Severe dehydration or shock.
- Marked hypertension.

TABLE 20.3 Nursing Diagnoses and Expected Outcomes

Nursing Diagnoses	*Expected Outcomes*
Altered urinary elimination patterns	The patient will have a urinary output greater than 1.0 ml/kg/hr (infant) and 0.5 to 1.0 ml/kg/hr (children and adolescents).
Potential for infection related to knowledge deficits of patient and/or parents	The patient will remain free of preventable infection. The patient and parents will verbalize an understanding of proper hygiene and protected sexual contact.
Knowledge deficits related to disease, treatment, complications, and prevention of reoccurrence	The patient and/or parents will verbalize an understanding of the underlying disease process, treatment, and prevention of reoccurrence.

- Anuria.
- Signs of an acute scrotum.

Urgent

- Fever.
- Pain or irritability.
- Mild dehydration.
- Hypertension and generalized edema.
- Hematuria.
- Penile edema and pain from possible paraphimosis.
- Excessive bleeding, pain, infection, or delayed healing following a male or female circumcision.
- Vaginal bleeding resulting in orthostatic blood pressure changes and a pale, weak appearance.

Nonurgent

- Burning with urination.
- General malaise.
- Normal vital signs for age.

Nursing Interventions

- Assess and maintain airway, breathing, and circulation (Chapter 6).
- Obtain venous access and initiate an intravenous infusion:
  - Obtain blood for laboratory studies, as needed.
  - Administer medications, as needed.
- Prepare for diagnostic studies, as needed.
- Reassess the child's neurologic and cardiopulmonary statuses.
- Insert an indwelling bladder catheter to measure urinary output, or perform a bladder catheterization, as needed:
  - Obtain a urine specimen for urinalysis, culture and sensitivity.
- Prepare the child for a genital or gynecologic examination.
- Provide psychosocial support to the child and family; inform the family frequently about their child's condition.
- Prepare for transfer and transport to a tertiary care facility (Chapter 10), hospitalization, or discharge and follow-up to the primary care physician.

Specific Genitourinary-Urinary Conditions

Urinary Tract Infections

Etiology

Urinary tract infection (UTI) is the presence of a significant amount of bacteria anywhere in the urinary tract. The bacterium that most commonly causes UTI is *Escherichia coli* (Ellis, 1997), which causes 80% of urinary tract infections. *Pseudomonas* or *Proteus* species are found infrequently and often are associated with abnormal genitourinary anatomy (Ellis, 1997) or urinary tract instrumentation, such as indwelling catheters and stents.

Urinary tract infections are a major concern in children. About 3 to 5% of all girls and 1% of boys will experience a symptomatic UTI before puberty. Females have more recurrences than do males, and 7- to 11-year-old girls are most susceptible because of bacterial ascension of the urethra (Gilman & Mooney, 1998).

Risk factors contributing to UTIs include poor hygiene, lack of fluid intake, sexual activity, and infrequent bladder emptying. Disease severity is affected by bacterial virulence and existing anatomic abnormalities (reflux or obstruction) (Gilman & Mooney, 1998).

Neonatal UTIs usually arise from bacteremic spread, while UTIs in infants and children tend to arise from bacteria that travel up the urethra to the bladder (Pye & Soud, 1998). The location of the UTI is often difficult to detect. *Cystitis*, or bladder infection, leads to mucosal inflammation, detrusor muscle hyperactivity, and a decrease in bladder capacity (Gilman & Mooney, 1998). Characteristics of cystitis include acute onset of fever, vomiting, dysuria, suprapubic pain, and urinary sediment (Ellis, 1997). Urinary reflux into the ureters can propel bacteria to the kidneys, leading to pyelonephritis.

Pyelonephritis, or kidney infection, results in renal edema and an enlarged kidney; renal scarring and abnormal kidney function can result (Pye & Soud, 1998). Repeated infections can lead to chronic renal failure. Signs of pyelonephritis include fever, chills, abdominal and flank pain, and an enlarged kidney (Gilman & Mooney, 1998; Pye & Soud, 1998).

The presence of UTIs should be considered in all febrile infants, especially in the first 2 weeks of age, even when meningitis, sepsis, or other infections are found (Ellis, 1997). Neonatal UTIs may be associated with bacteremia.

Focused History

- Patient history:
  - Foul-smelling urine.
  - Hematuria.

TABLE 20.4 Symptoms of Urinary Tract Infection in Infants and Children

Young Infants	*Older Infants/Toddlers*	*Children*
Lethargy.	Irritability.	Complaints of dysuria.
Poor appetite.	Abdominal pain.	Urinary frequency.
Irritability.	Vomiting.	Urinary urgency.
Presence or absence of fever.	Fever.	Abdominal or back pain.
	Incontinence in the toilet-trained toddler.	

- Prior episodes of UTIs or other urinary-related problems.
- Presenting signs and symptoms of UTIs in infants and children are variable (Table 20.4).

Focused Assessment

Physical Assessment

1. Assess the respiratory system:
   - Auscultate the chest for:
     - Respiratory rate. Tachypnea may be present with fever and infection.
2. Assess the cardiovascular system:
   - Auscultate the heart for:
     - Rate. Tachycardia may be present with fever and infection.
   - Assess skin and core temperature:
     - Fever may be present with infection and sepsis.
3. Assess the abdomen:
   - Palpate the abdomen and bladder for pain or tenderness.
   - Percuss the back:
     - Tenderness during costovertebral angle percussion may be elicited.
4. Assess the external genitalia:
   - Observe for mucopurulent or bloody vaginal discharge in young females.
   - Observe for mucopurulent penile discharge in males.

Psychosocial Assessment

- Assess the child's and family's understanding of UTIs.
- Assess for coping strategies if the UTI is recurrent.
- Assess the child's preparatory and coping strategies for invasive procedures, such as bladder catheterization.

Nursing Interventions

1. Assess and maintain airway, breathing, and circulation.
2. Obtain urine for diagnostic testing:
   - Urine for analysis and culture and sensitivity testing may be obtained through a clean-catch method, urinary bladder catheterization, or suprapubic bladder aspiration:
     - The clean-catch method (or bag method for infants) is not recommended for non-toilet-trained children because contamination from the surrounding tissues can affect the obtained specimen. However, in older children and adolescents, the clean-catch method may result in a reliable urine specimen.
     - Urinary bladder catheterization is the introduction of a catheter into the urinary bladder to obtain a sterile urine specimen.
   - Urine also may be obtained from an existing suprapubic catheter or indwelling urinary bladder catheter.
3. Perform diagnostic testing on the obtained specimen:
   - Urine dipstick tests detect nitrite and leukocyte esterase; when both are positive, the presence of a UTI is almost certain (Ellis, 1997).
   - Another method for diagnostic testing is enhanced urinalysis, which consists of counting white blood cells in a Neubauer hemocytometer and counting bacteria in a Gram-stained smear (Ellis, 1997).
   - Although a urinalysis does not detect the presence of bacteria, it does give information about other urinary components, such as the presence of white blood cells.
   - Urine culture analysis is based on the colony counts (Pye & Soud, 1998). Culture results generally are reported in 24 and 48 hours.

4. Administer prescribed antibiotics:
   - The antibiotics most commonly used for simple, uncomplicated UTIs are amoxicillin, ampicillin, trimethoprim (TMP)-sulfamethoxazole, co-trimoxazole, or a sulfonamide.
   - Cephalosporins and amoxicillin/clavulanate are expensive and rarely necessary unless sensitivities indicate their need.
5. Prepare for transfer or transport to a tertiary care center (Chapter 10) or for hospital admission:
   - Hospitalization may be required for infants and children with high fevers and suspected sepsis:
     - Intravenous antibiotics are administered.
     - Blood specimens are obtained for complete blood count and differential, cultures, and electrolytes.

Home Care and Prevention

The patient and family should receive directions for follow-up as well as discharge teaching. A urinalysis and culture are necessary after 48 hours of treatment to determine if the infection is resolving. This specimen may be tested by the child's primary care physician or at the ED.

The patient and family must have resources to obtain the prescribed antibiotic and to receive the follow-up urine cultures. Recurrent or partially treated UTIs can lead to health problems such as hypertension, renal calculi, and chronic renal failure (Pye & Soud, 1998).

Young children may have undetected or undiagnosed congenital abnormalities that predispose them to UTIs. The suspicion of such abnormalities indicates a need for future radiographic evaluations. Renal scanning with dimercaptosuccinic acid is finding popularity because it is more sensitive than the intravenous pyelogram for detecting renal lesions (Reynolds & Hoberman, 1995).

The patient and family should be taught strategies to prevent future UTIs (Ball, 1998):

- Drink at least six to eight glasses of water or noncarbonated, caffeine-free fluids daily.
- Urinate whenever the "urge" is felt; do not wait.
- Wipe from front to back after defecating; change the infant's diaper frequently.
- Use cotton underwear to absorb moisture.
- Avoid tight-fitting pants.
- Avoid bubble baths, scented and colored toilet paper, perfumed soaps, and nonprescription vaginal suppositories, sprays, and douches.
- Urinate before and after sexual intercourse.
- Change sanitary pads frequently during menstruation.
- Use condoms during sexual intercourse.

Glomerulonephritis

Etiology

Glomerulonephritis is an alteration of the glomeruli resulting from an immune response that causes a decrease in glomerular filtration. In glomerulonephritis, the capillary loops in the glomeruli become inflamed and infiltrated with leukocytes, resulting in a decreased blood supply to the glomeruli. Cellular proliferation and edema occlude the lumen of the affected glomeruli, causing a decrease in the glomerular filtration rate. This decreased ability to filtrate plasma results in excessive accumulation of water and retention of sodium, leading to expanded plasma volumes and clinical findings of circulatory congestion and edema (Kher & Makker, 1992).

Although forms of acute glomerulonephritis are associated with Henoch-Schönlein purpura and disseminated lupus erythematosus, the most common form follows infections from strains of group A beta-hemolytic *streptococci* infecting the pharynx or skin; other causes of glomerulonephritis include postpneumoccal glomerulonephritis, immunoglobulin A nephritis, and hemolytic-uremic syndrome (Ellis, 1997). Poststreptococcal glomerulonephritis follows a latent period of 10 to 14 days after the streptococcal infection before the onset of symptoms.

Glomerulonephritis is diagnosed in children between the ages of 3 to 12 years; the peak incidence is at 7 years of age. (Children with hemolytic-uremic syndrome can be younger.) Males are affected more often than females. Chronic glomerulonephritis is responsible for 53% of cases of renal failure in children and is the most common reason for renal dialysis and kidney transplantation in the school-aged and adolescent populations (Gilman & Mooney, 1998).

Focused History

- Patient history (Ellis, 1997):
  - Recent febrile illness (2 to 4 weeks prior) with painful pharyngitis for which treatment was not obtained.
  - Fever, malaise, and decreased appetite.
  - Sudden onset of oliguria with the production of dark brown, smokey, or tea-colored urine.
  - Headache.
  - Edema.

Focused Assessment

Physical Assessment

1. Assess the respiratory system:
   - Auscultate the chest for:
     - Respiratory rate.

- Adventitious sounds. Pulmonary congestion may be present.

2. Assess the cardiovascular system:
   - Auscultate the heart for:
     - Rate.
   - Measure the blood pressure:
     - Hypertension may be present.
3. Assess the renal system:
   - Observe for kidney failure:
     - Note the presence of periorbital edema; pitting edema in the sacrum.
   - Percuss the kidneys for tenderness.
   - Measure the urinary output.

Psychosocial Assessment

Assess the child's and family's coping strategies.

Nursing Interventions

1. Assess and maintain airway, breathing, and circulation.
2. Initiate blood pressure monitoring to observe for hypertension.
3. Obtain venous access and initiate an intravenous infusion at maintenance rate:
   - Restrict salt and fluids to maintain a normal intravascular volume.
   - Administer diuretics to control hypertension and fluid overload, as ordered.
   - Prepare to administer furosemide at 0.5 to 1.0 mg/kg.
   - Prepare to administer sublingual nifedipine (0.25 to 0.5 mg/kg), intravenous diazoxide (2.5 to 5.0 mg/kg), or intravenous hydralazine (0.5 mg/kg) if hypertension is noted.
   - Obtain blood for laboratory studies (Pye & Soud, 1998):
     - Complete blood count.
     - Electrolytes. Hyperkalemia or dilutional hyponatremia may be noted.
     - Blood urea nitrogen and creatinine. (Both will be elevated.)
     - Antistreptolysin titer. (May be elevated.)
     - Antideoxyribonuclease B (anti-DNAase B).
     - Immunoglobulin G (will be elevated).
     - C3 complement.
     - Total protein, albumin, and globulin.
     - Antinuclear antibody.
   - Administer antibiotics:
     - Penicillin will be prescribed if the streptococcal infection is still apparent.
4. Obtain urine for urinalysis and culture:
   - A urinalysis may show red blood cells and casts, polymorphonuclear neutrophil leukocytes, and proteinuria (Pye & Soud, 1998).
5. Obtain additional diagnostic information, as ordered:
   - Throat culture.
   - Skin culture (if pyoderma is present).
   - Chest radiograph.
6. Provide psychosocial support to the child and family.
7. Prepare for transfer or transport to a tertiary care center (see Chapter 10) or hospitalization if the child is oliguric or hypertensive.

Home Care and Prevention

Adequate follow-up and discharge teaching includes teaching the parents how to:

- Restrict fluid intake.
- Administer antihypertensive medications and be aware of their side effects.
- Measure their child's blood pressure. Parents may need a stethoscope and sphygmomanometer.
- Weigh the child each day.
- Recognize the signs of acute renal failure, such as a change in level of conscious, seizures, difficulty breathing, increase in weight, edema, and decreased urinary output.

Acute Renal Failure

Etiology

Acute renal failure (ARF), the sudden loss of renal function, occurs when bodily fluid homeostasis is disrupted and there is a sudden decrease in the glomerular filtration rate. Circulation to the kidneys may be impaired by arterial or venous obstruction, renal trauma, or obstructive processes. Decreased blood flow may cause tubular necrosis, the kidney may not be able to filtrate plasma, and there may be a loss of massive amounts of salt and water. The glomerular filtration rate decreases to prevent this water loss.

Causes of ARF

- Shock:
  - Hypovolemic.
  - Septic.
  - Anaphylactic.
- Dehydration.

- Diabetic ketoacidosis.
- Severe burns.
- Nephrotic syndrome.
- Renal vessel injury.

Diseases that contribute to ARF

- Henoch-Schönlein purpura (rare).
- Hemolytic-uremic syndrome.
- Systemic lupus erythematosus.
- Neoplasms.

Focused History

- Patient history (Flynn, 1999):
  - Dehydration from vomiting or diarrhea; burns.
  - Shock.
  - Diabetic ketoacidosis.
  - Nephrotic syndrome.

Focused Assessment

Physical Assessment

1. Assess the respiratory system:
   - Auscultate the chest for:
     - Adventitious sounds. Pulmonary congestion may be present with fluid overload, leading to pulmonary edema.
     - Respiratory rate. Tachypnea, and then bradypnea, may be present.
2. Assess the cardiovascular system:
   - Auscultate the heart for:
     - Rate. Tachycardia may be present with early shock and dehydration.
     - Rhythm.
   - Evaluate cardiac rhythm by initiating cardiorespiratory monitoring:
     - Dysrhythmias may be present with congestive heart failure or fluid overload.
   - Measure the blood pressure:
     - Blood pressure may be elevated with early shock.
     - Hypotension will be present with late shock.
   - Assess peripheral perfusion:
     - Palpate the peripheral pulses for quality; equality.
     - Measure core and skin temperature.
     - Inspect the skin for color (pallor present with poor perfusion); edema (may be present with fluid overload); turgor.
     - Measure capillary refill (> 3 seconds in shock states).
3. Assess the neurologic system:
   - Assess the child's level of consciousness with the AVPU method or Glasgow coma scale:
     - Lethargy may be present.
     - Seizures may be present.
4. Assess the gastrointestinal system:
   - Palpate the abdomen for a mass.
   - Observe for vomiting.
5. Assess the GU system:
   - Measure the urinary output:
     - Urinary output will be decreased (less than 0.5 ml/kg/hr) or there will be no urinary output.
6. Measure or estimate the child's weight:
   - An increase in weight may be observed with fluid overload.
   - A decrease in weight may be noted with weight loss from vomiting and dehydration.

Nursing Interventions

1. Assess and maintain airway, breathing, and circulation:
   - Administer supplemental oxygen, as needed.
   - Initiate cardiorespiratory monitoring.
   - Measure continuous oxygen saturation.
   - Observe for dysrhythmias:
     - Monitor for T-wave changes. Severe hyperkalemia causes dysrhythmias.
2. Obtain venous access and initiate an intravenous infusion at maintenance rate:
   - Obtain blood specimens for:
     - Hemoglobin and hematocrit.
     - Blood urea nitrogen and creatinine.
     - Electrolytes (sodium, potassium, chloride, phosphorus, calcium, and magnesium). Hyponatremia (less often, hypernatremia), hyperkalemia, hyperphosphatemia, and hypocalcemia may be found.
     - Venous blood gas.
     - Uric acid.

- Consider fluid restriction if fluid overload is present.
- Administer medications, as prescribed:
  - Diuretics may be needed if fluid overload is present.

3. Prepare for additional diagnostic tests:
   - Chest radiograph.
   - Electrocardiogram.
   - Echocardiogram.
4. Measure urinary output:
   - Insert an indwelling bladder catheter, as needed.
5. Prepare the patient for possible hemodialysis.
6. Continuously evaluate the patient for signs of fluid overload, such as congestive heart failure or pulmonary edema, and signs of septic shock.
7. Provide psychosocial support to the child and family.
8. Prepare for transfer and transport to a tertiary care facility, if indicated (Chapter 10), or hospitalization.

Home Care and Prevention

Emergency nurses can prevent or ameliorate ARF by anticipating it as a potential complication and by providing early treatment for signs of shock. On hospital discharge, the child may require frequent follow-up related to renal function as well as the predisposing health condition (e.g., burns) that resulted in the ARF.

Renal Transplantation

Children with kidney transplants may present to the ED with conditions that may or may not be related to their transplant, including rejection of the transplanted organ. Emergency nurses must be aware of the signs of kidney rejection. Selected considerations related to kidney transplantation are outlined in Table 20.5.

Specific Genitourinary Emergencies

Sexually Transmitted Diseases

Etiology

The incidence of sexually transmitted diseases (STDs) is highest in adolescents. Each year, 2.5 million teenagers are infected with a STD. This represents one of every six

TABLE 20.5 Considerations in Kidney Transplantation

Indications for Transplantation	*Physiologic Considerations*	*Signs of Rejection*	*Symptoms*	*Treatment*
Congenital anomalies. Vascular nephropathies. Cystic disease. Glomerular disease.	Organ function with graft revascularization. Donor kidney may be palpated in the lower abdomen; native kidneys may remain intact.	Fever. Decreased urinary output. Graft pain or tenderness. Increased blood urea nitrogen. Increased creatinine.	Hypertension. Signs of infection or rejection. Exposure to varicella.	Contact the transplant center; provide care as previously outlined in this chapter. For varicella exposure, administer varicella-zoster immune globulin. Obtain axillary or tympanic temperature measurements, because many transplant centers recommend avoiding rectal temperature measurement in immunosuppressed children. Review the child's complete medication list. Obtain blood and urine specimens.

Table compiled by: Sarah Martin, RN, MS, CCPNP, CPNP, CCRN

sexually active teens and one-fifth of all STD cases reported nationally. Adolescents who have sexual intercourse at younger ages are more likely to have multiple partners, increasing their chances of contracting a sexually transmitted disease. Adolescents frequently deny that they could be infected with a sexually transmitted disease. Other factors that increase the risk are the inconsistent use of protective and contraceptive devices and decreased healthcare options. Table 20.6 summarizes common STDs and their treatments.

Focused History

The patient history is obtained from the adolescent patient; if STDs are suspected in a younger child, a history is obtained from the child and the parent.

- Male and female patient history:
  - Frequency and type of sexual activity (oral, vaginal, anal).
  - Contraceptive use: type of contraceptive; frequency and regularity of use.
  - Number of prior sexual contacts.
  - Previous STD history and treatment: skin rashes, lesions, ulcers, and warts.
  - Fever, malaise, general illness.
- Female-specific history:
  - Vaginal discharge (amount, color, and odor).
  - Irregular or painful bleeding (dysmenorrhea).
  - Urinary complaints (dysuria, frequency, or urgency).
  - Abdominal or pelvic pain.
- Male-specific history:
  - Penile discharge (amount, color, and odor).

Focused Assessment

Physical Assessment

- Assess the abdomen:
  - Palpate the spleen. Hepatosplenomegaly may be present.
- Assess the skin:
  - Inspect the skin. Open and healing lesions or warts may be present.
  - Inspect the mucous membranes. Open and healing lesions may be present.
- Assess the immune system:
  - Palpate the cervical and femoral lymph nodes. Lymphadenopathy may be present.
- Assess the genitals:
  - Observe for lesions; open wounds; drainage.

Psychosocial Assessment

- Assess the adolescent's understanding of sexual activity and STDs.
- Assess interactions between the young child and the family:
  - Assess for psychosocial factors related to child sexual abuse (Chapter 47).

Nursing Interventions

- Assist with a pelvic examination and rectal examination:
  - Obtain specimens from the vagina, cervix, and rectum for culture and sensitivity.
- Assist with the male genital and rectal examination:
  - Obtain specimens from the meatus and rectum for culture and sensitivity.
- Obtain blood specimens to test for syphilis.
- Administer medications, as prescribed:
  - Antibiotics.
  - Antiviral agents.
- Arrange for an outpatient colposcopy if human papillomavirus is suspected:
  - The colposcope is a speculum with magnification for examination of the vagina and cervix.
- Report STDs to the health department.

Home Care and Prevention

Emergency nurses should take every opportunity to teach adolescents abstinence as well as safe sexual practices. Having literature available may help to engage adolescents in meaningful discussions. Making available family counseling and family practice clinic telephone numbers, as well as local hot lines, may encourage adolescents to seek further knowledge in preventing STD transmission.

Specific Male Genitourinary Emergencies

Acute Scrotum

Testicular torsion and epididymitis are common causes of acute scrotal conditions in young males. *Testicular torsion* is an emergency situation in which the blood supply to the testis is interrupted; *epididymitis* is an acute inflammation of the epididymis and is usually diagnosed in the adult male. Table 20.7 compares the clinical presentations of both entities.

TABLE 20.6 Overview of Sexually Transmitted Diseases

Disease	*Description*	*Incubation Period*	*Symptoms*	*Treatment: Older Children*	*Treatment: Younger Children*
Chlamydia	Caused by *Chlamydia trachomatis*, the most common bacterial STD, present in 5 to 15% of sexually active teenage females and 9% of teenage males	Variable; at least 1 week	*Males:* dysuria; urinary frequency; purulent urethral discharge *Females:* dysuria; mucopurulent discharge	Doxycycline, Azithromycin	Erythromycin or Azithromycin
Gonorrhea	Caused by *Neisseria gonorrhoeae*, a Gram-negative *diploccocus*	1 week	Usually occurs 2 to 7 days after exposure *Males:* dysuria; urinary frequency; and purulent urethral discharge *Females:* abnormal vaginal discharge; abnormal menses, dysuria; can be asymptomatic	Ceftriaxone or cefotaxime	Ceftrinxone or cefotaxime
Condylomata acyminata (genital warts)	Caused by human papilloma virus	Unknown; 3 months to 2 years	Single or multiple soft, fleshy painless growths on genital and/or anal areas	Podophyllum or Podofilox	Tretinoin
Herpes simplex	Caused by herpes simplex virus 1 and 2; present in approximately 20% of adolescents	*Neonates:* birth to age 4–6 weeks *Others:* 2 days to 2 weeks	Single or multiple vesicles that spontaneously rupture to shallow, painful ulcers Subsequent occurrences usually milder	Acyclovir	Acyclovir
Syphilis	Caused by *Treponema pallidum*, a spirochete; this disease is most common in adolescents	10–90 days	Three stages with overlapping symptoms: *Primary stage*—painless, indurated chancre at the site of infection *Secondary stage*—variable skin rash, lymphadenopathy, low-grade fever, and arthralgia *Tertiary stage*—no symptoms and not infectious, but cardiac, neurologic, opthalmic, and auditory lesions present	Penicillin G	Penicillin G or Benzamine Penicillin

From: Pickering, 2000. *Red book: Report of the committee on infectious diseases* (25th ed.). Elk Grove Village, IL: American Academy of Pediatrics.

TABLE 20.7 Comparison of Testicular Torsion and Epididymitis

Characteristic	*Testicular Torsion*	*Epididymitis*
Etiology	Under normal circumstances, the epididymis is posteriorly fixed with close approximation to the testes. The incomplete fixation by the tunica vaginalis allows mobility while providing stability of the testes. In cases of testicular torsion, there is no normal fixation of the testis to prevent rotation. Twisting of the testis results in occlusion of the blood supply, causing venous and arterial occlusion that lead to thrombosis and testicular infarction. The left testicle is affected twice as often as the right, probably because the left spermatic cord is usually longer.	Epididymitis is an acute bacterial infection. The most common causative agent is *Chlamydia trachomatis*, followed by *Neisseria gonorrhoeae*. Other causative agents include viruses and trauma.
Age group affected	Although the exact etiology is unknown, it is believed that congenital anatomic variations and a history of blunt trauma to the lower abdomen may predispose a male to the condition. Testicular torsion may occur at any age but is most common in adolescence. Unfortunately, this age group is least likely to present early for medical care because of concerns about modesty. About one in 160 males are affected. The prevalence is greater in teens with undescended testes.	Epididymitis is uncommon in prepubertal and non-sexually active males. When diagnosed in young males, it is usually a complication of congenital variations in anatomy.
History and physical assessment	Pain is almost always the presenting symptom and may be sudden or gradual in onset. Edema and swelling may be present in one or both sides of the scrotum. The scrotum is swollen and red. There is often a bluish hue to the affected side. Other symptoms include nausea, vomiting, and fever. Doppler examination reveals decreased pulsatile flow to the affected side. Technetium nuclear scanning is very reliable and also confirms decreased perfusion.	Symptoms include gradual onset of scrotal and groin pain with edema; epididymal swelling and tenderness; and urethral discharge. Findings may also include positive cultures for gonorrhea and/or chlamydia.
Treatment	Testicular torsion requires manual detorsion in early stages or, more commonly, surgical management to stop progressive necrosis. Although the chance of salvage may be remote after 6 to 8 hours, even patients with symptoms lasting greater than 12 hours should be explored surgically. There is great variability among patients in their arterial supply to the testicle and in the degree of torsion.	Treatment includes bed rest, scrotal support, and analgesics. Antibiotics such as ceftriaxone and doxycycline or tetracycline are indicated for treatment against gonorrhea and chlamydia.

From: Starr, 2000.

Nursing Interventions

- Prepare the patient for possible operative management or outpatient treatment, as needed:
  - Advise the patient not to eat or drink until it is determined that operative management will not be necessary.
- Provide privacy during examinations:
  - Provide continuity with physicians and nurses.
  - Provide male caregivers, if possible.
- Provide psychosocial support to the patient and family.
  - There may be uncertainty about long-term ramifications and questions of fertility with testicular torsion.

TABLE 20.8 Medical Conditions of the Penis

Characteristic	*Paraphimosis*	*Balanitis*	*Circumcision Complications*
Etiology	Occurs when the retracted foreskin of the uncircumcised male cannot be moved to its regular position. This results in venous congestion, swelling, inflammation, and engorgement. Vascular compromise may occur to the glans.	Inflammation of the foreskin, usually caused by poor hygiene.	Although there is no absolute indication for routine male newborn circumcision, it is the most commonly performed surgical procedure in the United States. Hemorrhage is the most common problem. The second most common complication is infection. Although most infections are localized, any generalized infections in a newborn are dangerous.
	Paraphimosis can be caused by any action that results in manipulation of the penis—including masturbation, intercourse, and irritation by clothing or other objects. Bacteria can also cause an inflamed penis. Occasionally a foreign body, such as hair, can act as a tourniquet.	Debris accumulates under the foreskin, leading to infection.	Poor surgical technique can result in severe complications such as necrosis or amputation during the procedure. Poor hygiene at home.
History/physical assessment	Penile pain and swelling; discoloration.	Inflamed and edematous foreskin with a collection of smegma. Older children may report pain and dysuria.	Recent circumcision; bleeding at the site; edema; signs of infection.
Treatment	The patient is given a sedative or a local penile dorsal block. Ice is then briefly applied in attempts to reduce the edema. This is followed by genital manual traction.	Warm soaks and local care are usually sufficient treatment.	Bleeding is usually controlled by direct pressure. For bleeding not controlled by direct pressure, other methods, such as silver nitrate application, epinephrine, fibrin, and suture placement, may be utilized. Infection may be treated with antibiotics.
Prevention	Although hair and clothing can accidentally restrict blood flow, some foreign bodies are placed purposefully; therefore, experimentation and abuse must always be considered. Although paraphimosis is frequently unpreventable, young uncircumcised males and their parents should be instructed in proper foreskin care.	A review of hygiene with the child and family is necessary.	Hygiene and signs and symptoms of infection should be reviewed. Parents may be concerned about the appearance of the penis. Surgical follow-up may be warranted.

Other Male Genitourinary Emergencies

Medical and minor traumatic conditions related to the penis may cause parents to seek emergency treatment. Although not life threatening, these conditions are frightening and painful to the child. Table 20.8 summarizes the medical conditions.

Minor traumatic injuries, such as zipper injuries, toilet-seat injuries, or tourniquet-type injuries, may result in an ED visit. In zipper and toilet-seat circumstances, the penis sustains a crush injury, resulting in edema and pain. Bleeding and hematuria may be present. In tourniquet-type injuries, magnifying lenses reveal a long hair or piece of string that is wrapped around the penis, resulting in edema and pain. Local anesthesia or analgesics may be required for the child to tolerate the procedures for removal of the zipper or tourniquet.

Patients and families should be taught prevention of zipper injuries by proper wearing of undergarments and careful closure of zippers. Toilet-seat covers should not be used with young children in the home because they can cause the toilet seat to fall forward onto the child's penis during urination. Parents and caregivers should keep their long hair secured away from their face during diaper changes and other infant/toddler care to avoid tourniquet-type injuries.

Specific Female Genitourinary Emergencies

Complications of Circumcision

Etiology

As the number of immigrants from Africa increases, emergency nurses must be aware of the practice of female circumcision or female genital mutilation. Female circumcision or genital mutilation involves cutting off the clitoris and sometimes the labia minora or labia majora. The sides may then be stitched together, leaving only a tiny opening. Besides the obvious risks of infection and severe pain, there are long-lasting ramifications:

- Irreversible damage to sexuality.
- Difficulty with GU examination, because normal landmarks are obliterated and tasks such as catheterization are almost impossible.

Female circumcision or female genital mutilation is practiced in as many as 26 countries, including Kenya, Gambia, Sudan, Somalia, Nigeria, Tanzania, Egypt, and Burkina Faso. The practice is performed outside of the hospital, by nonmedical practitioners. Female circumcision is not supported in the United States; some states have made this practice a felony, and other states have legislative bills pending.

The cultural meaning is part of the socialization of girls into womanhood. It is the marking of marriageability of women, and it symbolizes social control of sexual pleasure. The procedure is generally performed on girls between the ages of 4 and 10 years. Table 20.9 classifies the circumcision procedures.

Focused History

Patient history

- Recent immigration to the United States.
- Cultural beliefs and practices.
- GU complaints related to the length of time from the circumcision to ED presentation.
- Early complications:
  - Hemorrhage.
  - Severe pain.
  - Continued bleeding with anemia.
- Late complications:
  - Local and systemic infections.
  - Abscesses.
  - Ulcers.
  - Delayed healing.
  - Chronic pelvic infections.
  - Chronic UTIs.
  - Scarring.

Focused Assessment

Physical Assessment

- Assess the genitalia. Observe for age-related genital development:
  - Obliteration of normal genital landmarks may be present.
- Observe for signs of infection or trauma:
  - Bloody or purulent vaginal discharge.
  - Difficulty with urethral catheterization.
  - Scarring of the external genitalia.
- Perform or assist with a pelvic examination, as needed:
  - Pelvic examinations may be difficult or impossible to perform.

TABLE 20.9 Classification of Female Circumcision

Type	*Description*
Type I clitoridectomy	Removal of part or all of the clitoris.
Type II clitoridectomy	Excision of the clitoris and part of the labia minora. After healing, the clitoris is absent. The urethra and vaginal introitus are not covered.
Type III infibulation	Removal of the clitoris and labia minora. The labia majora are cut to allow raw surfaces that are stitched together. There is a large posterior opening for the passage of urine and menstrual blood.
Type IV infibulation	As above, but only a small opening remains for the passage of urine and menstrual blood.

From: Toubia, 1994.

Psychosocial Assessment

- Assess the child's and family's cultural beliefs:
  - It may be difficult to obtain a history of the female circumcision procedure unless the child is in severe distress because of complications.
  - Some cultures view this practice as normal; others may fear retribution or legal investigation if the practice is documented.

Nursing Interventions

- Assess and maintain airway, breathing, and circulation in the child with sepsis or shock (Chapter 17).
- Communicate a caring attitude to the patient:
  - Avoid forcing procedures, such as bladder catheterization or pelvic examination if pain and/or fear are elicited.
  - Prepare for a possible examination under anesthesia if necessary.
- Report the recent female circumcision to the local child protective agency:
  - This practice may constitute child maltreatment (Chapter 47).

Home Care and Prevention

Emergency nurses should know whether female circumcisions are performed in their ED's service area. Becoming involved in local or state efforts to end this practice is one strategy that emergency nurses can employ to prevent future episodes of female circumcision and genital mutilation.

Vaginal Bleeding

Vaginal bleeding may occur in prepubertal or adolescent females. It can have very different etiologies and treatments (Table 20.10).

Nursing Interventions

- Prepare the patient for a gynecologic examination:
  - The gynecologic examination can produce great anxiety in the patient. Positioning of the patient should take into consideration the patient's age and developmental level.
  - Sedation or general anesthesia may be necessary for internal examinations, suturing of lacerations, or removal of foreign bodies. The child should not be forced to participate in the examination.

Home Care and Prevention

Adolescents and their parents should be encouraged to investigate any irregular vaginal bleeding. To alleviate menstrual cramping, adolescents may try (Ball, 1998):

- Placing a heating pad or hot water bottle on the abdomen to relax tight muscles.
- Taking over-the-counter medications, such as ibuprofen or acetaminophen, as directed.
- Walking for short distances and/or engaging in light exercises.
- Eating a well-balanced meal and avoiding caffeinated foods and beverages.
- Drinking six to eight glasses of water daily.

TABLE 20.10 Vaginal Bleeding in Prepubertal versus Pubertal Females

Characteristic	*Prepubertal Females*	*Pubertal Females*
Etiology	Vaginitis. Trauma—straddle injuries. Sexual abuse—masturbation; foreign bodies. Tumors. Blood dyscrasias. Precocious puberty. Infection.	Normal menstrual bleeding occurs in cycles varying from 21 to 45 days, lasting 2 to 8 days. Blood loss averages 35 to 40 ml. Blood loss greater than 80 ml is considered excessive. Although dysfunctional bleeding may occur during an ovulatory cycle, it usually occurs as abnormal bleeding during an anovulatory cycle. Anovulation may be brought on by stress, illness, extreme athletic activity, and conditions of significantly decreased body fat, such as that found in dancers.
History/physical assessment	General physical assessment Pelvic examination for: ■ Differentiation of vaginal, cervical, or uterine bleeding. ■ Diagnosis of cervicitis, trauma, foreign bodies, and malignancies. Bimanual and rectal exam to differentiate tumors, cysts, and verify that the source of bleeding is the vagina. Blood from the uterus, urethra, or rectum may initially be diagnosed as vaginal in origin.	General physical assessment Pelvic examination for: ■ Differentiation of vaginal, cervical, or uterine bleeding. ■ Diagnosis of endometriosis, cervicitis, trauma, foreign bodies, and malignancies. Bimanual and rectal exam to differentiate tumors, cysts, and pregnancy-related complications such as: 　■ Ectopic pregnancy. 　■ Threatened or incomplete abortions, hydatiform mole, menstrual history, including tampon/pad usage. ■ Sexual activity and form of contraception. ■ Previous infections. ■ Endocrine disorders. ■ Hematologic disorders. ■ Recent stressors. ■ Medications. ■ Family history. ■ Skin inspection for petechiae or bruising.
ED treatment	Laboratory studies such as: ■ CBC with differential and platelet count. ■ Sedimentation rate. ■ Thyroid function tests. ■ Blood glucose. ■ PT/PTT. ■ Cervical cultures. ■ PAP smear (may be deferred to follow-up appointment). Radiographic tests may include pelvic ultrasound to rule out masses or anatomic abnormalities.	Laboratory studies such as: ■ CBC with differential and platelet count. ■ Sedimentation rate. ■ Thyroid function tests. ■ Blood glucose. ■ PT/PTT. ■ Cervical cultures. ■ PAP smear (may be deferred to follow-up appointment). ■ Pregnancy test. Radiographic tests may include pelvic ultrasound to rule out masses or anatomic abnormalities.
Other treatment	Determine underlying cause of bleeding and follow-up accordingly.	Management of dysfunctional uterine bleeding is dependent on the source and severity of bleeding: *Mild dysfunctional bleeding* in patients with a stable hemoglobin level higher than 12 g/dl usually is monitored. Iron supplements are frequently prescribed to prevent anemia. Oral contraceptives may be considered. Patient education is crucial. The patient should start and maintain a menstrual calendar. *Moderate dysfunctional bleeding* in patients with a hemoglobin level between 10 and 12 g/dl may be treated with all of the aforementioned interventions. Prescribed oral contraceptives will have higher amounts of progestin and estrogen. Folic acid is usually added to iron supplementation. *Severe dysfunctional bleeding* in patients with a hemoglobin level of less than 10 g/dl usually requires hospital admission, blood transfusion, hormonal therapy, and, if medical therapy is not successful, surgical intervention (dilation and curettage).

Vulvovaginitis and Vaginal Discharge

Vulvovaginitis and vaginal discharges are common female complaints. Etiologies differ with age (Table 20.11). Other etiologies include leukorrhea, foreign bodies, poor hygiene, chemical irritation, tumors, dermatologic disorders, and STDs.

Home Care and Prevention

Patients should be taught proper personal hygiene. Teaching adolescents about abstinence as well as safe sexual practices may prevent future occurrences of these conditions.

Conclusion

Genitourinary conditions are fraught with anxiety for parents, children, and adolescents. Emergency nurses must temper the need for thorough treatment with consideration of the child's and adolescent's sexual issues and development. Understanding GU development and its effects on bodily fluid regulation as well as sexual identity assists emergency nurses in the provision of expert care to this patient population.

TABLE 20.11 Etiologies of Vulvovaginitis and Vaginal Discharges

Characteristic	*Vulvovaginitis*	*Vaginal Discharge*
Etiology	Allergies; poor hygiene; irritation	Multiple causes
Age	Prepubescent	Postpubescent
History and physical assessment	Presence of: ▪ Genital irritation, itching, pain, and inflammation. ▪ Vaginal discharge. ▪ Onset, duration, quantity, color, consistency, and odor. ▪ Urinary complaints. ▪ Recent medication (especially contraceptives and antibiotics). ▪ Hygiene measures (soaps, bubble bath, deodorant sprays, and douches). ▪ Underlying medical problems.	Presence of: ▪ Genital irritation, itching, pain, and inflammation. ▪ Vaginal discharge. ▪ Onset, duration, quantity, color, consistency, and odor. ▪ Urinary complaints. ▪ Recent medication (especially contraceptives and antibiotics). ▪ Hygiene measures (soaps, bubble bath, deodorant sprays, and douches). ▪ Underlying medical problems. ▪ Any symptoms in sexual partners.
Description of discharge	Thin, mucoid. Clear, sticky (physiologic leukorrhea at onset of puberty).	Yellow, green, purulent (gonorrhea, chlamydia). Thick, white, pruritic (*Candida albicans*). Thin, frothy, malodorous, yellow-green (*Trichomonas vaginalis*). Gray, clear, fishy odor (*Gardnerella vaginalis*).
Treatment	Symptomatic care with attention to hygiene, removal of foreign bodies, and use of antibiotics specific for a bacterial infection.	Symptomatic care with attention to hygiene, removal of foreign bodies, and use of antibiotics specific for a bacterial infection.

References

Ball, J. (1998). Genitourinary/reproductive. In J. Ball (Ed.), *Mosby's pediatric patient teaching guidelines* (pp. J-1BJ-20). St. Louis: Mosby—Year Book.

Starr, N. (2000). Genitourinary diseases, Gynecological conditions. In C. Burns, N. Barber, M. Brady, & A. Dunn (Eds.), *Pediatric primary care* (pp. 974-1058). Philadelphia: Saunders.

Barkin, R., & Rosen, P. (1999). *Emergency pediatrics* (pp. 661-665). St. Louis: Mosby.

Bellinger, M. (1997). Urologic disorders. In B. Zitelli & H. Davis (Eds.), *Atlas of pediatric physical diagnosis* (3rd ed. pp. 421-440). St. Louis: Mosby-Year Book.

Ellis, D. (1997). Nephrology. In B. Zitelli & H. Davis (Eds.), *Atlas of pediatric physical diagnosis* (3rd ed., pp. 397-420). St. Louis: Mosby—Year Book.

Flynn, J. (1999). Acute renal failure. In R. Barkin & P. Rosen (Eds.), *Emergency pediatrics: A guide to ambulatory care* (5th ed., pp. 809-815). St. Louis: Mosby—Year book.

Gilman, C., & Mooney, K. (1998). In K. McCance & S. Huether (Eds.), *Pathophysiology: The biologic basis for disease in adults and children* (pp. 1273-1287). St. Louis: Mosby—Year Book.

Kher, K., & Makker, S. (1992). *Clinical pediatric nephrology* (pp. 23-41; 1176-1177; 672). New York: McGraw-Hill.

Pickering, L. (Ed.), (2000). *Red book: Report of the committee on infectious diseases* (25th ed.). Elk Grove Village, IL: American Academy of Pediatrics.

Pye, T., & Soud, T. (1998). Genitourinary system. In T. Soud & J. Rogers (Eds.), *Manual of pediatric emergency nursing* (pp. 364-389). St. Louis: Mosby—Year Book.

Reynolds, E., & Hoberman, A. (1995). Diagnosis and management of phyelonephritis in infants. *Maternal-Child Nursing Journal, 20*, 78-94.

Toubia, N. (1994). Female circumcision as a public health issue. *New England Journal of Medicine, 331*, 712-716.

21

Musculoskeletal Emergencies

Laurel S. Campbell, RN, MSN, CEN
Donna Ojanen Thomas, RN, MSN

Introduction

Health conditions related to the musculoskeletal system are common occurrences in children presenting to the emergency department (ED) for treatment. These conditions include musculoskeletal trauma (Chapter 38), medical problems, and congenital disorders. Emergency nurses must be able to recognize and treat musculoskeletal conditions and be aware of the normal growth and development of the child to prevent future musculoskeletal disability. The purpose of this chapter is to discuss selected musculoskeletal conditions that may be seen in the pediatric patient, nursing care, and interventions.

Embryologic Development of the Musculoskeletal System

The development of the musculoskeletal system is complex and is summarized in Table 21.1.

Pediatric Considerations

- A child's bones are in a dynamic state that predisposes them to patterns of injury. Their greater porosity results in bones that bow, bend, or buckle without complete fracture.
- Abnormal patterns of bone growth associated with diseases such as osteogenesis imperfecta and osteoporosis can result in pathologic fractures.
- Damage to epiphyseal (growth) centers may lead to acute or chronic disruptions in growth of the affected extremity.
- Injuries to joints and ligaments are rare in children. Traumatic forces are more likely to result in injury to the physis (growth plate).
- Generally, the younger the child, the faster the rate of bone healing (England & Sundberg, 1996):
  - The rate of bone healing is more rapid in children because there is an abundant blood supply to the developing bone.
  - Pediatric bones have a thick periosteum with a higher bone-forming potential, contributing to faster healing.
  - Nonunion of a fracture is rare in children.
- Pathogenic defects are the result of:
  - *Malformation*—improper formation of a structure resulting from defective embryologic differentiation or development.
  - *Disruption*—retarded development resulting from *in utero* destruction of a normally formed part.
  - *Deformation*—an antepartum or postpartum alteration of a part that originally developed normally.
- Disruption of the complex blood supply within the bone can result in avascular necrosis.

Focused History

The following history is important in assessing a child with a musculoskeletal complaint (Melnyk & Schultz, 1998):

- Date of onset of complaint or illness.
- Severity.
- Extent of disability.
- Precipitating factors.

TABLE 21.1 Summary of Musculoskeletal Development in Children

Area of Growth	*Developmental Considerations*
Bone formation	Bone formation begins at 8 weeks of gestation and involves two phases: 1. Delivery of bone cell precursors to sites of bone formation. 2. Aggregation of cells at primary centers of ossification. Cellular aggregation and maturation occur in two types of fetal tissue: 1. Mesenchymal (cranium, facial bones, clavicles, part of the jaw)—grow by the process of intramembranous formation. 2. Endochondral—progresses at primary center of ossification and extends toward either end of the developing bone. Two regions of cartilage remain at the ends of long bones: 1. Auricular—over free ends of the bone. 2. Epiphyseal plate—layer between diaphysis and epiphysis. This plate retains ability to form and calcify new cartilage and deposit bone until the skeleton matures (about 18 years of age).
Bone growth	Growth in length of bone occurs at the epiphyseal plate until adult stature is reached: More growth takes place at one end of a long bone than at the other—the growing end. This area is more likely to sustain a growth disturbance with injury. The longitudinal growth rate of extremities is greater at birth than it is at any other time. Factors affecting the development, physiology, and rate of growth of the epiphyseal plate include: ▪ Growth hormone. ▪ Genetic makeup. ▪ Nutrition and general health. ▪ Other hormones (thyroid, adrenal and gonadal androgens, and estrogens). When the skeleton is mature, the epiphyseal plate is replaced by bone.
Skeletal development	In the newborn, the entire spine is concave anteriorly; the child's natural posture is curled up. In first 3 months of life, the cervical spine begins to arch or become convex. The appendicular skeleton (extremities) grows faster than the axial skeleton. By age 1 year, 50% of the total growth of spine has occurred.
Muscle growth	In the fetus, muscle tissue contains a large amount of water and intracellular matrix. At birth, this is reduced considerably as cells enlarge by accumulating cytoplasm. Muscle fibers reach their maximal size around the age of 10 years in girls and the age of 14 years in boys. Muscle accounts for 25% of total body weight in the infant, but 40% in the adult. Respiratory and facial muscles are well developed at birth. Other groups, such as pelvic muscles, take years to develop.

Data from: McCullough, 1998.

- Associated signs and symptoms (fever, rash, weight loss).
- Previous treatment and resulting effects.
- Recent trauma.
- New, increased, or repetitive activities that may have contributed to the condition.
- Current medications.
- Recent exposure to infections.
- Past history, including:
  - Prenatal and birth history.
  - Growth and development.
  - Similar signs and symptoms.
  - Previous orthopedic injuries or chronic conditions.
  - Recent immunizations.
  - Congenital problems.

Focused Assessment

Physical Assessment

- Posture, position, gait.
- Symmetry of motion.
- Range of motion in joints.
- Muscle tone.
- Deformities in limbs or trunk; abnormal prominences or indentations.
- Joint swelling and erythema.
- Use of orthopedic devices, such as braces.
- Pain or tenderness.
- Pulses in extremities; capillary refill time.

Psychosocial Assessment

- Significant pain may be present. Children should be assessed for physical signs of pain and response to pain medication.
- The child will generally have significant fear of the ED and any procedures.

Table 21.2 lists nursing diagnoses and expected outcomes.

Triage Decisions

Emergent

- Possible septic joint:
  - The child will have severe pain.
  - Complications of a septic joint include long-term damage to the joint.
- Complications of juvenile rheumatoid arthritis (JRA):
  - Signs and symptoms of respiratory distress or chest pain, which may indicate cardiac complications such as pericarditis.
  - Signs and symptoms of acute uveitis, an inflammation of the interior pigmented vascular structures of the eye; an opthamology consult is needed as soon as possible.

Urgent

- Suspected osteomyelitis:
  - Complications of delayed treatment can include loss of limb or limb function, septic shock, and death.
- Severe joint pain, rashes, or unexplained fevers in children who may not be currently diagnosed with JRA.

Nonurgent

- Nonspecific chronic pain; child is afebrile, alert, and active with full mobility.

Nursing Interventions

Actual and anticipated nursing interventions will be discussed with each of the specific orthopedic emergencies.

Specific Orthopedic Emergencies

Osteomyelitis

Osteomyelitis is an inflammation of the bone most commonly of infectious origin. It is more common in boys

TABLE 21.2 Nursing Diagnoses and Expected Outcomes

Nursing Diagnoses	*Expected Outcomes*
Impaired physical mobility	The child will regain mobility appropriate for condition without permanent damage as a result of proper interventions and treatment.
Pain	Pain will be reduced by appropriate pharmacologic and nonpharmacologic methods.
Risk of infection	The risk of infection will be decreased or minimized with the use of antibiotics, as appropriate.

and several studies have found the highest incidence among infants and preschool children (Jottee & Loiselle, 2000) Osteomyelitis requires an aggressive multidisciplinary approach to treatment and can be classified into three categories (Griffin, 1993):

- *Acute:* occurring after an acute injury, with relatively rapid onset of symptoms and acutely ill presentation.
- *Subacute:* insidious onset; the child does not appear to be ill, and symptoms increase and subside with activity. The child may not present for evaluation until symptoms have been present for weeks or months.
- *Chronic:* not common; can result from a delay in diagnosis or inadequate treatment.

Etiology and Epidemiology

Introduction of bacteria into the bone occurs via three routes (Sonnen & Henry, 1996; Jottee & Loiselle, 2000):

- Direct inoculation related to open wounds, open fractures, puncture wounds, or following open reduction and internal fixation of fractures.
- Local invasion of the bone from adjacent infected structures.
- Hematogenous infection: spread of infecting agent from another source of infection through the blood to the bone; most commonly seen in infants, children, drug abusers, and immunosuppressed patients.

The most common infecting agents are:

- *Staphylococcus aureus* (most common).
- *Pseudomonas aeruginosa* (often seen with puncture wounds).
- Fungal infections in immunosuppressed patients.
- Salmonella in patients with sickle cell disease.
- *Staphylococcus aureus* and group B beta-hemolytic streptococcus in neonates (Patzakis, 1993).

Pathophysiology

The pathophysiology of osteomyelitis depends on the type:

- Hematologous osteomyelitis:
  - The infectious agent travels through the arterial circulation to the end arteries in the metaphysis, where pus forms.
  - When under pressure, the pus travels through the Volkmann canals into the subperiosteal region and then into the epiphysis or the intramedullary cavity (Griffin, 1993).
- Hematogenous osteomyelitis:
  - This form usually occurs in the metaphysis, which has slower blood flow, allowing bacteria to get established.
- Complications:
  - Necrosis of bone occurs after blood flow is impaired, as a result of increased intraosseous pressure (Lew & Waldvogel, 1997).
  - If the infection occurs in the metaphyseal cortex, bacteria can break through and cause a coexistent joint infection (Sonnen & Henry, 1996).

Focused History

- Recent bone surgery, open reduction and internal fixation of a fracture.
- Puncture wound, open wound, or open fracture.
- Recent infection in another location that results in hematogenous spread to the bone via the circulatory system.

Focused Assessment

The standard pediatric assessment is done. The following may be present in the child who has osteomyelitis:

- Fever.
- Chills.
- Limp, or inability or refusal to bear weight.
- General malaise; irritability.
- Pseudoparalysis in infants, pain with movement in older children with upper extremity involvement.
- Tenderness, warmth, and swelling at the site, often in the metaphyseal region.
- Failure to thrive, increased irritability, or poor feeding in an infant.
- Children may not appear ill and may not have significant systemic symptoms.
- Because developing bones of neonates have a thinner cortex and are not as effective as barriers to infection, infants may present with fulminant sepsis (Sonnen & Henry, 1996).
- Laboratory assessment:
  - Complete blood count: leukocytosis with a shift to immature white cells (bands).
  - Elevated erythrocyte sedimentation rate.
  - Elevated C-reactive protein (Sonnen & Henry, 1996).

Nursing Interventions

- Assist with aspiration or needle biopsy of the affected area; test for Gram stain, culture, and sensitivity.
- Obtain samples for blood cultures.
- Obtain samples for complete blood count.
- Obtain radiographic studies. First signs visible on the radiograph may be swelling of the deep soft tissue.

- Obtain imaging studies (computerized tomography, magnetic resonance imaging, bone scans).
- Prepare for possible surgical debridement of necrotic bone or abscess; open wounds are often left open until secondary closure later.
- Ensure adequate pain control (pharmacologic measures; extremity positioning).
- Begin administration of antibiotic therapy. Long-term administration (often up to 6 weeks) of intravenous antibiotic therapy is common. Some may advocate use of implanted antibiotic beads after surgical debridement. Some commonly used antibiotics include (Griffin, 1993; Sonnen & Henry, 1996):
  - For *Staphylococcus aureus*: synthetic beta-lactamase–resistant penicillin; cephalosporins; vancomycin (used especially if methicillin-resistant *S. aureus* is suspected).
  - For *Pseudomonas aeruginosa*: aminoglycosides; cephalosporins.
  - For *Mycobacterium tuberculosis*: isoniazid; streptomycin; *p*-aminosalicylic acid.
  - For fungal infections: amphotericin B.

Septic Arthritis (Septic Joint)

Joint sepsis occurs when bacteria invade the synovial space. Signs and symptoms of septic joints are similar to those of osteomyelitis, and the diagnosis is more difficult to make when both conditions occur simultaneously. Septic joints usually occur secondary to bacteremia from osteomyelitis or other sources of bloodborne bacteria. It may be difficult to differentiate between reactive arthritis and septic arthritis based on history and physical examination alone (Sonnen, 1996).

Septic arthritis is a serious condition. Untreated joint sepsis results in permanent disability caused by destruction of the articular cartilage. Residual sequelae are rare if septic arthritis is diagnosed and treated within 2 days of onset. Outcomes are usually not as favorable if the joint is infected secondary to osteomyelitis.

Etiology and Epidemiology (Griffin, 1993; Sonnen & Henry, 1996)

- Peak incidence: between the ages of 1 and 2 years. Prognosis is worse in children less than 1 year of age, with involvement of the hip joint, with delay in treatment and when the infection is caused by *Staphylococcus aureus* (Jottee & Loiselle, 2000).
- Most common joint affected: hip in neonates and infants; knee in older children.
- Most common organisms: *Staphylococcus aureus*, group B beta-hemolytic streptococcus, and *Haemophilus influenzae*.
- Introduction of bacteria into the joint occurs via three routes (Sonnen & Henry, 1996):
  - Traumatic or surgical infection. Traumatic infection can occur as a result of an undetected penetrating injury, for example, a sewing needle in a crawling infant.
  - Local invasion of the bone from adjacent infected structures.
  - Hematogenous infection: spread of infecting agent from another source of infection through the blood to the bone.

Pathophysiology

- Bacteria in the blood deposit in the joint synovium, resulting in an inflammatory reaction.
- Blood products, white blood cells, and bacteria enter the synovial fluid.
- Stimulation of the release of enzymes (collagenase and proteases) results in destruction of the articular cartilage (Griffin, 1993).
- Complications from septic arthritis include bone destruction and hip dislocation (Sonnen & Henry, 1996).

Focused History

- Rapid onset of severe joint pain within 24 to 48 hours.
- Irritability.
- Refusal to use extremity or bear weight.
- Fever.
- Malaise.
- Possible recent upper respiratory infection or local soft tissue infection.
- Poor feeding in the infant.

Focused Assessment

Symptoms are usually more dramatic than those of osteomyelitis or other bone injuries:

- Swollen, hot joint: usually confined to the intracapsular space.
- Severe pain with joint motion: pain specifically in the joint, as opposed to pain affecting the metaphysis in osteomyelitis.
- Abducted and externally rotated hip position or slight flexion for comfort.

Nursing Interventions

- Assist with aspiration of the affected area (under fluoroscopy if hip or shoulder) and send specimens for:
  - Gram stain.
  - Culture and sensitivity.
  - White blood cell count and differential (usually will show more than 90% polymorphonuclear leukocytes).
  - Mucin clot test; the infected joint fluid will usually be cloudy (Griffin, 1993).
- Counter immunoelectrophoresis of the synovial fluid to determine presence of *H. influenzae*, *Streptococcus pneumoniae*, and *Meningococcus*.
- Obtain samples for blood cultures.
- Obtain samples for a complete blood count: white blood cell count and sedimentation rate will be elevated.
- Obtain radiographic studies.
- Obtain imaging studies (computerized tomography, magnetic resonance imaging, bone scans, sonography).
- Prepare for surgical drainage or debridement of the joint. This is generally indicated for all cases, including the hip joint.
- Begin administration of parenteral antibiotic therapy: beta-lactamase-resistant penicillin or cephalosporins for *S. aureus*, *Pneumococcus*, or group B beta-hemolytic streptococcus.
- Provide pain control measures (pharmacologic measures; positioning for comfort).

Juvenile Rheumatoid Arthritis

Juvenile rheumatoid arthritis (JRA) is the most common rheumatic disease in the pediatric population. The incidence is higher in females than in males and the onset is greatest during the ages of 1 to 3 and 8 to 12 years. There are three subtypes of JRA (Mann, 1997):

- Systemic onset. Also called Stills disease, least common. Child may feel stiff but joint pain is not a common symptom initially (Sundel, 2000).
- Pauciarticular—involves fewer than five joints.
- Polyarticular—involves five or more joints, causes symmetric synovitis in both large and small joints.

Etiology and Epidemiology

- Diagnosed in any child younger than 16 years with arthritis (joint pain) lasting more than 6 weeks in one or more joints (Sundel, 2000).
- Exact cause unknown:
  - Genetic disposition for the disease. It can also be triggered by trauma, stress, or infection.
  - Autoimmune process.

Pathophysiology

- Characterized by chronic inflammation of the synovial membrane, joint effusion, and vasculitis.
- Hyperplasia of the synovial lining occur when fibrin is deposited with disease progression.
- Destruction of cartilage occurs when thickened synovial membranes spread from the edges of the joint.
- Immobility of the joints result from adhesions between joint surfaces.
- Complications of JRA include (Melnyk & Schultz, 1997):
  - Cardiac involvement (pericarditis is common with systemic JRA).
  - Pulmonary involvement (history of chest pain, dyspnea, and cough might indicate a pleural effusion).
- Ophthalmic involvement (history of red eye, pain, photophobia, or decreased visual acuity may indicate uveitis, which is an inflammation of the vascular structure of the inner eye).
- Infections.
- Cervical spine involvement (more common in adults):
  - The risk of atlantoaxial subluxation is increased in children with JRA.
  - A history of trauma requires cervical spine precautions.

Focused History

Generally, children with JRA are not diagnosed in the ED, but a history of the following acute complaints of children with JRA may result in a visit to the ED (Faries & Johnston, 1992):

- Fever.
- Joint pain.
- Rash.
- Pericarditis.
- Cervical spine pain or injury.
- Neurologic complaints.
- Injury to involved joint.

Focused Assessment

The standard physical assessment is done, focusing on the chief complaint and area affected by the disease. The following signs and symptoms in children who have not previously been diagnosed may be indicative of JRA:

- Prolonged fevers

- Rash
- Uveitis
- Pain and swelling in joints lasting more than 6 weeks.
- Signs and symptoms of complications.
- Signs and symptoms of concurrent illnesses, such as respiratory infections

Nursing Interventions

- Objectives:
  - Pain relief.
  - Early identification and intervention for complications and underlying illnesses.
  - Preservation of joint function.
  - Psychosocial support.
- Specific interventions:
  - Observe for and treat signs and symptoms of respiratory distress (tachycardia, tachypnea, and irritability or restlessness).
  - Provide supplemental oxygen.
  - Monitor heart rate and rhythm. Observe for signs and symptoms of pericarditis or pleural effusion (see Chapter 17). Pleural effusion could lead to cardiac tamponade.
  - Provide pain control through both pharmacologic and nonpharmacologic methods.
  - Use positioning, bed rest, and splints, as ordered, to decrease inflammation and prevent further joint damage.

Other Musculoskeletal Conditions

Several other orthopedic conditions, acquired and congenital, may be found in the pediatric ED patient. These conditions are summarized below, along with nursing considerations for caring for children with these conditions in the ED (Melynk & Schultz, 1997).

Toxic Synovitis

Description

Toxic synovitis is an inflammation of the hip, mainly affecting children between the ages of 18 months and 12 years. The etiology is unknown, but it is thought to be a viral, traumatic, bacterial, or allergic process. Toxic synovitis is the most common cause of acute hip pain in children 3 to 10 years of age (Jottee & Loiselle, 2000).

ED Considerations

The child presents with an acute onset of a painful limp. If the condition is severe, the child will refuse to walk. Diagnosis consists of ruling out other serious conditions, such as septic arthritis and JRA.

Nursing care consists of pain management. The child is generally managed at home with bed rest and analgesics.

Legg-Calvé-Perthes Disease

Description

Legg-Calvé-Perthes disease is an avascular necrosis of the femoral head, occurring in children between the ages of 4 and 9 years, but primarily affects boys. It is rare in African-Americans.

The etiology is unknown, but temporary interruption of the blood supply to the femoral head may play a role. The history may include a recent trauma or stress fracture.

ED Considerations

The child presents with a history of a painless limp that occurs intermittently after activity. The limp becomes constant and may be associated with hip, groin, thigh, or knee pain (most commonly on arising and at the end of the day). Behavioral disorders, such as hyperactivity, are common in children with this condition.

Diagnosis in the ED is confirmed by hip radiographs. A bone scan is done to determine the degree of avascularity. Other infections must be ruled out, especially acute emergencies such as septic arthritis and osteomyelitis.

An orthopedist must be consulted after the diagnosis is made. Generally, children younger than 6 years of age can be managed at home. Hospitalization and Buck's traction may be required. Teaching and emotional support are priorities.

Slipped Capital Femoral Epiphysis

Description

Slipped capital femoral epiphysis is a sudden or gradual displacement of the proximal femoral epiphysis on the femoral neck. It occurs in obese, inactive male adolescents between the ages of 13 and 15 years. It can also occur in rapidly growing, tall, thin youths between the ages of 10 and 16 years. The etiology is unknown, but genetic predisposition, defective growth plate, obesity, and hormonal factors have been implicated. This condition has also been associated with endocrine disorders and growth hormone therapy.

ED Considerations

In the chronic condition, there is a gradual onset of dull pain in the groin, thigh, and knee, resulting in intermittent limping. Acute conditions result in the sudden onset of severe groin, thigh, or knee pain and inability to bear weight. The diagnosis is based on examination and radiography.

Immediate treatment is necessary to prevent permanent damage. Orthopedic referral is necessary. Nursing care includes restricting the child from weight bearing and preparing the child for hospitalization for surgical pinning.

Osgood-Schlatter Disease

Description

Osgood-Schlatter disease is a painful enlargement of the tibial tuberosity at the insertion of the patellar tendon. It results from repetitive pulling of the quadriceps in children between 10 and 16 years of age. Male athletes are primarily affected when activities such as running and jumping pull on the patellar tendon, causing detachment of cartilage fragments from the tibial tuberosity. The disease typically resolves in late adolescence, when the bone becomes stronger than the inserted ligament.

ED Considerations

The child presents with pain in the anterior aspect of the knee that is aggravated by activity or direct pressure and relieved by rest. Symptoms are often first noted when the child is kneeling or after minor trauma. Diagnosis is made solely by physical examination.

Generally this condition is diagnosed and treated in the outpatient setting. Nursing care consists of the standard examination to rule out systemic illness and education regarding the disease, exercises to stretch and strengthen the muscles, and follow-up.

Osteogenesis Imperfecta

Description

Osteogenesis imperfecta (OI) is a connective tissue disorder and a primary etiology of osteoporosis in children. It is characterized by fractures and skeletal deformities. This is an inherited condition, characterized by immature collagen formation affecting all connective tissue. The bones are primarily involved. The signs and symptoms depend on the type of osteogenesis imperfecta (there are four types) and range from frequent long-bone fractures to stillbirth or perinatal death.

ED Considerations

ED presentation is usually for signs and symptoms of fractures resulting from an unknown etiology or minor trauma. It is important to distinguish osteogenesis imperfecta from child maltreatment.

ED management is generally concerned with maintaining airway, breathing, and circulation; taking cervical spine precautions; and providing care for fractures. The nurse must be careful when taking vital signs or positioning or transferring the child with osteogenesis imperfecta, and the parents will be helpful in suggesting ways to do this. If protective braces are removed to allow the examination, they should be replaced as soon as possible. Radiographs will be taken to evaluate fractures.

The parent and child need support because they will have frequent ED visits. Because osteogenesis imperfecta is an inherited condition, parents may have feelings of guilt.

Duchenne-type (Pseudohypertrophic) Muscular Dystrophy

Description

Duchenne-type muscular dystrophy is an inherited disorder that almost exclusively affects male children. It is the most common and severe form of muscular dystrophy; a progressive myopathy resulting in increasing hypotonia and muscle weakness. The specific mechanisms that cause muscular dystrophy are unknown. Duchenne-type muscular dystrophy usually becomes evident in affected boys by the age of 4 years; it is characterized by delayed walking, frequent falls, a waddling gait, and compensatory lumbar lordosis. With increasing impairment, the child eventually needs braces and crutches to aid in standing and, later, a wheelchair for continued mobility.

ED Considerations

Common health problems in children with this condition include fall-related injuries, pulmonary conditions (the most serious problem), pain, and anxiety. Weakness of respiratory muscles results in hypoventilation and decreased pulmonary function. Some children may require ventilatory support.

Nursing care depends on the illness or injury and involves the standard assessment and management of pain and acute symptoms because there is no effective treatment or cure for muscular dystrophy. It is vital to listen to the parents, because they know what usually helps their child. Braces should be removed during assessment and treatment, under the direction of the parents. The family will need support, because this is a progressive and terminal condition.

Home Care and Prevention

- Prevention of hematogenously acquired osteomyelitis is reliant on timely treatment of bacterial infections located at other sites.
- Aggressive treatment of open fractures, puncture wounds, and open wounds with thorough cleaning and administration of antibiotics, as indicated, can reduce the incidence of osteomyelitis.
- There are few measures that can be taken to prevent septic joints. Rapid diagnosis and treatment of osteomyelitis can reduce the incidence of subsequent joint sepsis.
- Provide the family of the child with JRA with information to prevent complications, relieve pain, and preserve joint function:
  - Signs and symptoms of medication toxicity.
  - Signs and symptoms of serious complications of the disease.
  - Pain relief: warm baths, heating pads, range-of-motion exercises, swimming, and bicycling.
  - Routine eye examinations to prevent uveitis.
  - Referral to support groups.

Conclusion

Musculoskeletal conditions can be caused by trauma, infections, and congenital and acquired conditions. The goals in treatment are to preserve function, control pain, and prevent damage to joints or other musculoskeletal structures. A knowledge of common musculoskeletal conditions and normal pediatric growth and development will assist the nurse in caring for pediatric patients with musculoskeletal complaints and reduce future disability.

References

England, S., & Sundberg, S. (1996). Management of common pediatric fractures. *Pediatric Clinics of North America, 43*(5), 991-1012.

Faries, G., & Johnston, C. (1992). Allergic and immunologic diseases. In R. M. Barkin (Ed.), *Pediatric emergency medicine: Concepts and clinical practice* (pp. 556-565). St. Louis: Mosby.

Griffin, P. (1993). Bone and joint infections in children. In M. Chapman & M. Madson (Eds.), *Operative orthopedics* (pp. 3251-3262.). Philadelphia: Lippincott.

Jottee, D., & Loiselle, J. (2000). Orthopedic emergencies. In G. Fleisher & S. Ludwig (Eds.), *Textbook of Pediatric Emergency Medicine* (pp. 1595-1612). Philadelphia: Lippincott, Williams & Wilkins.

Lew, D., & Waldvogel, F. (1997). Current concepts: Osteomyelitis. *New England Journal of Medicine, 336*(14), 999-1007.

Mann, R. (1997). Orthopedic emergencies. In E. F. Crain & J. C. Gershel (Eds.), *Clinical manual of emergency pediatrics* (3rd ed., pp. 493-497). New York: McGraw-Hill.

McCullough, F. L. (1998). Alterations of musculoskeletal function in children. In K. L. McCance & S. E. Huether (Eds.), *Pathophysiology—The biologic basis for disease in adults and children* (3rd ed., pp. 1486-1516). St. Louis: Mosby.

Melnyk, B. M., & Schultz, A. W. (1998). Musculoskeletal system. In T. E. Soud & J. S. Rogers (Eds.), *Manual of pediatric emergency nursing* (pp. 290-312). St. Louis: Mosby.

Patzakis, M. (1993). Management of osteomyelitis. In M. Chapman & M. Madison (Eds.), *Operative orthopedics* (pp. 3335-3356). Philadelphia: Lippincott.

Sonnen, G., & Henry, N. (1996). Pediatric bone and joint infections. Diagnosis and antimicrobial management. *Pediatric Clinics of North America, 43*(4), 933-947.

Sundel, R. (2000). Rheumatologic emergencies. In G. Fleisher & S. Ludwig (Eds.), *Textbook of Pediatric Emergency Medicine* (pp. 1191-1228). Philadelphia: Lippincott, Williams & Wilkins.

22

Dermatologic Emergencies

Julie Briggs, RN, BSN, MHA

Introduction

Rashes and skin disorders are frequent complaints of parents and children presenting to the emergency department (ED) and are cause for concern. An estimated 1 in 40 visits to pediatric health care providers is for a skin-related disorder (Fioravanti, 1998). Dermatologic conditions range from a mild irritation to the manifestation of a more serious underlying systemic illness that requires immediate attention or even hospital admission. Treatment modalities are generally focused on eliminating the underlying cause of the skin condition and related discomfort or symptoms rather than treating the actual skin condition. Many skin conditions are self-limiting and require only symptomatic relief, but these can be of a more serious nature in the immunosuppressed or chronically ill child.

A thorough assessment of the skin condition and other related symptoms is necessary to determine the urgency of the problem. The purpose of this chapter is to review common dermatologic conditions and outline their ED treatment.

Embryologic Development of the Integumentary System

The skin begins its development during the 11th week of gestation (Engel, 1997). Integumentary vascular disorders (vascular nevi) occur during embryologic development, when the angioblastic tissue fails to communicate with adjacent blood vessels (Nicol & Huether, 1998) (Table 22.1).

The skin is the largest organ of the body, accounting for 20% of the body's weight (Huether, 1998). Its primary functions are to protect against environmental forces, including microorganisms, ultraviolet radiation, and mechanical (trauma) energy; prevent fluid loss; sense pain, heat, cold, and touch; and assist with thermoregulation (Engel, 1997; Huether, 1998). The skin's appearance contributes to the child's body image (Dickerson, Gordon, & Walter, 1998).

The skin comprises the epidermis, dermis, hypodermis (subcutaneous layer), and dermal appendages. Table 22.2 describes each of these features.

Pediatric Considerations

Skin thickness is variable, depending on the child's age, gender, and the body location (Dickerson et al., 1998). Although skin thickness is proportionally similar in each body area in children and adults, the skin thickness of an infant may be less than half that of the adult (Dickerson et al., 1998). The skin's normal pH is acidic, presumably to ward off bacterial invasion, but the pH of the infant's skin is higher (Engel, 1997). This high skin pH, coupled with their thinner skin and minimal secretion of sweat and sebum, predisposes infants to dermatologic infections and conditions (Engel, 1997). The dermis and epidermis of infants and young children are not tightly attached, causing their skin to easily blister (Engel, 1997).

Etiology

Some of the most common dermatologic conditions presenting to the ED are caused by:

- Infections:
  - Viral.
  - Bacterial.
  - Fungal.
- Infestations.
- Insect bites (Chapter 43).

TABLE 22.1 Common Vascular Nevi

Condition	*Description*
Strawberry hemangioma	Raised, vascular lesion that is bright red with minute capillary projections. Can be present at birth or evolve at 3 to 5 weeks of age. Usually located on the head, neck, or trunk. Begins to involute at age 12 to 16 months, with 90% resolving without sequelae by 5 to 6 years of age.
Cavernous hemangiomas	Composed of larger and more mature vessels with a bluish red color and less distinct borders than the strawberry hemangiomas. Present at birth. Usually located on the head and neck. Grow rapidly up to age 6 months; involution completed at 2 to 3 years (20%) or 9 years (80%). May require surgical or laser treatment.
Port-wine stain	Flat lesions, ranging from pink to dark red, that do not fade with age. Present at birth or within a few days. Usually located on the face and may be large. Laser surgery may be helpful to lighten the color.

From: Nicol & Huether, 1998.

Focused History

1. Patient history:
   - Exposure to potential allergen (drugs, poison oak, ivy, sumac, foods soaps, perfumes, clothing not washed before use).
   - Recent exposure to persons with an infectious illness and rash.
   - Appearance of the skin lesions:
     - Description.
     - Manner of progression.
     - Distribution.
   - Associated symptoms:
     - Pain, itching, numbness.
     - Fever or chills.
     - Difficulty breathing, chest tightness, or swelling of the back of throat and/or tongue.
     - Headache.
     - Neck pain.
     - Change in level of consciousness.
     - Change in appetite or fluid intake.
     - Noisy respirations or tachypnea.
     - Sore throat or cough.
     - Joint pain.
     - Vomiting or diarrhea.
   - Pertinent health history:
     - Medications (prescribed and over-the-counter).
     - Allergies (food, medication, and environmental).
     - Immunization status.
   - Home treatments and their effectiveness (e.g., application of calamine lotion).
2. Family history:
   - Other family members or close contacts with similar illness and rash.
   - History of anaphylaxis, atopy, or skin disorders.

Focused Assessment

Physical Assessment

1. Assess the respiratory system:
   - Auscultate the chest for:
     - Respiratory rate. Tachypnea may be present with fever.
2. Assess the cardiovascular system:
   - Auscultate the heart for:
     - Rate. Tachycardia may be present with fever or pain.
   - Measure the blood pressure.
   - Assess peripheral perfusion:
     - Palpate peripheral pulses.
     - Measure capillary refill.
     - Inspect skin color and temperature.
3. Assess the neurologic system:

TABLE 22.2 Components and Functions of the Integumentary System

Component	*Function*
Epidermis	Serves as a barrier to the environment forces.
Stratum basale (basal cell layer)	Produces new cells (keratinocytes).
Stratum spinosum (spinous layer)	Produces the stratum germinativum with the basal layer.
Stratum germinativum	Represents the germinative layer of the skin.
Stratum corneum (composed of keratinocytes and melanocytes)	Protects the body's internal homeostasis.
Dermis	
Blood vessels	Forms the strength and elasticity of the skin regulate heat loss and temperature.
Nerve endings	Provide sensation.
Lymphatic vessels	Remove cells and proteins into the larger lymphatic ducts.
Hypodermis (subcutaneous tissue)	Provides cushion and contour as well as insulation to the body.
Dermal appendages	
Hair	Provides warmth
Nails	Provide protection to the digits
Sebaceous glands	Provide oils to the skin to prevent skin drying
Sweat glands (eccrine and apocrine)	Promote thermoregulation and body cooling through evaporation

From: Engel, 1997; Fioravanti, 1998; Huether, 1998.

- Assess the child's level of consciousness with the AVPU or Glasgow coma scale.

4. Assess the integumentary system:
   - Inspect and describe the lesions (Table 22-3) or skin condition:
     - Size.
     - Location.
     - Color.
     - Blisters, whiteheads, or pimples.
     - Hard or soft centers or borders.
     - Fluid or drainage.
     - Crusting or healing.
     - Configuration and distribution of lesions.
       - Flat, raised, or rough.
       - Circles with clear centers.
       - Diffuse or blotchy.
       - Bleeding or bruising under the skin.
   - Inspect the condition and color of surrounding skin and appendages:
     - Red streaks.
     - Edema.
     - Discoloration.
     - Turgor.
     - Nails.
     - Hair.
   - Note any skin odor.
   - Note the presence of scars, wounds, or bruises in varying stages of healing:
     - Unexplained surface trauma or bruises in varying stages of healing may be indicative of child maltreatment (Chapter 46).
   - Note the presence of keloids or surgical scars.

Psychosocial Assessment

- Assess the child's and parents' understanding of the child's health condition.
- Assess the child's and parents' coping strategies:
  - Parents are usually concerned about the cause of the affliction, the contagiousness of the condition, and the potential seriousness of the problem. They may be concerned about the child's appearance

TABLE 22.3 Skin Lesions Encountered in Children

Lesion	*Description*	*Example*
Raised lesions		
Papule	Small, discolored lesion.	Wart
Plaque	Raised, scaly lesion > 2–3 cm.	Eczema
Wheal	Elevated lesion with circumscribed and changing borders resulting from dermal edema.	Hives; insect bite
Vesicle/bulla	Fluid-filled, thin-walled elevated lesion; bullae are > 0.5 cm in diameter.	Varicella; impetigo
Pustule	Vesicle with purulent exudate.	*Staphylococcus* infection
Cyst	Accumulation of dried blood or serum.	Sebaceous cyst
Tumor	Circumscribed lesion > 2 cm in diameter.	Hemangioma
Flat lesions		
Macule	Circumscribed, discolored lesion.	Purpura
	Pinpoint, red-purple discoloration that does not blanch.	Petechia

From: Engel, 1997; Fioravanti, 1998; Huether, 1998.

and want relief from the uncomfortable or disfiguring symptoms.
   - Children may have concerns about how others will react to their physical appearance.
   - Because of the contagious nature of some dermatologic conditions or underlying systemic illness, children may have to cope with feelings of isolation and rejection.
- Assess for pain with age-appropriate pain scales and techniques (Chapter 13).

Table 22.4 lists nursing diagnoses and expected outcomes.

Triage Decisions

Emergent

- Patients with signs of respiratory failure and shock or altered level of consciousness.

Urgent

- Patients with lesions that are:
   - Red, blue, or purple.
   - Purpuric.

TABLE 22.4 Nursing Diagnoses and Expected Outcomes

Nursing Diagnoses	*Expected Outcomes*
Impaired skin integrity related to viral, bacterial, or fungal infection or infestation.	The patient's skin lesions will resolve with appropriate treatment.
Potential for infection related to transmission of infectious agent of disease and knowledge deficit related to immunizations.	Family members will be free of the infectious agent through: ▪ Proper handwashing. ▪ Proper hygiene (clean clothing, using one's own comb and makeup). The patient and family members will verbalize the understanding of techniques for preventing the spread of infection.
Body image disturbance related to perception of appearance.	The affected older child will verbalize an understanding of the disease and will be taught measures for coping with the skin condition (e.g., participating in own care, counting the number of lesions). The patient will express his or her feelings as encouraged and will experience pain relief, as evidenced by improvement in the age-appropriate pain scale and pain assessment techniques.

- Petechial.
- Burnlike (scalded skin).
- Tender to touch (cellulitis).
- Red streaked.
- Pustular.

- Patients with lesions and rashes with an infectious origin.

Nonurgent

- Patients with lesions that are not infectious or are not associated with a life-threatening illness.

Nursing Interventions

- Assess and maintain airway, breathing, and circulation:
  - Administer supplemental oxygen, as needed.
  - Initiate cardiorespiratory and oxygen saturation monitoring, as needed.
- Obtain venous access and initiate an intravenous infusion, as needed:
  - Obtain blood for laboratory studies as needed, such as complete blood count and differential; cultures; sedimentation rate.
- Administer medications, as prescribed:
  - Administer topical agents for relief of pain, itching, or discomfort.
  - Administer oral analgesics for relief of pain and discomfort (Chapter 13).
  - Administer oral or intramuscular antihistamines, as needed.
- Obtain other laboratory studies, as needed:
  - Skin culture.
  - Mucous membranes culture.
- Inform the family frequently of their child's condition; provide emotional and psychosocial support.
- Prepare for hospitalization or discharge to home.

Home Care and Prevention

- The child and family should be taught the proper home management of the skin lesions, including the application of topical agents.
- Proper handwashing to prevent the spread of infection should be demonstrated and discussed.
- Other methods for preventing the spread of infectious or contagious infestations, such as proper hygiene, should be reviewed.

Specific Dermatologic Conditions

Viral Infections of the Skin

Etiology

Viruses are intracellular parasites that are unable to sustain themselves or reproduce. Therefore, they are dependent on host cells to meet their metabolic needs. After they penetrate a host cell wall, the host is able to create additional virus material. The epidermal cells react to the viral infection through inflammation and vesiculation or may reproduce and form growths.

Common viral skin conditions treated in the ED are herpes simplex virus, varicella, rubeola, rubella, and roseola infantum. The physical assessment, nursing interventions, home care, and prevention for each viral condition are outlined in Table 22.5.

Herpes Simplex Virus

There are two types of herpes simplex virus: type 1–a cold sore or fever blister; and type 2–a genital lesion. These classifications are not mutually exclusive. For example, a type 2 lesion can appear on the mouth, and a type 1 lesion can appear on the genitals. The virus affects children, adolescents, and adults and remains in the body after the first infection. Repeated outbreaks can occur after a cold, fever, or exposure to the sun, or during stressful times or menstruation. Sometimes lesions appear for no apparent reason. The virus may be fatal in children with depressed immunity.

Symptoms of herpes simplex occur 2 to 30 days after contact with an infected person, and the lesions heal in 1 to 2 weeks.

Varicella (Chicken Pox)

Varicella, one of the most highly contagious infectious diseases, is transmitted through the respiratory route. Varicella is caused by the herpes zoster virus and affects the skin and mucous membranes. It is believed that the virus resides in the roots of nerves near the spinal cord and may cause shingles later in life. Although the virus is most common in childhood, it affects all age groups. Children who are immunosuppressed as a result of chemotherapy, steroid therapy, or human immunodeficiency virus (HIV) infection are at high-risk for complications and fatality.

General malaise, fever, cough, abdominal pain, or cold symptoms may occur 3 days before an outbreak of lesions. The symptoms include a progressive rash, pruritus, and low-grade fever; these symptoms are less severe in children, more problematic in adolescents, and can

TABLE 22.5 Summary of Viral Skin Conditions

Viral Condition	*Physical Assessment Findings*	*Nursing Interventions*	*Home Care and Prevention of Future Outbreaks or Complications*
Herpes simplex	*History of onset:* Stinging or prickling 1–2 days before lesion appears. *Physical assessment:* Vesicular clusters on mucous membranes, lip, or outer edge of mouth weep clear fluid and then form a scab.	Apply petroleum jelly to ease cracking and dryness. Apply Blistex® or Campho-Phenique® to ease discomfort. Consider acyclovir therapy for frequent outbreaks or an outbreak lasting more than 2 weeks. Acyclovir is effective if used early.	*Prevention of future outbreaks:* Apply ice when the first sign of outbreak appears, to reduce severity. Use sunscreen and wear a hat if sun exposure triggers outbreak. Avoid direct skin contact. Observe for complications: corneal ulceration, encephalitis, neonatal viremia with encephalitis.
Varicella	*History of onset:* 10–14 days after exposure. Lesions follow 3 days of fever, myalgia, chills, and arthralgia. *Physical assessment:* Lesions progress through several stages of raised red areas, blisters, and then scabs. Lesions appear mainly on trunk, face, and extremities, but can occur anywhere on the body.	Administer tepid baths with half cup of oatmeal (placed in a sock), baking soda, or Aveeno powder to reduce itching (Ball, 1998). Apply cool compresses to reduce discomfort. Administer acyclovir for severe or complicated cases. Trim the child's nails short and wash the child's hands frequently to discourage scratching and possible secondary infection; consider applying socks to the child's hands to prevent scratching associated with severe itching (Ball, 1998). Maintain isolation for 5–7 days after lesions appear until all lesions are crusted over. Instruct the caregiver in the above recommendations for home management of symptoms.	*Prevention of future outbreaks:* Avoid exposing high-risk children (steroid use, chemotherapy, immunodeficiency problems), pregnant women, infants, and immunocompromised adults to infected children (Ball, 1998). *Prevention of complications:* Consider administration of Varicella-zoster immune globulin with 72–96 hours after exposure to help prevent disease. *Observe for complications:* pneumonia, secondary bacterial infections, cellulitis, bacterial pneumonia, encephalitis, myelitis, hepatitis, Reye's syndrome. Permit the child to return to school after all lesions are scabbed over. Do not give aspirin because of its association with Reye's syndrome.
Rubeola	*History of onset:* 7–14 days after exposure. Rash follows 1–4 days of high fever, fatigue, loss of appetite, sneezing, runny nose, cough, red eyes, tiny bluish white spots in mouth and throat (Koplik's spots), light sensitivity. *Physical assessment:* Generalized red rash on forehead and ears, spreading to trunk and extremities. May be blotchy, irregular, flat or raised.	Use a cool mist humidifier. Measure temperature regularly. Treat a fever > 103°F with acetaminophen and tepid baths. Do not administer aspirin because of its association with Reye's syndrome. Administer decongestants for relief of upper respiratory tract infection symptoms. Maintain isolation for 4 days after rash appears. Encourage oral fluids to prevent dehydration. Consider administering vitamin A. Instruct caregiver in symptomatic management, as outlined above.	*Prevention of future outbreaks:* Immunize according to recommended immunization schedule. *Prevention of complications:* Administer gamma globulin injection if exposure occurs and immunizations are not obtained or are incomplete. Immunize unvaccinated, exposed children 8 weeks after contact. Observe for complications: otitis media, pneumonia, encephalitis, meningitis, thrombocytopenia, pneumothorax, orchitis, hepatitis.

(continued)

TABLE 22.5 (continued)

Viral Condition	*Physical Assessment Findings*	*Nursing Interventions*	*Home Care and Prevention of Future Outbreaks or Complications*
Rubella	*History of onset:* Onset occurs 14–21 days after exposure. Rash follows 2–3 days of fever, muscle aches, fatigue, swollen lymph nodes at base and sides of neck, and pain with lateral and upward eye movement. *Physical assessment:* Generalized reddish rash starting on the face and spreading to the trunk and extremities. Rash rapidly changes in appearance over the course of a few hours to a few days.	Administer acetaminophen for fever and discomfort. Refer the exposed pregnant woman to physician if exposed 1 week prior to onset of rash, during rash, or 1 week after rash resolves.	*Prevention of future outbreaks:* Repeat measles-mumps-rubella vaccine at 4–6 years of age. Obtain immunization at 15 months unless the child is immunosuppressed, taking cortisone or anticancer drugs, receiving radiation, or has an illness with fever. Observe for complications: arthritis, encephalitis, thrombocytopenia.
Roseola infantum (human herpes virus 6)	*History of onset:* 5–15 days after exposure. Rash follows 3–4 days of high fever, irritability, and drowsiness. *Physical assessment:* Flat, reddish rash, most prominent on the back and trunk.	Measure temperature frequently. Administer acetaminophen for fever >103° F; administer tepid baths. Do not give aspirin because of its association with Reye's syndrome. Encourage oral fluids to prevent dehydration. Instruct caregiver in management of symptoms, as outlined above.	*Prevention of future outbreaks:* Avoid exposure to infected persons. *Prevention of complications:* Complications include febrile seizures, which are difficult to prevent because they usually occur with the first fever spike. Measure the temperature frequently and administer acetaminophen as indicated to prevent sudden temperature spikes.

From: Goodman & Brady, 2000.

result in pneumonitis. Symptoms may persist for 1 to 3 weeks. The infected child is considered contagious 1 to 2 days prior to the onset of the rash and until all lesions are scabbed over (usually 10 days to 2 weeks) and no new lesions appear.

Rubeola (Red Measles)

Rubeola is a serious and highly contagious illness caused by a paramyxovirus affecting the skin, eyes, and upper respiratory tract. The virus is most common in children, but all age groups are affected. Preexisting conditions that increase the risk of infection include crowded or unsanitary living conditions, unimmunized population groups, and measles epidemics.

A cough, congestion, conjunctivitis, fever, and Koplik's spots on the buccal mucosa occur 1 to 4 days before the rash appears. Symptoms may last 3 to 4 days. Rubeola is no longer contagious after the rash is resolved.

Rubella (German Measles; 3-day Measles)

Rubella is a mild, contagious viral illness involving the skin on the face, trunk, and extremities and the lymph glands behind the ears and in the neck. It is most common in springtime. This virus can cause serious birth defects if a pregnant woman is infected with the virus during the first 3 to 4 months of pregnancy.

Enlarged lymph nodes, fever, sore throat, headache, and malaise occur 1 to 3 days before the onset of the rash. The rash lasts 2 to 3 days, and the infected child is contagious 1 week prior to the onset of the rash and 1 week after the rash fades.

Roseola Infantum

Roseola infantum (human herpesvirus 6) is a common contagious viral illness affecting infants and children younger than 3 years. The virus involves the skin and the central nervous system, including the brain, meninges, spinal cord, and peripheral nerves. Roseola is most common in spring and autumn. Generally, the child has a high fever 3 to 4 days before the onset of the rash. The rash lasts for 1 to 2 days.

Bacterial Infections of the Skin

Etiology

The skin normally harbors bacterial flora, including staphylococci and streptococci. The ability for these organisms to cause infection is related to the specific portal of entry, the number of microorganisms, the virulence of the organism, and host resistance. Children who are immunosuppressed or who have debilitating conditions or a generalized malignancy are a risk for bacterial infections. Infections affecting the skin range from a localized and self-limiting lesion to a generalized systemic illness that manifests skin lesions or problems. Common bacterial dermatologic conditions among children presenting to the ED are outlined below. Assessment, nursing interventions, and preventive measures for each bacterial infection are discussed in Table 22.6.

Abscess

An abscess is a localized collection of pus under the skin that causes fluctuant soft tissue swelling surrounded by erythema. The abscess may be accompanied by local cellulitis, lymphangitis, and fever. Cutaneous abscesses most commonly occur when *Staphylococcus aureus*, *Staphylococcus epidermidis*, or Streptococcus (group A) enter the skin through a hair follicle or break in the skin. The causative organism is determined by the location of the abscess and is reflective of the type of microflora of the skin and mucous membranes (Arndt, Wintroib, Robinson, & LeBoit, 1997). Predisposing factors to abscess formation include diminished host defense mechanisms; trauma; foreign bodies; tissue ischemia or breakdown; hematoma or excessive fluid accumulation in the tissue; sharing of needles, licking of needles, and use of poor injection technique, and by intravenous drug users (Arndt et al., 1997; Berkow & Fletcher, 1999).

Abscesses are located most often in the axillary, vulvovaginal, perirectal, head and neck, and buttock areas. A widespread abscess involving several pus-draining ports is usually located in the axilla or groin and involves the sweat glands. Such abscesses respond well to antibiotic therapy.

Boils (Furuncles)

Boils are common, contagious inflammatory nodules that arise from hair follicles. They occur only in hair-bearing parts of the body, but are most prevalent on the head, neck, axillae, buttocks, and groin. The red, hard lesion becomes tender and fluctuant over a couple of days. Pain subsides after the lesion discharges pus and a central plug of necrotic material. The infection is usually caused by *Staphylococcus aureus* that begins in the hair follicle and spreads to the skin's deeper layers. Predisposing factors include friction, moisture, obesity, immunosuppression, colonization by *S. aureus*, poor nutrition, diabetes mellitus, and diminished host defense mechanisms.

Without treatment, the boil may heal in 10 to 20 days. If the boil opens spontaneously, the draining pus may contaminate surrounding skin and cause new boils. Incision and drainage of the boil and administration of antibiotics is the recommended treatment. Symptoms should resolve within 3 to 4 days after treatment.

Cellulitis

Cellulitis is a noncontagious acute infection of the skin and subcutaneous tissues that may occur spontaneously or may secondarily complicate a preexisting wound or other inflammatory process. Cellulitis occurs most commonly on the face and lower legs. The infecting organisms are usually staphylococcal and streptococcal organisms or oral-based organisms, such as anaerobic streptococci or *Pasteurella multocida*. Predisposing factors for cellulitis include the use of immunosuppressive or cortisone medications, chronic infection, diminished host defense mechanisms, or any injury or condition that breaks the skin barrier.

Symptoms resolve within 7 to 10 days after antibiotic treatment.

Impetigo

Impetigo is a common, highly contagious bacterial infection, caused by group A streptococci or *S. aureus*, that affects the superficial layers of the skin. It is most prevalent in infants and young children, and it primarily affects the face, arms, leg, or areas of trauma. Predisposing factors for impetigo include a fair complexion, skin sensitive to sun and irritants, poor nutrition, unsanitary living conditions, warm and moist weather, poor hygiene, and diminished host defense mechanisms.

The symptoms resolve in 10 days after oral or topical treatment; however, scarring may result. Lesions are considered contagious until 24 hours from completion of antibiotic treatment.

Scarlatina (Scarlet Fever)

Scarlatina is a contagious bacterial infection caused by group A beta-hemolytic streptococci. This condition is preceded by a streptococcal throat infection and is characterized by a bright red rash. The infection is spread through respiratory secretions. Scarlatina is most prevalent in children between the ages of 2 and 10 years. Predisposing factors include a family history of recurrent streptococcal infections or impetigo, unsanitary living conditions, and exposure to others with sore throats.

Staphylococcal Scalded Skin Syndrome

Staphylococcal Scalded Skin Syndrome is an acute bacterial infection that causes the skin to separate and peel

TABLE 22.6 Summary of Bacterial Skin Conditions

Bacterial Skin Condition	*Physical Assessment Findings*	*Nursing Interventions*	*Home Care and Prevention*
Abscess	*History of onset:* Tender cutaneous mass. *Physical assessment:* Redness, heat, swelling, fever if surrounding cellulitis is present, and red streaks.	Assist with incision and drainage, followed by irrigation and possibly packing in severe cases. Prepare to administer conscious sedation or other forms of analgesia. Obtain a specimen for Gram stain, culture, and sensitivity. Instruct the child and family in wound care, application of warm compresses, signs of infection, and follow-up care.	*Prevention of infection:* Clean the skin surface well after skin trauma. Observe for complications, including bacteremia and, rarely, endocarditis, osteomyelitis, or brain abscess. If fluctuance is not present, administer antibiotics and heat over a 24- to 48-hour period to either resolve the boil or result in fluctuance responsive to incision and drainage.
Boils (furuncles)	*History of onset:* Sudden, painful, tender lesion that ripens within 24 hours. Fever and lymph node swelling may be present. *Physical assessment:* Red, hard lesion with pus, 1.5 cm to 3.0 cm in diameter, fever, and swelling of the closest lymph nodes.	Assist with incision and drainage, if necessary, followed by irrigation. Instruct in wound care, application of warm compresses, daily cleansing with antimicrobial solution, signs of infection, and follow-up care. For facial boils, treat with compresses and antibiotics to prevent infectious drainage through the veins into the cavernous sinus, leading to cavernous sinus thrombosis or meningitis.	*Prevention of infection:* Use separate towels for each family member. Wash towels frequently. Observe for complications, including bacteremia, endocarditis, osteomyelitis, and brain abscess.
Cellulitis	*History of onset:* Sudden tenderness, swelling, and reddened area rapidly growing over 24 hours. *Physical assessment:* Fever, chills, malaise, and swollen lymph glands near the affected area. Diffuse area of erythema and warmth, 5–20 cm initially; red streaks extending from the area toward the heart. Elevated white blood count.	Administer oral, intramuscular, or intravenous antibiotics. Prepare for hospitalization when there is systemic involvement; when the patient is immunosuppressed, has lowered resistance, or has a chronic disease; when the face is affected; or when there is an animal or human bite to the hand or foot. Instruct the child and family in wound care, applications of warm compresses, elevation of the affected area, and follow-up care.	*Prevention of infection:* Keep skin clean. Avoid skin damage. Take antibiotics for entire course, even after symptoms are resolved. Observe for complications, including bacteremia, infection of the underlying joint or bone, and sepsis.
Impetigo	History of onset: up to 20 days after exposure to the bacteria and rapid spread. *Physical assessment:* Red rash with many small blisters. Honey-colored crusts after blisters break.	Soak the affected area in warm water or warm, wet compresses to soften and remove crusts. Gently scrub the lesions with gauze and antiseptic soap, and break any pustules. Apply a dressing. Administer oral and topical antibiotics as prescribed. Treat all infected household members.	Minimize sharing of towels and linens. Wash with antibacterial soap. Bathe daily. Keep fingernails short to prevent secondary infection. Take full course of antibiotics, even after lesions disappear. Observe for complications, including acute glomerulonephritis, cellulitis, bacteremia, septic arthritis, osteomyelitis, or extensive streptococcal infection in the deep layers of the skin.

(continued)

TABLE 22.6 Summary of Bacterial Skin Conditions (continued)

Bacterial Skin Condition	*Physical Assessment Findings*	*Nursing Interventions*	*Home Care and Prevention*
Impetigo (cont.)		Instruct the child and parent in removing crusts, cleaning sores, and applying dressing. Instruct the child and parent to clean all clothing and linens in contact with the sores.	
Scarlatina	*History of onset:* 3–5 days after exposure. Rash progresses rapidly over 24 hours. *Physical assessment:* Sore throat, chills, fever, headache, vomiting, strawberry tongue, swollen tonsils, enlarged lymph nodes in the neck, and tachycardia precede rash by 24 hours. Diffuse pinkish red flush of skin, starting on the face except around the mouth, progresses to body creases, the neck, chest, back, and then entire body. Blanches on pressure. Looks like a sunburn with small bumps. Peeling skin on palms and soles for 10–14 days.	Administer antibiotics. Administer acetaminophen or ibuprofen for fever and discomfort. Encourage older children to use throat lozenges for sore throat. Obtain a throat culture.	Isolate the child until 24 hours of antibiotic treatment is completed. Administer the full course of antibiotics, even after symptoms resolve. Avoid contact with others who have sore throats. Observe for complications, including otitis media, adenitis, sepsis, rheumatic fever, and acute glomerulonephritis.
Staphylococcal scalded skin syndrome	*History of onset:* Lesion rapidly progresses with 24 hours. Systemic symptoms occur within 36–72 hours. *Physical assessment:* Crusted lesion on the face, neck, axilla, or groin, surrounded by tender, scarlet rash. Progresses into large, flaccid blisters that break easily, producing erosions. Skin separates with minor trauma and may peel off in large sheets.	Administer oral or intravenous fluids to prevent dehydration and maintain fluid and electrolyte balance. Administer analgesics for discomfort. Apply warm compresses. (If there is a large area of skin separation, treat as a burn.) Administer antibiotics. Obtain blood and skin cultures.	Practice infection control techniques. Perform frequent handwashing. Minimize handling of the child. Observe for complications, including dehydration and sepsis.

From: Goodman & Brady, 2000.

off in sheets when touched. A widespread erythematous process that results in the loss of the protective skin barrier, it is caused by group II coagulase-positive staphylococci. The organism produces an exotoxin and colonizes without overt infection. The colonized person can spread the organism through direct contact. In this disease, the upper layer of the skin splits, allowing the toxin to enter the circulation and affect the skin systemically. Staphylococcal Scalded Skin Syndrome is most prevalent among infants, small children younger than 6 years of age, and immunosuppressed adults. The staphylococcus organism can pass from infant to infant in nurseries and usually affects the umbilical stump or the area under the diaper during the first few days of life. In young children, crusted lesions appear initially around the nose or ear. Healing occurs 5 to 7 days after treatment with antibiotics.

Fungal Infections of the Skin

Etiology

Superficial fungal infections are classified as dermatophyte infections and yeast infections. Chronic cutaneous fungal infection occurs in approximately 20% of the population; greater than 90% of the male population is afflicted with one or more of these conditions at some point in life (Arndt et al., 1997).

Candidiasis and tinea (ringworm) are two of the most common fungal infections. Both conditions require a suitable environment for infection to occur. Decreased resistance, immunosuppression, diabetes, antineoplastic agents, corticosteroids, and use of potent antibiotics all contribute to the incidence of infection. A moist, warm environment and skin irritation lead to increased susceptibility to infection.

Common fungal infections of the skin are outlined. Table 22.7 addresses the nursing interventions for fungal infections.

Candidiasis (Moniliasis)

Candidiasis is a contagious yeast infection caused by *Candida albicans*, which is found in the intestinal tract and vagina. Candidiasis affects folds of contiguous skin or adjacent areas of skin that come in contact with each other. The yeast changes from its spore form to the mycelial phase when the skin is damaged and the environment is moist and warm. Its incidence is greatest among infants wearing wet and soiled diapers for prolonged periods of time. However, candidiasis affects older children and adolescents in folds of skin. Oral lesions (thrush) are also common in infants. Common locations for candidiasis are the diaper area, the groin, under the breasts, the folds of skin in scrotal, vaginal, and axillary areas, the inner thighs, the base of the spine, and webs between fingers and toes. It easily spreads to other areas of the body and from person to person with direct contact. Predisposing factors include thumb sucking, obesity, an uncircumcised penis, antibiotic and steroid use, diabetes, poor nutrition, excessive sweating, and crowded and unsanitary conditions.

Symptoms resolve after 2 weeks with treatment and in 4 to 5 years without treatment.

Tinea

Tinea is a contagious infection that varies in presentation, depending on anatomic location. In general, tinea infections are red, with well-defined margins and a clear center. The name, tinea, followed by the anatomic location, is used to identify the type of infection:

- Tinea corporis—chest, back, neck, and shoulders.
- Tinea capitis—scalp.
- Tinea pedis—foot (athlete's foot).
- Tinea cruris—groin (jock itch).
- Tinea unguium—nails.
- Tinea barbae—skin and beard.

Tinea infections are caused by a group of closely related, filamentous fungi (Microsporum, and Trichophyton, Epidermophyton) that are transmitted from person to person or animal to person through direct contact. They live in the outer layers of the skin and must multiply rapidly for infection to occur before the dead cells are removed through the normal sloughing process. The infection may also spread from one area of the body to another. Transmission may occur through contact with infected surfaces, such as towels, shoes, hats, or shower stalls. Predisposing factors include prolonged exposure to dark, moist, and warm conditions, and overcrowded and unsanitary conditions, obesity, excessive sweating, and friction of the skin against skin with constant movement.

Symptoms resolve within 5 days to 6 weeks after treatment. Ringworm becomes chronic in 20% of cases (Griffith,1989).

Infestations of the Skin

Etiology

Lice and scabies are two of the most common contagious infestations. They cause severe itching and are at times difficult to eradicate. Treatment of the infected person, other family members with symptoms, and clothing and linens is essential to prevent reinfection after treatment. Pediculosis and scabies are treated commonly in the ED; their nursing interventions are outlined in Table 22.8.

Pediculosis

Pediculosis includes head lice and body lice (crabs), which are most prevalent in children 4 to 12 years of age. Lice are tiny (3- to 4-mm), blood-sucking parasites; while feeding, they discharge their products of digestion into the skin, causing a severe pruritic response (Jenkins & Loscalzo, 1990). Lice are difficult to see, except in the groin, where hair distribution is lighter. The presence of eggs (nits) on the hair shaft and complaints of itching are clues to infestation. The severity of itching correlates to the number of lice and their bites. Matted hair and scalp inflammation indicate a severe infection that may require the hair to be cut if the hair shafts cannot be separated for proper treatment. Lice can live up to 3 days without human contact and are transmitted person to person through direct contact or sharing of clothing, hats, brushes, and combs. Predisposing factors include crowded and unsanitary conditions, exposure to other household members with lice, and sexual contact with an infected person.

Symptoms should resolve within 5 days after treatment; however, lice frequently recur.

Scabies

Scabies is a contagious skin infection caused by the mite *Sarcoptes scabiel*. Scabies is transmitted through close

TABLE 22.7 Summary of Fungal Infections of the Skin

Fungal Infection	*Physical Assessment Findings*	*Nursing Interventions*	*Home Care and Prevention*
Candidiasis	*History of onset:* Dermatitis > 3 days followed by prolonged exposure to moisture and warmth. Pruritus. *Physical assessment:* Skin moist and crusted. Inflamed areas with pustules, peeling, and easy bleeding. Patches 6–12 cm with irregular borders. Smaller white blisters may surround larger patches. *Site-specific lesions:* ■ Mouth—white plaque on tongue, esophagus, or trachea (thrush) ■ Diaper area—red lesions with well-defined margins. ■ Skin folds—red, moist papules. ■ Vagina—thick, white, cheesy discharge. ■ Penis—red, round lesions on glans and shaft. ■ Nails—redness and swelling at nail base.	Administer antifungal topical medication. Instruct the child and parent in the use of medication—continue application for 7 days after symptoms subside. Instruct the parent and child in care of the rash: Keep skin clean, cool, and dry. Expose to sunlight and air as much as possible. Change diapers frequently. Avoid plastic pants. Wear loose cotton clothing.	Feed the child yogurt, buttermilk, or sour cream when he or she is taking antibiotics, to prevent yeast infections. Keep skin cool and dry. Observe for complications, including secondary bacterial infections and blood poisoning. Treat breast-feeding mothers of infants with thrush.
Tinea	*History of onset:* Lesions grow slowly and center clears as the patch increases in size. *Physical assessment by site:* Corporis—red, flat, circular, scaly patches with well-defined borders and lighter colored centers. Capitis—red, scaly patch on scalp, hairline, or neck; scaly patches of alopecia. Pedis—moist, soft, gray-white or red scales between toes or vesicles on plantar surface of foot; itching; dead skin between toes. Cruris—scaling patches on groin, thighs, and buttocks with well-defined borders; small blisters; itching.	*For all lesions:* Administer oral griseofulvin (usually for scalp lesions) at meal time or with fatty foods, such as peanut butter or milk, for better absorption (Ball, 1998). Instruct the child and parent in medication use and side effects of oral medication (headache, gastrointestinal upset, fatigue, insomnia, and photosensitivity). Apply wet compresses for itching. Apply topical antifungal preparations with griseofulvin (usually with other tinea lesions). Provide reassurance that hair loss is rarely permanent and that itching may persist several days after treatment. Keep the skin clean and dry.	*For all lesions:* Keep affected area clean and dry. Observe for complications, including secondary bacterial infections, contact or allergic dermatitis, or allergic immunologic response to the disease on the hands and face. Apply lotion as prescribed. Wash the child's hair with dandruff shampoos containing selenium sulfide (e.g., Selsun Blue) two to three times a week; after lathering, leave the shampoo on the scalp for 10 minutes, then rinse off (Ball, 1998). Avoid sharing combs, brushes, etc. Wear clean, light socks and well-ventilated shoes. Apply lotion as prescribed. Wear loose cotton or breathable clothing when exercising or sweating. Apply lotion as prescribed.

From: Goodman & Brady, 2000.

TABLE 22.8 Summary of Skin Infestations

Infestation	*Physical Assessment Findings*	*Nursing Interventions*	*Home Care and Prevention*
Pediculosis	*History of onset:* Insect bites causing inflammation and severe itching. *Physical assessment:* Red bite marks and hives, matted hair (in severe cases), nits (eggs) on hair shafts, and scalp inflammation. Tender cervical or occipital adenopathy. Small lice may be seen crawling in the groin area.	*Instruct the child and family in home care:* Apply pediculicide shampoo for all members of the household to kill the adult lice and remove the eggs. (A current strain of lice has become resistant to many of the current modalities; however, repeated applications can be toxic for the child.) Remove nits manually with a fine-toothed comb dipped in hot vinegar; apply petroleum jelly to eye lashes with a swab 4 to 5 times a day for 2–3 days. Wash clothes and linens used prior to and during treatment; wash in hot water. Dry-clean nonwashable items or seal in a plastic bag for 3–4 days or freeze to kill eggs and lice. Vacuum and throw away vacuum bag. Boil articles such as combs, brushes, and barrettes (Arndt et al., 1997; Griffith, 1989).	Bathe and shampoo often. Avoid sharing clothing, combs, and brushes with others. Avoid wearing the same clothing for more than 1 day. Change bed linens often. Avoid close contact with others infected with lice. Observe for complications, including secondary infection from scratches and subsequent scarring.
Scabies	*History of onset:* Rash and itching occur 3 weeks after infestation. *Physical assessment:* Affects the head, neck, palms, and soles of feet. Red blisters with S-shaped linear burrows; blisters break easily. Nocturnal itching.	Administer antihistamines or topical steroids as necessary to stop the itch-scratch cycle. Instruct the child and family in home care: Use a pediculicide: Apply to body from neck down; wait 15 minutes before dressing and 2 hours before bathing (or per instructions on the medication). Bathe thoroughly before the application of a pediculicide lotion. Clean clothing, linens, and toys used prior to and during treatment. Observe for signs of infection.	Avoid contact with persons infected with scabies. Do not share clothing and articles with infected persons. Bathe daily. Wash hands before eating. Launder clothes often. Keep fingernails short. Observe for complications, including secondary bacterial infection.

From: Goodman & Brady, 2000.

personal contact and causes severe pruritus because of acquired sensitivity to the organism. The scabies mite can live up to 3 days without human contact. The female mite burrows deep into the skin layers to deposit eggs. The eggs mature into mites in 15 to 60 days and can only be seen through a microscope. Scratching collects the mites and eggs under the nails and spreads the mites to other areas of the body. The skin of the fingerwebs, wrists, skin folds under the arms, breasts, elbows, genitals, and buttocks often are involved. Small, itchy blisters break, leaving a characteristic S-shaped distribution pattern or scratch marks and thickened skin. Predisposing factors include crowded and unsanitary conditions, infection with the human immunodeficiency virus, and Down syndrome (Arndt et al., 1997).

Symptoms usually resolve within 1 to 2 weeks after treatment. Retreatment may be necessary in 20 days if skin irritation persists.

Conclusion

The treatment of dermatologic conditions almost always requires the support and assistance of family members. Except for a few urgent conditions or complications, most dermatologic conditions are safely managed at home. The nurse plays a vital role in educating the child and parent about the condition, management of the treatment regimen at home, expected outcomes, and when to seek medical attention (if the condition worsens, complications occur, or the condition fails to improve with treatment).

Additionally, emergency nurses can teach self-care to older children and involve them in planning treatment schedules. Finally, children and families should be taught simple methods, such as handwashing, for preventing the spread of infection to other body parts or to other people.

References

Arndt, K., Wintroib, R., Robinson, J., & LeBoit, P. (1997). *Primary care dermatology*. Philadelphia: Saunders.

Ball, J. (1998). Integumentary. In J. Ball (Ed.), *Mosby's pediatric patient teaching guides* (pp. B-1BB-19). St. Louis: Mosby—Year Book.

Berkow, R., & Fletcher, B. (Eds.). (1999). *Merck manual of diagnosis & therapy* (17th ed.). Rathway, NJ: Merck Research Laboratories.

Dickerson, P., Gordon, M., & Walter, P. (1998). Burns. In M. Slota (Ed.), *Core curriculum for pediatric critical care nursing* (pp. 652–675). Philadelphia: Saunders.

Engel, J. (1997). *Pocket guide to pediatric assessment* (3rd ed.). St. Louis: Mosby—Year Book.

Fioravanti, J. (1998). Integumentary system. In T. Soud & J. Rogers (Eds.), *Manual of pediatric emergency nursing* (pp. 417–451). St. Louis: Mosby—Year Book.

Goodman, M., & Brady, M. (2000). Infectious diseases. In C. Burns, M. Brady, A. Dunn, & N. Starr (Eds.), *Pediatric primary care: A handbook for nurse practitioners* (pp. 580–619). Philadelphia: W. B. Saunders.

Griffith, H. (1989). *Complete guide to pediatric symptoms, illness & medications*. New York: The Body Press/ Perigee Books.

Huether, S. (1998). Structure, function, and disorders of the integument. In K. McCance & S. Huether (Eds.), *Pathophysiology: The biologic basis for disease in adults and children,* 3rd ed. (pp. 1517–1554). St. Louis: Mosby—Year Book.

Jenkins, J., & Loscalzo, J. (1990). *Manual of emergency medicine; Diagnosis & treatment* (2nd ed.). Boston: Little, Brown.

Nicol, N., & Huether, S. (1998). Alterations of the integument in children. In K. McCance & S. Huether (Eds.), *Pathophysiology: The biologic basis for disease in adults and children,* 3rd ed. (pp. 1555–1569). St. Louis: Mosby—Year Book.

23

Eye, Ear, Nose, and Throat Emergencies

Cherie Revere, RN, MSN, CEN, CRNP
Donna Ojanen Thomas, RN, MSN

Introduction

Children present to emergency departments (EDs) with a variety of eye, ear, nose, and throat (EENT) complaints. These conditions can be the result of:

- *Trauma.*
- *Exposure to a chemical.*
- *Infectious organisms.*
- *Congenital problems.*

Traumatic and infectious conditions are the most common EENT complaints treated in the emergency department. Depending on the presentation and diagnosis, children may be evaluated and treated in the ED or may require examination or evaluation by an EENT specialist. The purpose of this chapter is to discuss specific EENT conditions seen in the ED and their assessment and treatment.

Embryologic Development

Eyes

Eye formation is first evident at the beginning of the fourth week of development (Moore & Persaud, 1998). The eyelids meet and adhere by about the 10th week and remain adherent until the 26th week. Myelination of the optic nerve fibers, incomplete at birth, is completed after the eyes have been exposed to light for about 10 weeks. The normal newborn can see but not well; he or she is able to fixate points of contrast.

Because of the complexity of eye development, many anomalies may occur, but most of them are uncommon. The eyes and ears are sensitive to the teratogenic effects of infectious agents; the most serious defects result from disturbances of development during the fourth to sixth weeks. Most common anomalies of the eye are related to defects in closure of the optic fissure, which normally closes during the sixth week. Congenital ptosis (drooping) of the eyelid is a fairly common anomaly.

Ears

The ear consists of three anatomic parts: external, middle, and internal. The development of the ear begins in the fourth week of gestation. The internal (middle) ear is the first to develop and reaches its adult size and shape by the middle of the fetal period (20 to 22 weeks). Parts of the external and middle ear are not fully developed until puberty.

There are many minor abnormalities of the auricle of the ear, but they may be indicative of associated major anomalies (heart or kidneys). Low-set, severely malformed ears are often associated with chromosomal abnormalities, particularly trisomy 18 and trisomy 13 (Moore & Persaud, 1998). Congenital deafness can result from abnormal development of the membranous labyrinth and/or bony labyrinth as well as from abnormalities of the auditory ossicle (Moore & Persaud, 1998). Recessive inheritance is the most common cause, but a rubella virus infection near the end of the embryonic period is also known to cause defective hearing.

Structures of the Nose and Throat

Major structures of the face and palate develop between the fourth and eighth weeks of embryonic development. Because of the complicated development, congenital anomalies of the face and palate are common and result from an arrest of development and/or a failure of fusion of the prominences and processes involved.

Pediatric Considerations

Eyes

As was mentioned earlier, the newborn cannot see very well but can fixate points of contrast. Visual acuity has been estimated to be in the range of 20/600. Because the oculomotor system is immature in the newborn and vision and fixation are poor, strabismus is common and usually resolves by 4 to 5 months of age (Rogers, 1998). The lacrimal glands are small and do not function at birth; therefore, the newborn does not produce tears for about six weeks.

Ears

The external auditory meatus is short at birth, and care must be taken not to injure the tympanic membrane during examination of the ear. The shortness of this meatus also results in a greater likelihood of ear infections because bacteria can easily reach the inner ear and secretions cannot efficiently drain from the middle ear. The external acoustic meatus attains its adult length around the ninth year.

Structures of the Nose and Throat

Most of the paranasal sinuses are rudimentary or absent in newborn infants. The maxillary sinuses are small at birth; they grow slowly until puberty and are not developed until all the permanent teeth have erupted in early adulthood (Moore & Persaud, 1998). The frontal and sphenoidal sinuses are not present at birth. The ethmoidal cells are small before the age of 2 years and they do not begin to grow rapidly until 6 to 8 years of age. Around 2 years of age, the frontal sinuses are formed. They are visible in radiographs by the seventh year. Growth of the paranasal sinuses is important in altering the size and shape of the face during infancy and childhood and in adding resonance to the voice during adolescence. Adenoidal tissue is present in infants and young children and can obstruct the eustachian tubes when inflamed (Rogers, 1998). This tissue usually atrophies by puberty.

Focused History

For all EENT complaints, the following history should be obtained:

- Onset and duration of symptoms.
- Past history including current infections.
- Discharge from eyes, ears, nose.
- Recent exposure to infectious conditions.
- Preexisting conditions (congenital or acquired).

Focused Assessment

Physical Assessment

The standard pediatric assessment is done for all EENT conditions. Specific assessment findings are discussed in the sections on individual conditions.

Psychosocial Assessment

Children with EENT problems are difficult to assess and treat because of their anxiety and fear. Parents may be concerned about loss of function and permanent damage to the affected area. Explain treatment to the patient, parent, and caregiver. The patient may be very self-conscious about his or her appearance because some EENT conditions, especially those affecting the eye, can be disfiguring. Reassure the patient that symptoms will subside with treatment.

Nursing diagnoses and expected outcomes are listed in Table 23.1.

Triage Decisions

Emergent

Conjunctivitis (see "Specific Conditions of the Eye," next section). In the neonate, conjunctivitis is an emergent condition because of the risk of complications, such as permanent blindness or loss of the eye.

- Loss of vision or abrupt changes in visual acuity.
- Periorbital swelling with signs and symptoms of sepsis or restricted eye movement.

TABLE 23.1 Nursing Diagnoses and Expected Outcomes

Nursing Diagnoses	*Expected Outcomes*
Pain related to inflammatory process.	Pain will be relieved by treating the cause of infection and by use of appropriate medications.
Actual or risk for infection.	Infection will be treated by appropriate measures without loss of function.
Sensory or perceptual alterations (visual, auditory, or olfactory) related to condition.	Perceptual alterations will be eliminated or alleviated with proper treatment.

- Severe pain.
- Signs and symptoms of sepsis or respiratory distress with any EENT complaint.

Urgent

- Acute pain.
- Foreign body in the nose or ear.
- Periorbital swelling without signs and symptoms of sepsis.

Nonurgent

- Minor symptoms in a child who is awake, alert, and afebrile and without sensory deficits.
- Ear checks.

Specific Conditions of the Eye

Conjunctivitis

Red eyes in children are most commonly a form of conjunctivitis. Conjunctivitis is inflammation of the normally clear conjunctiva. There are a number of causes requiring different treatments. Causes of conjunctivitis include:

- *Bacterial infections*—Cause of a large number of cases in children beyond the neonatal period. Table 23.2 lists common bacterial causes of conjunctivitis.
- *Viral infections*—More common in older children. The course is usually self-limited and resolves in 10 days. Common pathogens include adenovirus, enterovirus, and herpes simplex virus.

Another form of viral conjunctivitis is known as epidemic keratoconjunctivitis. It is highly contagious and may be associated with photophobia, increased redness, and pain of the affected eye. Enlarged and tender ipsilateral preauricular lymph nodes are usually present a few days after symptoms begin. Keratitis appears approximately 1 week after the onset of symptoms and is characterized by scattered subepithelial infiltrates that may greatly reduce visual acuity (Clark, 1992). Epidemic keratoconjunctivitis may last up to 3 weeks (Bentley, 1996).

- *Allergies*—Noninfectious and seasonal conjunctivitis are caused by an allergy to an unknown allergen.
- *Other*—Other causes of conjunctivitis include:
  - Trauma.
  - Foreign body.
  - Chemical irritants.
  - Systemic infections, such as rubella, rubeola, and Kawasaki syndrome (Uphold & Graham, 1994).

Conjunctivitis in the neonate is called opthalmia neonatorum. The major causes are chemical, chlamydial, bacterial, and viral.

The time of onset of symptoms after birth can help identify the causative agent (Grover & Silverman, 2000).

- Chemical conjunctivitis—Usually occurs 12-24 hours after birth and is usually caused by eye drops instilled at birth.
- *Neisseria gonorrhoeae* conjunctivitis—Appears 2-5 days after birth.
- *Chlamydia trachomatis*—occurs between 5-14 days after birth.

Gonococcal conjunctivitis is considered a medical emergency because the infection can spread to the cornea, producing corneal ulceration and perforation (Grover & Silverman, 2000).

Pathophysiology

Conjunctivitis is an inflammation of the conjunctiva, a thick mucous membrane that lines the posterior surface

TABLE 23.2 Causes of Bacterial Conjunctivitis

Type of Bacteria	*Comments*
Streptococcus pneumoniae *Haemophilus influenzae*	Both of these are common pathogens in children.
Neisseria gonorrhea	Common cause of conjunctivitis in newborns. Occurs within 3-5 days of birth if it is contracted during the birth process. Adolescents who are sexually active can also develop this infection.
Pseudomonas	Common cause of conjunctivitis in contact lens wearers.
Chlamydia	Conjunctivitis caused by *Chlamydial trachomatis* is seen in neonates and infants and is usually acquired during the birth process. Fifty percent of infants born to women with vaginal chlamydia will develop conjunctivitis, which may lead to infections in the nasopharynx and lungs.

of the eyelids and the eyeball (excluding the cornea). Conjunctivitis causes vasodilation, migration of inflammatory cells to the affected eye, pain, and tearing. Complications can be severe if the cornea is infected. These complications can include corneal scarring, perforation, or necrosis, leading to permanent blindness or loss of the eye itself (Rogers, 1998). Conjunctivitis may be unilateral or bilateral.

Focused History

- Onset and duration of symptoms, such as tearing, itching, burning, and/or red eyes.
- Recent upper respiratory tract infection.
- Discharge from the eyes (varies with different causes).
- Recent exposure to "pink eye."
- Recurrent symptoms.

Focused Assessment

- Assess the eye for the following signs and symptoms:
  - Irritated, red eye or infected conjunctiva.
  - Tearing, discharge, and pain.
  - Involvement of one or both eyes.
  - Photophobia—May be present with infections involving the cornea.
- Assess visual acuity if necessary. (Vision is not generally affected.)

Table 23.3 lists signs and symptoms of conjunctivitis based on the cause.

Nursing Interventions

- Administer medications as ordered, such as antibiotics and pain medications:
  - Because conjunctivitis is so contagious, antibiotics should be instilled in both eyes, even if only one eye is involved, to prevent the transfer of the infection from one eye to the other.
  - Allergic conjunctivitis may also be treated with antihistamines and topical decongestants.

TABLE 23.3 Causes and Clinical Features of Conjunctivitis

Cause	*Common Pathogens*	*Signs and Symptoms*
Viral	Adenovirus	Mild to moderate pain, itching eyes, excessive tearing.
		Bilateral symptoms.
		Watery discharge.
	Herpes simplex virus	Fever blisters on lips or face.
		Vesicles on the eyelids and herpetic lesions on the cornea.
Allergic	Known or unknown allergens	Redness of eyes without pain.
		Bilateral, stringy white discharge.
		Clear, watery nasal discharge.
		Chemosis (edema of conjunctiva).
		Intense pruritus.
		No change in vision.
Bacterial	*Streptococcus pneumoniae* and *Haemophilus influenza* in children	Mild pain, redness, and irritation.
		Gritty sensation with tearing in one or both eyes.
	Neisseria gonorrhea in newborns	Mucopurulent discharge; can be unilateral or bilateral.
	Chlamydia trachomatis	Mild to moderate pain.
		Purulent discharge; can be unilateral or bilateral.
		In neonates, infection usually begins on day 5 to 14 of the child's life.

- Offer comfort measures, to include a darkened room or environment.
- If epidemic keratoconjunctivitis is suspected or diagnosed, an ophthalmologic consultation is indicated.

Home Care and Prevention

Instruct the parent on the following:

- Symptomatic treatment measures, such as warm compresses.
- The extremely contagious nature of the condition: Eye secretions are contagious for 24–48 hours after the patient begins taking antibiotics.
- How to cleanse matted eyelids by wiping from the inner corner to outer corner of eye with a wet cottonball and warm water.
- The proper method of instilling ophthalmic medications, to the inner aspect of lower lid.
- Proper hand-washing techniques and their importance to prevent further spread of infection.
- If the child has epidemic keratoconjunctivitis, he or she should be kept out of school.

Cellulitis

Cellulitis is an acute inflammatory process of the skin and subcutaneous structures. Generally, there is some type of trauma to the skin that provides a portal of entry for invading organisms, but cellulitis may develop in normal skin. There are two types of cellulitis that affect the face:

- Orbital (postseptal):
  - Deeper and more serious infection behind the septum, involving posterior eye structures.
  - May form an abscess and need to be surgically drained.
  - Generally seen in children 6 years old or younger; however, it can occur at any age (Corrall, 1996).
- Periorbital (preseptal):
  - Soft tissue infection of anterior eye structures, usually localized to the eyelids and conjunctiva.
  - Seen more commonly in children younger than three years and is more likely to be caused by a bacteria (Corrall, 1996).

Periorbital and orbital cellulitis are serious conditions because of the close proximity of the infection to the brain. The most common etiologic agents causing cellulitis are *Staphylococcus aureus*, *Streptococcus pneumoniae*, and *Haemophilus influenzae*. The risk of cellulitis caused by an anaerobic organism is increased if there is a history of a human bite. *Haemophilus influenza* type B is less common since the HIB vaccine. In infants, group B streptococcal infection should be considered (O'Rourke, 1994).

Pathophysiology

Direct spread of infection from ethmoidal sinusitis is often the cause of orbital cellulitis. As sinus pressure obstructs venous and lymphatic drainage from the periorbital area, edema occurs. Bacteria can enter the orbit either directly across the bone that separates the ethmoidal sinuses from the orbit or through the venous system.

In periorbital cellulitis, bacteria invade the periorbital tissues, resulting in the accumulation of inflammatory cells and fluid (Rogers, 1998).

Focused History

- Onset and duration of symptoms.
- History of sinus, dental, or upper respiratory tract infections.
- Trauma or a preexisting wound to the affected area.
- History of systemic symptoms, such as fever, chills, and/or malaise.

Focused Assessment

It is difficult to clinically distinguish between orbital and periorbital cellulitis in children. General signs and symptoms may include:

- Erythema, edema, and redness in the area around the eye.
- Pain.
- Malaise.
- Fever.
- Chills.
- Lymphadenopathy.

Table 23.4 compares the signs and symptoms of periorbital and orbital cellulitis.

Nursing Interventions

- Test visual acuity.
- Prepare patient for laboratory studies and possible computerized tomography scan (may reveal source of infection as sinusitis).
- Obtain intravenous access or saline lock to administer antibiotics as ordered.
- Explain any procedures such as laboratory tests or X-rays to the child in understandable terms.
- Anticipate surgical or ophthalmologic consult.

TABLE 23.4 Signs and Symptoms of Cellulitis

Type	*Signs and Symptoms*
Periorbital—Usually in children younger than 6 years of age.	Local eyelid symptoms, usually unilateral (swelling, redness). Occasional discharge. Fever. Leukocytosis. Normal pupillary reflexes and visual acuity. Point of entry or break in the skin.
Orbital—Usually in older children and adolescents.	Acute unilateral eyelid swelling; red or purple eyelid. Fever and systemic illness. Exophthalmos. Pain with extraocular movements; one of the most consistent findings (O'Rourke, 1994). May have decreased visual acuity.

Home Care and Prevention

Provide the following home care instructions:

- Maintain good general hygiene and carefully cleanse cuts and abrasions that occur near the orbit to prevent orbital cellulitis.
- Apply cool compresses every 3 to 4 hours to relieve discomfort and inflammation.
- Continue medication until gone.
- Discuss symptoms that would require the child to return to the ED:
  - Increased fever
  - Increased area of involvement
  - Vision changes

Chalazions and Styes

Chalazions (internal hordeolums) and styes (external hordeolums) represent blocked glands within the eyelid (Levin, 2000). Both may present acutely with localized lid swelling, erythema, and tenderness. Styes are associated with purulent drainage and swelling at or near the lid margin.

Pathophysiology

A chalazion usually results from obstruction of a meibomian gland duct. The surrounding tissues may become secondarily infected. Small chalazia may improve and resolve without any treatment. If the chalazion is not treated and continues to increase in size, it may cause pressure on the eye globe, causing astigmatism.

Focused History

- Previous episodes and treatment.
- Presence of pain and tenderness of the eyelid.
- Vision changes.
- Feeling of pressure on the eye globe because of the nodule.

Focused Assessment

Assessment findings include:

- A nontender, hard nodule (up to 8 mm) on the midportion of the tarsus, away from the border of lid (Sutherland & Steahley, 1994). If the opening of the duct is involved, a stye may develop on lid border.
- Pain and swelling of the entire lid if the chalazion is infected.

Nursing Interventions

If chalazia are small, chronic, and asymptomatic, they generally do not require treatment and spontaneously disappear within a few months.

Home Care and Prevention (Levin, 2000)

The treatment for both chalazions and styes is the same:

- Eyelash scrubs once or twice daily with baby shampoo will help to establish drainage. Baby shampoo should be applied to a washcloth and then used to scrub the base of the eyelashes.
- Warm compresses are useful but rarely tolerated by young children.
- Antibiotics usually are not helpful, but a topical antibiotic ointment may be prescribed.
- If the lesion has not improved in 4 weeks, an opthalmic consult may be necessary.

Specific Conditions of the Ear

Otitis Externa

Otitis externa is common in children but may affect all age groups. It is inflammation of the external ear canal. This inflammation can range from a mild, diffuse dermatitis to cellulitis of the ear canal.

Pathophysiology

Otitis externa is caused by frequent exposure of the ear canal to water (swimming), vigorous cleaning of the canal, and trauma. Repeated entry of water in the ear or vigorous cleaning alters the normal protective wax found in the ear and the acidic pH that usually protects the ear from bacteria. Otitis externa can be localized or diffuse. Localized external otitis is the result of an abscessed hair follicle in the outer two-thirds of the ear canal, caused by *Staphylococcus aureous*. Diffuse external otitis is caused by *Pseudomonas aeroginosa*, *staphylocci*, fungi, or a mixture of Gram-negative and Gram-positive organisms. Viral external otitis is usually caused by herpes simplex or herpes zoster (Potsic & Handler, 2000).

Focused History

- Gradual onset of pain.
- Sensation of obstruction or fullness of the ear.
- History of frequent swimming or vigorous cleaning of the ear canal.
- Otorrhea or discharge from the ear.
- Pulling on the ear.

Focused Assessment

- Increased pain with manipulation of the auricle or tragus.
- Erythema and swelling of the affected ear canal.
- Purulent drainage from the affected ear.
- Preauricular and postauricular lymphadenopathy.

Nursing Interventions

- Clean the ear to remove exudate and wax and to improve visualization of the ear canal and tympanic membrane.
- Instill topical medications, as ordered, such as acetic acid otic solution.
- Severe infections may require topical antibiotics, such as polymyxin B and neomycin.
- If otitis media is also present, oral antibiotics may be necessary.

Home Care and Prevention

Provide the following home care instructions:

- Apply warm, moist compresses to the affected ear.
- Keep the ear canal dry with the use of ear plugs while showering or swimming.
- Follow-up instructions and proper use of medications.
- Avoid vigorous cleaning of the ear canal.

Otitis Media

Otitis media is defined as inflammation of the middle ear. Otitis media can occur at any age but is more common in children. If otitis media goes untreated, complications that may develop include mastoiditis, intracranial abscess, meningitis, neck abscess, and permanent hearing loss.

The most common pathogens include *Streptococcus pneumoniae*, *Haemophilus influenzae*, and, less often, *Moraxella catarrhalis*, Group AB hemolytic streptococcus, and various upper respiratory viruses (Potsic & Handler, 2000). Certain factors predispose children to developing otitis media:

- Native American or Caucasian race.
- Family history of otitis media.
- Passive or active smoking.
- Congenital disorders, such as Down syndrome.
- Frequent upper respiratory infections.

Bottle-fed children who are put to bed with bottles are at increased risk of developing otitis media. Otitis media occurs most frequently during the winter months, most likely because of its association with upper respiratory infections, which are also more prevalent in winter (Rogers, 1998).

Pathophysiology

Otitis media is common in small children and infants because of the straight position of the eustachian tube. The middle ear drains poorly and fluid can collect. The fluid provides a medium for bacterial growth. Children with upper respiratory tract infections that cause congestion are at risk for infections caused by the collection of bacteria. As the child matures, the eustachian tube becomes more curved, and the child becomes better able to equilibrate negative pressures in the middle ear by swallowing.

Focused History

- Ear pain.
- Fever.
- Pulling at one or both ears.

- Upper respiratory tract infections (frequently precede otitis media).
- History of anorexia, vomiting, or diarrhea.
- Drainage from one or both ears.
- Prior ear infections and response to treatment.
- Inability to sleep at night.

Focused Assessment

- Fever.
- Possible decrease in hearing ability.
- Full or bulging tympanic membrane, distorted light reflex, or absence of landmarks.
- Decreased tympanic membrane mobility with insufflation and possible erythema of the tympanic membrane (An erythematous tympanic membrane is an inconclusive finding and may result from vascular engorgement, caused by fever or crying.)
- Lymphadenopathy in the preauricular, postauricular, and cervical areas.
- Purulent drainage, indicative of a ruptured tympanic membrane.
- If the child appears ill, further evaluation may be necessary to rule out other infectious conditions, such as sepsis and meningitis.

Nursing Interventions

- Administer antibiotics. Amoxicillin is often the drug of choice, but others may be necessary if the infection does not improve. Antibiotics should only be used if the infection is confirmed by visualization.
- Administer analgesics for pain, such as analgesic ear drops.
- Administer antipyretics for fever.

Home Care and Prevention

Provide the following home care instructions:

- Elevate the infant's head when feeding and do not prop the bottle.
- Do not allow smoking in the house.
- Use medications until gone and make a follow-up appointment to recheck the ears.
- Return to the ED if the child's condition worsens or does not improve.

Mastoiditis

Mastoiditis is inflammation and bacterial infection of the air cells of the mastoid area. With early treatment, prognosis is good. Complications include facial paralysis, meningitis, brain abscess, and suppurative labrynthritis. The most common causes are group A streptococcus, *Streptococcus pneumoniae*, *Staphylococcus aureus*, anaerobes, and *Haemophilus influenzae* (rare) (Barkin, 1997).

Pathophysiology

Mastoiditis is usually a complication of chronic otitis media but can occur after acute otitis media. As pus accumulates under pressure in the middle ear cavity, necrosis of adjacent tissue occurs. The necrosis allows extension of the infection into the mastoid cells.

Focused History

- Tenderness and dull ache in the area of the mastoid process.
- History of low-grade fever.
- History of otitis media.

Focused Assessment

- Swelling and erythema behind the mastoid process of the ear.
- Earlobe elevation in children older than 1 year; displacement of the pinna down and out in younger patients (Barkin, 1997).
- Thick, purulent discharge that becomes profuse.
- Conductive hearing loss resulting from the obstruction of the external ear canal by the pressure inside the edematous mastoid area.

Nursing Interventions

- Administer intravenous antibiotics as prescribed.
- Assist with obtaining specimens for culture and sensitivity.
- Administer antipyretics and analgesics, as prescribed.
- Prepare the patient for possible admission and surgical intervention to remove diseased bone and irrigate the affected area.

Foreign Body

Children younger than 4 years may attempt to place almost any object into the external ear canal. Local tissue irritation occurs when small items, such as beads or stones, are inserted in the ear canal. Sometimes small insects may crawl or fly into the ear canal, become trapped, and, if they are still alive, cause discomfort. If a child introduces a vegetable foreign body, such as a pea or dried bean, it generally absorbs moisture, enlarges, and begins to obstruct the ear canal. If the foreign body remains for a period of time, an offensive odor may be noticed. Inorganic objects in the ear may go undetected if they do not cause pain or discharge or interfere with hearing.

Pathophysiology

Objects inserted in the ear canal can cause bleeding as a result of tissue trauma. Tissue irritation and inflammation can occur if the object is retained for an extended period of time. Eventually, the mucosa may erode and an infection may occur.

Focused History

- Ear pain.
- Decreased hearing.
- Discharge from ear (bloody or purulent).
- Swelling or foul odor if the object has been retained for an extended period of time.
- Complaints of buzzing in the ear (usually indicative of an insect).

Focused Assessment

- Erythema and edema of canal.
- Visualization of the object.
- Foul odor, discharge, and bleeding.

Nursing Interventions

- Assist with removal of the foreign body. Removal techniques used include:
  - Direct instrumentation with alligator forceps.
  - Irrigation with warm water or normal saline if the tympanic membrane is intact and the object is not vegetable material.
  - Suction.
  - Insertion of mineral oil or 2% lidocaine (Xylocaine) solution in the ear canal to kill a trapped insect before removal (Rogers, 1998).
- Administer medications, antibiotics, or analgesics, as ordered.
- The foreign body may have to be removed under anesthesia.
- Treat for otitis externa.

Specific Conditions of the Nose

Sinusitis

Sinusitis is an inflammatory condition of the mucous membranes that line the paranasal sinuses. Sinusitis may be acute or chronic and can range from mild congestion to a progressive, severe infection with lethal complications. The ethmoid sinuses are more commonly involved in children younger than 10 years of age.

Pathophysiology

Drainage from the paranasal sinuses into the meatus facilitates the movement of secretions and particulate matter. Any condition that obstructs drainage from the sinuses can cause secretions to stagnate, causing an environment for bacteria to grow. Acute sinusitis is more commonly caused by *Streptococcus pneumoniae*, *Haemophilus influenza*, and *Moraxella catarrhalis* (Rogers, 1998). Chronic sinusitis is usually caused by anaerobic bacteria and *Staphylococcus aureus*. Sinusitis frequently follows an upper respiratory infection or allergy. Factors that may predispose a patient to develop sinusitis include:

- Recent upper respiratory infection.
- Allergic response to airborne allergens.
- Adenoidal hypertrophy.
- Diving and swimming.
- Anatomic abnormalities, such as polyps or a deviated septum.
- Dental abscess.
- Neoplasms.
- Cystic fibrosis.
- Foreign body.
- Trauma.

Focused History

- Fever, headache, and sinus pain that worsens when coughing or leaning forward.
- Purulent nasal discharge.
- Prior episodes of same symptoms.
- Recent upper respiratory tract infections or recurrent otitis media.
- Prolonged cough and nasal discharge (greater than 7–10 days).

Focused Assessment

The complaints of children with sinusitis are generally nonspecific. Children may present with the following signs and symptoms:

- "Puffy eyes" or periorbital swelling
- Purulent (yellow or green) nasal drainage with inflamed, swollen nasal mucosa
- Tenderness to palpation over involved sinuses

Nursing Interventions

Administer antibiotics as ordered. If periorbital cellulitis is present, intravenous antibiotics are indicated along with a probable hospital admission.

Home Care and Prevention

For patients who are discharged home, the following instructions should be given:

- Promote sinus drainage by keeping the head of the bed elevated.
- Use heat and warm compresses on the face to help relieve pressure.
- Use a room vaporizer, which may help relieve nasal congestion by liquefying secretions.
- Increase the child's fluid intake.
- Eliminate cigarette smoking in the house.
- Use saline nose drops as directed.
- Avoid swimming or diving during the acute phase of sinusitis.
- Follow up in 24 to 48 hours if there is no improvement; otherwise, follow up in 10 to 14 days.

Foreign Body

Children aged 4 years or younger are commonly seen in the ED with a foreign object in the nasal cavity. Generally, there is no pain; therefore, parents and caregivers may not be aware of the foreign object. Vegetable or organic substances may germinate and swell in the warm, moist environment of the nasal cavity. Inorganic objects, such as small stones, crayons, or beads, may cause aspiration if they become dislodged and progress to the pharynx.

Pathophysiology

The pathophysiology is the same as that of a foreign body in the ear. The foreign body causes trauma, inflammation, and infection. Most often children place objects in their noses intentionally, because of boredom or curiosity. However, accidental placement of foreign bodies can occur when a child is attempting to smell or sniff an object.

Focused History

- Chronic runny nose, often unilateral.
- History of pain in the nose, foul smell, and breath.
- Unilateral foul smelling, purulent nasal discharge when the object has been in the nose over a period of time (Rogers, 1998).
- Frequent sneezing.
- Recurrent epistaxis.

Focused Assessment

- Purulent nasal drainage, usually unilateral and foul smelling, depending on the length of time the foreign body has been retained.
- Edema of the nasal mucosa.
- Visualized foreign body.
- Unilateral bleeding from the nose.

Nursing Interventions

- Attempt to remove object with gentle suction or alligator forceps.
- Have the older child forcibly exhale through the affected nostril while occluding the nonaffected nostril.
- Refer to an ear, nose, and throat specialist if the child is uncooperative and the object cannot be removed.
- Caution the parent and patient about placing objects in the nose.

Epistaxis

Epistaxis (nosebleeding) is commonly seen in children. Episodes are usually mild, infrequent, and self-limiting. The source of nosebleeds in children is usually an anterior site on the nasal septum.

Pathophysiology

Bleeding of the nose occurs because of nasal mucosal disruption, which can result from trauma, neoplasm, or inflammation (Uphold & Graham, 1994). Traumatic events include nose picking, insertion of a foreign body, dry mucous membranes, and direct blunt trauma. Low humidity, which causes drying of nasal mucosa, is another cause of epistaxis. The majority of nosebleeds result from inflammation and trauma. Significant nasal trauma may result in the formation of a septal hematoma, in which the septal vessels bleed and the overlying mucous membrane stays intact (Rogers, 1998). If the hematoma is not treated, a septal abscess, cartilage destruction, and perforation can occur.

Focused History

- Frequency and duration of nosebleeds; amount of bleeding.
- Recent nasal surgery.
- Recent trauma or foreign body.
- Other signs and symptoms.

Focused Assessment

The standard pediatric assessment is done, especially focusing on signs and symptoms of shock, which require immediate treatment. The following signs and symptoms may be present:

- Obvious bleeding from one or both nostrils.
- Fresh blood in the oropharynx; hemataemesis.
- Active bleeding points on the nasal mucosa.
- Visualized foreign body.

Nursing Interventions

Rarely do children with nosebleeds require emergent treatment. However, if signs and symptoms of shock are present, they must be treated immediately. The following interventions may be performed:

- Stop bleeding by applying pressure to the soft part of the nose for 10 to 15 minutes. Have the child sit upright with his or her head tilted forward.
- Assist with cauterization or nasal packing if indicated.
- Monitor airway and be prepared for vomiting of swallowed blood.
- Administer medications, as ordered, for vasoconstriction or pain.
- Obtain laboratory analysis if a bleeding disorder is suspected or if the child may have lost enough blood to become hypovolemic (complete blood count, coagulation studies, and bleeding times).

Home Care and Prevention

Give the parents the following information:

- How to control and stop bleeding.
- How to use a humidifier, especially during the winter months.
- How to use a lubricant in nostrils to prevent drying and promote hydration.
- Reassurance that nosebleeds seldom indicate an underlying disease.

Specific Conditions of the Throat and Pharynx

Pharyngitis

Pharyngitis, an inflammation of the pharynx, is a common upper respiratory tract infection. The surrounding lymph tissues (tonsils) are commonly infected.

Pathophysiology

Pharyngitis is most often caused by viral infections (adenovirus, parainfluenza virus, rhinovirus, coronavirus, cytomegalovirus, Epstein-Barr virus, and coxsackie virus A) (Barkin, 1997). About 20% of cases are caused by group A beta-hemolytic streptococcus ("strep throat"). A potential complication of pharyngitis is peritonsillar abscess, which requires aggressive treatment to prevent airway compromise. This usually occurs in an adolescent who has not been treated with antibiotics, but it can occur even if antibiotics have been used.

Focused History

- Sore throat.
- Fever.
- Signs and symptoms of upper respiratory tract infection.
- Headache.
- Anorexia, fatigue, malaise, and dysphagia.
- Reduced fluid intake.
- Exposure to another child or family member with strep throat.
- Rash.
- Abdominal pain.

Focused Assessment

The physical signs of pharyngitis can mimic those of other disorders. Areas of assessment to evaluate during the standard examination include:

- Auscultate heart sounds for possible murmur.
- Palpate the abdomen for possible splenic enlargement.
- Assess for signs and symptoms of meningitis.
- Thoroughly inspect the skin for rashes.

Any child who has obvious stridor, drooling, or trouble breathing may have epiglottitis, and should be treated emergently without attempts to examine the pharynx (Chapter 16). The following signs and symptoms may be present in the child with pharyngitis:

- Enlarged and tender cervical lymph nodes.
- Labored respirations.
- Flushed skin.
- Enlarged tonsils, with erythema and/or exudate.
- If an abscess has formed, unilateral bulging and swelling of the affected tonsil with displacement of the uvula along with voice changes.

The child with streptococcal pharyngitis (strep throat) may present with the same complaints and symptoms as pharyngitis but with the following symptoms:

- Fever greater than 101°F (38.3°C).
- Dysphagia.
- Abdominal pain, headache, and vomiting.
- Sandpaper rash.
- Yellow or white exudate on tonsils and pharynx.

Nursing Interventions

- Obtain throat cultures and a streptococcal screen. Group A beta-hemolytic streptococcus is not excluded by a negative rapid streptococcal test and should always be verified by a throat culture (Fleisher, 2000).
- Administer antipyretics and antibiotics, as ordered.
- Prepare the child for hospitalization.

Home Care and Prevention

- Provide warm saline gargles, hard candy, and lozenges for pain as appropriate based on child's age.
- Ensure adequate bed rest and fluid intake.
- Do not allow the child to return to school until antibiotics have been given for 24 hours.
- Continue giving the child all antibiotics prescribed until they are gone. If antibiotics are not given until the culture results are obtained, call for results of culture.

Retropharyngeal and Peritonsillar Abscess

A retropharyngeal abscess is the accumulation of pus in the retropharyngeal space, which is located in the prevertebral soft tissue of the upper airway. This is uncommon and usually occurs in children less than 4 years of age (Fleisher, 2000).

A peritonsillar abscess is an infection in the potential space between the superior constrictor muscle and the tonsil. It is usually caused by group A beta-hemolytic streptococcus and is most common in older children and adolescents. The signs and symptoms, assessment, and interventions are similar for both conditions.

Pathophysiology

Before the age of 3 or 4 years, the retropharyngeal space harbors a chain of lymph nodes that drain portions of the nasopharynx and the posterior nasal passages. Conditions that produce an increased amount of drainage (otitis media, sinusitis, bacterial pharyngitis) increase a young child's risk of developing an abscess. The most common causative agents include *Staphylococcus aureus*, *Haemophilus influenzae*, and group A streptococci (Jenkins et al., 1995).

Focused History

- Dysphagia and unilateral throat and ear pain.
- Unilateral tonsillar swelling and deviation of the uvula (peritonsular abscess).
- A feeling of throat swelling.
- Decreased fluid intake.
- Fever.
- History of cough, headache, and malaise.

Focused Assessment

- Dysphonia.
- Dysphagia.
- Drooling.
- Trismus (inability to open the mouth).
- Extremely medially swollen, and erythematous tonsil (in peritonsilar abscesses).
- Swelling that displaces the soft palate and uvula to the opposite side (in peritonsilar abscesses).
- Swelling and erythema of the soft palate.
- Tender and enlarged cervical lymph nodes.
- Foul odor of breath.
- Resistance to neck movement (in retropharyngeal abscess).

Nursing Interventions

- Assist with X-rays or CT scan.
- Monitor the airway, as respiratory distress may be present.
- Administer intravenous antibiotics.
- Obtain a referral to an ear, nose, and throat specialist.
- Prepare the patient for admission and possible incision and drainage of the abscess.

Conclusion

Eye, ear, nose, and throat conditions are usually relatively minor. However, some conditions can be emergent and, if left untreated, can result in loss of function. ED nurses must be aware of common EENT conditions and know how to recognize and treat them in the ED.

References

Barkin, R. (1997). Ear, nose and throat emergencies. In E. F. Crain & J. C. Gershel (Eds.), *Clinical manual of emergency pediatrics* (3rd ed., pp. 117-138). New York: McGraw-Hill.

Bentley, B. II., (1996). Ocular emergencies. In D. Cline, O. J. Ma, J. E. Tintinalli, E. Ruiz, & R. L. Krone (Eds.), *Emergency medicine: A comprehensive study guide* (4th ed.). *Companion handbook*. New York: McGraw-Hill.

Clark, R. (1992). Ocular emergencies. In J. E. Tintinalli, R. L. Krone, & E. Ruiz (Eds.), *Emergency medicine: A comprehensive study guide* (3rd ed.). New York: McGraw-Hill.

Corrall, C. J. (1996). Skin and soft tissue infections. In D. Cline, O. J. Ma, J. E. Tintinalli, E. Ruiz, & R. L. Krone (Eds.), *Emergency medicine: A comprehensive study guide* (4th ed.). New York: McGraw-Hill.

Fleisher, G. (2000). Sore throat. In G. R. Fleisher & S. Ludwig (Eds.), *Textbook of pediatric emergency medicine* (4th ed., pp. 581-585). Philadelphia: Lippincott, Williams & Wilkins.

Grover, G., & Silverman, B. (2000). Problems in the very early neonate. In G. R. Fleisher & S. Ludwig (Eds.), *Textbook of pediatric emergency medicine* (4th ed., pp. 1229-1246). Philadelphia: Lippincott, Williams & Wilkins.

Jenkins, J. L., Loscalzo, J., & Braen, G. R. (1995). *Manual of emergency medicine*. Boston: Little, Brown.

Levin, A. (2000). Opthalmic emergencies. In G. R. Fleisher & S. Ludwig (Eds.), *Textbook of pediatric emergency medicine* (4th ed., pp. 1561-1568). Philadelphia: Lippincott, Williams & Wilkins.

Moore, K. L., & Persaud, T. V. N. (1998). *The developing human: Clinically oriented embryology* (6th ed., pp. 491-512). Philadelphia: Saunders.

O'Rourke, E. J. (1994). Antibiotics and infectious disorders. In J. W. Graef (Ed.), *Manual of pediatric therapeutics* (5th ed.). Boston: Little, Brown.

Potsic, W. & Handler, S. (2000). Otolaryngologic Emergencies. In G. R. Fleisher & S. Ludwig (Eds.), *Textbook of pediatric emergency medicine* (4th ed., pp. 1569-1583). Philadelphia: Lippincott, Williams & Wilkins.

Rogers, J. S. (1998). Eye, ear, nose and throat disorders. In T. E. Soud & J. S. Rogers (Eds.), *Manual of pediatric emergency nursing* (pp. 452-471). St. Louis: Mosby.

Sutherland, J. E., & Steahley, L. P. (1994). Selected disorders of the eye. In R. B. Taylor (Ed.), *Family medicine: Principles and practice* (4th ed.). New York: Springer.

Uphold, C. R., & Graham, M. V. (1994). *Clinical guidelines in adult health*. Gainesville, FL: Barmarrae Books.

24

Endocrine Emergencies

Christine Nelson, RNC, MS, PNP

Introduction

Aside from diabetic emergencies, endocrine emergencies are uncommon occurrences in the pediatric population. However, emergency nurses must be aware of the underlying developmental and physiologic processes associated with endocrine imbalances and their emergency department (ED) treatment. The purpose of this chapter is to present a basic overview of the endocrine system and highlight the emergency nursing care of children with endocrine-related imbalances.

Embryologic Development of the Endocrine System

The *pituitary*, *thyroid*, *parathyroid*, and *adrenal glands* are important endocrine organs in pediatric development. The nervous system and endocrine system are closely related in the development of the *pituitary gland*. The pituitary gland, located beneath the brain, is surrounded by the sphenoid bone. Embryologically, the pituitary gland develops from both the floor of the brain and the roof of the mouth (Spence, 1990).

The *thyroid gland* is the first endocrine gland to appear in the embryo and is noted about 24 days after conception (Roberts, 1995). It originates as an epithelial thickening in the floor of the pharynx. The thyroid forms during the seventh week of fetal development. Cellular differentiation occurs over the next 7 weeks and hormone synthesis begins at 14 weeks (Avery & Villee, 1994). The *parathyroid glands* develop from the dorsal halves of the pharyngeal pouches.

The *adrenal medulla* arises embryologically from the neural crest cells and is closely related to the function of the sympathetic nervous system. The adrenal cortex is derived from the same mesoderm that gives rise to the gonads.

Pediatric Considerations

The endocrine system is a feedback system that plays a key role in the body's response to external stimuli. The endocrine system uses hormones to respond to changes in temperature, stress, and traumatic injury. Hormones facilitate the communication network between the cells of the organs of the endocrine system. Alterations in hormone balances cause children to become too fat or too thin, or too short or too tall; distinctive physical features also result (Finegold, 1997). The endocrine system also responds to internal stimuli, such as electrolyte imbalance or changes in osmolality.

The endocrine system consists of endocrine and exocrine glands. *Endocrine* glands are ductless; they secrete hormones directly into the bloodstream. *Exocrine* glands secrete through a duct system.

Hormones circulate throughout the body and initiate responses after focusing on target cells. These hormones are responsible for:

- Maintenance of internal environment, such as extracellular fluid status, electrolyte regulation, and maintenance of bone, muscle, and body fat storage.
- Regulation of energy conversion and availability.
- Reproduction.
- Growth and development.

The organs and tissues are affected by the hormones that circulate throughout the body in a feedback system. Any alteration in the ability of the endocrine system to regulate these multiple functions may lead to a life-threatening emergency. Table 24.1 highlights selected endocrine imbalances in children.

Etiology

The etiology of endocrine imbalances is variable, depending on the involved endocrine glands and hormones. Endocrine gland dysfunction may result from the gland's failure to produce adequate amounts of hormones, synthesis or release of excessive amounts of hormones, or inappropriate response to a hormone (Huether & Tomky, 1998).

The hormones themselves may be involved in endocrine imbalances, from causes such as degradation of the hormone at an altered rate, inactivation by antibodies, or ectopic hormone release (hormones produced by nonendocrine tissues) (Huether & Tomky, 1998).

In other situations, the target cells may fail to respond to the hormones because of receptor-associated disorders associated with water-soluble hormones, (e.g., insulin) or intracellular disorders such as inadequate synthesis of a "second messenger" that transduces the hormone signal within the cell (Huether & Tomky, 1998).

Focused History

- Patient history:
  - Changes in activity levels.
  - Changes in dietary patterns.
  - Lack of or excessive physical growth.
  - Precocious or delayed puberty.
  - Genetic conditions.
  - Polyuria.
  - Polydipsia.
- Family history:
  - Endocrine disorders.
  - Genetic conditions.

Focused Assessment

Physical Assessment

- Assess the child's growth patterns:
  - Measure the child's height and weight; plot them on a growth chart. A change in growth patterns may be related to an endocrine imbalance.
  - Observe for secondary sexual characteristics. Observe for breast development and for axillary and pubic hair development. Inquire about the onset of menses.

TABLE 24.1 Selected Endocrine Imbalances in Children

Disease	*Description*
Panhypopituitarism	Absence of growth hormones, leading to short stature (dwarfism) and loss of secondary sex characteristics.
Hyperpituitarism: hypersecretion of growth hormone	Exposure to continuously excessive levels of growth hormone in children whose epiphyseal plates have not closed, causing gigantism.
Growth hormone deficiency	Normal body proportions with increased adipose tissue in the trunk and extremities; delay in height and bone age.
Thyroid gland disorders	Hyperthyroidism; hypothyroidism.
Turner's syndrome	Genetic in origin; suspect Turner's syndrome in short females with pubic or axillary hair and absence of breast development or menses onset.
Parathyroid gland imbalance	Hypocalcemia; Chvostek's sign (distortion of the face with stimulation of cranial nerve VII); Trousseau's sign (hand cramping with blood pressure measurement).
Adrenal gland imbalance	Cushing's syndrome; increased glucocorticoid action from endogenous or exogenous glucocorticoid exposure, causing a round face, central obesity, excessive fat on the lower cervical and upper thoracic spine, muscle weakness, and wasting in the extremities.

From: Finegold, 1997; Huether & Tomky, 1998.

- Measure vital signs. Increased blood pressure and heart rate may be noted.

Psychosocial Assessment

- Assess the child's and family's coping strategies.
- Assess the child's and family's knowledge of the child's current health condition.

Table 24.2 lists nursing diagnoses and expected outcomes.

Triage Decisions

Emergent

- Hemodynamic compromise.
- Altered level of consciousness.

Urgent

- Low or high blood glucose level, as tested by the patient at home or at triage.
- Increased thirst.
- Signs of mild dehydration.

Nonurgent

- Normal vital signs.
- Normal mental status for age and development.

Nursing Interventions

- Assess and maintain airway, breathing, and circulation in the child with hemodynamic compromise.
- Obtain venous access and initiate an intravenous infusion:
  - Obtain blood for laboratory studies, such as complete blood count; electrolytes; glucose; calcium; phosphorus; magnesium.
  - Administer medications, as needed.
- Prepare for diagnostic studies, as needed.
- Reassess the child's neurologic and cardiopulmonary status, as needed.
- Provide psychosocial support to the child and family:
  - Inform the family members frequently about their child's condition.
- Initiate referrals as appropriate (e.g., endocrinologist).
- Prepare for transfer and transport to a tertiary care center (Chapter 10) as needed, hospitalization, or discharge and subsequent referral.

Home Care and Prevention

The onset of an endocrine imbalance may be difficult for the child and family to accept. The child may feel different or have emotional difficulties if puberty is delayed or is precocious (Ball, 1998). The family should be encouraged to support the child throughout ongoing treatment.

For other endocrine imbalances, proper diet and exercise are needed to promote hormonal balances. Parents and children can be taught healthy food choices and appropriate exercises. Various web sites and voluntary organizations devoted to specific endocrine disorders are available and are listed throughout this chapter.

Specific Endocrine Emergencies

Diabetic Emergencies

Diabetes mellitus (type I, juvenile-onset) is the most common endocrine disorder of childhood and adolescence (Betschart, 2000). Five percent of all people with diabetes were diagnosed with this disease during their childhood (Avery & Villee, 1994). Seventy-five percent

TABLE 24.2 Nursing Diagnoses and Expected Outcomes

Nursing Diagnoses	*Expected Outcomes*
Fluid volume deficit, related to fluid shifts.	Patient will maintain a urinary output of 1 to 2 ml/kg/hr.
Impaired gas exchange, related to metabolic acidosis or glucose imbalance.	Patient will have a stable respiratory status.
	Patient will have vital signs in normal range for age.
	Patient will maintain a blood glucose level of 60–120 mg/dL.
	Patient will exhibit normal (or baseline) neurologic status.
Knowledge deficit, related to therapeutic regimen.	Patient and/or caregivers will verbalize an understanding of the disease process, treatment, and prevention.

of newly diagnosed diabetics are children and adolescents (Betschart, 2000).

The two conditions arising from diabetes mellitus are *hyperglycemia*, or *diabetic ketoacidosis* (DKA), in which the blood glucose level is higher than the norm for age, and *hypoglycemia*, in which the blood glucose level is lower than the norm for age.

Etiology

Diabetes mellitus is caused by insufficient insulin. This lack of insulin causes alterations in the metabolism of carbohydrates, lipids, and proteins. Without adequate insulin, glucose and amino acids cannot be adequately transported to the muscle and adipose tissue. Without sufficient glucose and amino acids, the tissue does not have adequate substances for energy production and protein synthesis.

Metabolic alterations allow for glucose production to occur in the liver. This increase in glucose production by the liver and the inability of the body to utilize energy in the normal method results in hyperglycemia, increased breakdown of fat and proteins, and metabolic acidosis.

Glycosuria occurs when the renal threshold for glucose is surpassed, causing osmotic diuresis and polyuria. The body attempts to compensate with polydipsia. When intake does not compensate for the significant losses, the result is dehydration. As ketones accumulate secondary to the increased breakdown of fats and proteins, vomiting occurs and leads to volume depletion and dehydration. Notable losses of sodium and potassium result from polyuria (Avery & Villee, 1994).

Although hyperglycemia usually is related to diabetes mellitus, hypoglycemia may arise from other causes. Generally, hypoglycemia may be the result of hormone deficiencies, hereditary metabolic errors, or neurologic disorders. Causes of persistent or frequent episodes of hypoglycemia in early infancy include inborn errors of metabolism involving the glyconeogenic enzymes and a defect in amino acid or fat metabolism. Causes of persistent or frequent episodes of hypoglycemia in older children include (Bacon, Spencer, Hopwood, & Kelch, 1990):

- Drug-induced hypoglycemia, caused by ingestion of ethanol, salicylates, or oral hypoglycemic agents.
- Reye's syndrome.
- Hepatitis.
- Insulin overdose.
- Extrapancreatic tumors, specifically fibrosarcoma, Wilm's tumor, hepatoma, or neuroblastoma.

Pediatric Considerations

Several factors influence management of diabetes in the pediatric population (Saladino, 1997):

- Greater susceptibility to infection than adults.
- Numerous emotional and environmental stressors.
- Additional caloric requirements because of ongoing physical maturation, growth, and greater physical activity.
- Unpredictable dietary patterns, especially in adolescence.
- Decreased adherence to prescribed medical management, most often among adolescents (Weissberg-Benchell et al., 1995), making this population especially at risk for complications from their illness.

Focused History

The patient history differs for new-onset diabetes, hypoglycemia, and hyperglycemia (DKA) (Table 24.3).

Focused Assessment

Physical Assessment

The comparison of physical assessment findings for hypoglycemia and diabetic ketoacidosis are outlined in Table 24.4.

Psychosocial Assessment

- Assess the child and family's understanding of the disease process.
- For the child previously diagnosed with diabetes, ascertain the child's and family's coping strategies.

Nursing Interventions

- Initiate measures to maintain airway, breathing, and circulation.
- Obtain venous access and initiate intravenous fluids.
- Obtain a quick-screen blood glucose level.
- Obtain blood specimens for:
  - Complete blood count.
  - Glucose.
  - Electrolytes.
  - Blood urea nitrogen; creatinine.
  - pH.
  - Phosphorus.
  - Magnesium.
- Interpret the screening results.
- Table 24.5 compares the laboratory data for hypoglycemia and hyperglycemia.
- Initiate treatment for hypoglycemia (Table 24.6) or DKA (Table 24.7).
- Reassess the patient's respiratory, cardiovascular, and neurologic systems frequently (Conte & Grumbach, 1991).

TABLE 24.3 Historical Findings in New-Onset Diabetes, Hypoglycemia, and Hyperglycemia

New-Onset Diabetes	*Hypoglycemia*	*Hyperglycemia*
All of these findings may have been present for weeks: ▪ Polyuria (more common in patients who are previously undiagnosed or who have been poorly managed for a considerable amount of time). ▪ Polydipsia (more common in those who are previously undiagnosed or who have been poorly managed for a considerable amount of time). ▪ Polyphagia. ▪ Weight loss. ▪ Abdominal pain. ▪ Flu-like symptoms (e.g., malaise, vomiting).	(Barkin & Rosen, 1999): ▪ Infections: viral or bacterial. ▪ Poor compliance with insulin. ▪ Use of steroids or birth control pills. ▪ Change in diet. ▪ Emotional stressors. ▪ Major trauma or surgery. ▪ Pregnancy, puberty, or thyroid problems. ▪ Usual insulin regimen and last dose. *Infants:* ▪ Tremors. ▪ Seizures. ▪ Cyanosis or apnea. ▪ Episodes of limpness or unresponsiveness. *Older children:* ▪ Anxiety. ▪ Tremors. ▪ Fatigue. ▪ Vomiting.	(Barkin & Rosen, 1999): ▪ Infections: viral or bacterial. ▪ Poor compliance with insulin. ▪ Use of steroids or birth control pills. ▪ Change in diet. ▪ Emotional stressors. ▪ Major trauma or surgery. ▪ Pregnancy, puberty, or thyroid problems. ▪ Usual insulin regimen and last dose. *Young children:* In very young children, signs and symptoms can be very vague and resemble those of sepsis: ▪ Irritability. ▪ Lethargy. ▪ Dehydration. ▪ Enuresis. ▪ Fatigue. ▪ Weight loss. ▪ Abdominal pain.

- Initiate consultations with other healthcare professionals, such as the child's primary care provider, endocrinologist, and social worker:
  - Education for the patient and family is essential for management of this condition.
  - The initial diagnosis of new-onset diabetes may cause feelings of shock, denial, anger, fear, and guilt in parents and patients.
  - Healthcare providers must encourage positive coping behaviors and facilitate use of appropriate resources to assure compliance with treatment regimens.
- Prepare for transfer or transport to a tertiary care center, if needed (Chapter 10).

Home Care and Prevention

Management of diabetes is a lifelong process that includes careful consideration of diet, exercise, stress management, and use of insulin. The patient and family are taught to monitor blood glucose and urinary ketone levels and administer the insulin. As the child grows older, the child's responsibility for his or her own management increases. Daily or weekly written records of the child's blood glucose levels, the dose and time of insulin injections, and possible reasons for high and low blood glucose levels are helpful (Ball, 1998).

The parents and child must learn the signs of hypoglycemia and hyperglycemia and know what to do if these situations occur. Even with minor illnesses, parents should still contact the child's primary care physician for directions or changes in the routine treatment regimen. Noncompliance with prescribed treatment regimens and risk-taking behaviors can lead to many ED visits for the child and family.

Support groups, counseling, and other venues may help children and adolescents to cope with their disease. The American Diabetes Association (800/ADA-3472), and the Juvenile Diabetes Foundation (800/JDF-CURE) have web sites (www.diabetes.org and www.JDF.org) where additional information can be obtained.

Diabetes Insipidus

Maintenance of the body's water balance is a complex process involving hormonal interaction among the pituitary gland, hypothalamus, and kidneys. The volume of urine is controlled by antidiuretic hormone (ADH), which is produced by the hypothalamus and transported by axons for storage in the posterior pituitary

TABLE 24.4 Comparison of Physical Assessment Findings in Hypoglycemia and Diabetic Ketoacidosis

Assessment Parameter	*Hypoglycemia*	*Diabetic Ketoacidosis*
Respiratory system.	Tachypnea.	Deep, rapid respirations (Kussmaul breathing). Tachypnea. Acetone or fruity-smelling breath.
Cardiovascular system.	Tachycardia.	Tachycardia. Signs of dehydration (increased capillary refill time, doughy skin, dry mucous membranes). Increased or decreased blood pressure.
Neurologic system.	Coma may be noted in severe cases. In infants; generalized symptoms, such as (Conte & Grumbach, 1991): ▪ Apnea. ▪ Breathing difficulties. ▪ Tremors. ▪ Lethargy. ▪ Seizures.	Altered mental status that may progress to coma, seizures.
Gastrointestinal and genitourinary systems.	Hunger.	Complaints of increased thirst.
Integumentary system.	Pallor. Diaphoresis.	Dry, brittle hair. Alopecia. Hot, dry skin.

TABLE 24.5 Comparison of Laboratory Findings in Hypoglycemia and Hyperglycemia

Laboratory Test	*Hypoglycemia*	*Hyperglycemia*
Serum glucose	Lower limit for children is 45 mg/dl of plasma glucose; premature and small-for-age infants and infants younger than 72 hours of age may have lower values (Conte & Grumbach, 1991).	Glucose may range from 300–1,200 mg/dl (Barkin, 1997).
pH	Normal.	Blood pH is frequently below 7.3, as extreme diuresis leads to poor tissue perfusion and an increase in lactic acid production.
Sodium	Normal.	Mild to moderate hyponatremia results from urinary sodium losses and osmotic dilution.
Potassium	Normal.	Potassium may vary widely, from slightly low to mildly elevated, depending on the serum pH (i.e., decreased pH results in increased potassium levels).
Phosphate/ bicarbonate	Normal.	Phosphate and bicarbonate may be depleted because of the extreme diuresis.
Blood, urea nitrogen; creatinine	Normal.	Levels are increased because of dehydration.

TABLE 24.6 Treatment for Hypoglycemia

Intervention	*Specific Treatment*
Administer intravenous fluid therapy and medications, as prescribed.	Administer oral high dextrose solution if tolerated and if able to take orally. Administer aqueous glucagon (0.03 mg/kg with a maximum dose of 1.00 mg) if intravenous access is not attainable (Bacon et al., 1990, p. 54).
Administer intravenous glucose therapy for patients with an altered level of consciousness.	Administer 1 to 2 ml/kg of 25% glucose over 2 to 4 minutes in children. Follow with an infusion of 10% dextrose in 0.25% normal saline at a rate sufficient to keep the blood glucose level between 50 and 120 mg/dl.
Monitor serum glucose.	Obtain serum glucose measurements on a regular basis to measure improvement.

TABLE 24.7 Treatment for Diabetic Ketoacidosis

Intervention	*Specific Treatment*
Administer intravenous fluid therapy and medications, as prescribed (Siberry & Iannone, 2000).	Initiate replacement of water and electrolytes: ▪ Assume that the child has 10% dehydration. ▪ Give 20 ml/kg bolus of normal saline solution over 20 to 30 minutes (Primary Children's Medical Center, 2000). After consultation with the ED physician, repeat a bolus of 10 to 20 ml/kg of normal saline solution if signs of shock are present (Primary Children's Medical Center, 2000). ▪ After the bolus, start an infusion of 0.45% normal saline with 20 mEq potassium acetate and 20 mEq potassium phosphate per liter at 1 1/2 times maintenance (Primary Children's Medical Center, 2000).
Administer insulin. Monitor serum glucose and electrolyte levels.	Begin an insulin drip after the first fluid bolus, if the child is hemodynamically stable. Measure the glucose level hourly. The rate of decrease in glucose level should not exceed 80 to 100 mg/dl/hr.
Monitor the patient for complications, such as (Bacon et al., 1990; Primary Children's Medical Center, 2000). Complications that may occur include: ▪ Hypokalemia/Hyperkalemia. ▪ Dysrhythmias. ▪ Hypernatremia. ▪ Cardiac arrest. ▪ Water intoxication. ▪ Cerebral edema (abrupt change in the level of consciousness). If increasing cerebral edema is undetected, herniation of the brain stem may occur, resulting in respiratory arrest. ▪ Hypoglycemia.	

gland (Bacon et al., 1990). Antidiuretic hormone functions to conserve body water by reducing the amount of water excreted in the urine.

Etiology

Diabetes insipidus is characterized by the impaired ability of the kidneys to conserve urine. There are two types of diabetes insipidus:

1. Central (neurogenic) diabetes insipidus:
   - Is caused by an absence or insufficient amount of circulating ADH.
   - May be caused by a disruption of three processes involving ADH:
     - Disruption in production.
     - Disruption in the process of neural pathway transport.
     - Disruption in the release of ADH.

- May be caused by the following health conditions (Bell, 1994):
  - Hypothalmic injury, surgery, or ischemia.
  - Pituitary injury, surgery, or ischemia.
  - Traumatic brain injury.
  - Central nervous system infection.
  - Cerebral edema.
  - Cranial neoplasms.
  - Intracranial hemorrhage.

2. Nephrogenic (or renal) diabetes insipidus:
   - Is less common.
   - Occurs when appropriate levels of ADH are synthesized but the kidneys' collecting ducts and distal tubules are resistant to the effects of ADH (Bacon et al., 1990).
   - Can be a congenital condition that may present symptomatically the first few weeks of life but not become apparent to healthcare providers until there are difficulties with toilet training.
   - Can also be caused by:
     - Chronic renal disease.
     - Pregnancy.
     - Sickle cell disease.
     - Multiple myeloma.

Focused History

- Patient history:
  - Irritability.
  - Fever of unknown origin.
  - Dehydration.
  - Complaints of extreme thirst.

Focused Assessment

Physical Assessment

1. Assess the respiratory system:
   - Auscultate the chest for:
     - Respiratory rate. Tachypnea may be present with fever.
2. Assess the cardiovascular system:
   - Auscultate the heart for:
     - Rate. Tachycardia may be present with fever.
   - Assess the peripheral vascular system:
     - Palpate the peripheral pulses for equality and quality. Pulses may be weak with dehydration.
     - Measure capillary refill. Capillary refill may be greater than 2 seconds with dehydration and early shock.
     - Assess core and skin temperature. Fever may be present.
     - Assess skin turgor. Turgor may be poor with dehydration.
     - Measure the blood pressure. Blood pressure may be elevated in early dehydration; hypotension may be evident in late shock or severe dehydration.
3. Assess the neurologic system:
   - Evaluate the child's level of consciousness with the AVPU method or Glasgow coma scale.
4. Assess the genitourinary system:
   - Measure the child's urinary output:
     - Polyuria is the hallmark symptom of diabetes insipidus, with urinary excretion of greater than 30 ml/kg/day. The urine is dilute (< 250 mOsm/kg).

Psychosocial Assessment

- Assess the child's and family's knowledge of the child's current health condition.
- Assess the child's and family's coping strategies.

Nursing Interventions

1. Assess and maintain airway, breathing, and circulation in the child with dehydration.
2. Obtain venous access and initiate an intravenous infusion:
   - Obtain blood specimens for diagnostic testing of:
     - Glucose. Monitor patients with anterior pituitary deficiency closely for hypoglycemia.
     - Blood urea nitrogen.
     - Creatinine.
   - Monitor the patient's fluid status to avoid fluid overload.
3. Reassess the child's neurologic and cardiopulmonary status.
4. Administer medications, as prescribed:

- Prepare for the administration of a diagnostic trial of aqueous vasopressin.
- Prepare to administer desmopressin acetate intranasally.

5. Prepare for transfer and transport to a tertiary care facility (Chapter 10), hospitalization, or referral and follow-up with the primary care physician.

Home Care and Prevention

The parents should be encouraged to follow up with the prescribed treatment for this condition. The parents and the child must be taught how to administer the intranasal medication. Consultation with the appropriate healthcare specialists is warranted.

Thyroid and Adrenal Disorders

Thyroid and adrenal disorders are relatively rare in the pediatric population. Three conditions that may be present in children presenting to the ED are *hypothyroidism*, *hyperthyroidism* (*Grave's disease*), and *acute adrenal insufficiency*. Table 24.8 compares the characteristics of thyroid and adrenal diseases in children.

Home Care and Prevention

Parents and children may require education regarding these endocrine disorders. In hyperthyroidism, for example, parents and children must learn about eating a well-balanced diet to promote growth and to limit calories to prevent excessive weight gain after the disease is under control (Ball, 1998).

Various agencies are available for additional information about these and other endocrine imbalances. The MAGIC Foundation (800-362-4423) provides information on hypothyroidism and hyperthyroidism. The National Graves' Disease Foundation (904-724-6744) also has information about hyperthyroidism. The Human Growth Foundation (703-883-1773) has information regarding short stature. Web sites include www.magicfoundation.org, www.ngdf.org, and www.ngfound.org.

Conclusion

The endocrine system is very complex and is frequently not studied in the depth afforded other body systems because of the relatively few pediatric endocrine emergencies that present to the ED. Because of the subtleties of many of the signs and symptoms of endocrine disturbances, it is crucial that emergency nurses have a basic knowledge of the anatomy, physiology, and diseases of the endocrine system. Such knowledge provides the nurse with greater confidence regarding the initiation of specific treatment modalities.

TABLE 24.8 Comparison of Thyroid and Adrenal Diseases

Characteristic	*Hypothyroidism*	*Hyperthyroidism (Grave's Disease)*	*Acute Adrenal Insufficiency*
Definition	Clinical state of thyroid hormone insufficiency.	Excessive levels of circulating thyroid hormone; thought to be autoimmune in basis.	Insufficient production of corticosteroids by the adrenal cortex (Saladino, 1997); has three forms: ▪ Primary. ▪ Secondary. ▪ Tertiary.
Incidence/Prevalence	One in 3500 to 4500 births (Bacon et al., 1990, p. 141).	Five to seven times more common in females (Betschart, 2000).	Rare in children, but life-threatening.

Causes	*Acquired:*
	▪ Iodine or radiation exposure.
	▪ Trauma to the neck.
	▪ Neck surgery.
	▪ Viral or (rarely) bacterial infections or neoplasms (Avery & Villee, 1994).
	Congenital:
	▪ Inborn errors of metabolism.
	▪ Autoimmune diseases.
	▪ Maternal ingestion of drugs or toxins while pregnant.
		Congenital:
		▪ Autoimmune disorder.
		▪ Transient congenital hyperthyroidism.
		Acquired:
		▪ Acute, subacute or chronic thyroiditis.
		▪ Thyroid tumors.
		▪ Other tumors.
		▪ Exogenous thyroid hormone excess. (Gotlin, Kappy, Slover, & Zeitler, 1999).
			Congenital:
			▪ Enzymatic defects.
			▪ Hypoplasia.
			▪ Birth defects.
			Acquired:
			▪ Infections, such as:
			  ▪ Waterhouse-Friderichsen syndrome (adrenal hemorrhage).
			  ▪ *Neisseria meningitis*; *Streptococcus pneumoniae*; tuberculosis; histoplasmosis.
			▪ Rapid withdrawal of steroid therapy
			▪ Unusual stress, such as surgery or infection, in a patient taking pharmacologic dosages of glucocortico-steroids (Saladino, 1997).

History	*Congenital:* ▪ Prolonged gestation. ▪ Feeding or sucking difficulties. ▪ Constipation. ▪ Lethargy. ▪ Respiratory problems. *Acquired:* ▪ Decreased appetite. ▪ Cold intolerance.	May be abrupt but is usually slow in developing. The average duration of symptoms prior to treatment is 1 year (Bacon et al., 1990, p. 126). Symptoms are usually noted in children between the ages of 10 and 14 years: ▪ Emotional lability. ▪ Increased sweating with heat intolerance. ▪ Increased appetite with or without weight loss. ▪ Insomnia. ▪ Tremors.	▪ Weakness. ▪ Nausea. ▪ Vomiting. ▪ Diarrhea. ▪ Other historical findings may be consistent with hypoglycemia, hyponatremia, and hypokalemia.
Physical assessment	*Congenital:* ▪ Respiratory distress. ▪ Abdominal distention. ▪ Hypotonia. ▪ Poor peripheral circulation. ▪ Hypothermia.	▪ Persistent tachycardia. ▪ Systolic hypertension with markedly widened pulse pressure. ▪ Mild exophthalmos. ▪ Eyelid retraction and stare. ▪ Tremors. ▪ Warm, moist skin.	▪ Nausea, vomiting, diarrhea, and abdominal pain. ▪ Dehydration leading to circulatory collapse. ▪ Fever initially, followed by hypothermia. ▪ Deteriorating level of consciousness progressing to coma.

(continued)

TABLE 24.8 (continued)

Characteristic	*Hypothyroidism*	*Hyperthyroidism (Grave's Disease)*	*Acute Adrenal Insufficiency*
Physical assessment (continued)	*Acquired:* ■ Goiter. ■ Tenderness of the anterior neck. ■ Weakness. ■ Cool, dry skin.	■ Thyroid "storm": rare occurrence in children. Sudden onset of hyperthermia, severe tachycardia, and restlessness ■ Neurologic status may deteriorate to coma. ■ Death is rare.	
Emergency treatment	*Perform serum analysis:* ■ Thyroxine (T4). ■ Free T4. ■ Thyroid-stimulating hormone levels.	*Serum analysis:* ■ Thyroid function tests. ■ Initiate oral antithyroid medication. ■ Administer propanolol IV, then PO.	■ Maintain airway, breathing, and circulation. ■ Initiate fluid resuscitation with normal saline solution; administer a bolus of 10 to 20 ml/kg over 20 minutes. ■ Administer 25% dextrose at 2 ml/kg if hypoglycemia is present. ■ Monitor cardiac rhythm and vital signs. ■ Obtain blood specimens and monitor for: ■ Hypoglycemia. ■ Hyponatremia. ■ Hyperkalemia. ■ Decreased serum cortisol levels. ■ Acidosis.
Management	Administration of levothyroxine (Synthroid).	■ Activity restrictions. ■ Medications such as propanolol and propyethiouracil. ■ Radiation (controversial). ■ Surgery if medical management is not successful.	Adrenal corticosteroid replacement therapy: ■ Hydrocortisone, 2 mg/kg per dose, every 4 to 6 hours intravenously. ■ Cortisone 1 to 5 mg/kg per 24 hours, divided every 12 to 24 hours to allow tapering of intravenous medications (Barkin & Rosen, 1999).

References

Avery M., & Villee, D. (1994). Endocrine disorders. In M. Avery & D. Villee (Eds.), *Pediatric medicine* (pp. 998–1011). Baltimore: Williams & Wilkins.

Bacon, G., Spencer, M., Hopwood, N., & Kelch, R. (1990). *A practical approach to pediatric endocrinology*. Chicago: Yearbook.

Ball, J. (1998). Endocrine. In J. Ball (Ed.), *Mosby's pediatric patient teaching guides* (pp. E1–E18). St. Louis: Mosby-Year Book.

Barkin, R., & Rosen, P. (1999). *Emergency pediatrics: A guide to ambulatory care* (5th ed., pp. 614–625). St. Louis: Mosby.

Bell, T. (1994). Diabetes insipidus. *Critical Care Nursing Clinics of North America, 6*, 675–684.

Betschart, J. (2000). Endocrine and metabolic diseases. In C. Burns, N. Barber, M. Brady, & A. Dunn, (Eds.), *Pediatric primary care* (pp. 662–688). Philadelphia: Saunders.

Conte, F., & Grumbach, M. (1991). Endocrine disorders. In M. Grossman & R. Dieckmann (Eds.), *Pediatric emergency medicine: A clinician's reference* (pp. 467–473). Philadelphia: Lippincott.

Finegold, D. (1997). Endocrinology. In B. Zitelli & H. Davis (Eds.), *Atlas of pediatric physical diagnosis* (3rd ed., pp. 265–285). St. Louis: Mosby—Year Book.

Gotlin, R., Kappy, M., Slover, R., & Zeitler, P. (1999). Endocrine disorders. In W. Hay, A. Hayward, M. Levin,

J. Sondheimer (Eds.), *Current Pediatric Diagnosis & Treatment* (14th ed). Norwalk, CT: Appleton & Lange.

Huether, S., & Tomky, D. (1998). Alterations of hormonal regulation. In K. McCance & S. Huether (Eds.), *Pathophysiology: The biologic basis for disease in adults and children* (3rd ed., pp. 656–706). St. Louis: Mosby—Year Book.

Primary Children's Medical Center. (2000). *DKA protocol: Emergency department*. Salt Lake City, UT: Author.

Roberts, A. (1995). Systems of life: The endocrine system. *Nursing Times, 91*(37), 33–35.

Saladino, R. (1997). Endocrine and metabolic disorders. In R. Barkin (Ed.), *Pediatric emergency medicine: Concepts and clinical practice* (2nd ed., pp. 755–773). St. Louis: Mosby.

Siberry G., & Iannone, R. (Eds.) (2000). *The Harriet Lane Handbook*. St. Louis: Mosby.

Spence, A. (1990). *Basic human anatomy* (p. 479). Menlo Park, CA: Benjamin/Cummings.

Weissberg-Benchell, J., Glascow, A., Tynan, W., Wirtz, P., Turek, J., & Ward, J. (1995). Adolescent diabetes management and mismanagement. *Diabetes Care, 18*, 77–82.

25

Hematologic and Oncologic Emergencies

Nancy A. Noonan, MS, APRN
Carol Bolinger, RN, MSN, CPNP, CPON
Beth Cohen, RN, MSN, CRNP

Introduction

Hematologic disorders can and do occur both in previously healthy children and in those who have preexisting conditions. The conditions can be congenital (such as sickle cell disease and hemophilia) or acquired (idiopathic thrombocytopenia, disseminated intravascular coagulation, malignancies) and can cause symptoms ranging from minor to life threatening. Nurses working in the emergency department (ED) must to be aware of the assessment and emergency interventions for these disorders. The purpose of this chapter is to address recognition and management of selected hematologic conditions and complications resulting from malignancies and their treatment in children who present to the emergency department.

The hematologic system includes red blood cells (RBCs), white blood cells (WBCs) and platelets. Table 25.1 describes these components and their purposes.

Embryologic Development of the Hematopoietic System

In the early few weeks of embryonic life, primitive nucleated red blood cells are produced in the yolk sac. During the middle trimester of gestation, the liver is the main organ for production of RBCs, although RBCs are also produced by the spleen and lymph nodes. By the time of delivery, the bone marrow is the only significant site of hematopoiesis (Kline & Mooney, 1998).

Production of RBCs is stimulated primarily by the hormone erythropoietin. During periods of hypoxia, erythropoietin stimulates an increase in RBC production. Before birth, erythropoiesis increases because of the relative hypoxia that is present *in utero* (Manley & Bechtel, 1998). During the first week of life, the lungs replace the placenta as the primary source of oxygenation, so erythropoiesis declines. In children with chronic hypoxic states resulting from congenital heart disease, erythropoiesis is continuous.

The production of blood cells, *hematopoiesis*, occurs secondary to the proliferation and differentiation of hematopoietic stem cells of the bone marrow. Stem cells are pluripotent, meaning they may have the potential to develop into many types of blood cells but are not necessarily committed to a specific cell line (McCance, 1998; Oakes & Rosenthal-Dicher, 1998). Eventually they develop a commitment to a specific cell line (unipotential stem cells) and are capable of forming only a particular type of cell in the myeloid or lymphoid line.

Platelets also arise from the pleuripotent stem cells that inhabit the bone marrow. They are necessary for hemostasis and wound healing. Platelets (also called *thrombocytes*) are fragments of a type of myeloid cell found in the bone marrow, the megakaryocyte (Guyton & Hall, 1996).

Pediatric Considerations

Red Blood Cells

The RBCs are most brittle in infants and survive for 60 to 80 days, as compared to 80 to 100 days in a child and 120 to 150 days in an adult. Because of the increase in fragility, anemic episodes are usually more acute in young children than in adults (Manley & Bechtel, 1998).

The bone marrow of essentially all bones produces red blood cells until a child is 5 years of age; but the marrow of long bones, except for the proximal portions of

TABLE 25.1 Comparison of Red Blood Cells, White Blood Cells, and Platelets

Component	*Function*	*Comments*
Red blood cells (erythrocytes)	▪ Transport hemoglobin, which carries oxygen to the lungs and tissues. ▪ Acid-base buffer—responsible for most of the buffering power of whole blood.	Red blood cells have a shorter life span than in the older child and adult: 60–80 days in the neonate, 80–100 days in the child, and 120–150 days in the adult.
White blood cells: ▪ Neutrophils ▪ Eosinophils ▪ Basophils ▪ Monocytes ▪ Lymphocytes ▪ Plasma cells	Mobile units of the body's protective system. They are transported in the blood to areas of serious infection and inflammation, providing a rapid and potent defense against infectious agents. Neutrophils, eosinophils, and basophils are called granulocytes, or "polys," because of multiple nuclei. Granulocytes and monocytes protect the body against invading organisms by phagocytosis. Lymphocytes and plasma cells function in connection with the immune system.	Each type of WBC has a specific function. WBCs have a short life span that is decreased when inflammation or infection is present.
Platelets (thrombocytes)	Platelets are fragments of megakaryocytes found in the bone marrow and function to activate the blood-clotting mechanism.	Platelets survive 7–10 days. About 30,000 platelets are formed each day for each microliter of blood. Normal platelet count is 150,000 to 400,000/mm^3.

Data from: Guyton & Hall, 1996.

the humeri and tibiae, becomes quite fatty and no longer produces red blood cells after about 20 years of age (Guyton & Hall, 1996). After 20 years of age, most red blood cells are produced in the marrow of the membranous bones, such as the vertebrae, sternum, ribs, and ilia.

Under conditions of disease, RBC production can also occur in extramedullary locations such as the spleen (Malatack, Blatt, & Pechansky, 1997). The marrow becomes less productive as age increases.

White Blood Cells

The half-life of WBCs is the same for all ages (except the elderly): 6 to 8 hours in circulating blood and 4 to 9 days in tissues. The infant has an immature immune system that develops as the child matures. The infant has fewer circulating phagocytes as well, leading to a poorer ability to fight infection.

Platelets

Platelets survive 7 to 10 days in all age groups except the elderly. Platelet survival time is decreased in the presence of viral or bacterial infection. The normal platelet count is 150,000 to 400,000 mm^3. A low platelet count (thrombocytopenia) results from either an inadequate production or an increased destruction or consumption of platelets. Causes of thrombocytopenia in children include (Manley & Bectel, 1998):

- Bone marrow failure or suppression.
- Idiopathic thrombocytopenia purpura (ITP).
- Disseminated intravascular coagulation (DIC).
- Leukemia.
- Acute infectious processes.

Focused History

The following history should be obtained for any child with a suspected or known hematologic disorder:

- Recent illnesses, especially history of fever.
- Exposures to infectious diseases or other illnesses.
- Past history, including family history.
- Recent immunizations.
- Events surrounding the current illnesses: onset, duration, and treatment.
- All current medications, including chemotherapy and over-the-counter medications.

Focused Assessment

Physical Assessment

The standard pediatric assessment is done. A hematologic or oncologic disorder can affect many different body systems, so a thorough assessment is necessary. If the child has a known coagulation problem or has undergone chemotherapy, a rectal temperature should not be taken because of the risk of bleeding caused by rectal trauma and by infection. Assessment findings that might indicate a hematologic or oncologic disorder include:

- Pallor.
- Weight loss or poor nutritional status.
- Generalized lymphadenopathy.
- Lack of energy.
- Frequent infections.
- Easy bruising.
- Bleeding that is difficult to control.
- Petechiae.
- Unexplained fever.

A child with a known hematologic or oncologic disorder may also present with pain and anxiety. Because these children are at risk for encephalopathy or intracranial hemorrhage, a thorough neurologic examination should be performed. The child should be assessed for either a totally or partially implanted venous access device, which could be a source of infection.

Psychosocial Assessment

The child and family are often fearful of anticipated procedures, treatment, and hospitalization because of unfamiliarity with or previous experiences in the ED. The following interventions may be helpful:

- Provide emotional support, because hematologic disease may be a chronic illness with the potential for frequent exacerbations.
- Anticipate expressions of concern, anger, and frustration if the child or family is frequently seeking treatment at the emergency department or primary care provider.
- Provide age-appropriate explanations for all procedures and treatments to both the child and family.
- Approach the child in a calm and reassuring manner and allow family members to be with the child.
- Offer age-appropriate distractions (e.g., toys or books) to the child.
- Offer adolescents an opportunity to discuss issues of concern (e.g., social isolation, loss of independence, "difference" from unaffected peers) in a nonjudgmental atmosphere.
- Address complaints of pain promptly and without judgment. Discussion of dependence or addiction to analgesics is not appropriate in the midst of pain.
- The family may come to the hospital frequently and appear demanding because they are familiar with the routine. Allowing them to participate and asking for their suggestions during treatment will be helpful. Consulting with a nurse from an inpatient unit who knows the child might also be helpful.

Triage Decisions

Emergent

- Fever (in a child with a known hematologic or oncologic disorder).
- Severe pain.
- Hypotension.
- Tachycardia.
- Hemorrhage.
- Altered mental status.

Urgent

- Fever; hemodynamically stable.
- Mild to moderate pain.
- Persistent but mild bleeding (no signs of hypovolemia).
- Bleeding into a joint.

Nonurgent

- No signs of active bleeding.
- No complaints of pain.
- Stable vital signs.

Nursing Interventions

Nursing interventions in a child with a suspected or known hematologic condition focus on the airway, breathing, and circulation:

- Maintain the airway.
- Provide oxygen and assist breathing, if necessary.
- Support the circulation. Administer intravenous fluids; stop bleeding.
- Prevent exposure of the immunocompromised child to other children with infectious diseases.
- Support the family and provide information.

Specific interventions for Home Care and Prevention are discussed under each condition.

Nursing diagnoses and expected outcomes are given in Table 25.2.

TABLE 25.2 Nursing Diagnoses and Expected Outcomes

Nursing Diagnoses	*Expected Outcomes*
Pain, related to decreased tissue oxygenation	Pain will be relieved by administration of analgesics or other nonpharmacologic measures.
Altered cerebral, cardiopulmonary, renal, hepatic, gastrointestinal, urinary, and/or splenic tissue perfusion, related to sickled red blood cells or other hematologic dysfunction	Adequate perfusion will be achieved, as evidenced by age-appropriate level of consciousness, vital signs, capillary refill time, warm skin, and urinary output of 0.5–1.0 ml/kg/h.
Fluid volume deficit, related to vomiting, decreased input, or bleeding.	Fluid volume deficit will be corrected by administration of fluids and control of bleeding and vomiting.

Specific Hematologic Emergencies

Sickle Cell Disease

Sickle cell disease (SCD) is a generic term used to describe an entire group of symptomatic disorders, the clinical, hematologic, and pathologic features of which are related to the presence of hemoglobin S (HbS). Although SCD is sometimes used to refer to sickle cell anemia (SCA), the terms are not interchangeable. Sickle cell anemia is one of a group of disease states collectively referred to as *hemoglobinopathies*. Sickle cell anemia is a disorder involving a predominance of HbS, when normal hemoglobin (hemoglobin A [HbA]) is partially or completely replaced by HbS. Other terms for SCA are *HbSS* and *homozygous sickle cell disease* (Kline & Mooney, 1998).

Sickle cell disease is an inherited disorder primarily affecting African-Americans; however, it is also seen in individuals of Mediterranean, Indian, and Middle Eastern descent. In the United States, SCD is most commonly observed in African-Americans and Hispanics from the Caribbean, Central America, and parts of South America (Kline & Mooney, 1998).

There appears to be a geographic variable in the incidence of SCD. Among African-Americans the incidence of sickle cell trait is 7 to 13%, whereas among East Africans, the incidence is as high as 45% (Kline & Mooney, 1998). It is thought that the sickle trait is a protective mechanism against the lethal forms of malaria in the endemic zones of the Mediterranean and Africa.

Pathophysiology

Sickle cell disease is an inherited, autosomal-recessive disorder. Depending on the mode of inheritance, the disease may be manifested in the following patterns:

- *Sickle cell anemia:* the homozygous form of the disease, HbSS. It is the most severe form of SCD.
- *Sickle cell trait:* the heterozygous form of the disease, HbA and either HbS or HbAS. It is referred to as the *carrier state* of sickle cell anemia. This form rarely exhibits clinical manifestations of SCD except when a child is extremely hypoxic.
- *Sickle cell—hemoglobin C disease*: a heterozygous variant of SCD, including both HbS and HbC or HbD.
- *Sickle cell—thalassemia disease*: a combination of sickle cell trait and beta-thalassemia trait.

When both parents possess the sickle cell trait (HbAS), there is a 25% chance of their producing an offspring with SCA. In the United States, it is estimated that the frequency of SCA is one per 400–500 in newborn African-Americans (Kline & Mooney, 1998).

The sickling of erythrocytes is secondary to a defect in the globin fraction of hemoglobin, which is composed of greater than 500 amino acids. The substitution of the amino acid, valine, for glutamic acid in the beta chains of the hemoglobin molecule is the basic defect of SCD. This structural change facilitates the sickling predisposition of HbS (Guyton & Hall, 1996).

In deoxygenated, dehydrated, hypoxic, and/or acidotic conditions, the HbS molecule assumes an irregular, "sickled" (crescent moon-shaped) appearance. This sickled shape is associated with increased blood viscosity. Increased blood viscosity impedes flow and further contributes to deoxygenation. Tissue deoxygenation continues and spreads, eventually leading to obstruction within the microcirculation, precipitating tissue ischemia, infarcts, and necrosis, if left untreated.

The clinical features of SCD are the results of obstruction caused by the sickled red blood cells and increased destruction of sickled and normal red blood cells caught in microcirculation obstructions. Chronic hemolytic anemia is present, subject to periods of acute exacerbation precipitated by dehydration, hypoxia, infection, and/or stress. The sickling, known as *sickle cell crisis*, may manifest in one or a combination of the following scenarios (Kline & Mooney, 1998):

- Vasocclusive crises: The dominant and most debilitating clinical complications associated with SCD may lead to permanent damage to any organ. There is marked variation in clinical presentation and course:
  - Acute chest syndrome: Identified as the leading cause of death and hospitalization among patients with SCD (Vichinsky et al., 2000), the cause is largely unknown and treatment is supportive. Pulmonary emboli develop, with or without concomitant infection. May present with respiratory distress and pain, and progress to respiratory failure.
  - Aplastic crisis: There is an acute, but transient, decrease in the rate of red cell production in the bone marrow. This crisis may be precipitated by infection with Human Parvovirus-19 (Fifth Disease) (Iannone, 2001). This severe anemia may spontaneously develop within hours and is a major cause of death during the first 5 years of life.
  - Cerebral stroke: Cerebral infarction causes a varied presentation of neurologic compromise.
  - Dactylitis (Hand-Foot syndrome): Characterized by pain and swelling of the soft tissue of the hands and feet of young children (6 months to 2 years of age). Seen less frequently in older children after the bone marrow of the small bones of the hands and feet loses hematopoietic activity.
  - Priapism (prolonged, painful, unrelieved penile erection): Penile erection that may persist for hours and cause severe discomfort.
  - Hyperhemolytic crisis: The rate of hemolysis is greater than normal.
  - Splenic sequestration crisis: Seen only in the young child, this crisis occurs as the spleen acutely pools large quantities of blood. The spleen can hold as much as one-fifth of the body's blood supply at one time (Kline & Mooney, 1998). Up to 50% mortality has been reported due to precipitous hypotension, poor perfusion, and ultimate cardiovascular collapse.
- Infection:
  - Children with SCD are at high-risk for infections with *Streptococcus pneumoniae*, *Haemophilus influenzae*, and, less commonly, *Staphylococcus aureus* and *Mycoplasma pneumoniae*.
  - Defective splenic function appears to be a major factor in susceptibility to infection.
  - After splenic engorgement occurs, the spleen becomes incapable of normal reticuloendothelial function and may become small, fibrotic, and ineffective.
- Pain crisis:
  - The pathophysiology of sickle cell disease precipitates moderate to severe pain secondary to the ischemia and compromised microcirculation and, at times, general circulation.
  - It is not uncommon for a child to present in the emergency department with generalized complaints of pain and localization of specifically painful areas.
  - Children old enough to understand the pathophysiology and treatment of their condition may also be able to verbalize a request for a specific analgesic and analgesic dose that has worked for them in previous visits or admissions to the hospital.

Focused History

Children with SCD may experience various complications of their illness that may result in a visit to the emergency department. The following history should be obtained:

- Past history:
  - Family history of sickle cell disease.
  - Newborn screening results yet unknown, although most children younger than 6 months of age do not present ill secondary to their high percentage of hemoglobin F.
  - Past hospitalizations.
  - Infections.
  - Failure to thrive.
  - Jaundice.
  - Anemia.
  - Previous sickling crisis.
  - Painful joints.
  - Use of penicillin. (Children with SCA often receive penicillin prophylaxis.)
- Present illness:
  - Dactylitis: Painful swelling of hands and feet present for up to 2 weeks before spontaneously resolving.
  - Joint pain.
  - Chest pain.
  - Infection: Fever, pain, malaise, and compromised activity.
  - Abdominal pain.
  - Headache.
  - Nausea or vomiting.

Focused Assessment

- Airway and breathing: Frequent assessment is essential to identify signs and symptoms of respiratory insufficiency because of the patient's increased susceptibility to infection and potential for acute chest crisis:
  - Increased respiratory rate (per age-appropriate baseline).
  - Increased respiratory effort (retractions, flaring).
  - Decreased oxygen saturation (< 90%).
  - Compromised chest expansion and complaints of chest pain (or abdominal pain—referred chest pain).
- Circulation: Findings of septic and/or hypovolemic shock can be present in forms of vasocclusive crisis and overwhelming infection:
  - Increased heart rate.
  - Hypotensive or normal blood pressure.
  - Decreased peripheral pulses.
  - Prolonged capillary refill time.
  - Pallor.
  - Cool extremities.
  - Increased respiratory rate or effort.
  - Poor urinary output and/or altered level of consciousness.
- Disability: Altered level of consciousness.
- Presence of pain: Investigate location, type, and intensity of pain (general and localized):
  - Evaluate joints for signs and symptoms of sickling: swollen, erythematous, painful, decreased range of motion; limping, changes in gait, and/or paresis.
  - Evaluate for abdominal tenderness (guarding and rebound pain), hepatosplenomegaly, and vomiting, because these findings may be indicative of sickling in mesenteric or abdominal organ microcirculation. Pain in the left upper quadrant may also be indicative of sequestration crisis secondary to splenic congestion.
  - Evaluate for priapism, which is reflective of obstructed microcirculation within groin.
- Hydration status. Monitor for signs of inadequate perfusion:
  - Altered level of consciousness.
  - Increased heart and respiratory rate (per baseline).
  - Hypotensive or normal blood pressure.
  - Decreased peripheral pulses.
  - Prolonged capillary refill time.
  - Cool extremities.
  - "Tacky" mucous membranes in infants.
  - Pallor.
  - Decreased urinary output.
- Eyes: Evaluate for the presence of increased scleral icterus (jaundice). Ask the parent or caregiver to describe how the eyes normally look, because these children may typically exhibit some jaundice.

Nursing Interventions

- Ensure airway patency.
- Provide supplemental oxygen in a manner acceptable to the child.
- Initiate intravenous access for administration of crystalloid and/or colloid intravenous fluids:
  - Crystalloid fluid resuscitation is followed by administration of one and one-half to two times maintenance rate.
  - Colloid replacement with 10 to 15 ml/kg of red blood cells may be indicated during aplastic or hemolytic crises.
- Administer analgesics and evaluate effectiveness:
  - Acetaminophen may be effective for mild pain.
  - Opiates will be necessary for moderate to severe pain.
  - The use of aspirin is contraindicated in children with G6PD deficiency.
- Administer antibiotics after obtaining blood and/or urinary cultures if infection is suspected.
- Immobilize and support painful joints.

Home Care and Prevention

- Discuss preventive strategies with family:
  - Ensure adequate fluid intake.
  - Avoid high altitude or an abrupt change to high altitude.
  - Avoid stressful situations.
  - Avoid cold stress.
  - Observe for signs and symptoms of infection and promptly initiate medical treatment.
- Encourage compliance with prophylactic antibiotic regimens.
- Promote compliance with all immunizations, including *Haemophilus influenzae*.
- Encourage age-appropriate behavior to avoid unnecessary trauma.
- Ensure that the child has a primary care provider for follow-up and routine care.
- Encourage the child and family to carry a medical information card.

TABLE 25-3 Characteristics of Hemophilia

Characteristic	*Hemophilia A*	*Hemophilia B*	*Hemophilia C*	*von Willebrand's Disease*
Factor deficiency	Factor VIII	Factor IX	Factor XI	vWF* Factor VIII
Inheritance	X-linked recessive: carried by mother and expressed in son.	X-linked recessive: carried by mother and expressed in son.	Autosomal recessive: expressed equally in males and females.	Numerous types: • Types I and II: autosomal dominant. • Type III: autosomal recessive. • Occurs in both males and females.
Symptoms	Symptoms may be mild, moderate, or severe, depending on factor levels.	Same as hemophilia A.	Bleeding is less severe than in hemophilia A or hemophilia B.	• Symptoms may be mild, moderate, or severe, depending on subgroup; Type I is associated with mild symptoms.

*vWF is a specific clotting protein that normally helps platelets adhere to the wall of a disrupted blood vessel.

Hemophilia

Until 1952, the term *hemophilia* was used exclusively to describe the bleeding disorder resulting from lack of factor VIII. *Hemophilia* is the term now used to collectively describe 90 to 95% of three distinct bleeding disorders resulting from deficiencies of factors VIII, IX, and XI. In this chapter, *hemophilia* will refer to hemophilia A and hemophilia B. Clinically, hemophilia A and B appear identical; diagnostic differentiation is dependent on laboratory testing. However, the treatment of these disorders is different.

Hemophilia is the most common inherited coagulation bleeding disorder (Cohen, 2000). The incidence of hemophilia is about 1 in 5,000 males, 85% being hemophilia A, and 15% hemophilia B. In about two-thirds of cases, a positive family history is present (Radel, 2001).

Pathophysiology

Table 25.3 compares the pathophysiology of the different types of hemophilia and the symptoms associated with each type.

Patients with hemophilia (A and B) are categorized by their potential to experience bleeding based on the amount of factor deficiency. Table 25.4 lists the descriptions of these classifications.

Partial thromboplastin time is prolonged in hemophilia. All other coagulation tests, prothrombin time, bleeding, and platelet count should be normal.

Patients with hemophilia often present during the newborn period at the time of circumcision, which results in prolonged bleeding (Malatack et al., 1997). Associated manifestations may include prolonged cord bleeding or the presence of cephalahematoma. As the child gets older, tooth eruption may cause submucosal hematomas to develop. With increasing mobility, the toddler may develop more than the usual amount of bruising. The presence of bruising is unusual on the buttocks, however. Child abuse should be suspected if this is present (Chapter 46).

Hemarthrosis, or bleeding into the joints, is the most common complication of hemophilia. Most commonly seen in the knees, elbows, and ankles, hemarthrosis causes pain and limitation of mobility, and predisposes the child to degenerative joint changes (Kline & Mooney, 1998). Intracranial bleeding or hemorrhage into the neck or abdomen can be life-threatening.

Focused History

- Past history:
  - Bleeding.

TABLE 25.4 Hemophilia Factor Level and Bleeding Severity

Classification	*Active Factor VIII*	*Potential for Bleeding*
Severe	<1%	May bleed spontaneously.
Moderate	1–5%	Bleed with mild trauma.
Mild	6–50%	Bleed with severe trauma or surgery.

- Trauma.
- Pain.
- Family history of bleeding disorders.
- Coagulopathy.
- Thrombocytopenia.
- Previous diagnosis of hemophilia.

- Present illness:
  - Manifested by hemarthroses and hematoma formation with minimal or no trauma (Radel, 2001).
  - Prolonged bleeding.
  - Spontaneous bleeding.
  - Easy bruising.
  - Hematuria.
  - Pain and swelling in joints.

Focused Assessment

- Airway and breathing:
  - The airway of a child experiencing bleeding as a result of hemophilia is intact unless the airway, oral cavity, chest, or neck is involved.
  - Tachypnea may be observed if the child is hypovolemic.
  - Spontaneous epistaxis is a relatively common finding.
- Circulation: Findings of hypovolemic shock can be present during overwhelming bleeding episodes.
- Neurologic system: Neurologic findings may indicate a variety of neurologic insults.
  - Altered level of consciousness, seizures, and headache may be observed in a patient with an intracranial bleed.
  - Paralysis, weakness, back pain, and asymmetric responses to a neurologic examination may be observed in a patient with a spinal cord hematoma.
- Gastrointestinal system:
  - In young children with hemophilia, bleeding in the oral cavity is relatively common, secondary to tooth eruption and injury from the bumps or falls from learning to crawl and walk. By the age of 3 to 4 years, 90% of hemophiliac children have experienced bleeding from relatively minor traumatic lacerations to the lip or tongue (Kline & Mooney, 1998).
  - Frank hemorrhage from the gastrointestinal tract is rarely severe (Cohen, 2000). A child who has swallowed blood from an oral bleeding episode may demonstrate hematemesis, melena, and nausea.
- Genitourinary system:
  - Non-traumatic painless hematuria is the most common manifestation of renal bleeding. If a child has experienced trauma, renal damage may present as frank hematuria.
  - Prolonged bleeding from circumcision may be the defining event for the diagnosis of hemophilia in an infant.
- Skin:
  - Subcutaneous bleeding, evidenced by ecchymosis and hematomas, is a common finding. Observe these lesions for changes in size and tenderness because an increase in either parameter may be indicative of continued bleeding.
  - Subcutaneous bleeding in the neck may be indicative of bleeding that could compromise the child's airway.
- Musculoskeletal system:
  - Hemarthrosis commonly occurs in moderate to severe hemophilia.
  - Signs of hemarthrosis in the affected joints range from tenderness to severe pain; fullness to marked edema; decreased range of motion to refusal to move joint; gait changes in the lower extremities to a limp.

Nursing Interventions

- Ensure airway patency:
  - Gently clear airway to prevent further trauma.
  - Assist with insertion of an artificial airway, if necessary, in life-threatening airway-bleeding episodes.
  - Provide supplemental oxygen in a manner acceptable to the child.
- Replace fluid volume deficits with crystalloid and/or colloid fluids.
- Administer missing coagulation factors and monitor for side effects and efficacy of factor replacement therapy:
  - *Hemophilia A:* Factor VIII via factor VIII concentrate, cryoprecipitate (factor VIII and fibrinogen), or fresh frozen plasma.
  - *Hemophilia B:* Factor IX via factor IX concentrate or fresh frozen plasma.
- Promote comfort via administration of analgesics and evaluate their effectiveness.
- Treat hemarthroses:
  - Provide rest, cold, immobilization, and elevation of affected joints.
  - Provide analgesia.
  - Avoid aspirin and salicylate-containing medications.

Home Care and Prevention

- Encourage child to wear medical alert identification.
- Ensure that parents are capable of understanding and executing instructions:
  - Parents should understand the risk for bleeding.
  - Parents can modify activities based on bleeding potential.
  - Parents can promptly recognize bleeding episodes and ensure access to interventions to control or arrest them.
  - "Watchful waiting" applies if there is a joint pain or swelling but is *not* appropriate for the child who has hemophilia (Radel, 2001).
- Develop a plan of home treatment of minor bleeding episodes in conjunction with primary care provider and supporting agencies.

Immune Thrombocytopenic Purpura

Immune thrombocytopenic purpura (ITP) is a relatively common pediatric disorder characterized by a sudden onset of profound thrombocytopenia in an otherwise healthy child. ITP is a disorder of platelet consumption, in which antiplatelet antibodies bind to the plasma membranes of platelets. This leads to platelet sequestration and destruction by phagocytes at a rate that exceeds the ability of the bone marrow to produce them (Kline & Mooney, 1998). The classic presentation of ITP occurs in children one to four weeks after a viral infection, with acute onset of petechial rash and bruising. Mucocutaneous bleeding, epistaxis, and hematuria can also be presenting symptoms. The child will otherwise appear well.

Immune thrombocytopenic purpura can be acute or chronic; for the purposes of clarification, this discussion will refer to the acute form.

Fortunately, spontaneous remission of ITP occurs. In general, about 60% of children recover in 4 to 6 weeks (Warrier et al., 1997) and more than 90% recover within 3 to 6 months of onset of symptoms (George et al., 1996).

Immune thrombocytopenic purpura occurs most frequently in children between the ages of 2 and 5 years and there is no gender predominance (Imbach, Kuhne, & Holländer, 1997). Viral illnesses have been hypothesized as the possible inciting stimulus for the development of platelet autoantibodies.

Pathophysiology

Immune response (involving the level of regulation and self-tolerance) may be altered in the presence of an inflammatory reaction. This alteration in immune response may result in the creation of autoantibodies (self-generated and directed) that attack platelets and precipitate thrombocytopenia and the resulting clinical signs and symptoms. The spleen plays a major role in the removal of the antibody-platelet complexes and often can be enlarged and exhibit overactive reticuloendothelial activity.

Focused History

- Past history: Treatment for ITP.
- Present illness:
  - Abrupt onset of mucocutaneous bleeding in a previously healthy child, with or without epistaxis.
  - Recent viral infection.
  - Current medication usage.

Focused Assessment

- Airway and breathing: The airway of a child experiencing bleeding from ITP is intact unless the airway or oral cavity is bleeding profusely.
  - Mucocutaneous lesions in the oral cavity rarely compromise the airway.
  - Tachypnea may be observed if circulation is compromised as a result of hypovolemia in overwhelming bleeding episodes.
  - Spontaneous epistaxis is also a relatively common finding.
- Circulation: Findings of hypovolemic shock can be present during serious hemorrhage. These symptoms have been listed previously.
- Neurologic system: Headaches, seizures, or altered level of consciousness may be indicative of an intracranial bleed (rare).
- Gastrointestinal system: Hemorrhagic bullae of the gums, lips, and other mucous membranes may be present, leading to melena.
- Genitourinary system: Hematuria is an occasional finding.
- Skin: Asymmetric bleeding is typical, with petechiae, purpura, and ecchymoses found over the trunk and bony prominences in the absence of trauma.

Nursing Interventions

- Ensure airway patency and provide supplemental oxygen in a manner acceptable to the child.
- Provide fluid for volume deficit:
  - Administer crystalloid to restore fluid volume.

- Administer platelets only in life-threatening bleeding situations (intracranial hemorrhage).
- Administer packed red bloods cells only if fluid crystalloid resuscitation is unsuccessful in restoring fluid volume or if hemorrhage is severe.

- Apply ice and gentle pressure to the bleeding site, as appropriate.
- Provide comfort measures and information to the child and family to decrease anxiety.
- Administer medications, as ordered:
  - Considerable controversy exists on the most appropriate intervention for non–life-threatening bleeding.
  - A range of therapies may be offered, including administration of oral or intravenous steroids; administration of intravenous immunoglobulin; observation without intervention.

Home Care and Prevention

- Address knowledge deficits and clarify misconceptions:
  - Injury prevention for patients with low platelet levels: Restrict activities to avoid trauma, particularly head injury (e.g., avoid bicycle riding, roller blading, and contact sports, and/or wear a protective helmet during activity). Avoid administering intramuscular injections. Reinforce use of soft toothbrush or sponge toothettes for oral hygiene to minimize oral bleeding.
  - Avoid aspirin and aspirin-containing products, as well as nonsteroidal anti-inflammatory medications.
- Explain follow-up care. Refer to primary care physician.
- Provide child and family with resources: ITP Society (http://www.ultranet.com/~itpsoc/chlddrft.htm), an organization within the Children's Blood Foundation.

Disseminated Intravascular Coagulation

Disseminated intravascular coagulation (DIC) is an *acquired* hemorrhagic syndrome, characterized by uncontrolled formation and deposition of fibrin thrombi and resulting in consumption of clotting factors, which lead to uncontrolled bleeding.

In the oncology population, DIC can result from:

- Acute nonlymphocytic leukemia (also known as *ANLL/AML*).
- Acute promyelocytic leukemia (APML).
- Intravascular lysis: acute tumor lysis syndrome.

In oncology patients and in the general pediatric population, DIC can also result from:

- Infection or sepsis: (Gram-positive and/or Gram-negative organisms).
- Hypoxemia or hypoperfusion (e.g., cardiac arrest).

Pathophysiology

Disseminated intravascular coagulation is a "consumptive disorder" caused by abnormal activation of the clotting mechanism, resulting in rapid depletion of platelets, prothrombin, and fibrinogen. It is a pathologic syndrome resulting from the formation of thrombin, subsequent activation and consumption of certain coagulant proteins, and production of fibrin thrombi. Disseminated intravascular coagulation manifests itself via diffuse microvascular coagulation secondary to depletion of clotting factors, resulting in impaired hemostasis (Buchanan, 1997; Cahill-Alsip & McDermott, 1996; Rohaly-Davis, & Johnston, 1996; Mansen, McCance, & Field, 1998).

Focused History

- Present illness:
  - Bleeding from single or multiple sites.
  - Dizziness, weakness.
  - Rash: petechiae, ecchymosis.
- Past and current medical history:
  - Neoplasm.
  - Repeated blood transfusions.
  - Myelosuppression secondary to chemotherapy.
  - Medications, including anticoagulants and aspirin.

Focused Assessment

1. Airway and breathing:
   - Signs and symptoms consistent with hypovolemia, hemorrhage, and/or sepsis may be present.
   - The airway may be subject to compromise from compression of soft tissue secondary to bleeding of the neck, oral cavity, and chest:
     - Increased respiratory rate and effort (retractions or flaring).
     - Cyanosis.
     - Hemoptysis, nasopharyngeal bleeding, or epistaxis.
     - Pulmonary hemorrhage.
2. Circulation: Signs and symptoms consistent with cardiovascular compromise secondary to hypovolemic and/or septic shock may be present:
   - Increased heart rate.
   - Hypotension or normal blood pressure.
   - ST segment changes on the electrocardiogram.

- Cool, mottled extremities.
- Decreased peripheral pulses.
- Prolonged capillary refill time.
- Acrocyanosis.

3. Neurologic system: Signs and symptoms consistent with altered perfusion and/or cerebral bleeding may be present:
   - Restlessness or change in mood or affect.
   - Confusion or disorientation.
   - Alteration in level of consciousness, headache, and/or seizures.
4. Gastrointestinal/genitourinary system:
   - Melena or frank GI bleeding.
   - Oliguria or anuria.
   - Hematuria; urethral bleeding.
   - Flank pain (secondary to deposition of renal microvascular fibrin).
5. Skin:
   - Petechiae.
   - Purpura.
   - Ecchymosis.
   - Oozing from venipuncture sites; wound hematoma.
   - Pallor.
6. Musculoskeletal system:
   - Severe muscle pain secondary to ischemia.
   - Decreased range of motion in areas with active bleeding.

Nursing Interventions

- Monitor vital signs and assess for shock.
- Maintain airway patency and provide supplemental oxygen in a manner tolerable to the child.
- Establish intravenous access for administration of crystalloid and/or colloid fluids.
- Maintain adequate hydration to prevent renal failure (secondary to hemoglobinuria).
- Monitor:
  - Tissue perfusion, including color, temperature, capillary refill, and peripheral pulses.
  - Overt or covert bleeding: urine, stool, emesis, and needle puncture sites.
  - Laboratory values: fibrinogen, prothrombin time, partial thromboplastic time, d-dimer assay, hemoglobin, hematocrit, and platelet count.
  - Urinary output.
- Administer blood products as ordered. IV Heparin infusion may be indicated.
- Protect the child from further injury: Handle gently, avoid repeated venipunctures or invasive measures, decrease environmental stimuli, and promote rest.
- Monitor therapeutic response of precipitating conditions.

Home Care and Prevention

- Monitor the patient with APML for potential development of DIC. Early intervention may decrease morbidity.
- Recognize early signs and symptoms of shock and seek prompt treatment.

Specific Oncologic Emergencies

Annually, 139 individuals per million in the population younger than the age of 15 are diagnosed with a malignancy (Landis, Murray, Bolden, & Wingo, 1998). The most common pediatric malignancy is acute lymphoblastic leukemia, followed by tumors of the central nervous system. Pediatric cases account for only about 2% of all cancers. Pediatric cancer is the second-leading cause of death in children in this age group. Overall, 72% of these children will enjoy a long-term, disease-free survival after effective treatment. By the year 2000, it was estimated that 1 in every 900 adults between the ages of 15 and 45 years is an adult survivor of childhood cancer (Bleyer, 1990).

The majority of children with cancer are treated by a tertiary care center with a pediatric department dedicated to their care. When complications arise, they do not always present to the center providing their therapy. This presents emergency departments around the country with the challenge of caring for children whose current treatment is unknown.

The anticancer therapy selected depends on the disease process. Most therapies include a combination of multiagent chemotherapy, radiation, and surgery. Each of these treatments carries known toxicities and morbidity. Escalating-dose chemotherapeutic agents, known to cause cytopenias, metabolic imbalance, nausea, and vomiting, have improved long-term, disease-free survival. Side effects caused by increased doses of chemotherapy are a frequent cause for presentation to the ED.

Patients who are unaware of an underlying malignancy or who have progressive disease may present with compression or obstruction of vital organ structures. These instances represent emergent situations for patients. The purpose of this section is to describe the effects of malignancies (mechanical, systemic, hematopoietic, renal, metabolic) and specific conditions that are side effects of chemotherapy and ED considerations. The pertinent history and assessment findings are summarized under each condition.

Mechanical Effects of Malignancy

Superior Vena Cava Syndrome and Superior Mediastinal Syndrome

Superior vena cava syndrome (SVCS) refers to the signs and symptoms of compression or obstruction of the superior vena cava. *Superior mediastinal syndrome* (SMS), which occurs more frequently in children, refers to compression on the trachea resulting from the presence of a mediastinal mass. The trachea and bronchus in children are relatively rigid, compared to the superior vena cava, but may be compressed by a mediastinal mass. The relatively small intraluminal diameter of the child's trachea does not accommodate much compromise before the child begins to exhibit symptoms of respiratory distress.

The most common cause of SVCS is compression secondary to:

- Thrombosis after cardiovascular surgery for congenital heart disease.
- Shunting for hydrocephalus.
- Thrombosis caused by central venous catheters, especially implanted venous access devices (Merrill, 2000).

Malignant tumors are the most common primary cause of SVCS and SMS in children. Tumors that may present in the mediastinum, causing SMS, include:

- Leukemia.
- Non-Hodgkin's lymphoma.
- Neuroblastoma.
- Hodgkin's disease.

Nonmalignant causes of SMS may include infectious processes such as histoplasmosis or granuloma.

ED Considerations

Symptoms arising from malignancy often have a rapid, insidious course because of the doubling time of tumors responsible for SMS. Patients will often present with a brief history of increasing respiratory compromise, including cough, hoarseness, dyspnea, orthopnea, and chest pain.

Assessment findings may include swelling, plethora, and cyanosis of the face, neck, and upper extremities; engorged vessels of the chest wall; erythema and edema of the conjunctiva; diaphoresis; coughing and wheezing; chest pain; headache; and visual changes (Hinkle & Schwartz, 2001).

Care is focused on supporting the airway, breathing, and circulation. Patients with a new or progressive mediastinal neoplasm will be admitted for observation, diagnosis, supportive care, and initiation of therapy.

Presentation of SVCS related to thrombosis is treated with fibrinolytic therapy, along with anticoagulation.

Spinal Cord Compression

Spinal cord compression occurs as a result of rapid tumor growth within or surrounding the spinal column.

Spinal cord compression develops in approximately 5 to 10% of patients with cancer. It is the second most common neuroligic complication of cancer, surpassed only by brain metastases (Camp-Sorrell, 1998). Although spinal cord compression occurs infrequently in children, cord compression must be ruled out in children with cancer who present with a complaint of back pain.

Of children presenting with true cord compression, the primary diagnosis is most commonly Ewing's sarcoma (18%), neuroblastoma (8%), lymphoma (2%), and leukemia. Many pediatric solid tumors may result in cord compression, including Wilm's tumor, osteosarcoma, and rhabdomyosarcoma.

ED Considerations

Rapid recognition, evaluation, and treatment of spinal cord compression may prevent permanent neurologic complications. Pain is the most common complaint (80%) in children experiencing cord compression.

The pain may be local, described as a dull ache, or radicular, which may be constant or initiated with movement (Merrill, 2000).

Progression may be rapid or variable, depending on the underlying disease process. Cord compression should be a high consideration for any child with back pain until the cause is proven to be otherwise.

Assessment findings include:

- Localized tenderness to percussion in affected area.
- Unilateral or bilateral muscle weakness.
- Increased or decreased tendon reflexes.
- Loss of sensation, numbness, or paresthesias.
- Later symptoms may include loss of bowel function or bladder control.

Treatment must be immediate and aggressive to prevent further impairment of permanent loss of function. Nursing measures are mainly supportive in maintaining airway, breathing, and circulation and observing for progression of symptoms. IV access for administration of high-dose corticosteroids should be initiated.

Systemic Manifestations of Malignancy

Acute Tumor Lysis Syndrome

Tumor lysis syndrome (TLS) is an oncologic emergency resulting from the massive necrosis of rapidly dividing tumor cells, usually due to administration of combination chemotherapy. TLS may occur prior to the diagnosis of cancer, but occurs most frequently during the initial phase of treatment while the child is hospitalized. Laboratory findings include hypocalcemia, hyperuricemia, hyperkalemia, hyperphosphatemia, azotemia, and metabolic acidosis. Acute renal failure can result from the precipitation of uric acid, xanthine, and phosphate in the renal tubules. Severe renal dysfunction may further develop if the patient is experiencing dehydration and oliguria (Woodwood & Hogan, 1996).

Tumor types that commonly result in TLS include Burkitt's lymphoma and T-cell leukemia lymphoma. Either of these malignancies can present with a large intra-abdominal component, representing a large tumor "burden." Patients with rapidly growing chemotherapy-sensitive malignancies, such as myelogenous leukemias or solid tumors, may also be at risk for TLS (Woodward & Hogan, 1996).

Rapid cellular death is characterized by the release of intracellular contents. Intracellular components (uric acid, phosphorus, and potassium) are normally excreted by the kidney. Patients with inadequate renal function are unable to excrete ample amounts of these salts. Formation of uric acid crystals in the renal collecting duct or calcium phosphate precipitates in the microvasculature of the kidney may result in renal failure. Hypocalcemia may cause seizures. Hyperkalemia may result in ventricular arrhythmia and death.

ED Considerations

The child may present to the ED with complaints of abdominal pain or fullness, back pain, change in the amount of urine production, shortness of breath, fatigue, pallor, and bruising. Assessment findings include abdominal fullness, decreased urinary output, hypoxia, adenopathy; petechiae, hyperkalemia, uremia, hyperphosphatemia, and hypocalcemia. Treatment includes:

- Hyperhydration with intravenous sodium bicarbonate fluids to provide urinary alkalinization.
- Monitoring of urine for crystal deposits and pH. An indwelling bladder catheter is necessary.
- Analysis of blood for uric acid potassium, calcium, and phosphorus.
- Administration of oral allopurinol to decrease uric acid production.

The child will be admitted for ongoing management and diagnosis of underlying disease.

Hyperleukocytosis

Hyperleukocytosis occurs when a peripheral white blood cell count is greater than 100,000 cells/mm^3. Hyperleukocytosis can cause death secondary to central nervous system hemorrhage, pulmonary leukostasis with respiratory failure, central nervous system thrombosis, or metabolic change secondary to tumor lysis syndrome.

Hyperleukocytosis occurs in previously well children with a short duration of nonspecific complaints. Hyperleukocytosis is seen in 10% of patients with acute lymphocytic leukemia, 20% of patients with acute nonlymphocytic leukemia, and 100% of patients with chronic myelogenous leukemia in the acute phase (Wilson, 1998). Cytopenias frequently accompany these diagnoses of leukemia, further contributing to metabolic abnormalities and blood coagulopathies.

The viscosity of the blood is increased in patients with hyperleukocytosis because of the presence of white blood cell aggregates and thrombin in the microcirculation. Myeloblasts, responsible for acute myelogenous leukemia, are relatively large. The blast cells are not easily deformable and do not pass readily through the microvasculature, resulting in thrombi. Their anaerobic metabolism contributes to lactic acidosis. The blasts, trapped in the microvasculature of the brain or pulmonary parenchyma, may degenerate and release intracellular contents, resulting in tissue damage. Tumor lysis syndrome, described in the previous section, occurs when the cells release their intracellular contents.

ED Considerations

Clinical signs can include dyspnea, tachypnea, blurred vision, agitation, confusion, or stupor. Assessment findings include hypoxia, cyanosis, papilledema, ataxia, and a white blood cell count greater than 100,000 cells/mm^3 (Wilson, 1998).

Nursing interventions include:

- Initiation of venous access—hyperhydration and alkalinization:
  - Assess the patient's urine output and pH.
- Blood product support (exchange transfusions, platelets), as well as leukopheresis and chemotherapy administration.
- Monitoring of blood gases and chemistries.
- Ongoing neurologic assessment.

- Admission for further diagnostic evaluation and treatment.

Hematopoietic Effects of Malignancy

Infections are the leading cause of morbidity related to treatment in the pediatric oncology population (Frenck, Kohn, & Pickering, 1991; Weintraub, 1993). A number of coexisting conditions contribute to the increased risk of infection:

- Treatment-related alterations in taste, nausea, vomiting, and food aversion contribute to compromised nutritional status and depleted protein stores.
- Impaired chemotaxis, a defective macrophage-monocyte system, and immunologic dysfunction result from chemotherapy and steroid administration as well as disease.
- The presence of an indwelling venous catheter further compromises the patient's status by providing an additional portal of entry for bacteria.
- Neutropenia (discussed in the next section).

Neutropenia

The greatest risk factor for development of infection is treatment-related neutropenia—an absolute neutrophil count less than 500. Patients receiving marrow-suppressive chemotherapy develop treatment-related myelosuppression approximately 7 to 10 days after administration. The duration and degree of neutropenia are known risk factors for the development of infection. Neutropenia lasting greater than 10 to 14 days and/or an absolute neutrophil count of less than 500 cells/mm^3 greatly increase the risk of infection. The greatest source of bacterial infection is the patient's own microbial flora.

Radiation therapy may have an impact on the production of white blood cells, red blood cells, and platelets. In young children, marrow production occurs primarily in the bones of the extremities. As children mature, marrow production becomes more central. Lymphocytes are exquisitely sensitive to radiation. Irradiation directly to an area of marrow production has the greatest effect. Cells that pass through the area of radiation during treatment are also affected. The effect on platelet count is variable.

The life span of circulating white blood cells is approximately 6 to 8 hours. When bone marrow production is interrupted by cytotoxic chemotherapy, a brief period of neutropenia develops. Neutropenia may be minimized by the administration of granulocyte colony-stimulating factor (G-CSF), a cytokine responsible for the stimulation of granulocyte development. When given after chemotherapy or bone marrow transplantations, G-CSF enhances neutrophil recovery and thus reduces the risk of infections (Naparstek, 1995).

ED Considerations

Fever is often the only sign of infection in the patient who is neutropenic; however, patients may be acutely ill, in septic shock, and require immediate attention. The majority of patients are febrile at home and are sent by their oncologist for a physical examination, blood cultures, and evaluation of blood counts. Patients who present apparently well should be evaluated within 1 hour of arrival. Their status can change quickly, and delay in evaluation and administration of broad-spectrum intravenous antibiotics can have a detrimental effect on their condition.

Prompt management is indicated to prevent the development of a life-threatening infection in the neutropenic patient presenting with fever. The following protocols should be developed by ED staff and the oncology department:

- Emergent triage of a known oncologic patient with fever.
- Prompt administration of antibiotics (after cultures are obtained).
- Isolation to protect from infectious patients or rapid admission to the oncology unit.
- Restriction of invasive procedures (avoidance of rectal temperatures, medications, examinations).

Thrombocytopenia and Bleeding

Thrombocytopenia is defined as a quantitative decrease in the number of circulating platelets, often interpreted as a platelet count of fewer than 100,000 cells/mm^3. Patients receiving marrow-suppressive chemotherapy develop treatment-related marrow-suppression approximately 7 to 10 days after administration of chemotherapy. The life span of platelets is approximately 7 to 10 days. When bone marrow production is interrupted by marrow-toxic chemotherapy, a brief period of thrombocytopenia develops.

Children rarely experience severe bleeding at platelet counts greater than 20,000 cells/mm^3. The incidence of serious intracranial bleeding increases with platelet counts fewer than 20,000 cells/mm^3 (Beutler, 1993). The administration of prophylactic platelet transfusion for children who are actively bleeding remains controversial. Frequent transfusion of blood products increases the potential for development of sensitization to foreign antigens found on the surfaces of random-donor platelets (alloimmunization). Each institution or practitioner must weigh the risks and benefits of prophylactic platelet administration.

ED Considerations

A child may present to the ED with sites of frank bleeding, dark stool, hematuria, bruising, petechiae, headache, vomiting, dizziness, weakness, or neurologic changes. The history may include recent chemotherapy, previous transfusions, the presence of an implanted venous access device, and fever.

Nursing interventions include:

- Observe for signs and symptoms of covert or overt bleeding.
- Apply local pressure after venipuncture or invasive procedures.
- Apply local pressure for epistaxis.
- Administer platelets as ordered:
  - Obtain a postinfusion platelet count.
  - Preferentially use leukocyte-depleted, irradiated, cytomegalovirus-negative blood products.

Home Care and Prevention

- Monitor platelet counts post chemotherapy.
- Implement "bleeding precautions" in patients with thrombocytopenia.
- Structure age-appropriate, quiet play activities.
- Restrict activities that could result in head trauma, (e.g., skateboarding, trampolines, or bicycling).
- Keep room air humidified to decrease the likelihood that epistaxis will result from dried mucous membranes.
- Discourage digital irritation of mucous membranes (nose picking).
- Restrict invasive procedures.
- Restrict use of medications that may interfere with platelet function (aspirin, ibuprofen).
- Use an extra-soft toothbrush or Toothette for oral care.
- Notify physician if new bleeding or oozing is noted.

Anemia

In children, the life span of circulating red blood cells is approximately 80 to 120 days. When bone marrow function is interrupted by marrow-toxic chemotherapy, a brief period of anemia may develop, requiring transfusion of blood products.

Risk factors related to transfusion of blood products include transmission of viral pathogens (e.g., cytomegalovirus, hepatitis, and human immunodeficiency virus), ABO incompatibility, alloimmunization, and volume overload. Unique to the immunodeficient host (neutropenic child) is the potential for graft-versus-host disease (Spector, 1995).

Transfusion reactions are more common in patients who receive multiple transfusions. Repeated exposure to minor blood group incompatibility causes patients to develop antibodies to leukocytes present in transfused products. Reexposure to antigens, to which patients have developed antibodies, results in nonhemolytic, febrile transfusion reactions. Leukocyte filtration removes 90 to 99% of leukocytes from transfused products. Because of the frequent need for transfusions, leukocyte filtration by blood banks or at bedside is a cost-effective method of reducing alloimmunization.

Graft-versus-host disease may develop when an immunologically compromised host is transfused with viable lymphocytes, present in minute amounts in all blood products. The transfused lymphocyte recognizes "nonself" cells present in the host and attempts to destroy cells. To prevent graft-versus-host disease, immunologically compromised patients should receive irradiated blood products. Irradiation at 1,500 to 5,000 rads eliminates the ability of T lymphocytes to proliferate. Red cell and platelet viability of the transfused product is unaffected.

ED Considerations

The number and severity of symptoms caused by anemia depends on the body's ability to compensate for the reduced oxygen-carrying capacity of the erythrocytes (Mansen et al., 1998). The child may present to the ED with complaints of dyspnea, a rapid, pounding heartbeat, dizziness, and fatigue, even at rest. Low-grade fever (less than 38.0°C) occurs in some anemic individuals, and may be the result of leukocyte pyrogens being released from ischemic tissues.

The history obtained should include primary diagnosis, recent chemotherapy, type of chemotherapy administered, previous transfusion reactions, necessary transfusion premedications, and all concurrent medications. The assessment may reveal:

- Gallop arrhythmia.
- Pallor.
- Cyanosis.
- Tachycardia.

Nursing interventions may include:

- Administration of oxygen.
- Obtain type and cross match for transfusion of blood products.
- Initiate intravenous access.
- Administer appropriate blood product, per hospital protocol.

- Monitor for side effects related to administration of blood.

Renal and Metabolic Effects of Malignancy

Hemorrhagic Cystitis

Hemorrhagic cystitis is characterized by painful urination with blood clots. The use of cyclophosphamide and ifosfamide as chemotherapeutic agents are the cause of hemorrhagic cystitis. The incidence of the side effect is related to the dosage and can be as high as 75% in patients who received high-dose therapy (Assreuy et al., 1999). Main features of hemorrhagic cystitis include urothelial damage, edema, necrosis, ulceration, hemorrhage, and leukocyte infiltration of the bladder wall. Acrolein, the urotoxic metabolite of cyclophosphamide and ifosfamide, is responsible for causing microhemorrhages of the bladder mucosa.

Patients receiving cyclophosphamide or ifosfamide therefore require hyperhydration. As many as 10% of patients receiving cyclophosphamide and 45% receiving ifosfamide developed hemorrhagic cystitis prior to the advent of a regimen of vigorous hydration and sodium-2-mercaptoethanesulfonate (Mesna®). A mucolytic agent, Mesna® (MeadJohnson Oncology), is administered with and after cyclophosphamide or ifosfamide infusions. Patients receiving high-dose cyclophosphamide or ifosfamide infusions may be discharged home to continue hydration and Mesna® dosing.

The use of diuretics, such as furosemide, is also indicated as part of the chemotherapy regimen to minimize statis of the metabolite in the bladder.

Patients who are unable to comply with post chemotherapy hydration parameters and the Mesna® dosing schedule after high-dose cyclophosphamide or ifosfamide therapy are at greatest risk of developing hemorrhagic cystitis. Hemorrhagic cystitis may occur hours or years after administration of chemotherapy. Radiation therapy to the pelvis may cause chronic hematuria, requiring long-term urology follow-up.

ED Considerations

The child may present to the ED with complaints of painful urination, frank blood in urine, fever, and recent administration of cyclophosphamide or ifosfamide. The child may be afebrile, may have dysuria, and clots or erythrocytes may be present in the urine.

Nursing interventions may include:

- Administer antispasmodics, as prescribed.
- Obtain intravenous access.
- Initiate oral or intravenous hydration.
- Bladder irrigation to remove clots.
- Administration of blood products to replace blood loss in the bladder.

Home Care and Prevention

- Provide adequate hydration immediately after administration of cyclophosphamide or ifosfamide.
- Anticipate the need to provide the patient with an intravenous hydration and Mesna® regimen if the patient is unable to tolerate an oral schedule because of nausea, vomiting, or compliance issues.

Hypomagnesemia

Nephrotoxicity may develop secondary to a number of chemotherapeutic agents, including cisplatin. The exact mechanism for cisplatin-induced hypomagnesemia is not known. Renal blood flow, glomerular filtration rate, and decreased distal renal tubular function are known to occur after administration (Lau, 1999).

ED Considerations

The child with hypomagnesemia may present to the ED with malaise, leg and foot cramps, "racing" heart, recent administration of cisplatin, and renal disease. Assessment findings include:

- Hyperactive deep tendon reflexes.
- Tachycardia.
- Disorientation.
- Visual or auditory hallucinations.
- Seizures.
- Decreased serum magnesium level.

Nursing interventions include the following:

- Administer magnesium supplements and monitor for side effects.
- Monitor serum magnesium levels.

Home Care and Prevention

- Comply with the oral magnesium supplementation regimen.
- Report to the child's physician for routine follow-up of serum magnesium levels.

Hypercalcemia

Hypercalcemia is defined as a serum calcium level of greater than 10.5 mg/dl. Children infrequently develop hypercalcemia. Pediatric tumors associated with hypercalcemia include acute lymphocytic leukemia, rhabdomyosarcoma, rhabdoid tumor, and hepatoblastoma.

Malignant hypercalcemia often occurs in the presence of bony metastases.

Normal calcium homeostasis is a balance between bone production and bone destruction. Two hormones control this process: parathyroid hormone and calcitonin. Release of parathyroid hormone increases serum calcium. Calcitonin decreases serum calcium by enhancing bone resorption of calcium. In concert, these hormones maintain serum calcium levels within a narrow margin of normal. The exact mechanism that results in elevated calcium levels is not known. Some propose that the tumor itself releases parathyroid hormone (Samson & Ouzts, 1996). The severity of symptoms reflects the degree of imbalance.

ED Considerations

Patients with moderately elevated calcium levels may be asymptomatic. Early symptoms of escalating serum calcium levels are nonspecific and commonly associated with cancer. Patients may complain of anorexia, nausea, vomiting, and diarrhea. These symptoms contribute to dehydration and further elevation of calcium. The kidney attempts to reduce the excess calcium, resulting in polyuria, which further exacerbates the situation. Treatment is directed at improving renal excretion of calcium and reducing bone resorption.

The child may also have symptoms of fatigue, lethargy, confusion, weakness, bradycardia, arrhythmia, thirst, and polyuria (Merrill, 2000).

Nursing interventions include:

- Administer calcium-excreting "loop diuretics," as prescribed.
- Monitor for side effects.
- Monitor serum calcium levels.
- Limit exposure to thiazide diuretics, oral contraceptives, tamoxifen, antacids, calcium carbonate, and lithium because of their potential to increase serum calcium levels.

Other Complications of Chemotherapy

Cardiomyopathy

Cardiomyopathy, a defect of the heart muscle resulting from damage to cardiac myocytes, may present as a late effect of cancer treatment (Ellingson, 1998). Chemotherapy that included anthracyclines (daunomycin, adriamycin, mitaxantrone), or other single agents such as cyclophosphamide, may be directly responsible. Risk factors for the development of cardiomyopathy related to cancer treatment include:

- Age 5 years or younger at time of exposure.
- Lifetime cumulative dose of anthracycline greater than 300 mg/m^2.
- Radiation therapy to the mediastinum.
- Combination of chemotherapy and radiation to chest area.
- Underlying cardiac disease.

ED Considerations

The child may present to the ED with shortness of breath, exercise limitations, fatigue, irregular heart rate, and cough. The history may include a neoplasm treated with anthracycline or radiation, or previous cardiac problems.

Assessment findings may include dyspnea, arrhythmia, rales, and cyanosis. Nursing interventions may include:

- Monitor airway, breathing, and circulation.
- Administer diuretics, as prescribed.
- Limit fluid intake, as directed.
- Admit the child for monitoring and further therapy.

Seizures

Seizures are transient involuntary changes in mentation, behavior, sensation, and motor or autonomic function. The pediatric oncology population experiences seizures as the same rate as the general population. Increased intracranial pressure as a result of a primary brain neoplasm with a mass effect, or the presence of diffuse metastatic disease to the CNS, can cause seizures. Additionally, seizures may be caused by certain metabolic crises inducted by therapy, including hypoglycemia and hyponatremia. Cranial irradiation may contribute to the development of seizures because of microvascular changes within the brain. Some chemotherapeutic drugs are also associated with producing seizures.

ED Considerations

Seizures are treated in the same manner as with any other patient. The cause of the seizures must be determined (and not necessarily assumed to be the result of chemotherapy). Acute management focuses on maintenance of airway, prevention of aspiration, and avoidance of injury (Woodword & Hogan, 1996). The history, assessment, and interventions are the same as described in Chapters 6 and 18.

Cerebrovascular Accident

A cerebrovascular accident (CVA) is an acute hemorrhage and formation of thrombosis within the brain, secondary to coagulation abnormality. Cerebrovascular accidents that occur during treatment may be attributed to l-asparaginase-related coagulopathy (Shapiro, Clarke, Christian, Odom, & Hathaway, 1993). Hyperleukocytosis, discussed earlier, may be a contributing factor. Children with an underlying diagnosis of myelogenous leukemia are also at risk. Procoagulants present in the immature white cells may be released, leading to DIC and CVA. Cranial irradiation may lead to early or late CVA secondary to vessel abnormalities (Musaffar, Collins, Labropoulos, & Baker, 2000).

ED Considerations

The child may come to the ED with complaints of dyspnea, blurred vision, irritability, confusion, stupor, and a history of treatment with l-asparaginase, cranial irradiation, or underlying acute myelogenous leukemia. The nursing assessment may show the following signs and symptoms:

- Motor function impairment.
- Speech impairment.
- Asymmetric pupils.
- Sensory changes.
- Ataxia.
- Altered level of consciousness.

Nursing interventions include:

- Administer oxygen.
- Obtain intravenous access.
- Perform frequent neurologic assessments.
- Perform coagulation studies.
- Administer corticosteroid or hyperosmolar agents, as prescribed.
- Prepare for admission.

Conclusion

A wide variety of hematologic and oncologic conditions can be observed in the pediatric patient. These conditions can have an impact on every body system. Rapid assessment and recognition of life-threatening conditions are as important as knowledge of common malignancies and the adverse effects of treatment. The ED nurse also should be aware of resources, such as the hematology and oncology specialists available in the area, and, in collaboration with these professionals, develop protocols for treating these patients.

References

Assreuy, A., Martins, G., Moreira, M., Brito, B., Cavada, B., Ribiero, R., & Flores, C. (1999). Prevention of cyclophosphamide-induced hemorrhagic cystitis by glucose-mannose binding plant lectins. *The Journal of Urology, 161*(6), 1988–1993.

Beutler, E. (1993). Platelet transfusions: The 20,000 cells/ml trigger. *Blood, 81*, 1411–1413.

Bleyer, W. A. (1990). The impact of childhood cancer on the United States and the world. *CA: A Cancer Journal for Clinicians, 40*, 355–367.

Buchanan, G. (1997). Hematologic supportive care of the pediatric cancer patient. In P. A. Pizzo & D. G. Poplack (Eds.), *Principles and practice of pediatric oncology* (3rd ed., pp. 1051–1068). Philadelphia: Lippincott-Raven.

Cahill-Alsip, C., & McDermott, B. (1996). Hematologic critical care problems. In M. A. Curley, J. B. Smith, & P. Moloney-Harmon (Eds.), *Critical care nursing of infants and children* (pp. 793–818). Philadelphia: Saunders.

Camp-Sorrell, D. (1998). Spinal cord compression. *Clinical Journal of Oncology Nursing, 2*, 112–113.

Cohen, A. (2000). Hematologic emergencies. In G. Fleisher & S. Ludwig (Eds.), *Textbook of pediatric emergency medicine* (4th ed., pp. 859–886). Philadelphia: Lippincott, Williams & Wilkins.

Ellingson, L. (1998). Cardiac and pulmonary complications. In M. Hockenberry-Eaton (Ed.), *Essentials of pediatric oncology nursing: A core curriculum* (p. 129). Glenview, IL: Association of Pediatric Oncology Nurses.

Frenck, R. Kohn, D., & Pickering, L. K. (1991). Principles of total care: Infection in children with cancer. In D. J. Fernback & T. J. Vietti, *Clinical Pediatric Oncology* (4th ed., pp. 249–271). St. Louis: Mosby.

George, J. M., Woolf, S. H., Raskob, G. E., Wasser, J. S., Aledort, L. M., Ballen, P. J., Blanchette, V. S., Bussel, J. B., Cines, D. B., Kelton, J. G., Lichtin, A. E., McMillan, R., Okerbloom, J. A., Regan, D. H., & Warrier, I. (1996). Idiopathic thrombocytopenic purpura: A practice guideline developed by explicit methods for The American Society of Hematology. *Blood, 88*, 3–40.

Guyton, A. C., & Hall, J. E. (1996). *Textbook of medical physiology* (9th ed., pp. 425–434). Philadelphia: Saunders.

Hinkle, A., & Schwartz, C. (2001). Cancers in childhood. In R. A. Hoekelmann (Ed.), *Pediatric Primary Care* (4th ed., pp. 1359–1384). St. Louis: Mosby.

Iannone, R. (2001). Contagious exanthematous diseases. In R. A. Hoekelmann (Ed.), *Pediatric Primary Care* (4th edition, pp. 1441–1442). St. Louis: Mosby.

Imbach, P. A., Kühne, T., & Holländer, G. (1997). Immunologic aspects in the pathogenesis and treatment of immune thrombocytopenic purpura in children. *Current Opinion in Pediatrics, 9*, 35–45.

Kline, N. E., & Mooney, K. H. (1998). Alterations of hematologic function in children. In K. L. McCance & S. E. Huether (Eds.),

Pathophysiology: The biologic basis for disease in adults and children (3rd ed., pp. 935-967). St. Louis: Mosby.

Landis, S. H., Murray, T., Bolden, S., & Wingo, P. A. (1998). Cancer Statistics 1998. *CA: A Cancer Journal for Clinicians, 48*, 6-29.

Lau, Alan H. (1999). Apoptosis induced by cisplatin nephrotoxic injury. *Kidney International, 56*(4), 1295-1298.

Malatack, J. Blatt, J., & Pechansky, L. (1997). Hematology and oncology. In B. Zitelli & H. Davis (Eds.), *Atlas of pediatric physical diagnosis* (3rd ed., pp. 305-341). St. Louis: Mosby.

Manley, M., & Bechtal, N. (1998). Hematologic and immune systems. In T. E. Soud & J. S. Rogers (Eds.), *Manual of pediatric emergency nursing* (pp. 390-416). St. Louis: Mosby.

Mansen, T. J., McCance, K. L., & Field, R. (1998). Alterations of leukocyte, lymphoid, and hemostatic function. In K. L. McCane & S. E. Heuther (Eds.), *Pathophysiology: The biologic basis for disease in adults and children* (3rd ed., pp. 899-934). St. Louis: Mosby.

McCance, K. L. (1998). Structure and function of the hematologic system. In K. L. McCane & S. E. Heuther (Eds.), *Pathophysiology: The biologic basis for disease in adults and children* (3rd ed., pp. 845-877). St. Louis: Mosby.

Merrill, P. (2000). Oncologic emergencies. *Lippincott's Primary Care Practice, 4*(4), pp. 400-409.

Muzaffar, K., Collins, S., Labropoulos, N., & Baker, W. (2000). A prospective study of the effects of irradiation on the carotid artery. *Laryngoscope, 110*(11), 1811-1814.

Naparstek, E. (1995). Granulocyte colony-stimulating factor, congenital neutropenia and acute myeloid leukemia. *The New England Journal of Medicine, 333*(8), 516-518.

Oakes, L. L., & Rosenthal-Dichter, C. (1998). Hematology and immunology. In M. C. Slota, (Ed.), *Core curriculum for pediatric critical care nursing* (pp. 461-550). Philadelphia: Saunders.

Radel, E. G. (2001). Hemophilia and other hereditary bleeding disorders. In R. A. Hoekelman (Ed.), *Pediatric primary care* (4th ed., pp. 1515-1520). St. Louis: Mosby.

Rohaly-Davis, J., & Johnston, K. (1996). Hematologic emergencies in the intensive care unit. *Critical Care Nursing Quarterly, 18*(4), 35-43.

Samson, L. F., & Ouzts, K. M. (1996). Fluid and electrolyte regulation. In M. A. Curley, J. Bloedel-Smith, & P. A. Maloney-Harmon (Eds.), *Critical care nursing of infants and children* (pp. 385-409). Philadelphia: Saunders.

Shapiro, A. D., Clarke, S. L., Christian, J. M., Odom, L. F., & Hathaway, W. E. (1993). Thrombosis in children receiving lasparaginase, determining patients at risk. *American Journal of Pediatric Hematology-Oncology, 15*, 400-405.

Spector, D. (1995). Transfusion associated graft versus host disease: An overview and two case reports. *Oncology Nursing Forum, 22*, 97-102.

Vichinsky, E. P., Neumayr, L. D., Earles, A. N., Williams, R., Lennette, E. T., Dean, D., Nickerson, B., Orringer, E., McKie, V., Bellevue, R., Daeschner, C., Manci-Gardener, E., Abboud, M., Moncino, M., Ballas, S., & Ware, R. (2000). Causes and outcomes of the acute chest syndrome in sickle cell disease. *New England Journal of Medicine, 342*(25), 1855-1865.

Warrier, I., Bussel, J. B., Valadex, L., Barbosa, J., Beardsley, D. S., & The Low-Dose IVIG Study Group. (1997). Safety and efficacy of low-dose intravenous immune globulin (IVIG) treatment for infants and children with immune thrombocytopenic purpura. *Journal of Pediatric Hematology/Oncology, 19*, 197-201.

Weintraub, M. H. (1993). Nursing management of the child or adolescent with infection. In G. V. Foley, D. Fochtman, & K. H. Mooney (Eds.), *Nursing care of the child with cancer* (2nd ed.). Philadelphia: Saunders.

Wilson, K. (1998). Oncologic emergencies. In M. J. Hockenberry-Eaton (Ed.), *Essentials of pediatric oncology nursing: A core curriculum* (pp. 147-154). Glenview, IL: Association of Pediatric Oncology Nurses.

Woodward, W. L., & Hogan, D. K. (1996). Oncologic emergencies: Implications for nurses. *Journal of IV Nursing, 19*(5), 256-263.

26

Communicable and Infectious Diseases

Cynde Rivers, RN, MN, CEN
Rachael Rosenfield, RN, BSN

Introduction

Communicable and infectious diseases are frequently encountered in the pediatric population seeking emergency care. Emergency nurses should be familiar with the basic functions of the immune system and should be knowledgeable about the common communicable and infectious diseases affecting infants, children, and adolescents. The purposes of this chapter are to discuss common communicable and infectious diseases and describe their associated care and prevention.

Embroyologic Development of the Immune System

Cellular components of the immune system arise from precursor cells within blood islands of the yolk sac. Multipotential stem cells arise in these islands and migrate to the liver and spleen and later to the bone marrow and thymus. Pre B cells are seen in the liver by 7 to 8 weeks; immature B lymphocytes with surface immunoglobulin M (IgM) receptors are found by 10 to 11 weeks in the fetal liver. By 12 weeks, B lymphocytes are found in the peripheral blood and bone marrow. Synthesis of immunoglobulin G (IgG), IgM, and immunoglobulin E (IgE) begins by 12 to 15 weeks; synthesis of immunoglobulin A (IgA) begins by 30 weeks. In the last trimester of pregnancy, the fetus may be capable of producing a primary immune response with IgM to antigenic challenges and to infections such as cytomegalovirus, rubella virus, and *Toxoplasma gondii* (Rote, 1998a). The fetus cannot produce a significant IgG response, and the IgA response is underdeveloped (Rote, 1998a).

In utero and neonatal protection against infectious agents occurs through the passage of maternal antibodies into the fetal circulation (Rote, 1998a). At birth, umbilical total IgG levels are similar to the adult level (Rote, 1998a).

The function of the immune system is to recognize self from nonself and to initiate responses to eliminate the foreign substance or antigen. The functions of the immune system are basically of two types: nonspecific and specific. Nonspecific immune defenses are activated on exposure to any foreign substance but react similarly, regardless of the type of antigen. The principal activity of this system is phagocytosis. Phagocytic cells include neutrophils and monocytes.

Specific (adaptive) defenses are those that have the ability to recognize the antigen and respond selectively. The cells responsible for this form of immunity are the lymphocytes, specifically B cells and T cells (Table 26.1).

The immune system provides immunity, an inherited or acquired state in which an individual is resistant to the occurrences or the effects of a specific disease. There are two types of immunity:

- Passive:
  - Temporary immunity is achieved by transfusing plasma proteins either artificially, from another human or an animal that has been actively immunized against an antigen, or naturally, from the mother to the fetus via the placenta.
- Active:
  - Immune bodies are actively formed against specific antigens, either naturally, by experiencing the dis-

TABLE 26.1 Function and Description of the Lymphocytes

Lymphocyte	*Function*	*Description*
B lymphocytes (B cells)	Concerned with the immune processes occurring outside of the cells, such as on cell surfaces or in bodily fluids. When challenged with an antigen, B cells divide and differentiate into plasma cells. The plasma cells in turn produce and secrete large quantities of antibodies specific to the antigen.	Five classes of antibodies of immunoglobulins (Ig) are: ▪ IgA: Viral protection. ▪ IgD: Function unknown. ▪ IgE: Involved in reaction to allergens and parasitic infestation. ▪ IgG: Bacterial protection. ▪ IgM: Bacterial protection.
T lymphocytes (T cells)	Pass through the thymus during the differentiation process. Cell-mediated immunity occurs within the cell. Specific functions of T cells include: ▪ Protection against most viral, fungal, and protozoan infections and slow-growing bacterial infections. ▪ Rejection of histo-incompatible grafts. ▪ Mediation of cutaneous delayed hypersensitivity reactions, such as tuberculosis. ▪ Probably immune surveillance for malignant cells.	T cells have a regulatory function within the immune system. For example, helper T lymphocytes assist B lymphocytes and other types of T cells to mount an optimum immune response

From: Whaley & Wong, 1999, pp. 1690–1692.

ease clinically or subclinically, or artificially, by introducing the antigen (vaccine) into the individual.

- Inappropriate immune responses are categorized as *hypersensitivity* and *immunodeficiency*. Hypersensitivity results in *autoimmunity*, *isoimmunity*, or *allergy*. Table 26.2 compares and contrasts these immune responses. Hypersensitivity reactions can be immediate or delayed; anaphylaxis is an example of the most immediate reaction to antigen reexposure.

Immunodeficiency is the failure of the immunologic system to function properly. These deficiencies are either *congenital* (primary), arising from genetic defects that disrupt lymphocyte function, or *acquired* (secondary), resulting from a disease or other physiologic condition (Rote, 1998b).

Immunosuppression occurs following organ transplantation to prevent rejection of the organ by the body's immune system or following chemotherapy to prevent cancer cell growth (Chapter 25). Common medications administered to children to provide immunosuppression, infectious disease prophylaxis, and antiviral activity following organ transplantation are listed in Table 26.3.

Pediatric Considerations

Neonates are immunologically immature. Although cell-mediated immunologic capabilities most likely are functional at this time, antibody production, phagocytic activity, and complement activity are deficient (Rote, 1998a).

Initially, the neonate passively receives immunity from the mother, because immunoglobulins can be passed from the mother *in utero* (IgG) or in breast milk (IgA) (Burke, 1998). When the infant is 3 to 5 months of age, passive immunity decreases as immunoglobulin production increases (Burke, 1998). By 5 to 6 months of age, immunoglobulins reach a minimum level (Rote, 1998a).

Etiology

The etiologies of conditions involving the immune system are communicable and infectious diseases, as discussed in this chapter.

Focused History

Patient history

- Recent exposure to a person with the suspected communicable or infectious disease

TABLE 26.2 Description of Hypersensitivity Immune Responses

Immune Response	*Description*	*Examples*
Autoimmunity	Inappropriate immune responses to the body's own tissues. Causes include: ▪ Exposure to a previously sequestered antigen. ▪ Development of a neoantigen. ▪ Complications of an infectious disease. ▪ Emergence of a lymphocyte clone. ▪ Alteration of suppressor T-cell function.	Hyperthyroidism Rheumatic fever Crohn's disease Autoimmune thrombocytopenic purpura
Isoimmunity	Inappropriate immune responses to a beneficial foreign tissue, such as a transplanted organ.	Graft (organ) rejection Graft versus host disease Transfusion reactions

Allergy	Exaggerated responses to environmental antigens.	Anaphylaxis, urticaria, serum sickness, reactive airway disease, contact dermatitis from:
		▪ Ingestion:
		  ▪ Foods (peanuts)
		  ▪ Medications
		▪ Inhalation:
		  ▪ Molds
		  ▪ Pollens
		▪ Injections:
		  ▪ Bee venom
		  ▪ Drugs
		▪ Topical:
		  ▪ Plants (poison ivy)
		  ▪ Metals (copper)

From: Rote, 1998b.

- Illness-specific symptoms that may include (Oakes & Rosenthal-Dichter, 1998):
  - Fatigue.
  - Weakness.
  - Headache.
  - Weight loss or failure to thrive.
  - Poor wound healing.
  - Night sweats.
  - Fever.
  - Diarrhea.
- Recent travel outside of the United States
- Sexual activity, consensual and nonconsensual (Oakes & Rosenthal-Dichter, 1998):
  - Sexual preference.
  - Safe-sex practices.
  - Single or multiple partners.
- Current medication usage:
  - Immunosuppressive agents.
  - Chemotherapeutic agents (Chapter 25).

Past health history

- Solid organ or tissue transplantation.
- Splenectomy.
- Autoimmune disorders.
- Allergies.

- Immunization history.
- Placement of an implantable venous access device.

TABLE 26.3 Posttransplant Medications

Medication	*Dosage*	*Action*	*Side Effects*	*Nursing Implications*
Immunosuppression				
Tacrolimus (Prograf®)	I.V.: 0.05–0.15 mg/kg/day via continuous I.V. infusion P.O.: 0.15–0.3 mg/kg/day ÷ 12 hours	Inhibits t-lymphocyte activation by inhibiting interleukin II synthesis.	Nephrotoxicity, hyptertension, nausea, vomiting, headaches, insomnia, tremors, paraesthesia, hyperkalemia, hyperglycemia	Monitor drug levels (therapeutic levels patient-specific 10–20 mg/mL). Monitor creatinine, glucose, and potassium levels.
Azathioprine (Imuran®)	Maintenance: I.V./P.O.: 1.0–3.0 mg/kg/day qd	Prevents cell division, limiting T-cell production.	Bone marrow suppression, GI symptoms, pancreatitis	Monitor WBC and amylase level.
Corticosteroids Methylprednisolone (Solumendrol®) Hydrocortisone (Solu-Cortef®) Prednisone	Variable, depending on agent used	Decreases the number of circulating B and T-lymphocytes.	Hypertension, edema, increased appetite, mood swings, depression, acne, glucose intolerance, osteoporosis, cataracts, ulcers	Monitor weight, blood pressure, and blood glucose levels, administer with antacids, avoid sudden discontinuation of the drug.
Infectious Prophylaxis				
Co-trimoxazole (Bactrim®)	variable	Antibiotic.	Blood dyscrasia, rashes, renal or hepatic injury, GI irritation, allergy, hemolysis in G6PD deficiency	Not recommended in infants younger than 2 months of age, monitor CBC.
Nystatin (Mycostatin®)	variable	Antifungal.	Diarrhea and gastrointestinal side effects	Usually discontinued when steroid therapy is discontinued; treat thrush until 48–72 hours after resolution of symptoms.
Antiviral Therapy				
Acyclovir (Zovirax®)	I.V./P.O.: 500 mg/m2/dose, q 8 hours	Inhibits viral DNA synthesis of herpes viruses. After uptake by an infected cell, Acyclovir is phosphorylated to the inactive monophosphate form by a virus-specific thymidine kinase and then to the triphosphate form.	Altered renal function, headache, elevated liver enzyme levels	Dose adjustments may be necessary with renal impairment. Keep patient hydrated to decrease risk of nephrotoxicity. Monitor BUN, creatinine, and liver enzymes.
Ganciclovir (Cytovene®)	variable	Inhibits DNA polymerase but is not dependent on a virus-specific thymidine kinase for phosphorylation; therefore, it is active against CMB.	Neutropenia, thrombocytopenia, confusion, nausea	Dose adjustments may be necessary with renal impairment; maintain chemotherapy precautions. Monitor CBC with platelets, BUN, Creatinine
Cytomegalovirus immune globulin intravenous (CytoGam®)	I.V.: 150 mg/kg within 72 hours of transplant and 100 mg/kg repeated 2, 4, 6, and 8 weeks and 50 mg/kg at 12 and 16 weeks posttransplant	Provides passive immunization by raising relevant antibodies sufficient to attenuate or reduce the incidence of serious CMV disease.	Flushing, chills, muscle cramps, nausea, fever, wheezing, hypotension	Side effects correlate with rate of infusion; have emergency equipment available.

I.V. = intravenous; P.O. = by mouth

Keating, M. R. Antiviral agents. *Mayo Clinic Proceedings.* 1992; 67:160–178.

Siberry, G., & Iannone, R. (2000). The Hornet Lane Handbook (15th ed.) St. Louis: Mosby.

Takemoto, C. K., Hodding, J. H., & Kraus, D. M. *Pediatric Dosage Handbook.* 4th ed. Cleveland, OH: Lexi-Comp Inc., 1997.

Family history

- Recent exposure to a person with the suspected communicable or infectious disease.
- Recent travel outside of the United States.
- Autoimmune diseases.

Focused Assessment

Physical Assessment

1. Assess the respiratory system:
   - Auscultate the chest for:
     - Respiratory rate.
     - Adventitious sounds.
2. Assess the cardiovascular system:
   - Auscultate the heart for:
     - Rate.
     - Rhythm.
   - Interpret electrocardiogram readings, as needed.
   - Palpate the peripheral pulses for:
     - Rate.
     - Equality.
   - Measure capillary refill.
   - Measure the blood pressure.
   - Measure core and skin temperature.
   - Palpate the sternum and ribs for tenderness.
3. Assess the neurologic system:
   - Assess the child's level of consciousness with the AVPU method or Glasgow coma scale (GCS).
   - Assess the pupillary responses.
   - Assess for signs of meningeal irritation, as indicated.
   - Assess for signs of muscle weakness.
   - Assess the infant for (Manley & Bechtel, 1998):
     - Quality of sucking.
     - Type of cry.
     - Muscle tone and movement.
     - Feeding patterns.
     - Anterior fontanelle fullness.
4. Assess the abdomen:
   - Palpate the abdomen for:
     - Organ enlargement.
     - Pain and tenderness.
5. Assess the integumentary system:
   - Observe the skin for:
     - Rashes.
     - Petechiae.
     - Color.
   - Observe the oral mucosa for disease-specific changes.
6. Assess the lymphatic system:
   - Palpate the cervical, axillary, and femoral lymph nodes for:
     - Size.
     - Tenderness.
     - Location.
     - Texture.
     - Fixation.

Psychosocial Assessment

- Assess the child and family's understanding of communicable or infectious diseases.
- Assess the child and family's coping strategies.
- Assess for the presence of family support systems.

Table 26.4 lists nursing diagnoses and expected outcomes.

Triage Decisions

Emergent

- Signs of airway compromise.
- Respiratory failure.
- Shock.
- Altered level of consciousness.
- Cutaneous manifestations, such as petechiae.

Urgent

- Signs of respiratory distress.
- Thermoregulatory lability.
- Abnormal vital signs for age.
- Decreased urinary output.
- Suspected contagious disease (e.g., varicella).

Nonurgent

- Low-grade fever.
- Ambulatory.
- Complaints of sore throat.
- Awake and alert.

Nursing Interventions

1. Assess and maintain airway, breathing, and circulation (Chapter 6):
   - Initiate maneuvers to maintain airway patency, such as positioning and suctioning, and prepare for insertion of an airway adjunct.
   - Prepare for endotracheal intubation in the child who cannot maintain airway patency.

TABLE 26.4 Nursing Diagnoses and Expected Outcomes

Nursing Diagnoses	*Expected Outcomes*
Potential for infection, related to decreased host defenses	Sources of fever and infection will be identified and treatment will be initiated, as evidenced by: ■ Early administration of antibiotics. ■ Implementation of effective precautions to avoid cross-contamination and exposure to infectious pathogens among patients and other staff.
Fever related to the infectious process	The patient's core temperature will return to normal, as evidenced by: ■ Normothermia. ■ Pink skin. ■ Absence of discomfort associated with fever.
Knowledge deficit, related to the care of a child with an infectious disease	Parents will demonstrate an understanding of the disease process by: ■ Verbalizing an understanding of all treatments and procedures. ■ Demonstrating preventive techniques for cross-contamination for the child's care at home.

- Administer 100% oxygen through a non-rebreather mask.
- Initiate assisted ventilation in the child who is not maintaining adequate respiratory effort.

2. Initiate cardiorespiratory and continuous oxygen saturation monitoring.
3. Obtain venous access and initiate an intravenous infusion at the prescribed rate:
   - Obtain blood specimens for laboratory analysis.
   - Prepare to administer medications, as prescribed:
     - Vasopressors.
     - Antibiotics.
4. Reassess neurologic status and cardiopulmonary status.
5. Measure intake and output.
6. Administer oral medications, such as:
   - Acetaminophen.
   - Aspirin.
   - Corticosteroids.
7. Prepare for diagnostic tests, as needed.
8. Obtain additional specimens for laboratory analysis, such as:
   - Throat cultures.
   - Urine cultures.
   - Cerebrospinal fluid cultures.
9. Inform the family frequently about the child's condition; provide emotional support to the child and family.
10. Initiate consultations with specialists (e.g., infectious disease specialists), as needed.
11. Inform the local health department of children with communicable and infectious diseases.
12. Prepare for transfer and transport to a tertiary care facility as needed (Chapter 10); prepare for hospitalization as indicated.

Home Care and Prevention

General home care instructions for children with communicable or infectious diseases include:

- Use good hand-washing techniques to avoid spreading the illness to other family members.
- Avoid using the same eating utensils, cups, and toothbrushes of an infected child to avoid family contamination.
- Administer medications for their prescribed duration.
- Follow up with the child's primary care physician to detect potential disease-associated complications.
- Provide adequate rest for the child to recuperate completely.

Staff must protect themselves from communicable and infectious diseases by using proper hand washing, universal precautions, and other protective measures to prevent contamination of themselves or other patients and families. Exposure to communicable or infectious diseases should be reported to the emergency department (ED) manager for proper follow-up. Emergency nurses should know the procedures to follow in the event that they are exposed (e.g., needle-stick injury) to an infectious or contagious patient.

Specific Immunologic Emergencies

Communicable Diseases: Vaccine-Preventable

Etiology

Communicable diseases are those diseases that are spread from infected to noninfected individuals. Many deadly pediatric communicable diseases are now prevented through immunizations; however, with international travel, children may be exposed to such diseases, or unvaccinated children may present to the ED for treatment. Table 26.5 lists common vaccine-preventable communicable diseases and their disease processes; Table 26.6 lists each disease's signs and symptoms, ED treatment, and home care and prevention. Chapter 22 provides further detailed information related to rubella and rubeola.

Home Care and Prevention

Because of the rising incidence of communicable and infectious diseases, universal precautions should be practiced for all patients presenting for ED treatment. Exposure to bodily fluids is common in the ED, and patients' immunologic status (e.g., human immunodeficiency virus [HIV], hepatitis B) may not be known. Appropriate barriers must be utilized for any patient contact. Hands and other skin surfaces should be washed thoroughly and immediately following exposure to any bodily fluids. EDs should have policies and procedures in place in case a staff member experiences accidental exposure.

Following the ED treatment of infectious children and families, ED staff must consider treatment for themselves. For example, rubella titers and booster immunizations may be necessary for staff exposed to a child with rubella. Varicella vaccine may be needed for a staff member who never had varicella as a child.

Parents should be encouraged to have their children immunized against the common communicable diseases of childhood (Chapter 5).

Emergency staff must report communicable and infectious diseases to the local health department, as required (Chapter 5).

Tuberculosis

Etiology

Tuberculosis (TB) has afflicted humans for thousands of years and remains a major public health concern throughout the world. The majority of children with tuberculosis are asymptomatic and are identified by routine tuberculin skin testing or following a TB infection investigation.

In the United States, nearly 20% of deaths in the early 1800s were attributed to tuberculosis. Mortality declined by midcentury because of improvement in living conditions and nutrition. From 1992 through 1999, TB cases among U.S.-born persons decreased by 49%, whereas cases among foreign-born persons increased 4% (Centers for Disease Control and Prevention, 1999). In the United States, approximately 2,300 children and adolescents are diagnosed with tuberculosis annually. Children of minority groups are especially at risk, constituting nearly 70% of the cases. Living in crowded or urban settings presents an additional risk factor (Centers for Disease Control and Prevention, 1994), as does medically induced immunosuppression.

Mycobacterium tuberculosis, the etiologic agent, is spread by inhalation of droplets produced by the disease. The period from exposure to a positive tuberculin skin test is usually 2 to 10 weeks. Most tuberculous infections resolve without clinical evidence of disease. Often the disease will appear within the first 6 months, although it can lay latent for a year or more. Although 80% of tuberculosis cases are classified as pulmonary, the remaining are classified as more serious diseases, known as tuberculous meningitis and miliary tuberculosis. Tuberculous meningitis results from infiltration of disease into the central nervous system, while miliary tuberculosis results from infiltration of disease into the systemic circulation.

Focused History

Patient history

- Exposure to a person infected with TB
- Cough (mild or absent) or cold symptoms that linger.
- Low-grade fever.
- Irritability.
- Poor appetite.
- Weight loss or poor weight gain.

Family history

- Presence of a TB-infected person in the home.
- Crowded home environment or homelessness.

TABLE 26.5 Vaccine-Preventable Communicable Diseases

Disease/Agent	*Route of Transmission*	*Incubation Period*	*Communicability Period*
Diphtheria/*Corynebacterium diphtheriae*	Person to person; spread from the respiratory tract	2 to 5 days	Transmission may occur as long as virulent bacilli are present in discharges and lesions. The time is variable, but organisms usually persist 2 weeks or less, and seldom more than 4 weeks, without antibiotics. Chronic carriers may shed organisms for 6 months or more. Effective antibiotic therapy promptly terminates shedding (Centers for Disease Control and Prevention, 1995a).
Measles/viral	Usually direct contact with droplets of infected person	10 to 20 days	Transmission may occur from 4 days before to 5 days after the rash appears, but mainly during the prodromal (catarrhal) stage (Whaley & Wong, 1999).
Mumps/paramyxovirus	Saliva contact with or droplet spread from an infected person	14 to 21 days	Transmission is most likely immediately before and after swelling begins. By the third day of the disease process, the parotid gland (either unilaterally or bilaterally) enlarges and reaches a maximum size in 1 to 3 days; swelling is accompanied by pain and tenderness (Whaley & Wong, 1999).
Rubella/rubella virus	Person to person; spread via bodily fluids	14 to 21 days	Transmission is from direct contact and is spread via an infected person. The virus may also be spread indirectly via articles freshly contaminated with nasopharyngeal secretions, feces, or urine (Centers for Disease Control and Prevention, 1995a).
Pertussis/*Bordetella pertussis* and *B. parapertussis*	Person to person; spread via respiratory secretions	7 to 14 days	Transmission is greatest during the catarrhal stage, during which the child has symptoms of an upper respiratory infection, and can extend for up to 6 weeks (Dworken, Alexander, Boase, DeBolt, Goldoft, Green, & Maruse, 1997). Most commonly seen in infants younger than 6 months of age.
Polio/enterovirus	Person to person; feces and oropharyngeal secretions	7 to 14 days	Transmission is from direct contact with persons with apparent or inapparent active infection. The virus is spread via fecal-oral or in pharyngeal-oropharyngeal routes (Whaley & Wong, 1999).

Focused Assessment

Physical Assessment

1. Assess the respiratory system:
   - Auscultate the chest for:
     - Respiratory rate.
     - Adventitious sounds. Cough or shortness of breath may be present.
   - Assess for chest pain:
     - Children with pleural involvement present more acutely, exhibiting fever, chest pain, shortness of breath, and evidence of pleural effusion.
2. Assess the cardiovascular system:
   - Auscultate the heart for rate.
   - Measure the blood pressure.
   - Inspect the skin for:
     - Capillary refill.
     - Color.
     - Temperature.
   - Measure core and skin temperatures:
     - Fever may be present.
3. Assess the neurologic system:
   - Assess the level of consciousness with the GCS or AVPU method.

TABLE 26.6 Vaccine-Preventable Communicable Diseases

Disease	Signs/Symptoms/ Complications	ED Interventions	Home Care and Prevention
Diphtheria	*Pharyngeal*, including laryngeal and nasopharyngeal (most common): ■ Fever; sore throat; cervical lymphadenopathy; thick gray-white membranes; tachycardia. *Cutaneous* (common in the tropics) ■ Sharply demarcated ulcers (Barkin, 1997) (common in the tropics).	*Confirmed diphtheria:* ■ Rapid administration of intravenous antitoxin is recommended after the patient is tested for sensitivity (American Academy of Pediatrics, 2000). Antitoxin will not neutralize any toxins that have already fixed to tissues but will neutralize the unbound toxin and will prevent further progression of the disease. *Suspected diphtheria:* ■ Initiate parenteral erythromycin. ■ Initiate parenteral penicillin G. ■ Identify and treat close contacts, such as family members, regardless of their immunization status: 　■ Obtain a diphtheria culture. 　■ Administer either oral erythromycin or intramuscular penicillin G. 　■ Administer a booster dose of diphtheria in previously immunized contacts if they have not received one in more than 5 years. 　■ Prepare for hospitalization and respiratory isolation. ■ Institute respiratory isolation. 　■ Provide antibiotics to prevent secondary bacterial infection in high-risk children. 　■ Provide hydration for children with signs of dehydration (Centers for Disease Control and Prevention, 1995a).	*Suspected diphtheria:* ■ Continue parenteral erythromycin for 2 weeks ■ Continue daily parenteral penicillin G for 14 days, followed by a 10-day course of oral penicillin or erythromycin (Barkin & Rosen, 1999). ■ The disease is usually not contagious 48 hours after antibiotics are instituted (Centers for Disease Control and Prevention, 1995a). ■ Begin active immunizations, based on age, to nonimmunized persons or persons whose immunization status is unsure (American Academy of Pediatrics, 2000). ■ Prepare for hospitalization and respiratory isolation (Barkin & Rosen, 1999).
Measles	Fever and malaise, followed in 24-hours by coryza, cough, conjunctivitis, Koplik's spots (small, irregular red spots with a minute, bluish white center). *Cutaneous:* ■ Rash appears 3 to 4 days after onset of symptoms; begins as a maculopapular eruption on face and gradually spreads downward. *Other signs and symptoms:* ■ Anorexia; malaise; generalized lymphadenopathy. *Complications:* ■ Otitis media; pneumonia; bronchiolitis; encephalitis (Whaley & Wong, 1999).	Institute respiratory isolation. Provide antibiotics to prevent secondary bacterial infection in high-risk children. Provide hydration for children with signs of dehydration (Centers for Disease Control and Prevention, 1995a).	Maintain isolation until fifth day of rash. Maintain bed rest and provide quiet activity. Provide antipyretics; avoid chilling. Dim lights if photophobia is present; clean eyelids with warm saline solution to remove secretions or crusts; keep child from rubbing eyes. Use cool-mist vaporizer. Encourage fluids and soft, bland foods.

(continued)

TABLE 26.6 Vaccine-Preventable Communicable Diseases (continued)

Disease	*Signs/Symptoms/ Complications*	*ED Interventions*	*Home Care and Prevention*
Mumps	Fever, headache, malaise, and anorexia for 24-hours, followed by "earache" that is aggravated by chewing. *Parotitis:* By third day, parotid glands enlarge; accompanied by pain and tenderness. *Other signs and symptoms:* Submaxillary and sublingual infection. *Complications:* Sensorineural deafness; encephalitis; myocarditis; arthritis; hepatitis; sterility (orchitis) (Centers for Disease Control and Prevention, 1995a).	Maintain isolation during period of communicability; institute respiratory precautions during hospitalization. Provide analgesics for pain and antipyretics for fever. Intravenous fluids may be necessary for the child who refuses to drink or vomits.	Maintain isolation during period of communicability. Maintain bed rest until swelling subsides. Give analgesics for pain. Encourage fluids and soft, bland foods; avoid foods that require chewing. Apply hot or cold compresses to neck, whichever is more comforting (Whaley & Wong, 1999).
Rubella	Low-grade fever; headache; malaise; anorexia; mild conjunctivitis; sore throat; cough; lymphadenopathy. *Cutaneous:* Rash first appears on face and rapidly spreads downward; by the end of the first day the body is covered with a discrete, pinkish-red maculopapular exanthem.	Maintain respiratory and bodily fluid isolation. Provide analgesics for pain and antipyretics for fever. Isolate child from pregnant women (greatest danger is teratogenic effect on fetus).	Employ comfort measures, as necessary. Isolate child from pregnant women (Whaley & Wong, 1999).
Pertussis	*Catarrhal phase:* ■ Early symptoms include nasal congestion, tearing, mild conjunctival injection, malaise, and low-grade fever. ■ An initially mild and nonproductive cough develops. ■ These symptoms may last up to 2 weeks. *Paroxysmal phase:* ■ Cough increases in severity. ■ Severe coughing paroxysms may cause respiratory distress, cyanosis, or posttussive vomiting. ■ This may last for up to 2 months. *Convalescent phase:* ■ Decreased intensity of the paroxysms and increased time between spasms. *Complications:* ■ Pneumonia, atelactisis; otitis media; convulsions; hemorrhage (subarachnoid, subconjunctival, epistaxis); weight loss and dehydration; hernia; prolapsed rectum.	Institute respiratory and seizure precautions. Provide high humidity and oxygen. Suction gently but often. Encourage fluids; intravenous hydration may be necessary. Intubation may be necessary. Administer erythromycin for 14 days at a dose of 40 to 50 mg/kg/day (up to a maximum of 2 g/day) in 4 doses. Trimethoprim-sulfamethoxazole can also be used for treatment (trimethoprim, 8 mg/kg/day; sulfamethoxazole, 40 mg/kg/day). Household and other close contacts should receive medical evaluation for possible antibiotic prophylaxis to limit spread of disease.	Maintain isolation during catarrhal stage. Provide restful environment and reduce factors that promote paroxysms (dust, smoke, sudden change in temperature, activity, excitement). Encourage fluids. Provide humidified air; suction gently. Observe for signs of airway obstruction (increased restlessness, increased work of breathing, restlessness, apprehension, retractions, cyanosis) (Dworkin et al., 1997).

(continued)

TABLE 26.6 (continued)

Disease	Signs/Symptoms/ Complications	ED Interventions	Home Care and Prevention
Polio	*Abortive or inapparent:* Fever; uneasiness; sore throat; headache; anorexia; vomiting; abdominal pain; lasts a few hours to a few days. *Nonparalytic:* Same manifestations as abortive, but more severe, with pain and stiffness in neck, back, and legs. *Paralytic:* Initial course similar to nonparalytic type, followed by recovery and then signs of central nervous system paralysis. *Complications:* Permanent paralysis; respiratory arrest; hypertension.	Provide bed rest. Assist ventilation, if necessary. Provide analgesics. Provide sedatives, as necessary, to relieve anxiety and promote rest.	Maintain bed rest. Administer analgesics and sedatives. Participate in physiotherapy procedures (moist hot packs and range-of-motion exercises). Encourage child to move. Observe for respiratory paralysis (difficulty in talking; ineffective cough; shallow and rapid respirations) (Whaley & Wong, 1999).

- Assess for signs of meningeal irritation or increased intracranial pressure:
  - Children with tuberculous meningitis usually present with a gradual onset of symptoms, including irritability and lethargy, over 2 to 3 weeks.

4. Assess the child's overall appearance:
   - Observe the child's hygiene.
   - Measure the child's weight and height:
     - Weight loss may have occurred.

Psychosocial Assessment

- Assess the child and family's understanding of the disease process.
- Assess the child and family's living conditions and exposure to potential TB sources.

Nursing Interventions

- Administer supplemental oxygen, as needed.
- Initiate monitoring of oxygen saturation levels.
- Prepare for chest radiographs:
  - Pulmonary lesions are generally located in the right upper lobe and are subpleural. Segmental atelectasis is particularly common in infants (Vallejo, Ong, & Starke, 1994).
  - The chest radiograph of asymptomatic children is generally normal (Benenson, 2000).
- Isolate symptomatic children in negative-flow examination rooms. Staff members having contact with patient should have approved TB masks in place. As with all patients, universal precautions should be observed when handling bodily secretions.
- Perform tuberculin skin testing and arrange for the skin test to be read in 2 days:
  - Patients with a positive skin test who are asymptomatic should be started on preventive therapy with isoniazid (INH).
- Initiate treatment for uncomplicated pulmonary tuberculosis:
  - Prepare to administer INH, rifampin, and pyrazinamide. The treatment of drug-resistant strains of *M. tuberculosis* requires familiarity with local drug-resistance patterns (Starke, Jacobs, & Jereb, 1992).
- Prepare the patient and family for additional testing, which may include serologic sputum and urine testing to identify the specific TB bacteria (Ball, 1998).
- Report cases of TB to the local health department.

Home Care and Prevention

Prevention involves a high level of suspicion when children are assessed in the ED. Early identification and treatment are critical. Parents must be told of the importance of having the TB test read within 2 days. Remind the parents that this disease will be reported to the local health department and that other family members may need to receive TB testing.

Because the medication regimen may last daily for up to 18 months (Ball, 1998), parents must receive reinforcement about the importance of complying with the treatment and of having the proper amount of medication available for the child. Failure to comply with the treatment may result in a more serious infection as well as communicability to other family members (Ball, 1998).

Children may return to school or day care when the sputum is bacteria-free (Ball, 1998). Other teaching points include (Ball, 1998):

- Provide the child with a well-balanced, high-protein, and calcium-rich diet to promote immune function.
- Allow the child naps and sufficient sleep at night.

- Alternate periods of rest and activity to prevent exhaustion.
- Avoid exposing the child to others with infections, such as colds.
- Teach the child proper hand-washing techniques to prevent the spread of infection.
- Follow up regularly with the child's primary care physician.

Staff exposed to tuberculosis-infected patients must receive tuberculin skin testing to assure early detection and treatment of TB.

Infectious Mononucleosis

Etiology

Infectious mononucleosis is an acute viral syndrome. The infectious agent is most often the Epstein-Barr virus. Infectious mononucleosis occurs worldwide and is widespread among young children in developing countries and in socioeconomically depressed groups, where it is usually mild or asymptomatic. In young children, the disease is generally mild and more difficult to recognize; it is recognized most often in high school and college students. About 50% of those infected will develop clinical infectious mononucleosis, while the others are mostly asymptomatic.

The disease's duration is from 1 week to several weeks; it is rarely fatal. The incubation period is 4 to 6 weeks, and the period of communicability may be prolonged (up to a year or more after infection) (Barkin, 1997). Recovery usually occurs in a few weeks, but a very small proportion of individuals can take months to regain their former level of energy. There is no evidence that this is due to abnormal persistence of the infection in a chronic form.

Focused History

Patient history

- Fever.
- Sore throat (may be severe).
- Fatigue.
- Exposure to someone with infectious mononucleosis.
- Rash.
- Enlarged, nonpainful cervical lymph nodes.
- Myalgia.

Focused Assessment

Physical Assessment

1. Assess the respiratory system:
   - Auscultate the chest for:
     - Respiratory rate. Respiratory rate may be increased with fever.
2. Assess the cardiovascular system:
   - Auscultate the heart for:
     - Rate. Heart rate may be increased in the presence of fever.
   - Measure the blood pressure.
   - Measure core and skin temperature:
     - Fever may be present.
3. Assess the neurologic system:
   - Assess the child's level of consciousness with the GCS or AVPU methods.
   - Assess the child's motor strength:
     - Fatigue and weakness may be present.
4. Assess the lymphatic system:
   - Palpate the posterior cervical lymph nodes:
     - Enlarged nodes may be palpated.
5. Assess the abdomen:
   - Palpate the abdomen:
     - Splenomegaly may be present, occurring in 50% of patients.
6. Assess the integumentary system:
   - Observe the skin color:
     - Jaundice occurs in 4% of infected young adults.

Psychosocial Assessment

- Assess the child's and family's understanding of the disease process.
- Assess the child's coping strategies as it may be necessary to curtail activities.

Nursing Interventions

- Administer medications, as prescribed:
  - Administer antipyretics for fever control.
  - Prepare to administer nonsteroidal antiinflammatory drugs or steroids in small doses and in decreasing amounts over about a week in patients who have symptoms of toxicity or who have severe oropharyngeal involvement.
- Obtain blood specimens for laboratory testing:
  - Heterophile antibodies.
  - Epstein-Barr antibodies.
  - Liver function tests. In 95% of infected children, results of liver function tests will be abnormal.

Home Care and Prevention

Patients and families should receive home care instructions for infectious mononucelosis (Ball, 1998):

- Serve small, frequent meals of soft foods to patients with severe sore throats.
- Offer frequent fluids, such as water and fruit juices.
- Avoid medications that contain alcohol as well as alcoholic beverages.
- Avoid contact sports, heavy lifting, and strenuous activities to prevent splenic or liver injury.
- Employ hygienic measures to avoid salivary contamination from the infected patient, such as thorough hand washing, the avoidance of drinking from a common container, and the appropriate disposal of articles soiled with nasopharyngeal discharges (Benenson, 2000).

Acquired Immunodeficiency Syndrome

Etiology

Acquired immunodeficiency syndrome (AIDS) is a persistent and progressively debilitating viral infection that affects multiple systems. The AIDS virus commonly attacks the immune and nervous systems. The role of emergency nurses treating AIDS includes early diagnosis, management of acute complications, and implementation of universal precautions, as is the case with all patients. In 1981 AIDS was first recognized as a disease entity. The human immunodeficiency virus, the etiologic agent of AIDS, was first reported in 1984. It is estimated that there are nearly 1.1 million children living with the human immunodeficiency virus type 1 (HIV-1) infection worldwide. (Mueller & Pizzo, 2001, p. 447).

Children infected with HIV present with nonspecific signs and symptoms of HIV infections. The disease often progresses more rapidly and has a shorter incubation period in children than in adults (almost one half of all HIV-infected children are diagnosed at younger than 1 year of age), making early diagnosis critical. Only 35 to 55% of HIV-exposed children are identified before becoming symptomatic (Centers for Disease Control and Prevention, 1995c). More than 90% of pediatric HIV infections result from the transmission from mother to child. Infants born to HIV-infected mothers have approximately a 25–30% risk of acquiring the infection (Mueller & Pizzo, 2001). Other routes of HIV infection in children include sexual abuse, use of contaminated needles, and unprotected sexual intercourse (Mueller & Pizzo, 2001).

Human immunodeficiency virus is dependent on the cells it infects to reproduce. The AIDS virus attacks and infects the helper T cell or CD4 cell, major components in the immune response. A depletion in the number of CD4 T cells results in widespread immune dysfunction. The nervous system and other tissues have receptors similar to that on CD4 T cells and thus become targets for primary infections. Because the pathology of AIDS involves the immune system, children are extremely vulnerable to opportunistic infections by organisms, such as *Pneumocystis carinii*.

Focused History

1. Patient history for the child who is HIV positive:
   - Recurrent bacterial infections, such as bacteremia, otitis media, sinusitis, pneumonia, urinary tract infections, and meningitis.
   - Current medications and treatments.
2. Patient history for the child who is not HIV positive:
   - Risk factors (Reynolds & Kelley, 1994):
     - Maternal blood transfusions.
     - Intravenous drug use.
     - Sexual contact or sexual abuse.
     - Sexual contact with intravenous drug users or bisexual men.
     - Blood or blood product transfusion.
   - Non specific signs and symptoms, such as (Mueller & Pizzo, 2001):
     - History of failure to thrive or to gain weight.
     - Recurrent bacterial infections.
     - Chronic encephalopathy.

Focused Assessment

Physical Assessment

1. Assess the respiratory system:
   - Auscultate the chest for:
     - Respiratory rate. *Pneumocystis carinii* pneumonia is the most common infection in children with AIDS. Infants generally present with an acute onset of fever, cough, tachypnea, and dyspnea (Simonds & Orejas, 1998).
2. Assess the neurologic system:
   - Assess the child's neuromotor and neuromuscular capabilities:
     - Central nervous system dysfunction and developmental delay may be present (Reynolds & Kelley, 1994).
     - Encephalopathy, the most frequent presentation for HIV-infected children, is characterized by developmental delays, deterioration in motor

and intellectual skills, muscle weakness, ataxia, or seizures.

3. Observe the child's overall size and stature; measure the child's height and weight:
   - Small size and dysmorphic features may be observed in the young infant (Reynolds & Kelley, 1994).
   - Low percentile for height and weight may be found.
4. Assess the integumentary system:
   - Inspect the oral cavity:
     - Lesions may be observed.
   - Inspect the skin:
     - Nonhealing wounds may be noted.
5. Assess the lymphatic system:
   - Palpate the cervical and femoral lymph nodes:
     - Lymphadenopathy may be noted.
6. Assess the abdomen:
   - Palpate the abdomen:
     - Hepatomegaly and splenomegaly may be noted (Reynolds & Kelley, 1994).

Psychosocial Assessment

- Assess the HIV-positive child and family's coping strategies:
  - Children with AIDS may have feelings of fear, anxiety, anger, or denial, similar to other children with chronic or life-threatening illnesses.
  - Children and families may present frequently to the ED for treatment and may become well known to the staff, so they may be more likely to share their feelings and experiences.
- For those who are newly diagnosed, assess the child and family's understanding of the meaning of being HIV positive.
  - Support services may be needed to help the child and family cope with this new diagnosis.

Nursing Interventions

1. Administer supplemental oxygen and provide proper positioning for the child in respiratory distress.
2. Initiate cardiorespiratory and oxygen saturation monitoring.
3. Administer medications, as prescribed:
   - Administer antibiotics in the presence of infection.
4. Prepare the child for diagnostic testing:
   - Obtain a complete blood count, blood culture, urinalysis, and chest radiograph when a focus of infection cannot be readily diagnosed (e.g., middle ear infection) (Pinkert, Harper, Cooper, & Fleisher, 1993) and fever is present.
   - In children older than 18 months:
     - Obtain blood for enzyme immunoassay (EIA) to confirm a diagnosis of HIV. Any positive EIA must be repeated and confirmed by Western blot analysis.
   - In children younger than 18 months:
     - Obtain either an HIV viral culture or HIV polymerase chain reaction (American Academy of Pediatrics, 2000). A positive EIA in children younger than 18 months may be caused by maternal antibodies.
5. Prepare the child and family for hospitalization, if needed:
   - Evaluate febrile children who appear toxic for bacterial or opportunistic infections.
6. Provide psychosocial support for the child and family coping with a chronic illness.

Home Care and Prevention

Emergency nurses can teach children and families about ways to prevent opportunistic infections (Ball, 1998):

- Avoid exposing the HIV-positive child to people with infections, such as chicken pox, colds, or influenza.
- Contact the child's primary care physician if such exposure should occur.
- Continue with the regular immunization schedule, including the influenza vaccine.

Emergency nurses also can remind the child and family that HIV cannot be spread through common touch or play. All children and families, regardless of their HIV status, should teach their children to tell an adult if someone is bleeding and to avoid direct contact with other people's blood and bodily fluids (Ball, 1998).

On a personal or community level, emergency nurses can teach methods for prevention of HIV infection to school-aged children and adolescents (Ball, 1998):

- Do not have unprotected sexual intercourse. Condoms plus contraceptive foam or jelly containing nonoxynol-9 should be used. Condoms should be worn during sexual contact with other body orifices, such as the mouth or anus.

- Do not inject drugs and do not share needles and syringes. If drugs are injected, the person should use his or her own needles and syringes.

Meningitis and Meningococcemia

Etiology

Meningitis is caused by a bacterial or viral infection that results in inflammation of the meninges. *Streptococcus pneumoniae* and *Neisseria meningitidis* are common bacterial agents causing meningitis after 2 months of age. With the initiation of the *Haemophilus influenzae* type b vaccine, *H. influenzae* meningitis is much less common. More than 90% of meningitis cases result from infections with fever organisms: S. pneumoniae, N. meningitides, E. coli, group B streptococcus, and H. influenzae (Fleisher, 2001). These bacteria are transmitted by droplets, gaining entry into the cerebrospinal fluid via the vascular system. The incubation period is 1 to 7 days. Long-term effects of meningitis include seizure disorders; speech; hearing, and visual impairments; mental retardation; and behavior changes.

Meningococcemia is a potentially life-threatening disorder in which *N. meningitidis* gains access to the bloodstream. Septic shock is often associated with meningococcemia; more than one-third of patients who develop septic shock die. Children with meningococcemia may develop meningitis, pericarditis, hypotension, and disseminated intravascular coagulation. During the early 1900s, the mortality rate of children infected with *N. meningitidis* was near 80%. The overall mortality rate has decreased to less than 7%, because of improvements in antibiotic and supportive therapies.

Both meningitis and meningococcemia are true emergencies and can be fatal within a few hours, making rapid assessment and immediate action critical.

Focused History

Patient history

- Recent illness: rapid onset of fever, chills, malaise, and a rash.
- Decreased intake.
- Vomiting and diarrhea.
- Seizures.
- Respiratory distress.

Family history

- Family member or close acquaintance recently diagnosed with meningitis or meningococcemia.

Focused Assessment

Physical Assessment

Signs and symptoms of meningitis vary by age and may be difficult to diagnose in the neonate or infant. Table 26.7 compares physical findings in infants and children.

Psychosocial Assessment

- Assess the child and family's understanding of the disease process.
- Assess the child and family's exposure to potential infectious sources.

Nursing Interventions

1. Assess and maintain airway, breathing, and circulation (Chapter 6):
   - Initiate maneuvers to maintain airway patency, such as positioning and inserting an airway adjunct.
   - Prepare for endotracheal intubation.
   - Administer 100% oxygen through a nonrebreather mask; initiate assisted ventilation in the child who is not maintaining adequate respiratory effort.
   - Prepare for mechanical ventilation if endotracheal intubation is required (Chapter 16).
   - Initiate cardiorespiratory and continuous oxygen saturation monitoring.
2. Obtain intravenous access and initiate an intravenous infusion:
   - Administer a rapid fluid bolus of 20 ml/kg of a crystalloid fluid (normal saline solution or lactated Ringer's solution) in the child with signs of septic shock (Chapter 17) or poor perfusion.
   - Administer second and third boluses of 20 ml/kg of a crystalloid fluid (normal saline solution or lactated Ringer's solution) if improvement is not observed.
   - Prepare to administer vasopressor agents.
   - Administer antibiotics, as prescribed.
   - Obtain blood specimens for:
     - Complete blood count and differential.
     - Platelets.
     - Electrolytes, blood urea nitrogen, creatinine, and glucose.
     - Cultures.
     - Prothrombin time and partial thromboplastin time.
3. Reassess the child's neurologic status and cardiopulmonary status:

TABLE 26.7 Comparison of Physical Assessment Findings in Infants and Children

Body System	*Infants*	*Children*
Central nervous system	Irritability	Headache
	High-pitched cry	Altered level of consciousness
	Bulging anterior fontanelle	Nuchal rigidity
	Seizure activity	Photophobia
	Nuchal rigidity	Positive Kernig's sign
	Lethargy	Seizure activity
	Altered sleep pattern	Coma
		Positive Brudzinski's sign
Thermoregulation	Fever	Fever
Integumentary status	Petechiae below the nipple line	Petechiae
	Purpura	Purpura
Gastrointestinal status	Poor feeding	Vomiting
	Vomiting	
Respiratory status	Apnea	
Overall appearance	"Looks septic"	"Looks sick"

- Observe and monitor for signs of increased intracranial pressure, including changes in level of consciousness, irritability, sluggish pupillary responses, and decreased movements of extremities.

4. Assist with a lumbar puncture if there are no signs of increased intracranial pressure:
   - Obtain cerebrospinal fluid specimens for laboratory analysis:
     - Culture and sensitivity.
     - Glucose.
     - Protein.
     - Cell count and differential.
     - Gram's stain.
   - Note the color of cerebrospinal fluid.
   - Record the opening and closing pressures in older children.
5. Insert an indwelling gastric tube and bladder catheter:
   - Obtain a urine specimen for laboratory analysis:
     - Urinalysis.
     - Culture.
6. Monitor fluid and electrolytes for evidence of syndrome of inappropriate antidiuretic hormone, in which decreased serum sodium and serum osmolarity are found.
7. Inform the family frequently about the child's condition; provide emotional support to the child and family:
   - Initiate referrals to social services and hospital spiritual services.
8. Prepare for transfer and transport to a tertiary care facility, as indicated (Chapter 10), or prepare the child and family for admission to the intensive care unit.

Home Care and Prevention

Precautions must be taken by ED staff and family to avoid possible exposure to meningitis. Children suspected of having meningicoccemia should be isolated from other patients. Gowns, masks, and gloves should be utilized by anyone having direct contact with the child.

Of greatest concern is cross infection of siblings younger than 6 years old and those attending the same day care facility. Adults and children who have close contact with the patient should receive rifampin. Prophylaxis of hospital personnel is usually not necessary. Staff who have prolonged, close contact with the child (prior to the administration of antibiotics) and those who have provided mouth-to-mouth resuscitation should consider treatment (Reynolds & Kelley, 1994).

Encephalitis

Etiology

Encephalitis involves an inflammatory process of the brain, spinal cord, and meninges, producing altered function of various portions of the brain and spinal cord. The disease process occurs as a result of invasion of the central nervous system by a variety of organisms, including bacteria, spirochetes, fungi, protozoa, and viruses, or as a complication of infectious processes. Direct invasion of the causative agent generally results from the bite of infected mosquitoes. In the United States, the four major types of encephalitis are (Benenson, 2000):

1. Eastern equine encephalomyelitis, found in eastern and north central United States.
2. Saint Louis encephalitis, found in most of the United States with exception of the Northeast.
3. Western equine encephalomyelitis, found in the western United States and Canada and some areas further east.
4. California encephalitis, found throughout the United States.

Measles, mumps, varicella, rubella, enteroviruses, and herpes simplex virus may cause encephalitis as a complication of the disease process. Residual effects of encephalitis may include (Reynolds & Kelley, 1994):

- Developmental delays.
- Neurologic sequelae (variable frequency, depending on age and infecting agent).
- Seizure disorders.
- Hemiplegia.
- Hemiparesis.
- Hearing loss.

Focused History

- Patient history in mild cases of encephalitis:
  - Asymptomatic.
  - Afebrile headache.
  - Aseptic meningitis.
- Patient history in severe cases of encephalitis with a rapid onset:
  - Headache.
  - High fever.
  - Meningeal signs.
  - Stupor.
  - Disorientation.
  - Coma.
  - Tremors.
  - Convulsions (especially in infants).

Focused Assessment

Physical Assessment

- Assess the neurologic system:
- Assess the child's level of consciousness with the GCS or AVPU method:
  - Irritability or a decreased level of consciousness may be noted.
- Observe for meningeal signs:
  - Headache.
  - Difficulty or refusal to move head and neck.
  - Fever.
  - Seizure activity.

Psychosocial Assessment

- Assess the child and family's understanding of the disease process.
- Assess the child and family's coping strategies.
- Assess the availability of emotional support systems, such as family or neighbors.

Nursing Interventions

1. Assess and maintain airway, breathing, and circulation (Chapter 6).
2. Initiate cardiorespiratory and oxygen saturation monitoring.
3. Obtain venous access and initiate an intravenous infusion at maintenance rate:
   - Prepare to administer osmotic diuretics, as needed, to control increased intracranial pressure.
   - Obtain blood specimens for laboratory analysis:
     - Viral studies.
4. Perform initial and serial neurologic assessments to detect increases in intracranial pressure, including:
   - Cranial nerve assessments.
   - Level of consciousness.
   - Pupillary response.
   - Fontanelle assessments (infants).
5. Assist with a lumbar puncture if there are no signs of increased intracranial pressure:
   - Obtain cerebrospinal fluid specimens for laboratory analysis:
     - Culture and sensitivity.
     - Viral studies.

    - Glucose.
    - Protein.
    - Cell count and differential.
    - Gram's stains.
  - Note the color of the cerebrospinal fluid.
  - Record the opening and closing pressures.
6. Obtain pharyngeal and stool samples for viral cultures to identify the infecting organism.
7. Administer antipyretics to the febrile patient.
8. Antibiotics are not administered, because they are of no value in viral infections. However, the infecting organism may not be diagnosed initially in the ED.
9. Reassess the child's neurologic status and cardiopulmonary status.
10. Inform the family frequently about the child's condition; provide emotional support to the child and family.
11. Prepare for transfer and transport to a tertiary care facility (Chapter 10) or hospital admission.

Home Care and Prevention

Prevention of encephalitis begins with the community education regarding the mode of spread and control. Mosquito larvae must be destroyed, and breeding grounds (such as standing pools of water) must be eliminated. Children should avoid exposure to mosquitoes by avoiding outdoor play during hours of biting or by judicious use of repellents. Sleeping and living quarters should be screened. In endemic areas, domestic animals should be immunized or housed away from living quarters.

Infectious Diseases

Rabies

Etiology

Rabies is a rare, fatal viral infection with a 10-day to several months incubation period (Barkin & Rosen, 1999). Manifestations predominantly involve the central nervous system. The frequency of animal bites and the rising incidence of rabies in wild animals make evaluation for treatment a major consideration. The incidence of rabies varies greatly among geographic areas.

Transmission of the rabies virus occurs following a bite or scratch or after contamination of the mucous membranes or an open wound by an animal infected with the rabies virus. Sources of rabies in the United States include wild and domestic animals. The occurrence of rabies in domestic animals is very low; fully vaccinated dogs and cats are rarely infected with the virus (Centers for Disease Control and Prevention, 1991). Wild animals represent the most significant source of rabies in the United States. The highest incidence is among skunks, raccoons, foxes, and bats. Rodents are rarely infected. The diagnosis of rabies in an animal requires examination of the brain tissue for the virus (Centers for Disease Control and Prevention, 1991).

Focused History

Patient history

- Animal involved in the exposure:
  - Type (domestic or wild).
  - Whereabouts (stray, pet, or wild).
  - Animal's rabies status.
  - Animal's owner.
  - Animal's present location (i.e., caught and detained or unknown).
  - Where the bite occurred (indoors, street, or forest).
- Type of wound:
  - Bite (puncture, laceration, or avulsion).
  - Scratch.
- Location of the wound .
- Time of occurence.
- Provoked or unprovoked attack or contact.
- Cleansing or treatment measures prior to ED presentation.

Focused Assessment

Physical Assessment

1. Assess the neurologic system:
   - Assess the child's level of consciousness with the GCS or AVPU method.
   - Assess for neurologic findings indicative of rabies, such as (Barkin & Rosen, 1999):
     - Apprehension, followed by seizures, delirium, and lethargy.
     - Hydrophobia.
     - Paresthesia at the wound.
2. Assess the wound:
   - Observe the type of wound (puncture, scratch, or bite).
   - Note the location of the wound.
   - Observe the depth of the wound.
   - Determine if underlying structures are involved.

Psychosocial Assessment

- Assess the child for fear or apprehension:
    - Following an animal bite, the child may be fearful or apprehensive.
    - The child may have been warned about avoiding the particular animal, or the child may have been teasing the animal.
    - In unprovoked attacks, the child may become fearful of animals in the future.
- Assess the child and family's coping strategies.

Nursing Interventions

1. Initiate thorough wound cleansing:
    - Irrigate punctures and lacerations thoroughly with normal saline solution.
    - Wash the area with povidone iodine or antimicrobial soap.
    - Wash scratches with povidone iodine or antimicrobial soap and normal saline solution.
    - Prepare for suturing, if needed:
        - Prepare for conscious sedation (Chapter 13) in the child with facial or extensive lacerations.
    - Apply an antibacterial ointment and bandage the wound.
2. Administer medications, as prescribed:
    - Administer intravenous or oral antibiotics.
    - Administer tetanus prophylaxis if the wounds are extensive or if a booster is required based on age at last tetanus vaccine.
    - Administer human rabies immune globulin if rabies exposure is suspected or confirmed:
        - Administer as a single dose of 20 IU/kg, with up to one-half the dose infiltrated around the wound, if possible, and the remainder given intramuscularly.
    - Administer the human rabies vaccine:
        - Administer the vaccine intramuscularly (1 ml) in the deltoid of older children because this is the only acceptable site for the human rabies vaccine.
        - Administer the vaccine in the outer aspect of the thigh of younger children; the vaccine should never be administered in the gluteal area (Barkin, 1997).
3. Prepare the child with severe wounds for operative management and hospitalization.
4. Report the animal bite and suspected rabies cases to the local health department.
5. Report the animal bite to the animal control authorities if the animal is a stray or cannot be located, or if the owners are unknown:
    - Although wounds inflicted by dogs and cats that appear healthy represent the lowest rabies risk, the animal should be observed for 10 days for any unprovoked attacks or behavioral changes.

If the animal appears rabid or becomes ill during the period of observation, the child should begin rabies prophylaxis immediately.

Unprovoked attacks or behavioral changes in the animal should be interpreted as possible signs of rabies.

Other considerations should include the type of exposure (bite or nonbite) and the prevalence of rabies in the specified region.

All carnivores, bats, and woodchucks should be initially regarded as having the rabies virus, and prophylaxis should begin. Treatment should be discontinued after laboratory tests confirm that the animal tested negative for the rabies virus (Centers for Disease Control and Prevention, 1991).

Arrange for the child and family to return to the ED or to their health care provider on days 3, 7, 14, and 28 for injections of the human rabies vaccine.

Home Care and Prevention

Prevention of animal bites is both an individual and a community responsibility. The community should require that all domestic pets be licensed and leashed, under verbal control, or confined. Regular vaccination and immunization programs should be mandated for all domestic pets. Children should be taught to avoid reservoirs of rabies, particularly skunks, foxes, and bats. All homeless or stray animals should be rounded up and confined, and efforts should be made to find them homes. Shelters that put homeless animals up for adoption should require that pets received through them be sterilized to decrease the number of unwanted animals. ED staff should explore patterns of rabies susceptibility in their local areas.

Parents should be advised about bite-prevention measures and animal safety (Chapter 5), provided with instructions for reporting bites, and instructed in proper guidelines for pet selection and care. Parents and children may be concerned about the cosmetic outcomes of facial wounds; they also may fear undergoing rabies vaccination. Parents will have to work with the animal's owner and local health authorities regarding quarantine, rabies status, or euthanasia.

Kawasaki Disease

Etiology

Kawasaki disease (KD) is an acute, self-limiting multisystem disorder of unknown etiology. The disease affects mostly young children. Early diagnosis is vital because Kawasaki disease results in serious cardiac disorders in 20% of untreated patients. The disease was first recognized in Japan by Kawasaki in 1967. The disease is now recognized worldwide. In the United States, an estimated 3,000 to 3,500 cases occur annually (American Academy of Pediatrics, 2000).

Eighty percent of cases of KD occur in children younger than 4 or 5 years of age; the peak incidence is 18 to 24 months. Males are affected more often then females. The disease appears year round, but incidence is higher during late winter and early spring. Person-to-person contact has not been demonstrated.

Clinically and epidemiologically, KD behaves as an infectious disease. A number of viral, bacterial, and environmental associations have been made, but no causative factor has been identified (Barkin, 1997). In the early phase of KD, inflammation of the small blood vessels occurs, and within 12 to 25 days the medium-sized arteries are involved (Reynolds & Kelley, 1994). Aneurysms develop in the coronary arteries (rarely in the cervical, iliac, or renal arteries) and then heal, resulting in scarring and stenosis of the vessel walls (Reynolds & Kelley, 1994). Thrombus development may lead to myocardial ischemia or infarction (Reynolds & Kelley, 1994). Infants and children with prolonged fevers are at greatest risk for developing cardiac complications (Reynolds & Kelley, 1994).

Cardiovascular manifestations of KD are the major complication in the pediatric population. Patients with KD have approximately a 20% risk of developing coronary aneurysms without treatment. Patients younger than 1 year of age have an even greater risk. Most aneurysms develop after the acute phase of the disease between days 15 and 45.

The diagnosis of Kawasaki disease is based on clinical findings. Not all symptoms have to occur simultaneously, and symptoms may vary in duration, time of onset, and severity. Also, cases of atypical or incomplete KD have been reported; thus, KD should not be ruled out if a level of suspicion is present (Sundel, 2000).

Focused History

Patient history:

- Fever persisting at least 5 days.
- Rash.
- Irritability.
- Poor appetite and oral intake.
- Decreased urinary output.
- Decreased activity level.

Focused Assessment

Physical Assessment

1. Assess the respiratory system:
   - Auscultate the chest for:
     - Respiratory rate.
   - Adventitious sounds:
     - Cough may be present.
     - Pulmonary infiltrates may be detected on radiograph.
   - Inspect the nose for rhinorrhea.
2. Assess the cardiovascular system:
   - Auscultate the heart for:
     - Rate. Gallop rhythm may be present.
     - Rhythm. Pericardial effusion and valvular insufficiency may be present.
   - Interpret electrocardiogram readings for:
     - Dysrhythmias. Myocardial infarction and dysrhythmia are the most common causes of sudden death and occur in 1 to 2% of patients (Rosenfeld, Corydon, & Shulman, 1995).
3. Assess the central nervous system:
   - Assess the level of consciousness with the GCS or AVPU method.
4. Assess for neurologic changes:
   - Irritability.
   - Signs of meningeal irritation.
   - Photophobia.
5. Assess the gastrointestinal system:
   - Observe for:
     - Diarrhea.
     - Nausea and vomiting.
   - Palpate the abdomen for pain.
6. Assess the integumentary system:
   - Observe the skin color:
     - Color may be pale as a result of anemia.
     - May be jaundiced.
   - Observe for a rash.
   - Observe for induration of hands and feet and desquamation of fingers or toes.
7. Assess for changes in the oral cavity:
   - Erythema and cracking of lips.
   - Strawberry tongue.
   - Diffuse injection of oral and pharyngeal mucosae.
8. Assess the lymphatic system:

- Palpate the cervical lymph nodes for adenopathy (usually unilateral).

Psychosocial Assessment

- Assess the child and family's knowledge of the disease process.
- Assess the child and family's coping strategies.

Nursing Interventions

- Assess and maintain airway, breathing, and circulation (Chapter 6):
  - Initiate cardiorespiratory and oxygen saturation monitoring.
- Obtain vascular access and initiate an intravenous infusion at a maintenance rate:
  - Administer intravenous fluids cautiously to prevent congestive heart failure.
- Obtain blood specimens for laboratory analysis:
  - Complete blood count (elevated) and differential.
  - Platelets (elevated).
  - Erythrocyte sedimentation rate (elevated).
  - Alanine amino transferase (elevated).
- Administer medications, as prescribed:
  - Initiate aspirin therapy: Aspirin therapy inhibits platelet function and may decrease the associated coronary artery disease:
  - Begin aspirin therapy with 100 mg/kg/day orally, divided into four doses daily, and continue until fever has resolved.
  - Continue with low-dose aspirin at 3 to 5 mg/kg/day, orally, once daily (maximum, 40 to 80 mg in 24 hours) for 2 to 3 months or until the platelet count has normalized.
  - Monitor salicylate levels during high-dose aspirin therapy.
  - Administer intravenous gamma globulin as a single dose of 2 g/kg, infused over 8 to 12 hours. Observe for reactions such as flushing, chills, headache, nausea, and vomiting.
- Reassess the child's neurologic status and cardiopulmonary status.
- Monitor intake and output carefully:
  - Obtain a urine specimen; observe for white cells with no bacteria.
- Prepare for diagnostic testing:
  - Prepare for echocardiography to determine baseline cardiac function (American Academy of Pediatrics, 2000).
- Initiate a cardiology consultation.
- Inform the family frequently of the child's condition; provide emotional support to the child and family.
- Prepare for transfer and transport to a tertiary care facility, as needed (Chapter 10), or hospitalization:
  - Hospitalization and cardiorespiratory monitoring are required to detect cardiac complications such as congestive heart failure, pericardial effusions, and dysrhythmias.

Home Care and Prevention

The prognosis for patients receiving treatment within the first 10 days of illness is good. However, long-term morbidity is profound in patients who are not diagnosed and treated early in the course of the disease. Children diagnosed with KD require follow-up for several years; special attention should be paid to the development of coronary artery disease. Children and parents must be taught about the complications of KD.

Parents are instructed to provide bed rest during the first few weeks of the disease; therefore, parents and children will need suggestions for quiet activities, such as reading, board games, videos, or puzzles (Ball, 1998). Remind parents that the desquamation that occurs during the second and third weeks is painless, even though it looks distressing (Reynolds & Kelley, 1994). Advise the child that the discomfort associated with arthritis may persist for several weeks and may be relieved with passive range-of-motion exercises in warm water (Reynolds & Kelley, 1994).

Reye's Syndrome

Etiology

Reye's syndrome is a disorder characterized by fatty infiltration of the liver and mitochondrial damage. Reye's syndrome was first described in 1963. Reported cases rose during the 1970s, peaking at 555 cases in 1980. From 1974 to 1985, the mean fatality rate was 32%. During the 1980s, the incidence of Reye's syndrome began to decline as aspirin use in children was linked to the disorder. In 1982, the Surgeon General recommended that parents avoid using aspirin for treating fevers in children. In the late 1980s, cases of confirmed Reye's syndrome declined to fewer than 50 per year (Arrowsmith, Faich, Kennedy, Kuritsky, & Faich, 1986).

The etiology of Reye's syndrome is unknown; however, widespread mitochondrial damage is found in all parts of the body. This produces a disruption in urea synthesis, gluconeogenesis, and the Krebs' cycle, which leads to elevated ammonia levels, hypoglycemia, lipid accumulation in the cells, and lactic acidosis. The liver enlarges, and the brain swells. Laboratory data demonstrate elevated ammonia levels, decreased serum glucose, and a prolonged prothrombin time.

During the clinical course of the disease, within 3 to 5 days of a recent viral illness, persistent vomiting develops. The child then becomes listless or drowsy. Disorientation may lead to delirium and convulsions. The child may become confused or lethargic or can experience hallucinations. Behavioral changes develop into symptoms of combativeness and delirium. Rapid deterioration follows with signs of hyperventilation, coma, and decorticate posturing, followed by decerebrate posturing and deeper coma.

Focused History

Patient history

- Recent viral infection, such as varicella virus or a cold.
- Administration of aspirin or aspirin-containing medications:
  - Medication usage is an important history point when attempting to diagnosis Reye's syndrome.
  - Salicylate exposure is common and may occur through over-the-counter medicines with "hidden" salicylates (Chapter 44).
- Changes in level of consciousness, such as irritability or drowsiness.
- Vomiting.

Focused Assessment

Physical Assessment

- Assess the neurologic system:
  - Assess the child's level of consciousness with the GCS or AVPU method.
- Test the pupils for:
  - Size.
  - Reactivity.
  - Response to light.
- Test the cranial nerves.
- Assess the integumentary system for signs of dehydration.

Psychosocial Assessment

- Assess the child and family's coping strategies.
- Assess the child and family's understanding of the disease:
  - Parents may have guilt after innocently administering salicylates to the child.

Nursing Interventions

- Assess and maintain airway, breathing, and circulation (Chapter 6).
- Obtain venous access and initiate an intravenous infusion:
  - Administer dextrose to prevent hypoglycemia.
  - Titrate fluid administration to signs of cerebral edema.
- Obtain blood specimens for laboratory analysis, including (Barkin, 1997):
  - Liver enzymes.
  - Ammonia.
  - Prothrombin time and partial thromboplastin time.
- Initiate measures to control intracranial pressure, such as providing adequate oxygenation and osmotic diuretic agents.
- Insert an indwelling bladder catheter; measure intake and output.
- Inform the family frequently of the child's condition; provide emotional support to the child and family.
- Prepare for transfer and transport to a tertiary care center (Chapter 10) or for hospital admission. Depending on the severity of the symptoms, admission to the intensive care unit may be warranted.

Home Care and Prevention

Parents must be educated regarding the use of salicylates in children presenting with viral symptoms. Several over-the-counter medications may include "hidden" salicylate dosages. Parents should be instructed to carefully read labels or speak to a pharmacist before providing their children with any medication.

Acute Rheumatic Fever

Etiology

Rheumatic fever is an inflammatory disease that affects the connective tissue of the heart, joints, central nervous system, and subcutaneous tissue. Generally, the disorder presents in children between the ages of 5 and 17 years. A strong association with a preceding group A streptococcal infection of the nasopharynx has been found. Carditis is the most serious complication, resulting in severe congestive heart failure, myocarditis, valvulitis, dysrhythmias, renal disease, and death.

Acute rheumatic fever is thought to be an immune reaction to antigens of certain strains of group A streptococcus (Barkin, 1997). Antibody reactions produce triggers that affect the myocardium and joints. Involvement of the heart produces endomyocarditis and valvulitis involving the mitral and aortic vales. Joint involvement produces edema of the synovium and periarticular tissues.

Focused History

Patient history

- Streptococcal pharyngitis infection that occurred in the prior 2 to 6 weeks.
- Low-grade fever.
- Malaise.
- Joint pain:
  - Arthritis is the most common symptom of acute rheumatic fever, occurring in 60 to 80% of first attacks.
  - Generally, two or more large joints (ankle, knee, wrist, or elbow) are involved.
- Abdominal pain.
- Weight loss.
- Hair loss.

Focused Assessment

Physical Assessment

1. Assess the cardiovascular system:
   - Auscultate the heart for:
     - Rate. Tachycardia may be present.
     - Murmurs.
     - Gallop rhythm.
     - Friction rub: Signs of congestive heart failure and carditis may be found.
     - Symptoms of carditis can be variable in severity and occur in 35 to 40% of new cases. Carditis is most important to recognize and treat in the acute phase, because it can have potentially serious or fatal complications.
2. Assess the neurologic system:
   - Assess the child's level of consciousness with the GCS or AVPU method.
   - Observe for chorea:
     - Chorea is seen in about 10% of patients and is defined as a series of sudden movements that are involuntary.
     - Movements typically involve the facial and extremity muscles. The child may complain of an inability to write, uncontrolled grimacing, and weakness (Special Writing Group, 1992).
3. Assess the musculoskeletal system:
   - Palpate the joints for pain or tenderness.
   - Inspect the joints for edema or redness.

Psychosocial Assessment

- Assess the child and family's understanding of the disease process.

Nursing Interventions

1. Assess and maintain airway, breathing, and circulation (see Chapter 6):
   - Initiate cardiorespiratory and oxygen saturation monitoring.
   - Initiate treatment for shock, congestive heart failure, and dysrhythmias (Chapter 17).
   - Obtain venous access and initiate an intravenous infusion.
2. Obtain blood specimens for laboratory analysis:
   - Erythrocyte sedimentation rate.
   - C-Reactive protein.
   - Antistreptolysin O titer.
3. Administer medications, as prescribed:
   - Administer penicillin:
     - For patients who are allergic to penicillin, erythromycin may be substituted.
     - Prophylactic therapy should be started as soon as treatment for an acute attack is completed.
     - Generally, prophylactic therapy is continued intermittently for 5 to 10 years, depending on the amount of cardiac involvement (Barkin, 1997).
   - Administer steroids, such as prednisone, if carditis or congestive heart failure is present.
   - Administer aspirin:
     - Aspirin is generally prescribed in high doses to produce a serum salicylate level in the range of 20 to 30 mg/dl.
4. Reassess neurologic status and cardiopulmonary status.
5. Initiate consultation with a cardiologist.
6. Prepare for hospital admission, as needed.

Home Care and Prevention

Streptococcal infections trigger this disease, as well as its recurrences. Treatment of streptococcal pharyngitis is critical in preventing the occurrence of the disease, and prophylactic treatment for streptococcal disease after an attack of rheumatic fever will assist in preventing a recurrence of the disorder.

The child and family should be reminded that this disease lasts 2 to 8 weeks (Ball, 1998). Encourage parents to (Ball, 1998):

- Provide rest.

- Encourage quiet activities, such as board games, reading, videos or puzzles.
- Administer acetaminophen for fever.
- Administer aspirin for joint pain.
- Administer antibiotics, as prescribed by the physician.
- Observe for symptoms of carditis and arthritis.

Parents must be reminded that penicillin or sulfa drugs must be administered to the child for a prolonged period of time. Parents are encouraged to report the child's history of rheumatic fever to their primary care physician and dentist for the purpose of initiating prophylactic antibiotic therapy prior to invasive procedures (Ball, 1998). This action prevents the onset of endocarditis (Chapter 17). Should the child develop another sore throat despite current antibiotic therapy, a throat culture is needed to determine whether a different strain of bacteria is involved (Ball, 1998).

Lyme Disease

Etiology

Lyme disease (LD) is the most common tick-borne disease in the United States. It is a systemic infection that causes dermatologic, neurologic, cardiac, and musculoskeletal symptoms. Lyme disease is named after the town of Old Lyme, Connecticut, where it was discovered in 1975; however, evidence suggests that the disease dates back several years (Persing et al., 1990).

The etiologic agent of Lyme disease, *Borrelia burgdorferi*, is a bacteria that is transmitted by the bites of infected ticks. In the Northeast and in the north central states, the deer tick is the predominant carrier. In the West, it is the black-legged tick. Ticks that transmit LD can and do infect dogs, cats, and horses. Although pets do not directly transmit the disease, loose ticks may pose a threat to pet owners (Centers for Disease Control and Prevention, 1995b).

The *Borrelia burgdorferi* bacteria enters the human body through the wound made during the tick's feedings. The organism then invades local blood or lymph vessels and disseminates to various organ systems. Although later symptoms of untreated Lyme disease can occur anytime throughout the year, the onset of the disease most commonly occurs during the summer months.

Nearly every state in the United States has reported cases of Lyme disease. The age range of patients reported to have Lyme disease is 2 to 88 years; the peak age incidence is in the 9- to 12-year-old range (Centers for Disease Control and Prevention, 1995b). During the early stages of Lyme disease, if the child is treated with appropriate antibiotic therapy, the recovery is usually quick and the disease is completely curable. Unfortunately, the response of patients to treatment for chronic Lyme disease is variable. Damage to the nervous system or joints may require a prolonged period of repair after the infection has been treated. If treatment has been postponed for an extended period of time, treatment may have little or no beneficial effect (Centers for Disease Control and Prevention, 1995b). There is presently no vaccine available for protecting humans against Lyme disease.

Focused History

Patient history

- Flu-like symptoms appearing 2 to 21 days following a tick bite:
  - Fever.
  - Headache.
  - Lethargy.
  - General aches and pains.
  - Rash at the tick-bite site.
  - Outdoor activity, such as camping or hiking.
  - Tick exposure.

Family history

- Outdoor activity, such as camping or hiking.
- Tick exposure.

Focused Assessment

Physical Assessment

1. Assess the cardiovascular system:
   - Auscultate the heart for:
     - Rate.
2. Interpret electrocardiogram recordings for dysrhythmias:
   - Cardiac manifestations are present in 8 to 10% of patients.
   - Cardiac abnormalities clear in 1 to 6 weeks.
     - In rare cases, serious damage to heart muscle may lead to heart failure (Centers for Disease Control and Prevention, 1995b).
3. Assess the neurologic system:
   - Assess the child's level of consciousness with the GCS or AVPU method.
   - Assess for signs of meningeal irritation or infection:

- Headache.
- Stiff neck.
- Irritability.
- Photophobia.
- Nausea and vomiting: Progression of Lyme disease can also involve seventh cranial nerve palsy and weakness of the limbs caused by nerve inflammation, which generally appear within 4 weeks of the tick bite and occur in 15 to 20% of patients. Infections of the nervous system can progress to meningitis.

4. Assess the integumentary system:
   - Inspect the skin for a rash:
     - The most common feature of Lyme disease is a large, red skin rash called erythema migrans, affecting up to 80% of patients.
     - The rash expands outward from the site of the tick bite, beginning 3 to 30 days after the bite.
     - The Lyme disease rash is flat, circular, and generally at least 2 inches in diameter.
     - As the rash progresses, it may appear to have a "bulls-eye" appearance, as the central portion partially clears and the outer margins redden.
     - The single rash can become quite large.
     - One or more rashes may be present on other areas of the skin.
5. Assess the musculoskeletal system:
   - Inspect the joints for redness and edema; palpate for fluid:
     - Arthritis is the second most common finding in Lyme disease, after erythema migrans, and is present in up to 50% of patients.
     - Arthritis most often affects large joints, most often the knee.
     - Unlike most forms of arthritis, chronic Lyme arthritis usually does not attack the same joint on both sides of the body at once and usually only affects a few joints.
     - Lyme arthritis usually responds to antibiotic treatment; however, if severe joint damage has occurred, complete recovery may not be likely.

Psychosocial Assessment

- Assess the child and family's understanding of the disease.
- Assess the child and family's coping strategies.

Nursing Interventions

- Patients with a tick bite and no evidence of disease are not routinely treated because of the low-risk of infection, even in endemic regions.
- Patients with a tick bite and evidence of disease:
  - Administer oral antibiotics, as prescribed (American Academy of Pediatrics, 2000):

    Amoxicillin is the drug of choice for children younger than 8 years of age.

    Doxycycline or erythromycin is the drug of choice for children older than 8 years of age.
  - Obtain blood specimens, as needed, to isolate the bacteria or detect antibodies that have developed against the bacteria in the blood.
  - Prepare for a biopsy of the skin lesions (Centers for Disease Control and Prevention, 1995b) to confirm the diagnosis of Lyme disease.

Home Care and Prevention

The only certain way to prevent Lyme disease is to avoid situations where tick exposure may be possible. Instructions for families and children who may be in situations where tick exposure is a possibility include (Ball, 1998):

- Dress appropriately for the outdoors:
  - Wear long pants and long-sleeved shirts.
  - Tuck pant legs into long socks and tuck the shirt into the pants.
- Avoid tick-infested areas.
- Apply a repellant containing the compound N,N-diethyltoluamide (DEET) to exposed skin areas (except the face):
  - Follow label directions carefully, and be especially cautious when using any form of DEET on children.
  - Do not apply DEET to infants, because it may cause seizures.
  - It should be applied several times a day (approximately once every 1 to 2 hours).
- Wash children's clothes immediately on entering the house to prevent entry of ticks into the home.
- Inspect children carefully for ticks twice a day, including close inspection of the neck, scalp, axillae, and groin after all outdoor activities. A fine-toothed comb may be used to comb the hair for ticks.
- Inspect pets for ticks:
  - Contact the veterinarian for the appropriate pet insect repellant.

- Use tweezers to remove ticks found on the pet.
- Mow the lawn frequently.

- Remove attached ticks from skin immediately with fine-tipped tweezers by grasping the tick's head as closely as possible to the exposed skin.
  - Apply slow and steady pressure to remove the entire tick.
  - Do not attempt to burn or coat the tick; this may only force the tick to burrow deeper into tissue (McIntire, 1987).
  - Cleanse the skin afterward with isopropyl alcohol.
  - Place the tick into a plastic bag with a blade of grass for inspection by the primary care physician.

Conclusion

Although there are many types of communicable and infectious disease emergencies, the initial emergency nursing care generally remains the same. Emergency nurses should work closely with local health departments to determine endemic diseases in their hospital's geographic area. Prevention of transmission to other staff and family members is essential.

References

Advisory Committee of Immunization Practices. (1991). Rabies prevention—United States, 1991. Recommendations of the Advisory Committee on Immunization Practices. *Morbidity and Mortality Weekly Report, 40*, (RR-3): 1-19.

American Academy of Pediatrics. (2000). *Red book 2000: Report of the Committee of Infectious Diseases.* (25th ed.) Elk Grove Village, IL: American Academy of Pediatrics.

Arrowsmith, J., Kennedy, D., Kuritsky, J., & Faich, G. (1986). National patterns of aspirin use and Reye syndrome reporting, United States, 1980-1985. *Pediatrics, 77*, 598.

Ball, J. (1998). Integumentary section; hematologic and immunologic; and cardiovascular section. In J. Ball (Ed.), *Mosby's pediatric patient teaching guides* (pp. B1-B19; F1-F5; G1-G16). St. Louis: Mosby—Year Book.

Barkin, R. (1997). *Pediatric emergency medicine: Concepts and clinical practice.* St. Louis: Mosby.

Barkin, R., & Rosen, P. (1999). *Emergency pediatrics: A guide to ambulatory care.* (5th ed.). St. Louis: Mosby.

Benenson, A. (2000). *Control of communicable diseases manual.* Washington, DC: American Public Health Association.

Burke, S. (1998). Neonatal topics. In T. Soud & J. Rogers (Eds.), *Manual of pediatric emergency nursing* (pp. 660-685). St. Louis: Mosby—Year Book.

Centers for Disease Control and Prevention. (1991). Rabies prevention, United States, 1991. Recommendations of the Immunization Practices Advisory Committee. Morbidity and Mortality Weekly Report, 40, 1-19.

Centers for Disease Control and Prevention. (1993). Summary of notifiable disease, United States, 1993. *Morbidity and Mortality Weekly Report, 42*(53), 1-73.

Centers for Disease Control and Prevention. (1995a). *Epidemiology & prevention of vaccine-preventable diseases.* Washington, DC: Department of Health and Human Services (pp. 35-46).

Centers for Disease Control and Prevention. (1995b). Lyme disease surveillance—United States. *Morbidity and Mortality Weekly Report, 44*, 459-462.

Centers for Disease Control and Prevention. (1995c). Revised guidelines for prophylaxis against *Pneumocystis carinii* pneumonia for children infected with or perinatally exposed to human immunodeficiency virus. *Morbidity and Mortality Weekly Report, 44.*

Centers for Disease Control and Prevention (1999). Summary of notifiable diseases, United States, 1998. *Morbidity and Mortality Weekly Report, 47*(53), 91-92.

Dworkin, M., Alexander, E., Boase, J., DeBolt, C., Goldoft, M., Green, D., & Marcuse, E. (1997). *Pertussis: What Washington State health care providers need to know.* Seattle: Washington State Department of Health.

Fleisher, G. (2000). Infectious disease emergencies. In G. Fleisher & S. Ludwig (Eds). Textbook of pediatric emergency medicine (4th ed., pp. 725-793). Philadelphia: Lippincott, Williams & Wilkins.

Gersony, W. (1991). Diagnosis and management of Kawasaki disease. *Journal of the American Medical Association, 265*, 2699-2703.

Manley, L., & Bechtel, N. (1998). Hematologic and immune systems. In T. Soud & J. Rogers (Eds.), *Manual of pediatric emergency nursing* (pp. 390-416). St. Louis: Mosby—Year Book.

Mueller, B. & Pizzo, P. (2001). Acquired immunodeficiency syndrome in the infant. In J. Reminton & J. Klein (Eds). *Infectious diseases of the fetus and newborn infant* (5th ed., pp. 447-475). Philadelphia: W. B. Saunders Co.

Oakes, L., & Rosenthal-Dichter, C. (1998). Hematology and immunology. In M. Slota (Ed.), *Core curriculum for pediatric critical care nursing* (pp. 461-550). Philadelphia: Saunders Co.

Persing, D., Telfor, S., Rys, P., Dodge, D., White, T., Malawista, S., & Spielman, A. (1990). Detection of *Borrelia burgdorferi* DNA in museum specimens of Ixodes dammini ticks, *Science* 249, 1420-1423.

Pinkert, H., Harper, M., Cooper T., & Fleisher, G. (1993). HIV-infected children in the pediatric emergency department. *Pediatric Emergency Care 9*, 265-269.

Reynolds, E., & Kelley, S. (1994). Infectious disease emergencies. In S. Kelley (Ed.), *Pediatric emergency nursing* (pp. 423-452). Norwalk, CT: Appleton & Lange.

Rosenfeld, E., Corydon, K., & Shulman, S. (1995). Kawasaki disease in infants less than one year of age. *Journal of Pediatrics, 126*, 524-529.

Rote, N. (1998b). Infection and alterations in immunity and inflammation. In K. McCance & S. Huether (Eds.), *Pathophysiology: The biologic basis for disease in adults and children* (3rd ed., pp. 237-285). St. Louis: Mosby—Year Book.

Rote, N. (1998a). Immunity. K. McCance & S. Huether (Eds.), *Pathophysiology: The biologic basis for disease in adults and children.* (3rd ed., pp. 174-204). St. Louis: Mosby.

Simonds, R., & Orejas, G. (1998). *Pneumocystis caunii* pneumonia and toxoplasmosis. In: P. Pizzo & C. Wilfert (Eds.), *Pediatric AIDS: The challenge of HIV infection in infants, children and adolescents* (pp. 251-265). Baltimore: Williams & Wilkins.

Special Writing Group. (1992). Guidelines for the diagnosis of rheumatic fever. *Journal of the American Medical Association, 268*, 2069-2073.

Starke, J., Jacobs, R., & Jereb, J. (1992). Medical progress: Resurgence of tuberculosis in children. *Journal of Pediatrics, 120*, 839-855.

Sundel, R. (2000). Rheumatologic emergencies. In G. Fleisher & S. Ludwig (Eds). Textbook of pediatric emergency medicine (4th ed, pp. 1191-1228). Philadelphia: Lippincott, Williams & Wilkins.

Vallejo, J., Ong, L., & Starke, J. (1994). Clinical features, diagnosis and treatment of tuberculosis in infants. *Pediatrics, 9*, 1-7.

Whaley, L., & Wong, D. (1999). Nursing care of infants and children (6th Ed.), St. Louis: Mosby—Year Book.

27

Psychiatric Emergencies

Kathryn R. Puskar, RN, DrPH, CS, FAAN
Kathleen Sullivan, RN, PhD

Introduction

Psychiatric emergencies are sudden or severe changes in behavior or emotions that cause distress and concern for the patient as well as the family and community (Urbanitis, 1983). These emergencies include an acute disturbance in thought, behavior, mood, or social relationship that requires immediate intervention (American Psychiatric Association, 1995). Although pediatric psychiatric emergencies are not a routine occurrence, emergency nurses must be able to recognize, evaluate, and intervene with these children, adolescents, and their families. Children with ongoing psychiatric conditions may present to the emergency department (ED) with health problems not related to their conditions (Table 27.1).

The purpose of this chapter is to describe selected psychiatric emergencies affecting the pediatric population and to outline the related emergency nursing care. Emergency nurses should possess general knowledge of the American Psychiatric Association's (1995) psychiatric diagnostic classification system, the Diagnostic and Statistical Manual of Mental Disorders, Fourth Edition *(DSM-IV). The DSM-IV categorizes mental disorders based on certain defining characteristics, epidemiology, incidence, symptoms, assessment, treatment, and referral. Knowledge of developmental phases and age-appropriate behavior (Chapter 4) also is requisite.*

Pediatric Considerations

Preadolescent and adolescent patients with psychiatric disturbances are approached differently during the initial interview and history (Table 27.2).

Psychiatric Conditions

Etiology

The etiology of psychiatric conditions arises from developmental issues, traumatic events, and other situations as described in this chapter.

Focused History

- Obtain the history from the parent first, then from the preadolescent (Barkin & Rosen, 1994), and then from both together (Urbanitis, 1983); the adolescent can be interviewed alone (Barkin & Rosen, 1994).
- Patient history (Urbanitis, 1983):
  - Chief complaint or main concern.
  - History of symptoms.
  - Child's school adjustments.
  - Peer and sibling relationships.
- Parent and family history. (The parents may be referred to a social worker or mental health counselor for further history taking.) (Urbanitis, 1983):
  - Chief complaint or parents' main concern.
  - History of symptoms.
  - Child's health history.
  - Behaviors leading to the emergency department visit.
  - Family health history and mental health history.

Focused Assessment

Physical Assessment

1. Assess the patient's physical health to determine whether the psychiatric symptoms are caused by an underlying health condition (i.e., organic).
2. Assess the respiratory system:
   - Auscultate the chest for:
     - Respiratory rate.
3. Assess the cardiovascular system:
   - Auscultate the heart for:
     - Rate.
     - Rhythm.
   - Measure the blood pressure.

TABLE 27.1 Selected Pediatric Psychiatric Conditions

Condition	*Description*
School avoidance/school phobia	Long-standing fear of school or reluctance to attend school that is most common in children older than 9 years of age. School absences occur most frequently in the first grade and in the middle school grades (Ball, 1998). It generally occurs with the initial school entrance, after a change in schools, or at the beginning of the school year (Barkin & Rosen, 1994). These children stay at home and generally have one or more physical complaints, such as a stomachache, headache, nausea, dizziness, or feeling tired, that resolve throughout the day (Ball, 1998). They fear school because it is a scary place, they believe the parent will abandon them, or they have separation anxiety. Treatment includes obtaining a physical examination and identifying ways to help the child feel safe when leaving home (Ball, 1998).
Conduct disorders	Chronic behaviors that violate others' rights and society's rules. It is usually observed in preadolescent children. Four major behaviors of conduct disorders are: *aggression* (hurting people or animals, stealing, forced sexual activity, bullying others, and using weapons); *damaging property* (starting fires or destroying others' possessions); *stealing or being dishonest* (shoplifting or breaking and entering); and *breaking established rules* (curfew violations, truancy, or runaway behavior). Drug, tobacco, and alcohol use, precocious sexual behavior, and inability to empathize with others can occur. Treatment includes intensive, long-term mental health counseling for both the patient and family. Placement in a school or other facility geared to these children may be needed (Ball, 1998).
Attention-deficit hyperactivity disorder (ADHD)	A short attention span, poor impulse control and/or hyperactivity, usually observed in children before 7 years of age. A very short attention span is noted when the child makes careless mistakes in schoolwork, is easily distracted, has difficulty maintaining focus, and other behaviors. Poor impulse control or hyperactivity is observed in the child who fidgets and squirms, talks too much or interrupts others, runs around and climbs in inappropriate situations, among other behaviors. Treatment includes behavior management and medication, such as Ritalin, Dexedrine, Tegretol, clonidine, and imipramine (Ball, 1998).
Anorexia nervosa	Self-starvation, characterized by very strict dieting, excessive exercising, and an intense fear of becoming fat (Ball, 1998). Adolescent females (especially those in white, upper-middle-class families) are most often affected, usually between 14 and 18 years of age (Sciera, 1998). Signs of an eating disorder include constant dieting and concern about food, rapid weight loss, excessive concern about body size and weight, loss of menstrual periods, long-term continuous exercising, and physical and psychosocial changes (Ball, 1998). Physical changes, such as cardiac dysrhythmias, fluid and electrolyte disturbances, and extreme fatigue, may herald an emergency department visit. Treatment includes recognizing this disorder, treating underlying physiologic disturbances, and counseling for the child and family.
Bulimia	An eating disorder in which abnormal methods are used for weight maintenance, such as binging (eating a large amount of food in a short time period) and then purging (taking laxatives or diuretics or inducing vomiting) (Ball, 1998). Adolescent females usually are affected; the onset of bulimia occurs later in adolescence than anorexia (Sciera, 1998). Signs include an excessive concern about food, secret binge eating, fear of loss of control over food intake, self-induced vomiting after eating, bad breath and tooth decay, and physical and psychosocial changes (Ball, 1998). Treatment includes attending to immediate health needs, counseling for the child and family, and perhaps medications.
Depression	A mood disorder that can occur in children and adolescents (Ball, 1998). Depression is common in adolescents. Its prevalence is estimated to be 4.7%. It is equally common in males and females prior to puberty but is approximately four times more common in females after the onset of puberty (Brent, 1993). Recent research has shown that some individuals who are depressed have changes in brain chemicals, such as reduced amount of serotonin. The most important risk factor for depression appears to be having at least one parent with an affective disorder (Sciera, 1998). Thus, depression may have both genetic and environmental components (Sciera, 1998). Symptoms include frequent physical complaints of illness; irritability or frequent crying; a sad mood lasting most of the day, every day; changes in sleeping, eating, schoolwork and activity; verbalization of thoughts about death and dying or hurting self; and feelings of uselessness, worthlessness, and guilt (Ball, 1998). Treatment includes counseling for the patient and family, medication administration, hospitalization if the patient threatens to harm self or others, and a long-term commitment to achieving a healthy outlook on life (Ball, 1998; Varicolis & Colson, 2002).

TABLE 27.2 Comparison of Approaches with Preadolescent and Adolescent Patients with Psychiatric Disturbances

Preadolescents	*Adolescents*
Obtain a history from the parents first; then obtain a history from the child, usually alone, unless the child has separation anxiety.	Obtain a history from the adolescent first and alone; then talk with the parents, if present.
Ascertain the child's understanding of the evaluation and reason for being in the emergency department.	Be honest and objective with the adolescent to build trust. Avoid projecting one's own values onto the adolescent.
Reserve the use of drawings and toys for the end of the interview.	Not needed with adolescents.
Observe the child's interaction with the parents and the evaluator as well as the child's activity level.	Note the adolescent's interaction with the evaluator and the parents, if present.
Ask the child and family, "How do you get along with your friends?". This is probably the most effective screening question to identify major psychopathology. If the child has difficulty with peer relationships or is isolated from them, psychological problems can be expected.	Focus on concerns related to family emancipation, peer pressure, and heterosexual and homosexual exposure; these issues usually are an underlying reason for the adolescent's psychiatric disturbance.

- Assess peripheral perfusion:
  - Palpate peripheral pulses.
  - Measure core and skin temperature.
  - Inspect the skin color.
  - Measure capillary refill.

4. Assess the neurological system:
   - Assess the level of consciousness with the AVPU method or the Glasgow coma scale (GCS).
   - Assess pupillary responses.
5. Assess other body systems, as needed.

Psychosocial Assessment

Assess the patient's underlying psychiatric-related condition as follows (Urbanitis, 1983).

1. Determine the severity of the psychiatric symptoms:
   - Ascertain if the current condition is a social problem or a health problem.
   - Conduct a mental status examination with an established scale to further understand the child's mental health development:
     - Behavioral Checklist (Jarvis, 1996) for children aged 7 to 11 years.
     - Reynolds Adolescent Depression Scale (Reynolds, 1987) for adolescents.
2. Identify the child's and family's resources:
   - Child's resources:
     - Coping skills.
     - Family support.
     - Social support.
   - Family's resources:
     - Coping skills.
     - Social support.
     - Financial capacity.

Triage Decisions

Emergent

- Patients who are a threat to themselves or others.
- Patients who exhibit violent behavior.
- Patients with an altered level of consciousness.
- Patients in cardiopulmonary arrest or hypovolemic shock from suicide attempt or anorexia/bulimia.
- Patients with cardiopulmonary instability from a drug or alcohol overdose.

Urgent

- Patients who committed suicidal acts (e.g., minor lacerations) that are not life threatening.
- Patients who cannot converse rationally.
- Patients who are agitated or aggressive.

Nonurgent

- Patients who exhibit nonthreatening behavior to self or others.

TABLE 27.3 Nursing Diagnoses and Expected Outcomes

Nursing Diagnoses	*Expected Outcomes*
Risk for violence, self-directed or directed at others	The patient will be safe, as evidenced by: ▪ An environment free of weapons. ▪ The display of safe behaviors.
Anxiety	The patient and family will be free of or have decreased anxiety, as evidenced by: ▪ The acceptance of psychiatric counseling. ▪ The acceptance of community referrals. ▪ Verbalization of reduced anxiety.
Sensory or perceptual alterations	The patient will be free of or have decreased sensory or perceptual alterations, as evidenced by: ▪ Absence of auditory and visual hallucinations. ▪ Coherence in thought.

Nursing Interventions

1. Assess and maintain airway, breathing, and circulation (Chapter 6).
2. Remove potential weapons, medications, and unsafe objects:
   - The presence of such implements may lead to suicidal or homicidal gestures.
3. Administer medications to abate or relieve psychiatric symptoms.
4. Apply physical restraints according to hospital policy:
   - Apply soft restraints to the wrists and/or ankles.
   - Apply leather restraints to the wrists and/or ankles:
     - Physical restraints may be needed to prevent the patient from harming self or others.
5. Initiate a referral for psychiatric treatment:
   - Initiate outpatient psychiatric treatment for the stable child who is not a threat to self or others:
     - Initiate a referral to a child or family psychiatrist; the initial evaluation can take place in the ED or on discharge.
   - Initiate inpatient psychiatric treatment for the unstable child who is a threat to self or others:
     - Informal commitment allows a competent adolescent to admit or to discharge himself or herself from an institution without fear of involuntary commitment (Constantino, 1996).
     - Voluntary commitment, under the 1983 Mental Health Act (301 commitment), allows an adolescent 18 years of age and older to voluntarily seek inpatient treatment. Certain requirements may have to be satisfied prior to the patient's discharge; the admitting institution reserves the right to involuntary commitment instead of discharging the patient (Constantino, 1996).
     - Third-party commitment (involuntary) hospitalization under the 1983 Mental Health Act (302 commitment) allows 72 hours for hospitalized assessment without the child's consent. The Mental Health Act defines the rights of the child and adolescent and legitimizes the actions of the healthcare professional who overrides the wishes of the child and adolescent when their insight or judgment is impaired. Third-party involuntary commitment is sought when the child or adolescent refuses hospitalization or is harmful to self or others.
6. Inform the family frequently of the child's condition; provide emotional support to the child and family.
7. Prepare for transfer and transport to a psychiatric or tertiary care facility for voluntary or involuntary treatment, hospitalization with a psychiatric referral, or discharge from the emergency department with a psychiatric referral.

Home Care and Prevention

Emergency nurses should be familiar with the local community agencies that support mental health activities for children and adolescents. Emergency nurses can be involved in programs that promote the mental health of youth, such as the Teaching Kids to Cope© program, a 10-week psychoeducational group intervention designed to enhance the coping repertoire of adolescents (Puskar, Lamb, & Tusaie-Mumford, 1997). Emergency nurses can obtain continuing education on pediatric psychiatric emergencies to be prepared for treating these patients and families. Emergency nurses should acknowledge their own values and beliefs while empathizing with the patients and families.

Selected Psychiatric Emergencies

Suicide

Etiology

A suicide is a sudden, impulsive reaction to a stressful action (Wilson & Kneisel, 1992). Suicide is the third-leading cause of death among young people 15 to 24 years of age. Experts estimate that each year nearly 5,000 teens commit suicide (American Psychiatric Association, 1995). Suicidal behavior has become increasingly common; about 4% of high school students have made a suicide attempt within the previous 12 months and 8% have attempted suicide in their lifetime (Brent, 1993). Ten percent of high school students have reported depressive symptomatology (Puskar, Tusaie-Mumford, Rohay, Lamb, Boneysteel, & Sereika, 1996). Although females attempt suicide more often, males are more successful (Barkin & Rosen, 1994). Suicide attempts are rare in young children (Sciera, 1998).

Adolescent suicide occurs either without warning or in planned detail. The suicide event may be triggered by a minor or trivial incident. Children and adolescents either have expressed suicidal ideation (thoughts) or suicide gestures or attempts (actions). Suicide attempts include the ingestion of medications, ingestion of alcohol or other toxic substances, inhalation of toxic fumes, or self-inflicted trauma, ranging from minor lacerations to severe gunshot wounds or asphyxiation. Many times the suicide gesture is masked by other behavior, such as acting out, truancy, withdrawal, changes in school performance, promiscuity, and unrecognized or untreated depression.

Focused History

- History taking may be difficult because of the patient's reluctance to discuss the suicidal ideations or actions.

Patient history

- Mood changes.
- Irritability.
- Change in school performance.
- Withdrawal from friends.
- Associated risk factors:
  - Hopelessness.
  - Male gender (more successful in suicide attempts).
  - Female gender (more suicide attempts).
  - Previous suicide attempts.
  - Substance abuse. Forty percent of completed suicides are alcohol-related. Alcohol or other drugs have an impact on the adolescent's mood, may alter thought processes, and may increase impulsivity.
  - Availability of lethal weapons, such as guns.
  - Life event change (e.g., breakup with boyfriend or girlfriend; pregnancy).
  - A recent loss or anniversary or reminder of a loss (Barkin & Rosen, 1994).
  - Depression (Puskar et al., 1999).
  - Low self-esteem.
  - Homosexuality issues.
  - Chronic illness (Barkin & Rosen, 1994).
  - History of incest, child abuse, runaway behavior, or incarceration (Valente, 1989).
  - Other risks (exposure of vulnerable youth to suicide messages in hard rock music or to satanic cults) (Valente, 1989).

Family history

- Risk factors:
  - History of suicide attempts by a family member.
  - Family history of psychiatric illness.
  - Family discord.
  - Availability of lethal weapons, such as guns.

Focused Assessment

Physical Assessment

1. Assess the respiratory system:
   - Auscultate the chest for:
     - Respiratory rate.
   - Assess for signs of respiratory distress.
   - Assess breath odor:
     - Alcohol or other substance may be detected (Chapter 44).
2. Assess the cardiovascular system:
   - Auscultate the heart for:

- Rate. Early tricyclic antidepressant ingestion or ingestion of stimulants increases the heart rate.
- Rhythm.

- Palpate the peripheral pulses.
- Measure the capillary refill.
- Measure the blood pressure.
- Observe the skin color.
- Measure core and skin temperature.

3. Assess the neurological system:
   - Assess the level of consciousness with the GCS or AVPU method:
     - Assess for lethargy, agitation, or somnolence. These behaviors may be symptoms associated with poison exposure (Chapter 44).
   - Assess pupillary response.
4. Assess the integumentary system:
   - Assess skin integrity:
     - Open wounds or other trauma may be present.

Psychosocial Assessment

1. Assess the patient's risk for suicide:
   - Suicide intent scales (e.g., Reynolds, 1987) are useful for adolescents. These scales may be given to the adolescent or family members to complete.
2. Assess the patient's current psychosocial situation for factors such as:
   - Depressive symptoms:
     - In adolescents experiencing mood swings, explore other symptoms such as insomnia, loss of appetite, fatigue, or somatic complaints.
   - Anxiety symptoms:
     - Anxiety sometimes coexists with depression.
   - Stressful event that triggered the suicidal act.
3. Assess the patient's and family's coping strategies and resources.
4. Assess the suicide attempt itself (Barkin & Rosen, 1994):
   - Determine the lethality of the attempt and the use of one or more suicide methods (e.g., ingestion followed by wrist-slashing):
     - High-lethality plan: precise plan for the upcoming 24 to 72 hours; a lethal means for suicide act; available means to enact the plan; an intent to die; poor impulse control; no rescue plan (Valente, 1989).
     - Moderate-lethality plan: a less immediate or less lethal method and plan (Valente, 1989).
     - Low-lethality plan: vague, imprecise plans; methods are generally nonlethal, such as wrist cutting; rescue plans are in place.
   - Ask the patient directly about the suicidal intent and plan—premeditated or impulsive; prior suicide attempts.
   - Determine the circumstances of the suicide attempt, such as being alone or being found prior to dying and the presence of a suicide note.
   - Assess the patient's intent to repeat the attempt.
   - Determine the patient's feelings about surviving or being rescued from the suicide attempt.
   - Determine whether the adolescent was involved in autoerotic asphyxia:
     - Autoerotic asphyxia is the use of ropes, ligature, or belts that are self-applied to enhance pleasure during masturbation by producing cerebral anoxia (Kirksey, Holt-Ashley, Williamson, & Garza, 1995). Young, white males are most often the victims.
     - Autoerotic asphyxia should be considered when asphyxia-producing items, such as plastic bags, are found near the victim. The ligature may be padded to prevent marks to the neck during the act. Materials to enhance sexual arousal, such as pornographic material or objects, may be present (Kirksey, et al., 1995).

Nursing Interventions

1. Assess and maintain airway, breathing, and circulation (Chapter 6).
2. Initiate cardiorespiratory and oxygen saturation monitoring.
3. Initiate diagnosis-specific treatment:
   - Initiate trauma resuscitation measures for the severely injured patient.
   - Initiate poison-specific treatment for poison exposures (Chapter 44):
     - Consider screening for acetaminophen and acetylsalicylic acid levels regardless of the presence or absence of a suicidal history. Many adolescents attempting suicide are untruthful about what medications have been ingested (Chapter 44).
   - Assist with suturing of minor lacerations.
   - Obtain a urine or blood pregnancy test.
4. Assure safety for the staff, patient, and family:
   - Take all suicide threats seriously:

- Suicidal children and adolescents may share their suicide plan with friends and family; most do give suicide messages (Valente, 1989).
- Suicidal youths may request that the emergency nurse keep their suicidal thoughts or attempts confidential. These patients must be told by the emergency nurse that he or she cannot hold any secrets that may endanger the patient's health or safety (Valente, 1989).

- Implement suicide precautions:
  - Assess the patient every 15 minutes.
  - Assign a nurse or qualified healthcare provider to remain with the patient at all times.
  - Be empathetic and nonjudgmental.
- Apply physical restraints, as necessary.
- In the presence of hospital security officers, search the patient's belongings for harmful objects (such as medications, drugs, glass, or razor blades).
  - Remove harmful objects from the patient's bedside area.
- Educate the family members about these safety precautions, their rationale, and the need for their enforcement.

5. Reassess cardiovascular status and neurological status.
6. Initiate a psychiatric consultation. A referral to family counseling may be beneficial to the parents and family members (Sciera, 1998).
7. Inform the family frequently of the child's condition; provide emotional support to the child and family.
8. Prepare for transfer and transport to a psychiatric facility or hospital admission.

Home Care and Prevention

Suicidal behavior may be prevented by acute attention to its warning signs and risk factors. Family, school, and community personnel must be educated about early signs of depression and subsequent suicide acts. Children who appear to be depressed should be asked about suicidal ideation (Barkin & Rosen, 1994). Families and friends must take seriously any suicide-related comments, threats, and jokes before these ideas escalate into suicide attempts (Valente, 1989). Family may erroneously believe that asking the child or adolescent about suicide will "put the idea into their heads," which is not true. Families and friends should maintain an open dialogue about the child's or adolescent's suicide-related thoughts.

On the child's discharge from the emergency department, family members should remove medications, toxic substances, and weapons from the home. The legal ramifications of emergency department discharge followed by another suicide attempt should be considered.

Psychosis

Etiology

Psychosis is an impairment with reality testing. The limbic system in the brain serves as the central integrating system or the gateway through which most incoming stimuli must pass. Impairment of this system affects the unifying functions by which all experiences are made congruent with reality. A breakdown in this system results in disorganized perceptual and behavioral responses. Problems in the integrating function of the brain are the inability to factor out minor or irrelevant stimuli, the inability to deal with complexity, and the inability to integrate perceptual activities. When the system is impaired, the result is sensory flooding and excessive attention to minor environmental details, distortion in thinking and perception, and altered sense of self and withdrawal. Table 27.4 lists examples of pediatric psychotic disorders.

A psychotic disorder may be related to a health condition such as a brain tumor or a substance-induced psychosis. Computerized tomograms of the brains of patients with psychoses have shown an increased size of the lateral ventricles and a decrease in brain volume of the frontal lobe. Dopamine, a major neurotransmitter in the brain, has been postulated to be a factor in development of schizophrenia, resulting in a hyperactivity of the dopamine system. Therefore, an organic cause for the psychosis, such as infections, metabolic disturbances, or brain injury, should be entertained.

Focused History

Patient and family history varies with each disorder (Table 27.4).

Focused Assessment

Physical Assessment

- Assess the patient's overall appearance:
  - Assess hygiene and grooming:
  - Hygiene may be poor; the patient may appear disheveled.
  - Clothing may be inappropriate for the weather conditions.
- Assess the neurological system:
  - Assess the level of consciousness with the Glasgow Coma Scale or AVPU method.
  - Assess the pupils for size and reactivity.

TABLE 27.4 Selected Categories of Psychotic Disorders

Disorder	*Description*
Infantile autism	Thought to result from physiologic (organic) factors within the child that lead to aberrant parenting behaviors (Barkin & Rosen, 1994). Diagnostic criteria (Barkin & Rosen, 1994, p. 690): ▪ Onset of symptoms occurs in children < 30 months of age. ▪ Unusual responses to the environment (e.g., need for sameness and routine); poor social interactions. ▪ Deficits in language development; abnormal speech patterns (echolalia, pronoun reversals). ▪ May have normal or precocious cognitive abilities. ▪ Abnormal auditory-evoked responses. Treatment includes: ▪ Multidisciplinary team approach. ▪ Medication administration.
Schizophrenia ▪ Rare in children. ▪ Increases in frequency in adolescence, with onset in middle to late adolescence. ▪ Incidence of schizophrenia in the general population is between 0.5% and about 1.0% (American Psychiatric Association, 1995).	Occurs in late adolescence but may develop in early childhood (Barkin & Rosen, 1994). Diagnostic criteria (American Psychiatric Association, 1995, pp. 285–286): ▪ Two of the following symptoms: delusions, hallucinations, disorganized speech, disorganized behavior, and negative symptoms. ▪ Social dysfunction. ▪ Duration of 6 months or more. ▪ Exclusion of mood disorder with psychotic features. ▪ Exclusion of general medical condition. ▪ Relationship to developmental disorders. Symptoms of schizophrenia are *positive* (an excess of neurologic functioning, resulting in distortions in thinking or delusions, hallucinations, and disorganized speech) and *negative* (a loss in functioning, such as restricted emotional expression or flat affect, lack of goals, and slowness in speech and thought). Treatment includes: ▪ Medication administration. ▪ Patient and family therapy.

Organic psychoses	Result from an organic cause, such as (Barkin & Rosen, 1994, p. 691):
	▪ Ingestion of medications or drugs (e.g., cocaine or amphetamines) (Chapter 44).
	▪ Systemic illness.
	▪ Endocrine disorder.
	▪ Renal, cardiac, or liver failure symptoms (Barkin & Rosen, 1994):
	  ▪ Hallucinations (usually visual).
	  ▪ Cognitive impairment.
	Treatment includes:
	  ▪ Focusing on underlying illness or ingestion; treating accordingly.

Manic-depressive psychosis	Rarely seen in children. Symptoms include (Barkin & Rosen, 1994): ▪ Heightened motor activity. ▪ Flight of ideas. ▪ Euphoric or dysphoric moods. Treatment includes: ▪ Hospitalization. ▪ Medication administration.

- Determine whether the patient is oriented to time, place, and person.
- Listen to the patient's speech patterns. Speech may be stuttering, fast, slow, or incomprehensible.

Psychosocial Assessment

- Assess the patient's thought content:
  - Listen to the topics of discussion and for flight of ideas.
  - Determine whether the patient is delusional.
- Assess for auditory or visual hallucinations.
- Assess for suicide intent—suicidal ideations or actions.

Nursing Interventions

- Apply physical restraints if the patient is extremely agitated.
- Administer antipsychotic medications, such as Haldol, to stabilize hallucinations or delusions.
- Obtain blood and urine specimens for toxicology screening to determine drug-induced psychosis (Chapter 44).
- Initiate a psychiatric referral.
- Inform the family frequently of the patient's condition; provide emotional support to the patient and family.
- Prepare for transfer and transport to a psychiatric facility, hospitalization, or discharge to home.

Home Care and Prevention

Unfortunately, there are no preventive measures for psychoses; however, observance of early warning signs is necessary to provide early treatment and referral. Education of the adolescent and family regarding importance of adherence to medication for prevention of future emergency department visits and hospitalizations is essential.

Posttraumatic Stress Disorder

Etiology

Posttraumatic stress disorder (PTSD) results when an individual either is witness to or is the victim of a violent crime that threatens the physical well-being of himself or herself or another. For children and adolescents, this violent act may be child physical and sexual abuse; rape or date rape; domestic violence (acts of terrorism, acts of war, gangs, drive-by shootings, sniper attacks); kidnapping; hostage situations; dog bites, life-threatening illness or injuries (e.g., severe burns); homicide; or natural and man-made disasters. The traumatic event results in significant injury and/or death and may result in a psychiatric emergency.

It is estimated that 1 to 14% of the population will develop PTSD, especially those exposed to sudden, unexpected, violence. Because trauma is the leading cause of death in children and adolescents, one can only presume that the incidence of PTSD will increase in children (Schwartz, 1994). Posttraumatic stress disorder is categorized as (McFarland, Wasli, & Gerety, 1997):

- Acute (symptoms last less than 3 months).
- Chronic (symptoms last more than 3 months).
- Delayed-onset (symptoms do not begin until at least 6 months after the stressor).

The short- and long-term effects of PTSD are listed in Table 27.5.

Focused History

Patient history (Carson & Arnold, 1996)

- Nature of the traumatic event (human, environmental, or loss of a loved one).
- Time elapsed since the event.
- Patient's personality prior to and after the event:
  - A happy, productive child or adolescent who becomes withdrawn and sad.
  - A child or adolescent becomes angrier, shows hostility, and/or destructiveness.
  - Excessive fear of others.
  - Inability to protect self/or assert self.
  - Avoidance behaviors.
- Patient's coping and support systems prior to event.
- Presence of risk factors:
  - Being exposed to *any* trauma to self, family, peers, school, or community/media; for children and adolescents in particular, experiencing domestic violence, child abuse, childhood sexual abuse, sudden death of a loved one, or violence in school, the community, or reported in the media.
  - Being hit or severely beaten.
  - Exposure to anything that is making the child or adolescent scared, nervous, or jumpy.
  - The number, severity, and duration of the traumas to which the child or adolescent was exposed.
- Symptoms indicative of sensory disruption, such as hyperactive behavior.
- Nonspecific complaints, including stomachaches, headaches, or back pain.

TABLE 27.5 Effects of PTSD

Short-term Effects	***Long-term Effects***
Sleep disturbances (frequency, duration, intensity of any nightmares)	Antisocial behavior
Persistent thoughts about the trauma	Vandalism
Fear that another traumatic event will occur	Psychosomatic complaints/illnesses
Hypervigilance	Truancy and other conduct disorders
Behavioral changes indicating the loss of previously mastered tasks	Mood disorders
Distractibility	Eating disorders (Antai-Otong, 1995 p. 198)
Expecting to die young (Merenstein, Kaplan, & Rosenberg, 1997, p. 211)	
Intense fear	
Attempts to avoid activities, people, feelings, and thoughts associated with the traumatic event (Carson & Arnold, 1996)	
Excessive silence, feelings of hopelessness and guilt, grief, fear, anger (Hazinski, 1992)	
Avoidance of physical contact or closeness	
Forgetfulness	
Loss of enjoyment in being a child	
Disorganized, agitated behavior (McFarland et al., 1997)	
Scholastic underachievement (Paquette & Roderick, 1997)	

- Life pattern deviations:
  - Functioning prior to the stress (Paquette & Roderick, 1997).
  - Nightmares.
  - Visual reliving of the event.
  - Flashbacks.
  - Play that takes on reenactment of the traumatic event.

Focused Assessment

Physical Assessment

1. Assess the respiratory system:
   - Auscultate the chest for:
     - Respiratory rate. Tachypnea may be noted.
2. Assess the cardiovascular system:
   - Auscultate the heart for rate. Tachycardia may be noted.
   - Measure the blood pressure. Elevated blood pressure may be noted.
3. Assess the neurological system:
   - Assess the level of consciousness with the GCS or AVPU method:
     - Irritability may be noted.
     - Hypervigilance may be noted.
   - Assess the patient's motor ability:
     - Increased motor activity may be noted, such as pacing, hitting, or other signs of agitation or aggression.

Psychosocial Assessment

- Assess for age-specific symptoms of PTSD (Table 27.6).

Nursing Interventions

- Administer antidepressant medications as needed, such as (Oakley & Potter, 1997; Schwartz, 1994):
  - Tricyclic and serotonin receptor inhibitors.
  - Clonidine.
  - Prozac.
- Use a calm, quiet approach to decrease anxiety.

TABLE 27.6 Age-Specific PTSD Symptoms

Age	Symptoms
Infancy	■ Excessive crying, eating, sleeping. ■ Overstimulated states. ■ Failure to thrive.
Preschool	■ Sleep disorders. ■ Repetitive play associated with the traumatic event. ■ Hyperalertness. ■ Regressive behaviors. ■ Fear. ■ Sadness. ■ Shame.
School-Age	■ Sleep disorders. ■ Anxiety. ■ Depression. ■ Hyperalertness. ■ Retelling the event. ■ Return of old fears or the onset of new fears. ■ Loss of interests.
Adolescents	■ Many of the PTSD symptoms experienced by adults. ■ Suicidal gestures. ■ Hypersexuality. ■ Substance abuse. ■ Truancy. ■ Minor self-injury.

- Assure the child's safety in situations of suspected child maltreatment or sexual abuse/assault (Chapter 47).
- Teach the child or adolescent anxiety-reducing strategies:
  - Deep breathing.
  - Relaxation.
  - Visualization or guided imagery.
- Focus on the child's ability to survive and heal.
- Offer reassurance of safety and support from family and peers.
- Initiate referrals for:
  - Individual psychotherapy.
  - Family counseling.
  - Therapy groups.
  - Play therapy.
  - Cognitive therapy.
- Discuss with the family the need for long-term treatment for the child and family, which may include peers, community, and a network of caregivers (Antai-Otong, 1995; Burgess, 1997; Carson & Arnold, 1996; Fortinash & Holoday-Worret, 1996; Schwartz, 1994).

Home Care and Prevention

Prevention of PTSD includes educating the public about strategies to decrease violence and children's and adolescents' exposure to violence. Emergency nurses can advocate for services needed by traumatized children, especially those affected by natural and/or community disasters or community violence. Emergency nurses can also participate in public education efforts regarding the effects of violence and trauma on children.

Substance Abuse

Etiology

Pediatric and adolescent substance abuse has increased during the last two decades. Today's youth mature in a society in which they are exposed to adults who use a variety of legal and illegal substances to cope with anxiety, stress, and depression. Teenagers with anger, depression, and low self-esteem may turn to substance abuse or may be driven to substance abuse by peer groups (Allender, 1998). Furthermore, substance abuse is a significant risk factor for suicide and other psychiatric disturbances (Barkin & Rosen, 1994).

The total number children and adolescents who abuse drugs and alcohol is not really known (Johnson, O'Malley, & Bachman, 1994). However, it is known that marijuana use among eighth graders has doubled since 1991 (Zimbler, 1997). Five percent of high school athletes report using anabolic steroids (Sefuentes, 1996). In one study of 231 injured adolescents presenting to a pediatric emergency department for treatment, 90 (39%) tested positive for alcohol in their urine (Mannenbach, Hargarten, & Phelan, 1997). The mean age of the alcohol-positive patients was 16 years. Positive urine alcohol tests were found in 33% of those injured as passengers in motor vehicle crashes, 38% who were motor vehicle drivers, 37% who attempted suicide, and 44% who were assaulted. Mannenbach et al. (1997) concluded that alcohol screening should be initiated during the emergency department treatment of injured adolescents.

Children and adolescents may begin consuming drugs or alcohol in response to peer pressure, family drug or alcohol abuse, or as a way of experimentation. Their consumption may progress from experimentation to recreational use, habituation, and finally abuse and dependence (Zimbler, 1997). Substance abuse may precede the emergency department visit and may be associated with unintentional or intentional trauma.

Focused History

Children and adolescents may not admit to using alcohol or drugs, and their parents may not be aware of their involvement in these activities. The child and parents are interviewed separately, and then together if needed.

Patient history (Use of H-E-A-D-S-S-S) (Busen, 1992, p. 196; Sefuentes, 1996, p. 426)

- H—Home:
  - Nutrition and dietary patterns:
    Nutrition history to identify anorexia
    High sugar intake (often seen in addiction)
- E—Education/employment:
  - Impaired attention.
  - Decreased concentration.
  - Chronic fatigue.
  - Decline or change in school or work performance.
  - Truancy.
- A—Activities:
  - Recreational activities.
  - Peer group and friends.
- D—Drugs:
  - Drug/alcohol use by peer group.
  - Favorable attitudes about drug use or abuse (Merenstein et al., 1997).
  - Young age at initial alcohol or drug use (Merenstein et al., 1997)
  - Injection or inhalation of any substance.
  - Specific agent used and its street name (Table 27.7).
  - Duration of use.
  - Frequency of use.
  - Feelings experienced following use.
  - Past episodes of intentional or accidental drug overdose.
- S—Sexual activity.
- S—Suicide/depression:
  - Low self-esteem.
  - Guilt.
  - Feelings of worthlessness.
- S—Safety.

Family history (Merenstein et al., 1997)

- Family history of alcohol/drug abuse.
- High levels of family conflict.

Focused Assessment

Physical Assessment

(Ball & Bindler, 1995; Allender, 1998; Fortinash & Holoday-Warrett, 1996; Sefuentes, 1996).

1. Assess the respiratory system:
   - Auscultate the chest for:
     - Respiratory rate. Respiratory depression or rapid, shallow respirations may be present. Chronic cough may be present.
   - Assess for chronic respiratory problems:

TABLE 27.7 Drugs, Street Names, and Overdose Symptoms

Drug	*Street Name*	*Symptoms*
Narcotics/analgesics ■ Opium/heroin ■ Morphine ■ Codeine ■ Demerol ■ Fentanyl ■ Percodan	White lady, stuff, smack, big Harry, horse, joy powder, stuff, morf	Respiratory depression leading to death Central nervous system Constricted pupils Bradycardia Hypotension Drowsiness Euphoria Symptoms of shock Seizures
Benzodiazepines ■ Valium ■ Ativan ■ Halcion ■ Xanax	Bennies	Disorientation Staggering Slurred speech Abrupt cessation lowers the seizure threshold and leads to seizures and status epilepticus Lethal when taken in combination with alcohol Respiratory depression leading to respiratory arrest
Barbiturates	Downers, goofers, barbs, idiot pills, sleepers, peanuts	Central nervous system depression (sluggish pupils) Slurred speech Disorientation Staggering
Stimulants ■ Amphetamines ■ Methamphetamines ■ Cocaine	Beans, berries, black beauties, dice, eye-openers, speed, zip	Euphoria, excitation Insomnia Anorexia Hypertension Tachycardia Hyperthermia Paranoia
Cannabis	Joint, bush, reefer, weed, hemp, hooter	Laughter Panic, confusion Drowsiness Red eyes

(continued)

TABLE 27.7 (continued)

Drug	*Street Name*	*Symptoms*
Hallucinogens ▪ LSD ▪ Mescaline	Acid, angel dust, elephant, magic mist	Hallucinations—auditory, olfactory, tactile, visual Delusions Labile emotions Psychosis Tremors; diaphoresis Increased blood pressure
Inhalants ▪ Glue ▪ Typing correction fluid ▪ Nail polish remover ▪ Gasoline ▪ Butane ▪ Paints (spray and acrylic)	Huffing (inhalation of these agents)	Giddiness Headache Nausea Drowsiness Fainting Loss of consciousness Respiratory arrest
Anabolic steroids		Euphoria Increased aggression Psychoses
*Illy** (A marijuana, phencyclidine [PCP], and embalming fluid mixture)	Purple rain, crazy Eddie, wet, no name fry, AMP, clickers, love boat	Violent behavior Auditory and visual hallucinations Euphoria Tachycardia Severe hypertension Seizures

*Symptoms may result from inhalation or contact through preparation of the drug (Moriarity, 1996).

Data from: Engel, 1997; McFarland et al., 1997; Oakley & Potter, 1997; Paquette & Roderick, 1997; Stanhope & Knollmueller, 1997).

- Chronic nasal congestion, frequent colds, allergies, or epistaxis (prolonged cocaine inhalation) may be observed.

- Assess the breath for alcohol odor.

2. Assess the cardiovascular system:
   - Auscultate the heart for:
     - Rate. Tachycardia or bradycardia may be present.
   - Measure the blood pressure:
     - Hypertension may be noted.
   - Assess skin color and temperature:
     - Skin may be cool and clammy.
3. Assess the neurological system:
   - Assess the level of consciousness with the GCS or AVPU method.
   - Assess for changes in orientation or level of consciousness:
     - Slurred speech.
     - Confusion.
     - Delirium.

- General apathy.
- Decreased level of consciousness.
- Sleepiness.
- Clumsy or unsteady gait.
- Restlessness.
- Irritability.
- Tremors.

- Assess pupillary responses:
  - Pupils may be sluggish, pinpoint, or dilated.
  - Conjunctiva may be red.

3. Assess the abdomen:
   - Nausea, vomiting, and diarrhea may be present.
4. Assess the integumentary system:
   - Observe for needle or track marks, abscesses, or cellulitis.
5. Assess the overall appearance:
   - Measure the patient's weight:
     - Note low weight for age and height.
     - Note symptoms of malnutrition, such as weight loss, dry skin, brittle hair, emaciated appearance.

Psychosocial Assessment

- Assess the patient's social support systems:
  - Observe the interactions between the patient and peers and/or family.
- Assess the patient's coping strategies:
  - Children and adolescents who are unable to effectively cope with the stresses of childhood and adolescence may be at risk for substance abuse.
- Assess the patient's behavior:
  - Children and adolescents who are aggressive and rebellious may be at risk for substance abuse (Merenstein et al., 1997).

Nursing Interventions for Acute Drug or Alcohol Overdose

- Assess and maintain airway, breathing, and circulation (Chapter 6).
- Initiate cardiorespiratory and oxygen saturation monitoring.
- Obtain venous access and initiate an intravenous infusion:
  - Obtain blood specimens for toxicology screening (Chapter 44).
  - Administer medications to control seizures, as needed (Chapter 18).
  - Prepare to administer 50% dextrose to decrease encephalopathy and alcohol-induced hypoglycemia.
  - Administer naloxone hydrochloride to reverse the effects of narcotics.
- Initiate interventions to eliminate the drug from the body (Chapter 44).
- Obtain urine and gastric samples, as needed for toxicology screening (Chapter 44):
  - Initiate screening if the patient identifies the substance.
  - Test for inhalants as indicated by history.
- Reassess neurological and cardiopulmonary status:
  - Observe for clinical findings indicative of alcohol intoxication versus alcohol withdrawal (Table 27.8).
- Inform the family frequently of the patient's condition; provide emotional support to the patient and family.
- Place the patient in physical restraints to promote patient safety, if needed.
- Initiate psychiatric and social service consultations.
- Prepare for transfer and transport to a tertiary care center or hospitalization.

Nursing Interventions for Substance Abuse

- Initiate psychiatric and social service consult.
- Encourage the patient to initiate contact with a rehabilitation unit for detoxification.

Home Care/Prevention

Emergency nurses can participate in the prevention of alcohol and drug use among youth by (Sefuentes, 1996; Stanhope & Knollmueller, 1997):

- Participating in education programs designed to assist the child and adolescent in making decisions about drug and alcohol use, to build self-esteem, and to improve communication skills.
- Promoting the inclusion of alcohol and drug use information in school curricula.
- Participating in community outreach programs for children, adolescents, and families (Appendix A).
- Providing positive reinforcement for children and adolescents who avoid drug/alcohol use.
- Encouraging and facilitating discussions among children and adolescents about peer pressure; practicing refusal behaviors.

TABLE 27.8 Comparison of Acute Alcohol Intoxication and Alcohol Withdrawal

Acute Alcohol Intoxication	*Alcohol Withdrawal*
▪ Decreased alertness	▪ Restlessness
▪ Slurred speech	▪ Anxiety
▪ Nausea	▪ Tachycardia
▪ Vertigo	▪ Vomiting
▪ Staggering gait	▪ Tremors
▪ Stupor	▪ Diaphoresis
▪ Unconsciousness	▪ Anorexia
	▪ Insomnia
	▪ Confusion
	▪ Hallucinations leading to convulsions
	▪ Delirium tremens (if treatment is not initiated within 72 hours of withdrawal): uncontrolled shaking, restlessness, and agitation
	▪ Disorientation, confusion, hallucinations
	▪ Potential grand mal seizures

Data from: Chulay, Guzzetta, & Dossey, 1997; Hazinski, 1992.

Conclusion

Caring for children with psychiatric emergencies is challenging. Updating emergency department policies and procedures for using restraints, initiating voluntary and involuntary commitments, and staffing for suicidal observation are imperative to avoid legal ramifications. Collaboration with community agencies helps emergency nurses to provide additional resources to these patients and families as needed.

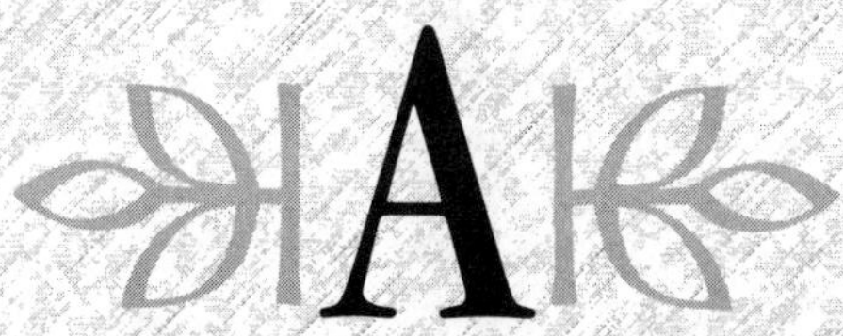

Patient Education Resources

Al-Anon Family Group Headquarters
P.O. Box 1862
Madison Square Station
New York, NY 10010

Alcohol Hotline
(800) ALCOHOL (252-6465)

Alcoholics Anonymous
P.O. Box 459
Grand Central Station
New York, NY 10017

Cocaine Anonymous
3740 Overland Avenue, Suite H
Los Angeles, CA 90034

Drugs Anonymous/Pills Anonymous
P.O. Box 473
Ansonia Station
New York, NY 10023

EN-CARE
Emergency Nurses Association
915 Lee Street
DesPlaines, IL 60016-6569

Nar-Anon Family Group
P.O. Box 2562
Palos Verdes Peninsula, CA 90274

Narcotics Anonymous
P.O. Box 9999
Van Nuys, CA 91409

National Clearinghouse for Alcohol and Drug Information
Center for Substance Abuse Prevention
P.O. Box 2345
Rockville, MD 20852

National Committee for the Prevention of Alcoholism and Drug Dependency
6830 Laurel Street, NW
Washington, DC 20012

National Council on Alcoholism and Drug Dependence
12 West 21st Street
New York, NY 10010

National Council on Drug Abuse
571 West Jackson Boulevard
Chicago, IL 60606

National Institute of Mental Health, National Institutes of Health
5600 Fishers Lane
Rockville, MD 20857

National Institute on Drug Abuse
5600 Fishers Lane, Room 10-05
Rockville, MD 20857

National Runaway Switchboard
(800) 621-4000

Runaway Hotline
(800) 231-6946

SADD—Students Against Destructive Decisions
P.O. Box 800
Marlboro, MA 01752
(800) 787-5777
SADD.org

Teaching Kids to Cope
University of Pittsburgh
School of Nursing/Puskar
3500 Victoria 415
Pittsburgh, PA 15261
(412) 624-6933

U.S. Public Health Service
Report of the Surgeon General's conference on children's mental health: A national action agenda. (2000).
Washington, DC

References

Allender, M. (1998). Adolescence. In C. Edelman & C. Mandle, (Eds.), *Health promotion throughout the lifespan* (4th ed., pp. 553-581). St. Louis: Mosby—Year Book.

American Psychiatric Association. (1995). *Diagnostic and statistical manual of mental disorders* (4th ed.). Washington, DC: Author.

Antai-Otong, D. (1995). *Psychiatric nursing: Biological and behavioral concepts*. Philadelphia: Saunders.

Ball, J. (1998). Psychosocial section. In J. Ball (Ed.), *Mosby's pediatric patient teaching guidelines* (pp. K-1-K-7). St. Louis: Mosby—Year Book.

Ball, J., & Bindler, R. (1995). *Pediatric nursing caring for children*. Norwalk, CT: Appleton & Lange.

Barkin, R., & Rosen, P. (1994). Psychiatric disorders. In R. Barkin & P. Rosen (Eds.). *Emergency pediatrics* (4th ed., pp. 688-695). St. Louis: Mosby—Year Book.

Brent, D. (1993). Depression and suicide in children and adolescents. *Pediatrics in Review, 14*, 380-388.

Burgess, A. (1997). *Psychiatric nursing: Promoting mental health*. Stanford, CT: Appleton & Lange.

Busen, N. (1992). Counseling the high-risk adolescent. *Journal of Pediatric Health Care, 6*, 194-199.

Carson, V. B., & Arnold, E. N. (1996). *Mental health nursing. The nurse-patient journey*. Philadelphia: Saunders.

Chulay, M., Guzzetta, C., & Dossey, B. (1997). *AACN handbook of critical care nursing*. Stamford, CT: Appleton & Lange.

Constantino, R. (1996). Legal issues in psychiatric-mental health nursing. In S. Lego (Ed.), *Psychiatric nursing: A comprehensive reference* (2nd ed., pp. 551-561). Philadelphia: Lippincott.

Engel, J. (1997). *Pocket guide to pediatric assessment*. St. Louis: Mosby—Year Book.

Fortinash, K. M., & Holoday-Worret, P. A. (1996). *Psychiatric mental health nursing*. St. Louis: Mosby—Year Book.

Hazinski, M. F. (1992). *Nursing care of the critically ill child* (2nd ed.). St. Louis: Mosby—Year Book.

Jarvis, C. (1996). *Physical examination and health assessment* (2nd ed.). St. Louis: Mosby—Year Book.

Johnson, L. S., O'Malley, P. M., & Bachman, J. G. (1994). *National survey results on drug use from the Monitoring the Future Study, 1975-1998* (Publication No. 94-3809). Rockville, MD: National Institute on Drug Abuse.

Kirksey, K., Holt-Ashley, M., Williamson, K., & Garza, R. (1995). Autoerotic asphyxia in adolescents. *Journal of Emergency Nursing, 21*(1), 81-83.

Mannenbach, M., Hargarten, S., & Phelan, M. (1997). Alcohol use among injured patients aged 12 to 18 years. *Academic Emergency Medicine, 4*, 40-44.

McFarland, G., Wasli, E., & Gerety, E. (1997). *Nursing diagnosis and process in psychiatric mental health nursing* (3rd ed.). Philadelphia: Lippincott.

Merenstein, G., Kaplan, D, & Rosenberg, A. (1997). *Handbook of pediatrics* (18th ed.). Stamford, CT: Appleton & Lange.

Moriarty, A. (1996). What's "new" in street drugs: "illy." *Journal of Pediatric Health Care, 10*, 41-43.

Oakley, L., & Potter, C. (1997). *Psychiatric primary care*. St. Louis: Mosby—Year Book.

Paquette, M., & Roderick, C. (1997). *Psychiatric nursing diagnostic care plans for DSM-IV*. Sudbury, MA: Jones & Bartlett.

Puskar, K., Tusaie-Mumford, K., Rohay, J., Lamb, J., Boneysteele, G., & Sereika, S. (1996). Computers link adolescent health research to rural settings. *Bringing Excellence to Substance Abuse Services in Rural and Frontier America, 20*, 101-108.

Puskar, K., Lamb, J., & Tusaie-Mumford, K. (1997). Teaching kids to cope: A preventive mental health nursing strategy for adolescents. *Journal of Child Adolescent Psychiatric Nursing, 10*(3), 18-28.

Puskar, K., Tusare-Mumford, K., Sereika, S., & Lamb, J. (1999). Screening and predicting adolescent depressive symptoms in rural settings. *Archives of Psychiatric Nursing, 13*(1), 3-11.

Reynolds, W. (1987). *Reynolds adolescent depression scale: Professional manual*. Odessa, FL: Psychological Assessment Resources.

Schwartz, E. (1994). The posttraumatic response in children and adolescents. *Psychiatric Clinics of North America, 172*, 1311-1326.

Sciera, M. (1998). Psychosocial and behavioral problems. In T. Soud & J. Rogers (Eds.), *Manual of pediatric emergency nursing* (pp. 727-740). St. Louis: Mosby—Year Book.

Sefuentes, M. (1996). Substance abuse. In C. Berkowitz (Ed.), *Pediatrics: A primary care approach*. Philadelphia: Saunders.

Stanhope, M., & Knollmueller, R. (1997). *Public and community health nurses' consultant*. St. Louis: Mosby—Year Book.

Urbanitis, J. (1983). *Psychiatric emergencies*. Norwalk, CT: Appleton-Century-Crofts.

U.S. Public Health Service. (2000). Report of the Surgeon General's conference on children's mental health: A national action agenda. Washington, DC.

Valente, S. (1989). Adolescent suicide: Assessment and intervention. *Journal Child Adolescent Psychiatric Nursing, 2*(1), 34-39.

Varcarolis, E., Colson, C. (2002). Disorders of children and adolescents. In E. Varcardis (Ed.), *Foundations of psychiatric mental health nursing: A clinical approach* (4th ed., Ch. 31, pp. 856-881, Cherrill Colson). Philadelphia: W. B. Saunders.

Wilson, H., & Kneisl, C. (1992). *Psychiatric nursing* (4th ed). Redwood City, CA: Addison-Wesley.

Zimbler, E. (1997). *Psychiatric nursing. Promoting mental health: Review and study guide*. Stanford, CT: Appleton & Lange.

28

Crisis Intervention and Management

Donna Ojanen Thomas, RN, MSN

Introduction

Caring for a critically ill or injured child in the emergency department (ED) is difficult, especially if death is the end result. As ED staff, nurses are trained to help people to get well, and death seems to be a failure. The death of a child seems unfair. People tend to view children as innocent and not having had a chance to live their lives. Often, nurses are unprepared to deal with the raw anguish of the family and the emotions it creates in themselves. No amount of training can prepare nurses for the indescribable sound of a parent's cry of disbelief at being told that his or her child has died or help nurses "get used to" it. However, information on how to better deal with the family and cope with their own emotions will help emergency nurses to face these situations in a way that is helpful to families and to themselves.

The reality of working in the emergency department is that people die, even children. Although children may die from congenital conditions, chronic illness, and from acts of violence, more than half of all childhood deaths are caused by injury. Each year, more than 20,000 children under 19 years of age die from trauma, and 80% of all trauma deaths occur either at the accident scene or in the ED (Ziegler & Gonzalez Del Rey, 2000).

The purpose of this chapter is to describe interventions to help families cope with crisis situations, such as sudden critical injury, illness, or death of a child; specific situations in the emergency department that may result in the need for crisis intervention; and methods of helping staff to cope with crisis situations. It is impossible to discuss crisis intervention and management without including how to help the ED staff cope with their own feelings created by these events.

Pediatric Considerations

There are several challenges in dealing with the critical illness, injury, or death of a child in the emergency department:

- Most medical and nursing education covers the clinical but not the emotional aspects of care.
- Staff and families have differing philosophies and beliefs concerning illness and death, based on past experiences and cultural influences. These cannot be fully explored during the brief ED interactions but need to be considered.
- Emotional situations are not straightforward, and it is not possible to write care process models or standards of care that will work in every situation.
- The fast pace of the emergency department allows nurses little time to care for families, let alone take care of their own needs. There is always another patient waiting.

Definitions

Many situations that families and staff experience in the emergency department can lead to stress, which can progress to a crisis. *Stress* is tension, strain, or pressure, such as the feelings that occur after a family has waited for extended periods of time in the emergency department or when the ED staff is overwhelmed by conflicting demands and stimuli. A *crisis* refers to an acute emotional upset arising from situational, developmental, or social sources resulting in a temporary inability to cope by one's usual problem-solving devices (Hoff, 1989). Examples include sudden illness, injury, or death. A crisis can result for both the families in the emergency department and the staff caring for them when one of these events occur. Although the terms *stress* and *crisis* refer to differing conditions, increasing stress with no relief can lead to a crisis for both families and staff.

Crisis management refers to the entire process of working through the crisis to its end point of resolution. *Crisis intervention* is a short-term helping process that focuses on the resolution of the immediate problem through the use of personal, social, and environmental resources. The positive or negative resolution of the crisis often depends on crisis intervention (Hoff, 1989). Whether a stressful event precipitates a crisis depends on the following:

- The family's (or staff member's) interpretation of the events.
- The coping ability and previous experience.
- Social and personal resources.

Several characteristics of an event may increase the level of stress experienced by a family or the ED staff:

- Onset of the event (sudden or gradual).
- Anticipation of the event—generally ED visits are precipitated by an unanticipated event.
- Control over the event. Feeling as if one has no control over an event can increase the stress of that event. This happens frequently in a busy emergency department, for both staff and families. Staff cannot control the number of patients seeking care, and families cannot control the situations that are occurring with their child.
- Previous experience.
- Other stressful events occurring in the family or in the emergency department.
- The meaning that the family attaches to the event. Some events are more stressful for families and staff because the situation may remind them of a similar situation that was hard to handle.

How staff members in the emergency department respond to a crisis will also depend on their own beliefs, experiences, and support systems.

Focused History

A brief history will aid in the diagnosis and treatment of the child. Providing a history can by a therapeutic experience for the family. By telling the medical team about their child, parents participate in the treatment and feel more in control (Frader & Sargent, 1993). The following are important components in the history (Emergency Nurses Association [ENA], 1998a):

- The family's perception of the event or situation.
- Availability of support systems.
- Previous illness or injury of the child.
- Concurrent maturational crisis within the family.
- Family's current level of functioning, past experiences, and usual coping mechanisms.
- Drug and/or alcohol use by the family, especially if associated with the child's injury.
- The family's religious preference.

Focused Assessment

During contact with the family members, the ED nurse should assess their interaction. Signs and symptoms demonstrated by family members in a crisis situation may be:

- Behavioral:
  - Withdrawal or isolation.
  - Demanding behavior.
  - Loud crying or shouting.
  - Self-destructive behavior.
  - Violence against other family members or the healthcare team.
- Physical:
  - Tachycardia.
  - Hyperventilation.
  - Chest pain.
  - Fainting.

Anger may be expressed toward other family members or toward the ED staff. Anger is a coping mechanism and can be allowed as long as it does not result in violent behavior that may cause injury to staff or others.

Provocation of a potentially hostile, angry family member in borderline control can increase the likelihood and frequency of violence in the emergency department. The ED nurse must assess for emotional distress and intervene on a corresponding level, averting unnecessary hostility while providing the most therapeutic response to the family's emotional needs (Bjorn, 1991).

Nursing diagnoses and expected outcomes are listed in Table 28.1.

Nursing Interventions

How the nurse approaches the family in the emergency department will positively influence their ability to cope with the crisis. The family needs to receive information on what is happening, to participate in the care, to receive compassionate support, and to maintain hope. The following are ways to meet these needs of the family:

- General approach:
  - Take the family to a private area to talk with them.
  - Assign one staff member (nurse or social worker) to communicate information about the child's condition.
  - Explain that the ED physician will talk with them as soon as he or she is able to do so.
  - Allow the family to ask questions and expect expressions of guilt, depending on the situation.

TABLE 28.1 Nursing Diagnoses and Expected Outcomes

Nursing Diagnoses	*Expected Outcomes*
Ineffective family coping	The family will be helped to accept the initial pain of the loss or potential loss of their child.
Powerlessness	The family will be given some control by being allowed to make decisions concerning the care of their child and by being informed of what is being done.
Risk for violence, self-directed or directed at others	The family will be able to grieve without harming themselves or others, with the assistance of the ED staff.

- Communicate with the family. Talking with a family whose child is seriously ill or injured is very difficult, but family members will appreciate the contact of someone who is involved in the care of their child. The following are suggestions for talking with the family:
  - Introduce yourself; use the family name and the name of the child.
  - Give accurate, honest information.
  - Meet the family's physical needs (bathroom, water, tissues, and telephone).
  - Do not eliminate hope while a resuscitation is still under way.
  - Ask about the need for clergy or religious rights. Many hospitals now have a chaplain to help families of any or no faith.
  - Give brief, frequent updates on the child's condition (e.g., "We are doing everything we know how to do to help him.").
- Avoid telling the family by telephone that a child has died. Tell them that the child is critically ill or injured and that they should have someone drive them to the emergency department immediately.
- Communicate with the child:
  - Assume that the child can hear what is being said.
  - Assign a staff member to talk to the child during the resuscitation, touching and holding the hand and letting him or her know what is being done. If family is present, encourage them to talk to the child.
- Let the family in during resuscitation efforts. Allowing family presence during a resuscitation is controversial, but experience has shown that this is helpful. In one study, 76% of families who were allowed in during a resuscitation said it was beneficial, and 64% felt that it was beneficial to the patient (Hanson & Strawser, 1992). The ENA believes that families should be given the option to be present during resuscitation efforts (ENA, 2001a). The most important needs identified by family members are (Molter, 1979):
  - To be with the patient.
  - To be helpful to the patient.
  - To be informed of the patient's condition.
  - To be comforted and supported by other family members.
  - To be accepted, comforted, and supported by the healthcare professionals.
  - To feel that the patient was receiving the best possible care.
- Family presence during resuscitation efforts allows the patient and family to support each other and facilitates the grieving process by bringing a sense of reality to the treatment efforts and the patient's clinical status (ENA, 2001a). Protocols for family presence should be developed, including the following concepts:
  - Give the family the choice of being present.
  - Prepare the family for what they will see and how the child will look.
  - Assign a support person for the family.
  - Be prepared to handle emotions (both the family's and your own).
  - Watch for signs from the family that show they need to leave the room.
  - Be aware as to when an invasive procedure, such as a thoracotomy, is about to take place and consider moving the family. A thoracotomy is an intensely stressful procedure and most family members would not fare well viewing this invasive, bloody procedure (Williams, 2002).
- Be prepared to deal with family emotions, including anger toward staff or other family members. Have a plan to summon help (should be part of a departmental security plan):
  - Remain confident and nonjudgmental.

- Maintain a path of easy escape and remain within shouting distance of help.
- Listen initially without interrupting the family member.
- Speak in a calm, quiet voice and be aware of what you say and how you say it.
- Set realistic limits. For example, "I really want to help you, but your shouting is upsetting to me and to other patients."
- Never attempt to restrain a physically abusive family member; make sure you have a plan to contact security personnel.

■ Support cultural differences. Emergency department staff should know about different cultures that exist in their area and be aware of language barriers and differing beliefs. Other suggestions for helping others from different cultures to cope include (Valk-Lawson, 1990):

- Provide an interpreter to translate.
- Ask the family what would be helpful.
- Watch family members, especially parents, for cues as to what is acceptable (body space, speaking of the dead).
- Help family identify resources within their culture in the community.

Specific Crisis Situations

Death of a Child in the Emergency Department

The sudden death of a child does not allow the family to evolve through the stages of accepting death and throws them into an acute grief reaction. *Grief* is defined as the reaction of the bereaved to a loss (Cork, Fuller, & Barnickol, 1991). Sudden death eliminates the family members' opportunity for the anticipatory grief that usually prepares survivors for death following a long illness (Frader & Sargent, 1993). *Anticipatory grief* is defined as the normal reaction in preparation for a loss and allows for absorbing the reality of the loss over time (Rando, 1984).

Sudden death of a child puts survivors at a much higher risk for *prolonged* or *complicated grief*, which can result in personal disability. Situations that may dispose survivors to the development of complicated grief include the sudden, unexpected death of an infant or child, death involving homicide or suicide, or death caused by the survivor (Walters & Tupin, 1991).

Expressions of grief vary from person to person and are almost always influenced by the person's cultural background. Assisting families through the expressions of grief is one of the hardest jobs of the ED nurse, but perhaps one of the most important in determining how the family copes with the loss.

Nursing Interventions

Telling the family

Perhaps nothing is more painful or stressful for an ED nurse than telling a family, or being present when a family is told, that their child has died. Medical and/or nursing education usually does not include information on how to do this. The discussion of emotional issues, such as organ donation and autopsy, further complicates the issue (Swisher, Nieman, Nilsen, & Spivey, 1993).

The physician in charge of the child's care should be the one to inform the family, but the nurse may be present or must be the one to inform the family. The family should be told as soon as possible after the child has died.

- Bring the family to a private area, preferably one that is away from the emergency department. If possible, all family members should be told together. In the midst of the medical turmoil and uncertainty that inevitably accompanies critical injury, illness, or death, family members cannot be expected to absorb, accurately recall, and then transmit information to spouses or other family members (Frader & Sargent, 1993).
- If all family members are not present, make sure someone is assigned to watch for arriving family members so that they can be told immediately and do not have to wander through the emergency department looking for someone to help them. Table 28.2 lists some "dos and don'ts" for informing a family of a child's death.

Communicating with siblings

Direct and honest communication concerning illness and death is critical to limiting long-term psychological consequences for children who have lost a loved one (Barakat, Sills, & LaBagnara, 1995). Siblings should be told of the death sensitively and promptly and be encouraged to share in the mourning (Serwint, 1995).

The approach to children should be matched to the child's developmental level:

- Children younger than 3 years of age may be affected by the loss of a sibling but have little or no understanding of the meaning of death.
- Children aged 3 to 5 years may believe that death is reversible or analogous to someone's going away.
- Children aged 5 to 9 understand that death is permanent but believe that it will not happen to them or

TABLE 28.2 Informing the Family of a Child's Death

DO:	*DON'T:*
■ Tell the family immediately. ■ Sit down with family—physically join them unless the situation is hostile. ■ Be kind, but direct. Speak directly to the person closest to the child (mother or father). ■ Give a brief explanation of what was done in the emergency department and the suspected cause of the death, if known. ■ Provide physical comfort (by touching the family, if you are comfortable doing this). ■ Allow the family to express pain. ■ Stay long enough to answer questions. ■ Say you are sorry.	■ Say, "I know how you feel." ■ Imply guilt (of parents, medical care, or others). ■ Use euphemisms "your child has passed away, or is "gone." ■ Offer meaningless comfort such as, "It was God's will" or "He is in a better place." ■ Tell them they can always have another child. This may not be true, and another child will not replace the one who has died. ■ Tell the family how they should or should not feel. Grief is individual. ■ Routinely offer sedatives, because this may delay some of the grieving process for later.

Data from: Frader & Sargent, 1993; Hamilton, 1988; Hoff, 1989.

affect them, and they are unprepared to encounter it in their own families.

- Children 9 years or older do understand that death is permanent and can happen to them and their family members.

The following suggestions may be helpful in communicating with siblings:

- Talk with the siblings to find out their perception of death.
- Reassure them that they were not to blame.
- Avoid using euphemisms, such as, "Your brother has gone to sleep." This will make the siblings fearful of going to sleep, afraid that they may die too.
- Children should be offered a chance to see their sibling in the emergency department, but should not be forced to see or touch the body after death.
- Parents should be encouraged to involve siblings in the funeral and burial. To be able to let go and reinvest in life, the children need a clear understanding of what has happened and some closure.
- Parents should not attempt to protect siblings from sadness, because children will know something is wrong by the way the parents are acting. Children excluded from the grief may believe that they somehow are at fault for the death. Normal responses to the loss of a loved one should be explained to children, and they should be told that it is permissible for them to be sad and to cry.
- Questions should be answered with honesty. Children have a need to talk to someone and to be reassured.

Viewing the body

The family should be given the choice of viewing the body. Evidence should be preserved as necessary by leaving tubes in place and following the hospital's guidelines for evidence preservation. Wrapping the baby in a warm blanket or quilt prior to having the parents view the baby will be comforting to the family. If the family is not present when death is declared, keep the child in the emergency department until they have a chance to see the body. Never allow the family to view the body in the hospital morgue, even if keeping the child in the emergency department may tie up a needed treatment room:

- Prepare the family for how the child will look and feel. Explain any tubes that are left in place.
- Provide privacy.
- Remain with the family if they ask you to do so.
- Allow the family ample time to be with the child.
- Give the family permission to leave.
- Have one nurse remain with the child when the family leaves.

Additional Interventions

- Provide information concerning funeral arrangements and autopsy:

- An autopsy is required in all cases of sudden and unattended death.
- The ED nurse must be familiar with local laws.
- Tell the family whom to contact for the results.

- Provide help with cessation of breast-feeding following an infant's death. The mother may need to use a breast pump or obtain information from her obstetrician, a lactation specialist, or from the LaLeche League.
- Provide mementos. Even if the parents do not want mementos, it is often wise to obtain them because the family may call back later and ask for them:
  - Handprints and/or footprints and a lock of hair: Kits are commercially available that contain plaster to make a hand or foot imprint.
  - A picture, if the parents request it. A Polaroid photograph of the baby wrapped in a blanket may be helpful to the family later, especially if the infant is very young and the parents have not had much time to take photographs.
  - The blanket or quilt that the baby was wrapped in when the family viewed and held the baby.
- Provide information about organ donation (Chapter 2):
  - Requesting organ donation is another identified area of stress for staff after the death of a child in the emergency department (Swisher et al., 1993).
  - Requesting organ donation is the law in all states, and every hospital should have policies concerning when and by whom this should be done.
- Provide follow-up:
  - Give the family names of local support groups or a social worker to call.
  - Some hospitals have a program in which follow-up calls are made by a social worker or nurse at intervals such as 2 weeks, 6 months, and 1 year.
  - The family can be provided with the name of a staff member who they can contact if they have any questions.
  - Give written material concerning the grieving process, support groups, and who can be contacted. Parents may not be able to process any information that has been discussed or given to them at the time, and written information will be useful to them later. Having a prepared "grief packet" with information and resources is helpful.
- Provide closure. Watching a family whose child has died leave the emergency department and knowing that they must go home and face all of their child's belongings is very emotional for ED staff:
  - If possible, ED staff should arrange transportation home for family members so that they will not have to drive.
  - The family will often have questions about what will happen to their child. Simply tell them that you will take care of their baby until he or she is picked up by the mortuary.
- Complete all necessary documentation:
  - Most hospitals have standard forms to fill out for any death in the emergency department.
  - Having a "death packet" that consists of a prepared envelope with all the necessary forms will make documentation easier and prevent omission of a needed form.

Sudden Infant Death Syndrome

Sudden infant death syndrome (SIDS) is the sudden death of an infant younger than 1 year of age for which postmortem examination, investigation of the death scene, and a review of the case history fails to establish a cause (Zylke, 1989). About one-third of all infant deaths involving children between the ages of 1 week and 1 year are attributable to SIDS (Valdes-Dapena, 1991). Sudden infant death syndrome is the third-leading cause of death in infants, after congenital anomalies and disorders relating to short gestation and unspecified birth weight (Guyer, Martin, MacDorman, Anderson, & Strobino, 1997). The death rate from SIDS has decreased since the American Academy of Pediatrics (1992) recommended that normal infants be placed on their sides or their backs instead of on their stomachs during sleep. In fact, postnatal mortality rate per 1,000 live births declined 29.8%, from 4.1 in 1980 to 2.9 in 1994; most of the decline resulted from reduced mortality from infections and SIDS (Scott, Iyasu, Rowley, & Atrash, 1998).

Most deaths from SIDS occur in the winter months. The peak age for a SIDS death is 2 months, and SIDS rarely occurs in a child younger than 1 month of age.

Pathophysiology

The exact cause of SIDS remains unknown, but studies underline a multiple-cause hypothesis, which involves (Kolhendorfer, Kiechl, & Sperl, 1998):

- Genetic predisposition.
- Immaturity in the first months of life.
- Environmental factors acting at various ages.

Theories that have been or are being researched include:

- Abnormal respiratory control.
- Small airway occlusion.
- Cardiovascular abnormalities.
- Defects of metabolism.

- Infection.
- Delayed neural development.
- Abnormal sleep and arousal states.

Risk factors for SIDS have been identified for both mother and infant. These are listed in Table 28.3.

Focused History

When an apneic and pulseless baby is brought to the emergency department, the following history may be indicative of SIDS:

- A healthy baby who was put to sleep for a nap or for the night.
- A child who had a slight cold and may have recently seen a physician for a minor illness.
- Pink, frothy drainage from the nose and mouth.

Focused Assessment

Generally, the child will be lifeless but still may be warm, depending on how long it has been since the arrest has occurred. The assessment is the same for any child who presents to the emergency department in cardiopulmonary arrest (Chapter 15). The ED nurse has to assess for signs and symptoms of other injuries that may be indicative of child abuse (Chapter 46).

Nursing Interventions

Nursing interventions for the child who is suspected to have died of SIDS are the same as for any death in the emergency department. The following are interventions specific to SIDS (Thomas, 1998):

- Explain the definition of SIDS and that the diagnosis is only probable until it is confirmed by autopsy.
- If possible, allow the family the option to say goodbye to the baby while the resuscitation is still being attempted.
- Provide literature on SIDS.
- Allay feelings of guilt as much as possible. Feelings of guilt are universal in most deaths but are especially prominent in SIDS parents because the child was previously healthy.
- Refer the family to a local SIDS support group.

Prevention

Although SIDS cannot be prevented entirely, the ED nurse can give families of neonates literature on the American Academy of Pediatrics' recommendations concerning placement of healthy infants in the supine position. The ED nurse can also inform parents of risk factors relating to SIDS, such as maternal smoking.

Violence

Violence and assault in the emergency department are recognized as significant occupational hazards for nursing professionals (Presley & Robinson, 2002). The emergency department is an area where care is provided 24 hours per day, 7 days per week, and 365 days per year. It is often the primary source of access of the public to the hospital, especially after hours. Because the emotional and physical reactions of patients and families cannot be predicted, especially when they are given bad news, it is impossible to know when violent acts against staff may occur. Factors that predispose to ED violence include:

- Long waiting times.
- Staff shortages and temporary staffing.
- Overcrowding in the emergency department.
- The availability of controlled substances and other drugs.
- Potential hostages.
- Easy hospital access through the emergency department.
- Increasing gang violence and changing gang culture.
- Use of the emergency department for medical evaluation of patients with psychiatric and substance abuse problems.
- Increasing number of patients needing care for injuries resulting from violence.

TABLE 28.3 Risk Factors for SIDS

Risk Factors for the Mother	*Risk Factors in the Infant*
■ Age less than 20 years	■ Prematurity and low birth weight
■ Poor prenatal and antenatal care	■ Male
■ Low social and educational levels	■ Sleeping in prone position
■ Smoking during pregnancy	■ Gestational age of less than 37 weeks
■ Narcotic or methadone use	■ Repeated episodes of apnea
	■ Family history of SIDS
	■ Exposure to smoking

Data from: Carroll & Loughlin, 1993; Elliot, Vullermin, & Robinson, 1998.

- Patients, family members, friends and staff in a crisis situation.

All emergency departments should develop protocols for both the prevention of violent behavior and for interventions when necessary (Thomas, 1998). The protocols should involve a team approach with hospital security, the local police, and ED staff.

The Emergency Nurses Association (2001b) believes that healthcare organizations have a responsibility to provide a safe and secure environment for their employees and the public. Emergency nurses have the right to take appropriate measures to protect themselves and their patients from injury caused by violent individuals who present to the emergency department.

Nursing Interventions

Preventing a situation from escalating into violent behavior is preferable, but not always possible. The following are suggestions to help deal with potentially violent situations:

- Contact security and notify them of the situation.
- Remain confident and nonjudgmental.
- Deal with the family one on one, but maintain a path of easy escape.
- Speak in a calm, quiet voice.
- Listen without talking initially.
- Set realistic limits (e.g., "I would like to help you, but can't help you when you are yelling at me.").
- Never attempt to restrain a patient or family member unless you have been trained to do so.
- Review protocols yearly so that all staff members are familiar with actions to take to recognize and prevent violent behavior.

Homicide

In 1996, homicide was the fourth-leading cause of death for children 1 to 4 years of age, the third-leading cause of death for children aged 10 to 14 years, and the second-leading cause for 15- to 19-year-olds (Guyer et al., 1997). Handgun injuries have increased dramatically in the pediatric age group. The number of pediatric gunshot wounds reported by urban trauma centers has increased by 300% since 1986 (Committee on Injury and Poison Prevention, 1992).

It is becoming more common in the emergency department to see the results of violence in the form of child abuse injuries and even death. Most childhood victims of homicide are injured by their parents. Death of a child by homicide creates special problems for both parents and ED staff.

Focused Assessment

As in most cases of death in the emergency department, the family becomes the patient. For the survivors of a homicide victim, grief is often overwhelming. Parents often feel guilty that they could not protect the child. The situation is compounded if the murder was committed by family members, friends, or acquaintances. The drive for revenge may be a central issue.

Nursing Interventions

Nursing interventions for the family of a homicide victim are the same as for other deaths in the emergency department. Evidence preservation and collection become crucial, and the ED nurse must be familiar with procedures for preserving and collecting evidence for the medical examiner. If the death is thought to be the result of gang violence, the following precautions should be taken to protect the staff, family, and other patients (Rollins, 1993):

- Notify security to provide surveillance.
- Disrobe the child entirely to check for weapons.
- Observe for signs of imminent violence by family members or visitors.
- Limit access to the patient and family.
- Develop reporting policies for the media to avoid publicizing information that could endanger the family or the victim.

The brutal death of a child will have an impact on ED staff, and critical incident stress management (CISM) is appropriate.

Critical Incident Stress Management

Critical incidents are defined as any events that have sufficient emotional power to overcome the usual coping abilities of ED staff (Mitchell, 1983). Emergency department staff face these situations (the death of a child, overwhelming numbers of critically ill patients, and demands from families and other staff members) on a fairly routine basis. Many times there is no opportunity to recover and process the event because other patients require care. The consequences of untreated stress can lead to absenteeism, sleep disorders, burnout, health problems, and emotional difficulties.

It is impossible for staff to not be affected by the emotional aspects of the job, but they must be able to contain their emotions while caring for patients so that they can deliver needed care. The Committee on Pediatric Emergency Medicine (1994) and the American Academy of Pediatrics (2001) believe that emergency departments should have written policies and procedures concerning support of staff members and coping with death in the ED.

The Emergency Nurses Association supports the use of critical incident stress management (CISM) to accelerate recovery of emergency nurses from acute incidents (ENA, 1998b). CISM provides care for the healthcare professional after an emotional or stressful event and consists of debriefings and defusings (ENA, 1995). A *defusing* is an informal gathering after an event and is shorter and less structured than a debriefing. An example might be getting staff together for 15 minutes after a death and allowing them to discuss their feelings concerning the death. A *debriefing* is an organized approach, ideally occurring 24 to 72 hours after an event and involves the use of trained personnel such as social workers and other healthcare professionals. Staff involved are allowed to describe the feelings and reactions to the event and are provided with information to lessen the impact of the stress.

Other suggestions for helping staff cope with death or other critical incidents in the emergency department include:

- Protocols that describe the treatment of patients or families following death.
- Education on the grieving process.
- Evaluation of one's feelings concerning death and available support systems.
- Recovery time after a death, even if only for a few minutes.
- Support of ED staff toward each other and support from the nurse manager.
- A sympathy card signed by all staff and sent to family members.
- Encouragement for ED staff to take care of themselves physically, mentally, and spiritually.
- Support from the hospital chaplain.
- Focusing on the positive. Most children do get better and go home.

Although it is not a popular topic, coping with death and critical incidents must be included in orientation programs for new employees. This should include not only the mechanical aspects of dealing with the body and the paperwork but also the emotional aspects, which are often the hardest to handle.

Conclusion

Caring for a critically ill or injured child in the emergency department is always difficult emotionally. Emergency nurses can have protocols and procedures and take classes on how to perform the perfect resuscitation. This is the easy part. The emotional part—helping the family cope when the resuscitation is unsuccessful—is hard. How nurses treat the family is critical and will determine, to a large extent, how they cope with their grief later on. Realizing that the grief response is different and cannot be dealt with in a cookbook manner will help nurses be more accepting and to provide support, which may involve simply saying "I am sorry."

Although the feelings of the staff are often attended to last, they should not be neglected. Teams for CISM should be developed and used as necessary. Staff members often provide the best support for each other. The long-term effects of dealing with the constant stressors in the emergency department will result in serious health and emotional problems for the staff if these traumas are not recognized and treated.

References

American Academy of Pediatrics. (1992). To lessen SIDS risk, AAP recommends infants sleep on side or back [News release]. Elk Grove Village, IL: Author.

American Academy of Pediatrics. (2001). Care of children in the emergency department: Guidelines for preparedness. Policy Statement. *Pediatrics, 107*, 777-781.

Barakat, L. P., Sills, R., & LaBagnara, S. (1995). Management of fatal illness and death in children or their parents. *Pediatrics in Review, 16*, 419-423.

Bjorn, P. (1991). An approach to the potentially violent patient. *Journal of Emergency Nursing, 17*, 336.

Carroll J., & Loughlin, G. (1993). Sudden infant death syndrome. *Pediatrics in Review, 14*, 83.

Committee on Injury and Poison Prevention. (1992). Firearm injuries affecting the pediatric population. *Pediatrics, 89*(4), 788-790.

Committee on Pediatric Emergency Medicine (1994). Death of a child in the emergency department. *Pediatrics, 93*(5), 861-862.

Cork, C. A., Fuller, H., & Barnickol, C. A., Eds. (1991): *Sudden infant death syndrome. Who can help and how.* New York: Springer Publishing Company.

Durch, J. S., & Lohr, K. N. (1993). *Emergency medical services for children*. Washington, DC: Institute of Medicine.

Elliot, J., Vullermin, P., & Robinson, P. (1998). Maternal cigarette smoking is associated with increased inner airway wall thickness in children who die from sudden infant death syndrome. *American Journal of Respiratory Critical Care Medicine, 158*, 802-806.

Emergency Nurses Association (1995). Psychosocial aspects of trauma care. In *Trauma nursing core course provider manual* (3rd ed.). Chicago: Author.

Emergency Nurses Association. (1998a). *Emergency nursing pediatric course, provider manual*. Park Ridge, IL: Author.

Emergency Nurses Association. (1998b). *Position statement: Critical incident stress management*. Park Ridge, IL: Author.

Emergency Nurses Association (2001a). *Position statement: Family presence at the bedside during invasive procedures and/or resuscitation*. Park Ridge, IL: Author.

Emergency Nurses Association. (2001b). *Position statements: Violence in the emergency care setting*. Park Ridge, IL: Author.

Frader, J., & Sargent, J. (1993). Sudden death or catastrophic illness: Family considerations. In G. R. Fleisher & S. Ludwig (Eds.), *Textbook of pediatric emergency medicine*. Baltimore: Williams & Wilkins.

Guyer, B., Martin, J. A., MacDorman, M. F., Anderson, R. N., & Strobino, D. M. (1997). Annual summary of vital statistics—1996. *Pediatrics, 100*, 905-918.

Hamilton, G. (1988). Sudden death in the ED: Telling the living. *Annals of Emergency Medicine, 17*, 382.

Hanson, C., & Strawser, D. (1992) Family presence during cardiopulmonary resuscitation: Foote Hospital emergency department's nine-year perspective. *Journal of Emergency Nursing, 18*, 104.

Hoff, L. A. (1989). *People in crisis. Understanding and helping* (3rd ed.). Redwood City, CA: Addison-Wesley.

Kolhendorfer, U., Kiechl, S., & Sperl, W. (1998). Sudden infant death syndrome: Risk factor profiles for distinct subgroups. *American Journal of Epidemiology, 147*, 960-968.

Mitchell, J. T. (1983). When disaster strikes. The critical incident stress debriefing process. *Journal of the Emergency Medical Services*, January 1983, p. 36.

Molter, N. (1979). Needs of relatives of critically ill patients: A descriptive study. *Heart and Lung, 8*, 332-339.

Presley, D., & Robinson, G. (2002). Violence in the emergency department. *Nursing Clinics of North America, 37*(1), 161-169.

Rando, T. (1984). *Grief, dying, and death*. Champaign, IL: Research Press.

Rollins, J. (1993). Nurses as gangbusters: A response to gang violence in America. *Pediatric Nursing, 19*(16), 559-567.

Scott, C. L., Iyasu, S., Rowley, D., & Atrash, H. K. (1998). Postneonatal mortality surveillance—United States, 1980-1994. *Morbidity and Mortality Weekly Report CDC Surveillance Summary, 1998, 47*, 15-30.

Serwint, J. (1995). When a child dies. *Contemporary Pediatrics, 12*(3), 55-76.

Swisher, L., Nieman, L., Nilsen, G., & Spivey W. (1993). Death notification in the emergency department: A survey of residents and attending physicians. *Annals of Emergency Medicine, 22*, 102.

Thomas, D. (1998). Crisis intervention and death. In T. E. Soud & J. S. Rogers (Eds.), *Manual of pediatric emergency nursing* (pp. 178-192). St. Louis: Mosby.

Valdes-Dapena, M. A. (1991). The phenomenon of sudden infant death syndrome and its challenges. In C. A. Cork, H. Fuller, C. Barnickol, & D. M. Corr (Eds.), *Sudden infant death syndrome. Who can help and how*. New York: Springer.

Valk-Lawson, L. (1990). Culturally sensitive support for grieving parents. *Maternal Child Nursing, 15*, 76.

Walters, D., & Tupin, J. (1991). Family grief in the emergency department. *Emergency Medicine Clinics of North America, 9*, 189.

Williams, J. (2002). Family presence during resuscitation. To see or not to see? *Nursing Clinics of North America, 37*(1), 211-220.

Ziegler, M., & Gonzalez, Del Rey (2000). Major trauma. In G. R. Fleisher & S. Ludwig (Eds.), *Textbook of pediatric emergency medicine* (4th ed., pp. 1259-1269). Philadelphia: Lippincott, Williams & Wilkins.

Zylke, J. (1989). Sudden infant death syndrome: Resurgent research offers hope. *Journal of the American Medical Association, 262*, 1565.

SECTION 6

Trauma

29

Mechanisms of Injury

Kathy Haley, RN, BSN
Nancy L. Mecham, APRN, FNP

Introduction

Injury is defined as "any intentional or unintentional damage to the body resulting from acute exposure to thermal, mechanical, electrical, or chemical energy or from the absence of such essentials as heat or oxygen" (National Center for Injury Prevention and Control, 2002). The injury may be primary, which occurs immediately on the transfer of energy (e.g., contusion or fracture) or secondary, which occurs as a consequence of a primary injury (e.g., cerebral edema) (Emergency Nurses Association, 2000).

Injuries are the leading cause of childhood mortality and disability in the United States. In 1991, 37,529 children and adolescents died from injuries in the United States alone (Ray & Yuwiler, 1994). Nearly 22 million children are injured each year; approximately 600,000 children require hospitalization following an injury, and 80,000 sustain permanent lifelong disability (Gallagher, 1996; Horwitz & Andrassy, 1994). Allen (1997) reported the leading causes of injury-related death for children from 1986 through 1992:

- Motor vehicle-related crashes
- Firearms
- Drowning
- Fire or flame
- Suffocation or hanging
- Cutting or piercing

The costs associated with fatal pediatric injuries are estimated to be more than $3 billion (Ray & Yuwiler, 1994), and the costs of pediatric injury are estimated to be more than $413 billion (Allen, 1997).

Pediatric trauma care requires the integration of knowledge related to mechanisms of injury, initial resuscitation, treatment of specific injuries, and injury prevention. The purposes of this chapter are to describe the incidence of pediatric trauma and to discuss common mechanisms of kinetic force injury.

Mechanisms of Injury

Mechanism of injury refers to the method by which energy is transferred from the environment to the child. The term *cause* is often used interchangeably with the term *mechanism*. Energy sources are:

- Mechanical or kinetic.
- Thermal.
- Chemical.
- Electrical.
- Radiant.
- Lack of oxidation.
- Lack of thermoregulation.

Mechanisms of injury related to kinetic energy are discussed in this chapter. Mechanisms of injury related to thermal, electrical, and radiant energy sources are discussed in Chapter 39; mechanisms of injury related to chemical sources are presented in Chapters 44 and 45 and mechanisms of injury related to a lack of oxidation and a lack of thermoregulation are discussed in Chapters 37, 41, and 42, respectively.

Kinetic Energy Sources and Injuries

The transfer of kinetic energy to the body structures arises from several sources: from blunt (injury to internal organs), penetrating (disruption to skin and organ integrity), acceleration-deceleration (abrupt, forceful, forward-and-backward movement), and crushing (direct compression onto body structures).

Blunt Force Trauma

Blunt force trauma constitutes approximately 80% of childhood trauma. In blunt trauma, external evidence of injury may be minimal, and energy is often absorbed by underlying structures; therefore, a high index of suspicion for potential injuries is required.

Falls

Falls are the most common cause of injury requiring hospital admission. Jumping on beds, falling downstairs, falling from a height of three stories or less, and child abuse are common scenarios for childhood fall-related injuries (Mosenthal, Livingston, Elcavage, Merrit, & Stucer, 1995). Injuries sustained during falls result from blunt forces and most often involve the extremities, head, and abdomen. The orientation of the body at the time of impact correlates with the pattern of injuries:

- Feet-first impact leads to injury of the ankles and lower extremities as well as to the lumbosacral spine.
- Buttocks-first impact is associated with pelvic and vertebral injuries.
- Head-first impact results in brain, head, face, and cervical spine injuries from axial loading. Young children have a large head in proportion to the body, placing them at greater risk for the head-to-feet orientation on impact and thereby explaining the higher incidence of skull fractures and head injury associated with falls in children (Kottmeier, 1995).

Deaths have occurred in children who have fallen short distances; however, lethal injuries are extremely uncommon with short falls, and child abuse must be suspected and investigated when a serious injury is reportedly due to a fall of less than 4 feet (Chadwick, Chin, Salerno, Landswerk, & Kitcher, 1991). A fall from a height two and a half to three times the child's height is considered a significant mechanism of injury.

Motor Vehicle Crashes

Motor vehicle crashes are the leading cause of death among children and account for about 10% of all traffic-related fatalities (Pautler, Henning, & Buntain, 1995). In 1994, 673 children younger than 5 years of age died while riding in motor vehicles; of those, 362 were unrestrained, and many more were restrained incorrectly (National Highway Traffic Safety Administration, 1995). Vehicular ejection accounts for approximately 27% of all motor vehicle-associated deaths (Orsborn & Hammond, 1995).

The distribution of motor vehicle-related fatalities is relatively equal among males and females until they reach 14 years of age. Males 14 years of age and older are two to three times more likely than females to be victims of motor vehicle–related trauma (Ray & Yuwiler, 1994).

Analysis of the biomechanics of a motor vehicle crash demonstrates that four collisions occur (Table 29.1). Injuries may be predicted from the type of safety restraint used (Table 29.2). Therefore, the passenger seating arrangements and the use of child restraint devices are key to the prevention of occupant deaths in children younger than 5 years of age (Rivara & Grossman, 1996). Data indicate that about 70% of motor vehicle-related deaths could be prevented through the use of an appropriate restraining device (National Highway Traffic Safety Administration, 1995). Chapter 5 details car seat usage and safety.

Motor Vehicle–Pedestrian Crashes

Motor vehicle–pedestrian crashes are a lethal form of pediatric trauma. Although there are fewer children hit by cars than child passengers involved in crashes, pedestrians are much more likely to be seriously injured (Rivara, 1990).

More than 60% of the deaths and injuries occur when pedestrians cross or enter streets. Of these incidents, more than twice as many occur between intersections than at intersections (National Safety Council, 1996). Preschool children often are struck while playing around parked vehicles. Older children are more likely to dart across the street unexpectedly.

The biomechanics associated with pedestrian–motor vehicle crashes are related to the speed and size of the vehicle and the height of the child. Left-sided injuries are more common because of impact with cars approaching from the right side of the road (Templeton, 1993). On occasion, the history of the event may include the child who was knocked "out of the shoes"; this history has been associated with a motor vehicle traveling about 40 mph on direct impact with a child (Templeton, 1993).

The most frequent injuries occur to the head, chest, abdomen, and lower extremities. Depending on the height of the child, contact with the vehicle is first made at the bumper and then the hood of the car. The point of impact with these car parts is at the child's lower extremity and the chest and abdomen, respectively. The child is then thrown onto the hood or windshield and is now moving with the vehicle. The driver usually responds by braking, and the car stops; however, the

TABLE 29.1 The Four Collisions of Motor Vehicle Injury

Collision	*Description*	*Impact*	*Pediatric Considerations*
First	Vehicle strikes another moving vehicle or a stationary object.	The collision creates a sudden change in the vehicle's velocity and direction.	The unrestrained child becomes mobile; force is exerted on the fixation points of the restraint device or seat.
Second*	The occupant collides with the interior of the vehicle.	Energy change causes the occupants to continue their velocity, until they are stopped by the steering wheel, dashboard, or airbag.	An unrestrained child involved in a front-end crash at 30 miles per hour hits the dashboard with the same force as in a three-story fall. The child's large head becomes a moving missile.
Third*	Internal organs collide with unyielding body wall structures.	The lung, brain, liver, spleen, and descending aorta are particularly susceptible to injury during this phase.	The brain may strike the cranium; white matter shearing injuries may occur or the descending aorta may pull forward, separating from the ligamentum arteriosum (rare).
Fourth	Loose objects become mobile.	Toys, groceries, purses, passengers, or other objects become missiles, causing additional injuries.	A car seat that is not appropriate for the vehicle or a car seat and child that are not properly restrained may become projectiles (Pautler et al., 1995; Templeton, 1993).

*From: Pautler et al., 1995; Templeton, 1993. The second and third collisions are magnified when the child is ejected from the vehicle. In this case, death is 25 times more likely than it is when the passenger remains in the vehicle.

child slides and rolls, usually head first, to the street. A recent study showed that rarely is the child injured in all three regions; however, an understanding of the biomechanics identifies body regions that are more commonly injured (Haley, Hammond, Osborn, & Falcone, 1997).

Prevention strategies for pedestrian injuries are discussed in Chapter 5.

Bicycle Crashes

The Consumer Product Safety Commission's National Electronic Injury Surveillance System (NEISS) ranks the bicycle as the leading hazardous product in the United States (Mofensen & Greensher, 2001). Bicycle mishaps occur most frequently between 3 P.M. and 9 P.M. (Pautler et al., 1995). A comparison of injury circumstance, severity, and outcome among young children (younger than 5 years of age) and older children (5 to 14 years of age) who sustained bicycle-related injuries found that young children constitute a very small percentage of this group (5%), but both groups have similar injuries, severity, and outcome (Powell, Tanz, & DiScala, 1997).

Head injury is the most frequent cause of morbidity and mortality associated with bicycle crashes. Approximately 60% of bicycle-related deaths result from head injuries and about one-third of bicycle-related nonfatal injuries treated in the emergency department (ED) are head injuries (Li, Baker, Fowler, & DiScala, 1995). Other bicycle-related injuries include fractures, lacerations, abdominal injuries, such as those caused by handlebars, and contusions. A recent study showed that helmets reduce the risk of head injury by 88% and brain injury by 88%; unfortunately, compliance with helmet use is generally poor (Committee on Accident and Poison Prevention, 2001). Among 4,041 patients sustaining bicycle-related injuries, only 126 were reported to be wearing helmets (Powell et al., 1997).

Prevention of bicycle crash-related injuries is detailed in Chapter 5.

Skateboarding

Skateboarding activity has surged in popularity among the nation's youth, resulting in 25,000 visits to the ED each year. There are about 4.9 million skateboarders in the United States (National Safety Council, 1996). The Consumer Product Safety Commission data from 1991 reported that 95% of skateboarders were persons 25 years and younger; of those, 87% were males (Retsky, Jaffe, & Christoffel, 1991).

Skateboarding falls among older children more commonly result in extremity fractures. Serious head injury is possible and related to collision with a motor vehicle or falling while moving at higher speeds. The American

TABLE 29.2 Restraint Devices and Associated Injuries

Device	*Energy Description*	*Anatomical Difference*	*Potential Injuries*
Two-point or lap belt	The center of gravity is above the restraint, allowing the child to jackknife forward on impact.	The young child's center of gravity is high (near T11 to T12 in the infant).	Flexion-distraction injuries to the lumbar spine; small-bowel contusion and perforation; hollow viscus injuries; pancreatic fracture; and external contusions
Loose-fitting restraints	Precrash braking may throw an unrestrained child against the dashboard at or near the passenger air bag location. The inflating air bag and its plastic cover can violently impact the child at a force of 200 mph.	The child's head is lower and thus sustains most of the airbag's impact.	High cervical spine injury, including dislocations; massive tissue lacerations; facial lacerations; and arm fractures.
Three-point restraints	The child may "submarine" under the belt.	Because of the child's anatomy, lap belts, two-point and three-point restraints should not be used in children less than 4 years of age.	Hyperflexion and hyperextension of the cervical spine; can result in spinal cord injury.
Air bag*	Shoulder belt with shoulder restraints worn incorrectly under the arm can result in injury.	The restraint is improperly fitted or used because the child is too small for the restraint to work properly.	Passenger-side patients': possible liver injuries; driver-side patients: possible splenic rupture; disruption of neck vasculature or tracheal fracture.

*From: Pautler, et al., 1995; Templeton, 1993. Federal safety standards require that all new passenger cars and light trucks be equipped with both driver- and passenger-side air bags.

Academy of Pediatrics advises that children younger than 5 years of age not use skateboards (Committee on Injury and Poison Prevention, 1995). Young children have a higher center of gravity, their neuromuscular system is not well developed, their judgment is poor, and they are not sufficiently able to protect themselves from injury.

All children who use skateboards should wear protective clothing, including a helmet, knee pads, and elbow pads, and should skate in designated, safe areas (Chapter 5).

Infant Walker–Related Injuries

Infant walkers are a common cause of nonfatal injury to younger children. Approximately 3 million baby walkers are sold each year. Approximately 25,000 children between the ages of 5 and 15 months were treated in hospital EDs during 1993 for injuries associated with infant walkers. Parents generally believe that walkers keep their infants and young toddlers safe, but data to support this theory are nonexistent. Recent data suggest that walkers either do not stimulate walking or that they may actually impede crawling and delay walking by several weeks (Committee on Injury and Poison Prevention, 2001).

The American Academy of Pediatrics recommends prevention activities aimed at banning the sale and use of infant walkers (Committee on Injury and Poison Prevention, 2001). Safety strategies for families who choose to use infant walkers are outlined in Chapter 5.

Sledding Injuries

Sledding injuries are common during the winter months when icy conditions entice children to sled in potentially dangerous areas. In one series of 224 children admitted to Pennsylvania trauma centers for injuries sustained from sledding, the average age was 11 years (Bernardo, Gardner, & Rogers, 1998). The majority of injured sledders were males, and most of the sledders were injured from hitting a tree or other stationary object. Head injuries and extremity fractures were common. Children struck by motor vehicles had higher proportions of head injuries than did those who hit stationary objects or trees. Seven children died as a result of sledding injuries; all were school-aged children struck by moving vehicles who had low Glasgow coma scale scores on ED arrival.

Prevention of sledding injuries includes selecting a designated safe sledding area that is free of trees and obstacles and clear of moving vehicles; a sledding surface that is not icy; a limited number of other sledders in the designated area; and a sledding slope of less than 30 degrees (Rowe & Bota, 1994). The sled should be well maintained, and the sledder should dress warmly to prevent cold injuries. Sledding in the feet-first position may decrease the risk of head injury compared to sledding in a prone, head-first position (Mofenson & Greensher, 2001). However, lumbosacaral spine injuries should be suspected when sledding feet first.

Penetrating Forces

Penetrating trauma includes gunshot wounds, stabbing injuries, and injuries from objects, such as toys. The severity of injury is related to the child's age, the environment in which the injury occurred, the wounding agent, and the presence or absence of intent (Long & Philippart, 1995).

Firearm Injuries

Between 1988 and 1992, 1,489 firearm injuries were reported to the National Pediatric Trauma Registry (1995). Males were victims four times more often than females, and adolescents had the highest rate of firearm-related injuries. Home was the most frequent place children were wounded or killed. Deaths represented 11% of the cases.

Firearms associated with injuries are handguns, rifles, and shotguns. Important features of firearms are found in Table 29.3.

Penetrating firearm injuries in children usually are unintentional; they occur when the child is at home and is the innocent victim of his or her own playing with guns or is caught between feuding family members (Long & Philippart, 1995). In adolescents, however, firearm injuries occur out of the home and usually are intentional from gang- or drug-related causes or from suicide attempts, resulting in injuries similar to those found in adult trauma patients (Long & Philippart, 1995).

Stabbing and Other Penetrating Injuries

Stabbing injuries occur infrequently in the pediatric population. The severity of a stab wound depends on the body system involved, the length of the knife blade, and the angle of penetration (Creel, 1997). In adolescents, stab wounds usually are intentional.

Toys or other objects also serve as sources of penetrating trauma. Lawn darts, although no longer manufactured, were associated with penetrating brain injuries. Air guns, toy musical instruments, wrought iron fencing, and other innocuous items, such as pencils, can cause serious injury to the affected body areas. Children should be taught to avoid running with objects in their mouths and to avoid climbing iron fencing. Dangerous toys should be kept away from young children to prevent the occurrence of these penetrating injuries.

Acceleration-Deceleration Forces

Acceleration-deceleration forces cause bodily injury from excessive forces applied during the injury event. For example, in a motor vehicle crash, the child passenger is thrown forward and is stopped by the restraining device. The internal organs, however, may continue to move forward and then abruptly return to their normal position after sustaining damage (Table 29.2). Acceleration-deceleration forces occur not only during motor vehicle crashes but also during other injury episodes, such as shaken impact syndrome and sledding, farming, or other occupational injuries. Prevention of acceleration-deceleration injuries is similar to the prevention of blunt force trauma.

Crush Injuries

Crush injuries occur when direct pressure is applied to a body area. Animal bites, entrapment in farm equip-

TABLE 29.3 Description of Firearm-Associated Features

Feature	*Description*
Caliber	Internal diameter of the weapon barrel; corresponds to the weapon's ammunition.
Ammunition	Case, primer, powder, and slug.
Bullet	Comprises a solid lead alloy and a jacket (copper or steel), configured into a shape (rounded, flat, conical, or pointed) with a soft or hollow bullet nose. The larger the bullet, the more tissue resistance. Hollow-point and soft-nose bullets flatten out on impact and cause a larger area of damage. The tumbling of the bullet causes more tissue damage. The bullet's yaw, its vertical and horizontal oscillation, causes additional tissue damage.

From: Creel, 1997.

ment, lawnmower injuries, and compression under a motor vehicle or other heavy object are examples of situations that result in crushing injuries. Degloving injuries occur when the skin, fascia, and perhaps the muscle and bone are torn from the body, usually from shearing forces, such as being struck and run over by a motor vehicle.

Farm-Related Injuries

Comprehensive data are not available on the incidence of farm-related injury among children who live or work on farms; however, it is estimated that 300 deaths occur and 27,000 children are injured each year in farm-related activities (Children's Safety Network, 1996).

Farming is the only occupation in which, under specific conditions, children are permitted to operate complicated industrial-type equipment. Additional risk factors include long working hours, lack of developmental and intellectual maturity to operate machinery, and the general isolation associated with the occupation.

Injuries are often caused by tractor runover, entrapment in harvesting equipment, silo entanglements, and animal kicks. The severity of injury varies and includes traumatic asphyxia, major lacerations or amputations, and multisystemic injuries.

Prevention strategies for farm-related injuries include a "no extra seat, no rider" policy for tractor riding; using developmental guidelines for age-appropriate work tasks; and wearing appropriate clothing. Children should not be near moving gears and belts. In some communities, though, children are expected to be involved in the farm work. If children are included in the barnyard activity, certain considerations must be entertained. Children should wear cotton clothing to enable quick extrication from machinery and to spare the child from further injury. The number of hours a child assists in farm activity should be limited. The use of safety devices such as machine guards and the employment of safe animal handling should be enforced (Stuelan, Lee, Nordstrom, Layde, & Wittmans, 1996). Parents should be encouraged to create safe barriers on farms to prevent children from entering hazardous areas.

Lawnmower Injuries

Lawnmower injuries can be life threatening as well as limb threatening. School-aged children and adolescents who operate power mowers may slip under the blade and sustain amputation of the foot or toes. Young children who are held on an adult's lap while positioned on a riding mower can fall from the vehicle and be run over by the moving blade. Adults who operate riding mowers cannot see small children as they are backing up and can run over a child. In one series of 190 children admitted to Pennsylvanian trauma centers for injuries from lawnmowers, 48% of the children were 5 years of age or younger (Bernardo & Gardner, 1996). Although power mowers were most often implicated (69%), the more severe injuries were sustained by young children who were run over by or thrown from riding lawnmowers. The most common injuries were traumatic amputation of the toes, fracture of one or more phalanges of the foot, amputation of the fingers, and amputation of the foot.

Prevention of lawnmower injuries includes keeping young children indoors during mower operation, forbidding passengers on riding mowers, and the use of protective equipment for adolescents who operate lawnmowers. The American Academy of Pediatrics recommends that operators of riding mowers follow guidelines similar to those required for all-terrain vehicle operation, such as a minimum of 16 years of age and completion of an established training program (Committee on Accident and Poison Prevention, 2001b).

Conclusion

Knowledge of mechanisms of injury allows emergency nurses to have a high index of suspicion for the resultant injuries in the child who presents to the ED for treatment. Efforts to reduce and prevent trauma-related morbidity and mortality are within the purview of emergency nursing.

References

Allen, K. (1997). *Preventing childhood emergencies: A guide to developing effective injury prevention initiatives.* Washington, DC: Emergency Medical Services for Children, National Resource Center.

Bernardo, L., & Gardner, M. (1996). Lawn mower injuries to children in Pennsylvania, 1989 to 1993. *International Journal of Trauma Nursing, 2*, 36–41.

Bernardo, L., Gardner, M., & Rogers, K. (1998). Pediatric sledding injuries in Pennsylvania. *Journal of Trauma Nursing, 5*, 34–40.

Chadwick, D., Chin, S., Salerno, C., Landswerk, J., & Kitchen, L. (1991). Deaths from falls in children: How far is fatal? *Journal of Trauma, 31*, 1353–1355.

Children's Safety Network (1996, September). *Rural Injury Prevention Resource Center fact sheet: Childhood agriculture injury*. No-2F, MCHB. Newton, MA: Author.

Committee on Accident & Poison Prevention. (2001a). Bicycle Helmets. *Pediatrics, 108*(4), 103–1032.

Committee on Accident and Poison Prevention. (2001b). Lawn mower-related injuries in children. *Pediatrics, 107*(b), 1480–81.

Committee on Injury and Poison Prevention. (1995). Skateboard injuries. *Pediatrics, 95*(4), 611–612.

Committee on Injury and Poison Prevention. (2001). Injuries associated with infant walkers. *Pediatrics, 108*(3), 790–792.

Creel, J. (1997). Mechanisms of injuries due to motion. In J. Campbell (Ed.), *Basic trauma life support: Advanced prehospital care* (3rd ed., pp. 1-20). Englewood Cliffs, NJ: Prentice-Hall.

Emergency Nurses Association. (2000). *Trauma nursing core course provider manual.* B. Jacobs & S. Hoyt (Eds.), Park Ridge, IL: Author.

Gallagher, S. (1996). *Injuries in the school environment: A resource packet.* Children's Safety Network, National Injury and Violence Prevention Resource Center, Education Development Center. Newton, MA: Children's Safety Network.

Haley, K., Hammond, S., Orsborn, R., & Falcone, R. (1997). *Pediatric pedestrian versus motor vehicle patterns of injury: Debunking the "myth."* Unpublished abstract.

Horowitz. J. R., & Andrassy, R. (1994). Considerations unique to children. In E. Ford & R. Andrassy (Eds.), *Pediatric trauma: Initial assessment and management* (pp. 3-19). Philadelphia: Saunders.

Kottmeier, P. (1995). Falls from heights. In W. Buntain (Ed.), *Pediatric trauma* (pp. 450-454). Philadelphia: Saunders.

Li, G., Baker, S., Fowler, C., & DiScala, C. (1995). Factors related to the presence of head injury in bicycle-related pediatric trauma patients. *Journal of Trauma, 38,* 871-875.

Long, J. & Philippart, A. (1995). Penetrating injuries. In W. Buntain (Ed.), *Pediatric trauma* (pp. 581-593). Philadelphia: Saunders.

Mofensen, H., & Greensher, J. (2001). Accident prevention. In R. Hoekelman, S. Friedman, N. Nelson, H. Seidel, & M. Weitzman (Eds.), *Primary pediatric care* (4th ed., pp. 260-284). St. Louis: Mosby—Year Book.

Mosenthal, A., Livingston, D., Elcavage, J., Merritt, S., & Stucer, S. (1995). Falls: Epidemiology and strategies for prevention. *Journal of Trauma, 38,* 753-756.

National Center for Injury Prevention & Control, Centers for Disease Control & Prevention Web Site available at: http://www.cdc.gov. Accessed 2/6/02.

National Highway Traffic Safety Administration, National Center for Statistics and Analysis. (1995). *Traffic safety facts 1994. A compilation of motor vehicle crash data from the Fatal Accident Reporting System and General Estimates System.* Washington, DC: U.S. Department of Transportation.

National Pediatric Trauma Registry. (1995, February). *Firearm injuries. Rehabilitation and childhood trauma.* Fact sheet #7. Boston, MA: Author.

National Safety Council. (1996). *Accident facts, 1996 ed.* (p. 30). Itasca, IL: Author.

Orsborn, R., & Hammond, S. (1995). Common childhood injuries. In A. Dietrich & S. Shaner (Eds.), *Pediatric basic trauma life support* (pp. 9-15). Oakbrook Terrace, IL: Basic Trauma Life Support International.

Pautler, M., Henning, J., & Buntain, W. (1995). Mechanisms and biomechanics of traffic injuries. In W. Buntain (Ed.), *Management of pediatric trauma* (pp. 10-27). Philadelphia: Saunders.

Powell, E., Tanz, R., & DiScala, C. (1997). Bicycle-related injuries among preschool children. *Pediatrics, 30,* 260-265.

Ray, L., & Yuwiler, J. (1994). *Child and adolescent fatal injury databook.* San Diego, CA: Children's Safety Network.

Retsky, J., Jaffe, D., & Christoffel, K. (1991). Skateboarding injuries in children: The second wave. *American Journal of Diseases of Children, 145,* 188-192.

Rivara, F. (1990). Child pedestrian injuries in the United States. *American Journal of Diseases of Children, 144,* 692-696.

Rivara, F., & Grossman, D. (1996). Prevention of traumatic deaths to children in the United States: How far have we come and where do we need to go? *Pediatrics, 97,* 791-797.

Rowe, B., & Bota, G. (1994). Sledding deaths in Ontario. *Canadian Family Physician, 40,* 68-72.

Stuelan, D., Lee, B., Nordstrom, D., Layde, P., & Wittmans, L. (1996). A population-based case-control study of agricultural injuries in children. *Injury Prevention, 2,* 192-196.

Templeton, J. M. (1993). Mechanism of injury: Biomechanics. In M. Eichelberger (Ed.), *Pediatric trauma* (pp. 20-36). St. Louis: Mosby—Year Book.

30

Initial Trauma Assessment and Intervention

Kathy Haley, RN, BSN

Introduction

Pediatric trauma resuscitation requires the skill and expertise of a trauma team dedicated to the care of injured children. The team uses systematic, prioritized assessments: the primary assessment identifies life-threatening injuries to the airway, respiratory, circulatory, and neurologic systems, whereas the secondary assessment identifies injuries to the remaining body systems. The purpose of this chapter is to discuss the initial assessment and interventions for the multiply injured child. The trauma team performs the assessment and interventions simultaneously; however, they are discussed separately for clarification.

Pediatric Trauma-Related Considerations

Although adults' responses to injury are often obvious, children's responses to serious injury are usually subtle. Normal pediatric anatomy and physiology related to multiple traumas must be understood to detect abnormalities and implement resuscitation measures.

Airway and Cervical Spine

- The airway comprises soft tissues that are compliant and susceptible to edema when traumatized following an injury or during insertion of an oral or nasopharngeal airway, suctioning, or placement of an endotracheal tube. Even minimal airway edema and/or secretions result in disproportionately higher resistance to airflow.
- The tongue is relatively large in comparison to the oral cavity and can easily obstruct the airway of an unconscious child. The large tongue and hypertrophied tonsils of 3- to 5-year-old children make visualization of the vocal cords difficult (Ludwig & Loiselle, 1993).
- When the young child or infant is in a supine position, the mouth, pharynx, and trachea form a more acute angle; for this reason, the neutral or sniffing position provides ideal alignment for optimal airflow.
- The trachea is pliable and easily obstructed when the head and neck are hyperextended or hyperflexed. When the young child is supine during spinal immobilization or diagnostic procedures, the relatively large occiput can cause neck flexion and subsequent airway obstruction as the head is tilted forward.
- Children have short, fleshy necks, making inspection for jugular venous distention and tracheal deviation difficult. Rarely are the jugular veins and the trachea visible.
- The cervical spine assumes similarity to that of the adult when the child is about 8 years of age. Infants and small children have proportionally larger heads and underdeveloped neck musculature that make them particularly susceptible to flexion and extension injuries of the cervical spine.

Breathing (Respiratory)

- Infants and children usually breathe with minimal effort. Respiratory rates and primary muscles used for respiration vary with age. Until a child reaches the age of 7 to 8 years, the diaphragm and abdominal muscles are used to breathe; thus it is important to observe abdominal excursion in addition to chest movement in this age group.

- Children commonly cry before, during, and after injury. The crying child swallows air, resulting in gastric distention. The stomach distends and restricts diaphragm movement and respiratory excursion.
- The chest wall in younger children is cartilaginous. Rib fractures rarely are observed in young children and, when present, reflect a powerful force and transfer of energy. Significant injury to the lungs and mediastinum can occur even without rib fractures (Moulton, 2000). Flail segments are uncommon in children and are associated with parenchymal injury (Reynolds, 1995). Because of the rarity and the subtleties of rib fractures in children and the risk for associated injury to underlying structures, there may be no external marks and few initial signs or symptoms in children with heart and great-vessel injuries.
- Breath sounds are easily transmitted through the thin chest wall, despite the presence of a pneumothorax or tracheal malpositioning. Therefore, it is dangerous to rely solely on breath sounds to determine the adequacy of ventilation in injured children.
- Children and infants have higher oxygen consumption needs than adults, 6 to 8 ml/kg/min versus 3 to 4 ml/kg/min, respectively (Chameides & Hazinski, 1997), accounting for children's higher respiratory rates and early fatigue.
- Children have fewer alveoli, creating less respiratory reserve than adults. The appropriate tidal volume of 7 to 10 ml/kg should result in symmetric chest rise.

Circulation

- Children have much higher metabolic demands on the cardiovascular system, requiring more fluid per kilogram of body weight (Golladay, Donahoo, & Haller, 1979). Their higher oxygen requirement and metabolic needs require a higher cardiac output per kilogram of body weight (Chameides & Hazinski, 1997).
- The average circulating blood volume in children is about 80 ml/kg. Small volumes of external or internal hemorrhage may result in shock; thus, rapid stabilization of any ongoing sources of blood loss is vital to successful resuscitation.
- Children can compensate for blood losses in excess of 15 to 20% with tachycardia and vasoconstriction. When blood losses are greater than 15%, signs of circulatory failure (tachycardia, decrease in intensity of peripheral pulses, delayed capillary refill, and cool extremities) will be observed. Blood pressure will be normal until about 20 to 25% of blood volume is lost (Chameides & Hazinski, 1997). Hypotension is a late, ominous sign of shock. Signs of shock may initially be subtle and it may be difficult to discern whether the tachycardia is related to fear, pain, or shock.
- The initial response to hypovolemia is tachycardia. In early hemorrhage, tachycardia and tachypnea become more readily apparent, and the rise in diastolic blood pressure results in a narrowed pulse pressure. When compensatory mechanisms fail, tissue hypoxia and hypercapnia occur, leading to bradycardia and hypotension (Chameides & Hazinski, 1997).

Disability (Neurologic)

- The cranial cavity of children younger than 2 years of age is somewhat more elastic than that of an adult. Limited increases in intracranial mass are tolerated better by younger children than by adults because of open fontanelles and the ability to reopen unfused sutures.
- Children are more susceptible to head injury because the head of the child represents a relatively greater proportion of mass and body surface area. The head is usually first to crash into a stationary object.
- The incomplete myelinization of the brain in children younger than 2 years of age enhances the susceptibility of neural tissue to traumatic injury.

Exposure (Thermoregulation)

- Children lose body heat rapidly. Infants younger than 2 years of age have a decreased ability for mature thermoregulatory control. They have a greater body surface area-to-mass ratio than adults, leading to greater transfer of body heat to the environment.
- Other developmental factors that influence thermoregulatory balance in children include their lesser quantity of subcutaneous fat; their thin skin with increased permeability; and their delayed shivering and inefficient ability to generate heat.

Etiology

The mechanisms of pediatric injury are discussed in Chapter 29.

Focused History

Children may be unable or unwilling to provide a history of injury. Therefore, witnesses, such as family members, neighbors, prehospital medical personnel, and police personnel, should be queried.

Injury History

- Time of the incident:
  - Comparison of emergency department (ED) presentation time with time of injury (delays in seeking treatment may be an indicator of child maltreatment) (Chapter 46).
  - Time required for extrication and transport.
- Description of the injury:
  - Mechanism of injury (see Table 30.1).
- Patient's response to the injury:
  - Vomiting or choking episode.
  - Apnea or difficulty breathing.
  - Length of time the response occurred.
  - Estimated blood loss.
  - Loss of consciousness, the length of time the child was unconscious, the presence of amnesia, seizure, and the child's level of consciousness after the injury event (e.g., crying, awake).
  - Ambulation after the injury.
- Child's age and developmental capabilities in relation to the injury (Chapter 4):
  - Child's developmental ability to sustain the injury based on the reported history.
- Credibility of witnesses.
  - Changes in the injury history to match the injuries as they are identified should raise suspicion.

TABLE 30.1 Mechanism of Injury and Pertinent Historical Findings

Mechanism of Injury	*Historical Findings*
Blunt forces	*Point of impact:*
▪ Motor vehicle crash	Rollover; front; side; rear; T-bone.
	Use of restraints/car safety seat:
	Car or booster seat properly affixed to car; two-point or three-point restraints; airbag deployment.
	Occupant position in car:
	Front- or back-seat passenger; driver; pick-up truck passenger.
	Other vehicle information:
	Vehicle speed (if unknown, posted speed for area of crash); object of collision (stationary or moving; object or vehicle).
	Other occupant information:
	Scene fatalities; entrapment and extrication required; unusual noises, odors, or sights occupants may have endured.
▪ Bicycle crash	*Bicycle information:*
	Object of collision (stationary or moving; object or vehicle); runover; speed of vehicle (if unknown, posted speed for area of crash); vehicle damage (spidered windshield, indentations).
	Cyclist information:
	Location of cyclist on impact (distance thrown from bicycle); use of bicycle helmet; condition of helmet; condition of bicycle.
▪ Pedestrian-versus-motor vehicle crash	*Vehicle information:*
	Speed of vehicle; location of crash (intersection, midblock, road, driveway); vehicle damage (spidered windshield, indentations).
	Pedestrian information:
	Run over or pinned under vehicle; type of surface; witness account of point of impact; location of pedestrian on impact (distance thrown from vehicle).

(continued)

TABLE 30.1 Mechanism of Injury and Pertinent Historical Findings (continued)

Mechanism of Injury	*Historical Findings*
▪ Farm machinery	*Machinery information:*
	Type of surface (soil, road, gravel, fertilized area); runover; length of blade; machine use at time of injury; potential chemical exposure (pesticide, gasoline).
	Patient information:
	Duration of entrapment before rescue; body areas involved (hands versus legs).
▪ Falls	*Fall information:*
	Height of fall; location of fall (tree versus second-story window); type of landing surface (concrete versus mulch).
	Patient information:
	Body areas that first hit the ground.
Penetrating forces	
▪ Gunshot wound	*Penetrating object:*
	Type of firearm; caliber of bullets; number of shots fired.
	Patient information:
	Distance of child from shooter; number of wounds; location of wounds.
▪ Stab wound	*Penetrating object:*
	Type of object (such as wrought iron fence, fork, or javelin); type of knife and length of blade.
	Patient information:
	Number of wounds; location of wounds; object impaled in child.
Crushing forces	
	Crushing object:
	Animal (type of animal, domesticated versus wild; rabies status); machinery (type of machinery, entrapment).
	Patient information:
	Number of wounds; location of wounds; preservation of amputated body parts.

Initial Care Rendered

- Level of prehospital care received (bystander first aid; advanced trauma life support). This level of support is variable, relative to bystander preparedness, access to 911, level of emergency medical services system response, and time to emergency medical services arrival:
  - Airway support.
  - Breathing assistance.
  - Application of pressure dressings or splints.
  - Preservation of amputated body parts.
  - Performance of cardiopulmonary resuscitation. Injured children receiving CPR at the injury scene have a higher survival rate compared to injured children receiving CPR in the ED (Li, Tang, DiScala, Meisel, Levick, & Kelen, 1999).
- Child's response to the interventions:
  - Compare the injury circumstances, the prehospital interventions, and the child's current status.

Patient's Health History (AMPLE mnemonic)

- **A**llergies to medications or environmental agents, including latex.
- Current **M**edications (over-the-counter, prescribed, or illicit).
- **P**resence of chronic illness, immunization status, and presence of hearing or visual aids.
- Time of the **L**ast meal; consumption of food or alcohol.
- **E**vents surrounding the injury, as described above.

Family History

- Involvement of other family members in the injury episode.
- Previous involvement in injuries (e.g., child maltreatment).

Focused Assessment

Physical Assessment

1. Assess the airway and cervical spine.
   - Inspect the airway for:
     - Patency.
     - The presence of foreign bodies (chewing gum, loose teeth, vomitus, secretions, and blood). Perform the jaw thrust maneuver and suction the oropharynx while maintaining the cervical spine in neutral alignment. Prevent flexion of the cervical spine to avoid airway compromise from an existing spinal cord injury. Prepare for endotracheal intubation if the child is unable to maintain a spontaneous airway.
     - Listen for the child's ability to speak or make age-appropriate sounds. Ask an age-appropriate question, such as What is your name? An appropriate verbal response indicates the level of consciousness, airway, and ventilation.
     - Note the smell of the breath (alcohol, marijuana, or fruity odor).
   - Inspect the anterior neck for:
     - Jugular vein distention.
     - Tracheal deviation. Inspect for these abnormalities prior to cervical collar placement; if the collar is in place, open the collar, inspect the neck, and close the collar. A trauma team member should be assigned to maintain the child's head and neck in a neutral position.
   - Maintain cervical and spinal alignment:
     - Apply a correctly sized and fitted cervical collar to prevent flexion and extension of the cervical spine.
     - Apply towel rolls or commercially available age- and size-appropriate blocks to prevent lateral head movement.
     - Apply a commercially available spinal immobilization board to prevent spinal movement. Limit the duration of spinal immobilization to 30 minutes or less.
2. Assess the respiratory system (breathing).
   - Observe the chest for:
     - Deformity.
     - Surface trauma.
     - Penetrating wounds.
     - Spontaneous chest rise and fall.
     - Presence or absence of expired air.
     - Quality and equality of chest expansion.
     - Use of accessory muscles.
     - Signs of respiratory distress.
   - Auscultate the chest high in the axillae and anterior chest for:
     - Presence of breath sounds.
     - Respiratory rate.
   - Palpate the rib cage for:
     - Tenderness.
     - Crepitus.
     - Flail segments.
   - Palpate the sternum for:
     - Tenderness.
     - Deformity.
   - Administer supplemental oxygen by a nonrebreather mask (100% oxygen).
   - Provide assisted or complete ventilation.
3. Assess the cardiovascular system.
   - Inspect quickly for areas of open hemorrhage or amputation:
     - Control open hemorrhage with pressure dressings.
   - Auscultate heart sounds for:
     - Rate. Initiate chest compressions if the pulse is absent or if pulseless electrical activity is present (Chapter 15).
     - Rhythm.
     - Quality. Observe for Beck's triad (muffled heart tones, distended neck veins, and general signs of shock), which may indicate cardiac tamponade.
   - Palpate central and peripheral pulses for:
     - Presence.
     - Quality.
     - Equality.
   - Assess the adequacy of peripheral circulation:
     - Palpate a radial or brachial pulse.
     - Assess skin color and temperature.
     - Measure capillary refill.
   - Establish one or two intravenous lines based on assessment findings.
4. Assess the neurologic system (disability).

- Assess the level of consciousness with the **A**lert, Unresponsive-to-**V**erbal-Stimulus, Responds -to-**P**ainful-stimulus, **U**nresponsive (AVPU) mnemonic:
  - Responsiveness may be difficult to evaluate in the nonverbal child.
  - Observe for alterations in developmentally expected behaviors, such as inability to focus and follow objects in a 6-month-old infant
- Assess the pupils for:
  - Size.
  - Shape.
  - Reactivity to light.
  - Accommodation.

5. Expose the patient to continue the assessment.
   - Remove, rather than cut, remaining clothes to further identify other potential injuries:
     - Scissors and the cutting of clothes can be frightening to the child and especially distressing to adolescents who may have invested valuable allowance in their prized clothing.
     - Cutting of clothing may damage or destroy physical evidence in cases of child maltreatment, homicide, or other acts of violence.
   - Initiate warming measures to prevent radiant heat loss:
     - Warm the ambient air by increasing the room temperature.
     - Apply overhead warming lights.
     - Apply warmed blankets to prevent convective heat loss, provide comfort, and assure modesty.
6. Involve the family.
   - Assign a member of the resuscitation team to provide emotional support to the parents.
   - Facilitate the process for the parent or child to be together during the initial resuscitation (Emergency Nurses Association, 1996).
7. Obtain or measure vital signs (heart rate, blood pressure, respiratory rate, temperature, estimated weight in kilograms).
   - Monitor vital signs for trends and changes.
8. Obtain a head-to-toe assessment:
   - Palpate the head for:
     - Depressions.
     - Step-off defects.
     - Pain.
     - Hematomas.
     - The condition of the anterior and posterior fontanelles in children younger than 2 years of age. A tense, raised fontanelle in the calm or comatose young child may indicate increased intracranial pressure.
   - Inspect the head for:
     - Lacerations.
     - Abrasions.
     - Puncture wounds.
     - Foreign bodies, such as glass and metal.
   - Assess the neurologic system:
     - Assign a Glasgow coma scale (GCS) score or Pediatric Glasgow coma scale score. Changes of two points in the GCS score are significant clues of hypovolemia, hypoxia, or increased intracranial pressure. Sudden changes in GCS score may demand immediate interventions.
   - Inspect the face and oral cavity for:
     - Deformity. Midfacial fractures, which are described using the Le Fort classification system, occur less commonly in children younger than 12 years of age (Beals, 1994) (Chapter 33).
     - Lacerations.
     - Symmetry. Ask the child to smile and grimace and open and close the mouth; note any deviations. Irregular mouth and tooth positioning or inability to close the mouth may be indicative of a fractured mandible.
     - Impaled objects.
     - Raccoon's eyes.
   - Palpate the forehead, orbits, maxilla, and mandible for:
     - Tenderness.
     - Pain.
     - Step-off deformities.
     - Crepitus.
     - Stability.
   - Inspect the oral cavity for:
     - Lacerations.
     - Loose, chipped, or missing teeth. In children, missing teeth may be a normal finding unrelated to the trauma. Parents can usually give a reliable dental history.
     - Orthodontia apparatus. Observe for damage, including loose or penetrating wires.
   - Inspect the pupils of the eyes for:
     - Size. An irregular pupil or blood in the anterior chamber (hyphema) should be reported immediately.
     - Equality. Unequal pupils may be indicative of increased intracranial pressure on the cranial

nerves and may be an early indication of brain stem herniation.

- Reaction to light. Nonreactive or sluggish pupils may be associated with head injury, drug or alcohol intoxication, or other pathology.

- Inspect the eyes for:
  - Extraocular movements. Entrapment of ocular muscles from a blowout fracture may inhibit upward eye movement. "Sundowning" may indicate increased intracranial pressure.
  - Visual acuity. Request the younger child to point to a familiar object. Ask the older child about the quality of vision.
  - Scleral deformity and hemorrhages. Scleral hemorrhages may indicate compression injury, such as traumatic asphyxia.
  - Remove the child's contact lenses, if present.
  - Secure penetrating objects and lightly patch both eyes, avoiding direct pressure on the eyes.
- Assess the ears:
  - Inspect the external canal for otorrhea, which may be cerebrospinal fluid; hematotympanum.
  - Inspect the tympanic membrane for hematotympanum.
  - Inspect the mastoid process for ecchymosis (Battle's sign). Although usually not evident until several hours after an injury, Battle's sign usually indicates a basilar skull fracture.
- Inspect the nose for:
  - Deformity.
  - Septal deviation or septal hematoma.
  - Rhinorrhea. Clear rhinorrhea may indicate a cerebrospinal fluid leak.
- Assess the neck:
  - Open the cervical collar, always maintaining neutral positioning and alignment; secure the cervical collar once the neck is assessed.
- Inspect the anterior neck for:
  - Edema.
  - Lacerations.
  - Abrasions.
  - Avulsions.
  - Puncture wounds.
  - Jugular vein distention.
- Palpate the anterior neck for:
  - Pain.
  - Subcutaneous emphysema or crepitus (indicates disruption of the trachea or bronchial tree).
  - Tracheal deviation. Normal tracheal position is midline. In the young child with a thick, short neck, tracheal deviation is assessed at the sternal notch. If the trachea is deviated, it is a sign of potential life-threatening injury or complication (tension pneumothorax) and should be reported immediately.
- Palpate the cervical spine (posterior neck) for:
  - Tenderness. Children with cervical spine injury commonly complain of tenderness when the cervical vertebrae are palpated. Remind the verbal child to answer "yes" about tenderness rather than to nod or shake the head for confirmation. For the nonverbal child, palpate while using distraction methods; observe for facial grimace or crying.
  - Pain.
  - Malaligned vertebrae. Maintain cervical spine stabilization by using a rigid spinal immobilization board with additional devices to prevent head-spine movement. Successful cervical immobilization includes restriction of lateral, flexion, and extension movements of the head and cervical spine and restraint of the head, shoulders, hips, and legs. The efficacy of common immobilization techniques was examined, and it was found that no single immobilization device or technique is ideal in consistently protecting the cervical spine from angulation (Curan, Dietrich, Bowman, Ginn-Pease, & King, 1995).
- Assess the child's voice for:
  - Quality.
  - Phonation. A hoarse, muffled voice may indicate laryngeal injury; anticipate potential airway compromise.
- Inspect the chest for:
  - Abrasions. Linear ecchymosis may indicate seat belt and shoulder belt injury.
  - Lacerations.
  - Symmetry during inspiration and expiration.
  - Open wounds.
  - Scars.
  - Paradoxic movements during inspiration and expiration.
  - Use of accessory muscles.
- Auscultate the entire chest for:
  - Equality, quality, and characteristics of breath sounds.
  - Respiratory rate, depth, pattern, and effort.
- Palpate the anterior rib cage and clavicles for:
  - Tenderness.
  - Crepitus.

- Deformity. Children are particularly ticklish in these areas, so anticipate and prepare for additional movement.

■ Percuss the chest for:
- Tympany.
- Resonancy.

■ Auscultate heart sounds for:
- Rate.
- Rhythm.
- Quality.

■ Inspect the abdomen for:
- Surface trauma (lacerations, abrasions, ecchymoses, and contusions).
- Impaled objects.
- Exposed abdominal contents.
- Scars.
- Distention.

■ Auscultate the abdomen for the presence of bowel sounds:
- Suspect a paralytic ileus in the absence of bowel sounds.

■ Palpate the abdomen gently in all four quadrants for:
- Tenderness.
- Rigidity.

■ Palpate the lower abdomen gently for:
- Bladder distention.
- Tenderness. Ask the verbal child to point with one finger to the painful area to localize symptoms.

■ Inspect the pelvis for:
- Surface trauma (contusions, lacerations, and abrasions).

■ Palpate the pelvis for:
- Stability.
- Tenderness. Any pain or displacement on palpation is indicative of a pelvic fracture.

■ Inspect the external genitalia, urinary meatus, perineum, and rectum for:
- Surface trauma (contusions, lacerations, and abrasions).
- Bleeding. Blood at the urinary meatus may signify a urethral injury; therefore, an indwelling bladder catheter is not inserted.
- Bruising.
- Foreign objects.
- Priapism, indicating spinal cord injury.

■ Assist with testing of rectal sphincter tone (usually completed by the trauma surgeon) by preparing the child for the examination.

■ Inspect the musculoskeletal extremities for:
- Surface trauma (abrasions and contusions).
- Deformities.
- Edema.
- Open wounds.
- Bleeding.
- Impaled objects.

■ Assess the neurovascular status:
- Skin temperature.
- Color.
- Capillary refill.
- Equality and amplitude of peripheral pulses compared to central pulses.
- Sensation. Ask the verbal child to describe if the toes and fingers are being touched. Observe the nonverbal child for withdrawal on touch to the toes and fingers to validate neuromotor integrity.

■ Assess neuromotor integrity and strength.
- Ask the verbal child to wiggle the fingers and toes.
- Perform hand grips and foot flexion and extension with the verbal child.

9. Inspect the back.

■ Cautiously logroll the child to the side as a single unit.
- One member of the trauma team should be assigned to maintain neutral cervical immobilization.
- Assess motor and neurovascular status before and after the back inspection.

■ Inspect the posterior surface of the body for:
- Deformity.
- Surface trauma (abrasions, lacerations, contusions, and ecchymoses). Bruising in the flank area may indicate renal trauma.
- Impaled objects.
- Open wounds.
- Entrance or exit wounds.

■ Palpate each vertebra for:
- Stability.
- Tenderness.

■ Palpate the entire surface of the back for:

- Deformity.
- Tenderness.
- Inspect the posterior aspect of each extremity for:
  - Surface trauma (abrasions, lacerations, contusions, and ecchymoses).
  - Impaled objects.

Table 30.2 lists nursing diagnoses and expected outcomes.

Psychosocial Assessment

- Assess the child's and family's coping strategies.
- Assess the child's and family's understanding of the injury and its treatment.

Triage Decisions

The injured child may be triaged several times and by several different methods, guidelines, or scoring tools immediately following the injury. Fundamental to trauma care is a triage process to ensure that the right patient goes to the right place at the right time. Matching trauma resources with patient need is essential and potentially lifesaving.

Optimal triage for appropriate pediatric trauma care requires established guidelines, which vary among hospitals, regions, and states. Established triage guidelines are required for:

- Prehospital transport decisions (Chapter 10).

TABLE 30.2 Nursing Diagnoses and Expected Outcomes

Nursing Diagnoses	*Expected Outcomes*
Ineffective airway clearance related to: ■ Edema of the airway, vocal cords, epiglottis, and upper airway. ■ Laryngeal spasm. ■ Altered level of consciousness, secondary to hypoxia. ■ Inability to remove oropharyngeal secretions. ■ Fatigue. ■ Pain.	The child will maintain a patent airway, as evidenced by: ■ Regular rate, depth, and pattern of breathing. ■ Bilateral chest expansion. ■ Effective cough/gag reflex. ■ Absence of signs and symptoms of airway obstruction. ■ Normal amount of clear sputum without abnormal odor. ■ Absence of signs and symptoms of retained secretions.
Ineffective breathing pattern, related to: ■ Pain. ■ Injury.	The child will have an effective breathing pattern, as evidenced by: ■ Regular rate, depth, and pattern of breathing. ■ Clear and equal bilateral breath sounds. ■ Symmetric chest wall expansion. ■ Arterial blood gas values within normal limits.
Fluid volume deficit, related to: ■ Hemorrhage. ■ Alteration in capillary permeability.	The child will have an effective circulating volume, as evidenced by: ■ Stable vital signs appropriate for developmental age. ■ Urinary output 1 to 2 ml/kg/hr. ■ Urine specific gravity within normal limits. ■ Strong, equal peripheral pulses. ■ Improved level of consciousness. ■ Pink, warm, and dry skin and pink and moist mucous membranes. ■ A hematocrit of 30 ml/dl. ■ Controlled external hemorrhage.
Hypothermia, related to: ■ Rapid infusion of intravenous fluids. ■ Decreased tissue perfusion. ■ Exposure.	The child will maintain a normal core body temperature, as evidenced by: ■ Core temperature measurement of 36.0°C to 37.5°C (96.8°F to 99.5°F). ■ Absence of shivering, cool skin, and pallor. ■ Pink, warm, and dry skin.

- Interfacility transfer (Chapter 10).
- Trauma team activation.
- ED triage.
- Disaster management (Chapter 1).

Trauma scoring is an objective method for determining injury severity. Based on the trauma score and according to established guidelines, the injured child may be admitted to a trauma center. The two most common trauma scores used in pediatrics are the Revised Trauma Score (RTS) and the Pediatric Trauma Score (PTS). Both the RTS and PTS should be obtained at the scene and on arrival at the ED:

- The RTS is an adult score that can be used in children. It comprises the respiratory rate, systolic blood pressure, and GCS score.
- The PTS is exclusive to pediatrics.
  - It combines physiologic and anatomic measures to assess the severity of injury (airway, systolic blood pressure, central nervous system status, skeletal fractures, and cutaneous injuries).
  - The PTS values range from −6 to 12; injured children with a PTS of 8 or less should be transferred to a Level I trauma center (Eichelberger, Gotschall, Sacco, Bowman, Mangubat, & Lowenstein, 1989).

Emergent

- Life-threatening injuries
- Cardiopulmonary resuscitation in progress

Urgent

- Potential for shock if not treated immediately

Nonurgent

- Minor injuries without signs and symptoms of shock

Nursing Interventions

1. Assess and maintain airway and cervical spine stabilization.
   - Open and maintain the airway while the cervical spine is manually immobilized in a neutral position:
     - Ask the conscious child to open the mouth.
     - Open the unconscious child's mouth with the jaw thrust maneuver while maintaining cervical spine stabilization.
     - Place a small pad under the upper back and shoulders of the younger child to balance the flexion created by the child's large occiput.
     - Avoid neck traction or movement of the neck, because spinal cord injury may occur.
   - Suction the mouth and upper airway with a large, rigid tonsilar suction in the presence of debris, blood, or secretions.
     - Avoid deep oral suctioning, because stimulation of the posterior pharynx, larynx, or trachea may cause vagal stimulation with resultant bradycardia.
   - Insert an airway adjunct in conjunction with the jaw thrust maneuver in the unconscious child who is unable to maintain a patent airway.
     - Insert an oropharyngeal airway.
     - Insert a nasopharyngeal airway in the absence of head injury. A nasopharyngeal airway is better tolerated in the conscious patient but generally is not used in the pediatric trauma patient when a basilar or cribiform plate fracture is suspected because of the risk of entry in the cranial vault.
   - Prepare for oral endotracheal intubation while maintaining cervical spine stabilization. The nasotracheal route is contraindicated because:
     - It is difficult to insert an endotracheal tube blindly through the pediatric vocal cords.
     - It is associated with adenoid tissue trauma.
     - There is a risk of insertion into the cranial vault through a cribiform fracture.
   - Endotrachael intubation is indicated in the pediatric trauma patient when (Chameides & Hazinski, 1997):
     - A functional or anatomic airway obstruction is present.
     - The GCS or modified GCS score is 8 or less.
     - There is a need for prolonged ventilatory support.
     - Respiratory arrest occurs.
     - Respiratory failure results from hypoventilation.
     - Hypoxemia occurs despite administration of supplemental oxygen.
   - Prepare for rapid-sequence induction; when indicated, it is a useful adjunct for the skilled, trained clinician.
   - Insert an orogastric tube or a nasogastric tube (in the absence of basilar skull fracture) to prevent gastric distention and restricted ventilation.
   - Prepare for needle cricothyrotomy or tracheostomy for children in whom airway control is not possible because of craniofacial injuries.
   - Maintain cervical and spinal stabilization until evaluation of the cervical spine is completed.
     - Recent data suggest that children immobilized on flat backboards are not in the recommended

neutral position but rather in a position of dangerous flexion (Treloar & Nypaver, 1997).

- Because of the young child's large head-to-torso ratio, either elevation of the back from a commercially available pediatric spinal immobilization board or placement of a towel under the shoulders will enhance the optimal head and neck position for cervical neutrality.
- Maintain immobilization of the infant or child arriving restrained in an infant car seat. Carefully remove the infant or child, maintaining spinal alignment. Infants and children can be transported in their car seats if they are in no distress and their car seats are not damaged (Dietrich & Shaner, 1995).
- Maintain complete spinal immobilization. Commercially available rigid cervical collars (available in sizes to fit children 6 months of age and older) are used to prevent cervical flexion and extension. Proper fit is achieved by following the manufacturer's directions; the chin should rest securely in the chin holder, the ears should not be covered by the collar, and the bottom of the collar rests on the upper sternum (Bernardo & Waggoner, 1992).
- Towel rolls or commercially available immobilization devices are used to prevent lateral cervical movement.
- Commercially available immobilization devices for pediatrics provide complete spinal immobilization in young children; long backboards or short backboards also can be used to complete the immobilization process.

- Obtain radiographs of the cervical spine with lateral, odontoid, and anterior-posterior views:
  - Obtain lateral radiographs to assess for gross malalignment or distraction; C1 through C7 should be included, as well as the C7-T1 junction.
  - Obtain anterior-posterior and lateral views of the thoracic and lumbar spine, as indicated.
  - Obtain flexion and extension radiographs to determine the stability of the bony canal, as indicated, *only when spinal cord integrity and absence of injury are confirmed.*

2. Initiate measures to assess and maintain breathing.
   - Administer supplemental 100% oxygen through a nonrebreather mask to the patient who has a patent airway and effective respiratory effort (adequate bilateral, symmetric chest rise and air entry without central cyanosis).
   - Obtain and monitor oxygen saturation measurements to determine the adequacy of oxygenation (95%). Detect percent of oxygen saturation in the blood and then trend to assess breathing effectiveness.
   - Initiate artificial ventilation with a bag-valve-mask and 100% supplemental oxygen in the presence of apnea or ineffective respiratory effort. Maintain oxygen saturation levels at better than 95%.
   - Prepare for endotracheal intubation in the patient whose respiratory effectiveness has not improved with administration of supplemental oxygen.
   - Prepare for mechanical ventilation when a prolonged need for control of airway and breathing is anticipated.
   - Prepare for thoracostomy and chest tube insertion in the presence of hemothorax, pneumothorax, or hemopneumothorax.
3. Initiate measures to maintain circulation.
   - Ensure universal blood and bodily fluid precautions.
   - Perform continuous cardiorespiratory, oxygen saturation, and blood pressure monitoring.
   - Apply direct pressure to control external hemorrhage.
   - Obtain vascular access with one or two short, large-bore intravenous catheters, preferably in the upper extremities, in the child with suspected moderate to major trauma:
     - Prepare for intraosseous infusion if vascular access is not obtained in the unconscious child within three attempts or 90 seconds.
     - Prepare for central venous access or venous cutdown by an experienced clinician if intravenous and intraosseous attempts are unsuccessful.
     - Obtain blood specimens for laboratory analysis. Individualize the tests to match patient assessment:
       - Hemoglobin, hematocrit, and platelet count.
       - Blood urea nitrogen and creatinine.
       - Amylase, lipase, serum glutamic oxaloacetic transaminase, and serum glutamic pyruvic transaminase (for patients with suspected abdominal trauma).
       - Type and crossmatch or type and screen (if blood will be administered or operative procedure is probable).
       - Toxicology screening (if suspected).
       - Pregnancy testing (postmenarchal females).
     - Administer lactated Ringer's solution, the recommended isotonic crystalloid solution for fluid resuscitation in the injured child. Normal saline is the alternative. Warm the fluid if large volumes will be delivered.

- Provide rapid volume replacement in the child with signs of compensated or uncompensated shock:
    - Administer a bolus of 20 ml/kg of lactated Ringer's solution. Reassess the child for signs of improvement (heart rate, mentation, capillary refill, and blood pressure).
    - Administer a second bolus if symptoms of shock persist. Reassess the child for signs of improvement.
    - Consider administration of a bolus of warmed O-negative packed red blood cells (10 ml/kg). Blood transfusion is a lifesaving measure in the presence of significant blood loss. Results of compatibility studies for blood should not delay transfusion of blood. Rapidly administered O-negative packed red blood cells will suffice until type-specific blood is available (Chameides & Hazinski, 1997).
- Begin cardiopulmonary resuscitation in the child whose pulse is absent or inadequate:
    - Thoracotomy and open cardiac massage are rarely indicated in the pediatric victim of blunt trauma arrest; prognosis is poor (Clemence, 2000).
- Consider use of pneumatic antishock garments, recognizing that they have limited usefulness in the treatment of traumatic shock (Chameides & Hazinski, 1997):
    - These garments can be used to splint lower extremity fractures and unstable pelvic fractures.
    - The abdominal compartment may impair respiratory effort and is never inflated for children.
- Control external hemorrhage with pressure dressings.
- Insert an indwelling urinary bladder catheter in the absence of genitourinary trauma:
    - Measure urinary output.
    - Perform a urinalysis.

4. Assess and maintain neurologic functioning.
    - Perform ongoing neurologic assessments to identify signs of increasing intracranial pressure in head-injured children:
        - Changes in level of consciousness.
        - Vomiting and irritability.
        - Disorientation.
    - Maintain the $PaCO_2$ at approximately 30 to 35 mm Hg in the severely head-injured child.
    - Continue to administer intravenous fluids in the head-injured child with signs of hypovolemic shock:
        - Prepare for the administration of osmotic agents to decrease intracranial pressure if the blood pressure is adequate.
5. Promote thermoregulation.
    - Obtain ongoing core temperature measurements (aural, rectal, or bladder).
    - Initiate passive warming measures:
        - Apply warming blankets.
        - Increase ambient room temperature.
        - Apply overhead heating lights.
    - Initiate active warming measures:
        - Administer warmed intravenous fluid.
6. Provide ongoing psychosocial support to the injured child and family (Chapter 4).
    - Have the family accompany the child to other hospital areas, such as the computerized tomography scan or radiology department. Even a few moments together provides much needed reassurance to the child and family.
    - Prepare the child and family for transfer to a trauma center, as needed (Chapter 10).
7. Perform additional interventions as needed.
    - Prepare to splint or cast deformed and fractured extremities:
        - Monitor motor and neurovascular status before and after splinting and casting.
    - Prepare for suturing and wound care.
    - Begin treatment of the amputated wound and part:
        - Amputations are either *partial* (limb or digit attached) or *complete* (limb or digit removed). Complete amputations are either the guillotine type (clean, well-defined edges that enhance reattachment) or the crush-avulsion type (irregular separation with additional soft tissue, bone, nerve, and vascular trauma that may contraindicate reattachment). The amputated part is wrapped in sterile gauze moistened with normal saline solution, placed in a labeled container, and then placed in an ice water bath. Amputated parts can be reimplanted up to 24 hours postinjury.
        - Assess the stump for neurovascular integrity and bleeding. The parent and child may not want to view the wound; however, if the child and family do want to view the wound, emotional support should be provided.
    - Prepare for peritoneal lavage.
    - Prepare for diagnostic testing:
        - Radiographs.

- Computerized tomography scan.
- Other tests (angiography, xenon studies).

8. Administer medications, as prescribed.
   - Tetanus immunization.
   - Antibiotics.
   - Analgesics (Chapter 13).
9. Initiate consultations with other health care professionals.
   - Social services.
   - Chaplain services.
   - Child life specialists.
   - Medical subspecialists.
10. Prepare for transfer and transport to a trauma center (Chapter 10) or hospital admission.
11. Initiate support measures for the family whose child dies in the ED (Chapter 28).
12. Arrange for staff debriefing following a pediatric trauma resuscitation, as needed (Chapter 28).

Conclusion

Timely assessment of and interventions for the injured child may mean the difference between a functional or devastating outcome. Emergency nurses must be prepared to care for multiply injured children and their families. Participation in ongoing educational activities, such as mock trauma codes, may help to sharpen assessment and intervention skills.

References

Beals, D. (1994). Head and neck trauma. In E. Ford & R. Andressy (Eds.), *Pediatric trauma* (pp. 310-335). Philadelphia: Saunders.

Bernardo, L., & Waggoner, T. (1992). Pediatric trauma. In S. Sheehy (Ed.), *Emergency nursing: Principles and practice* (3rd ed. pp. 683-690). St. Louis: Mosby—Year Book.

Chameides, L., & Hazinski, M. (1997). *Textbook of pediatric advanced life support.* Dallas, TX: American Heart Association, American Academy of Pediatrics.

Clemence, B. (2000). Emergency department thoracotomy: Nursing implications for pediatric cases. *International Journal of Trauma Nursing*, *6*, 123-127.

Curan, C., Dietrich, A., Bowman, M., Ginn-Pease, M., & King, D. (1995). Pediatric cervical-spine immobilization: Achieving neutral position? *Journal of Trauma*, *39*, 729-732.

Dietrich, A. & Shaner, S. (1995). *Pediatric basic trauma life support.* Oakbrook Terrace, IL: Basic Trauma Life Support International, Inc.

Eichelberger, M., Gotschall, C., Sacco, W, Bowman, L., Mangubat, E., & Lowenstein, A. (1989). A comparison of the Trauma Score, the Revised Trauma Score, and the Pediatric Trauma Score. *Annals of Emergency Medicine*, *18*, 939-942.

Emergency Nurses Association. (1996). Presenting the option for family presence. Park Ridge, IL: Author.

Golladay, E., Donahoo, J., & Haller, J. (1979). Special problems of cardiac injuries in infants and children. *Journal of Trauma*, *19*, 526-531.

Li, G., Tang, N., DiScala, C., Meisel, Z., Levick, N., & Kelen, G. (1999). Cardiopulmonary resuscitation in pediatric trauma patients: Survival and functional outcome. *Journal of Trauma*, *47*(13), 1-7.

Ludwig, S., & Loiselle, J. (1993). Anatomy, growth and development: Impact on injury. In M. Eichelberger (Ed.), *Pediatric trauma* (pp. 39-58). St. Louis: Mosby—Year Book.

Moulton, S. (2000). Early management of the child with multiple injuries. *Clinical Orthopaedics and Related Research*, *376*, 6-14.

Nakayama, D. (1991). *Pediatric surgery: A color atlas.* Philadelphia: Lippincott.

Reynolds, M. (1995). Pulmonary, esophageal and diaphragmatic injuries. In W. Buntain (Ed.), *Management of pediatric trauma* (pp. 238-247). Philadelphia: Saunders.

Soud, T., Pieper, P., & Hazinski, M. (1992). Pediatric trauma. In M. Hazinski (Ed.), *Nursing care of the critically ill child* (2nd ed., pp. 829-873). St. Louis: Mosby.

Treloar, D., & Nypaver, M. (1997). Angulation of the pediatric cervical spine with and without cervical collar. *Pediatric Emergency Care,* 13(1), 5-7.

SECTION 7

Specific Injuries

31

Head Trauma/Traumatic Brain Injury

Kathy Haley, RN, BSN
Christine Nelson, RNC, MS, PNP

Introduction

Traumatic brain injury is the leading cause of death among injured children. Most deaths occur within the first 4 hours after injury. It has been reported that 60 to 80% of children with multiple injuries sustain head injuries (Vernon-Levett, 1998). Children may require care that ranges from overnight observation to operative management to relieve intracranial bleeding. Table 31.1 outlines common pediatric head injuries.

There are two phases of brain injury:

1. Primary injury occurs at impact when traumatic forces are applied to the brain, and the brain comes into contact with the interior skull (Greenes & Madsen, 2000). Resulting injuries include contusions, skull fractures, and diffuse axonal injury (Greenes & Madsen, 2000).
2. Secondary injury occurs as the sequela of the injured brain and includes injuries such as cerebral edema, hypoxia, or increased intracranial pressure (Greenes & Madsen, 2000).

Guidelines for treating children with head injury are controversial and are evolving. The decisions made during the initial minutes of management often influence the child's outcome.

Pediatric Considerations

Selected anatomic and physiologic features affect injuries to the brain:

- Children up to approximately 3 years of age have skulls that are pliable, thinner, and have nonfused cranial sutures. Therefore, blunt forces applied to the skull cause more local brain injury (Greenes & Madsen, 2000) because energy is absorbed by the brain and not the skull:
  - The nonfused sutures allow intracranial expansions in the presence of increased intracranial pressure (ICP).
  - Management of increased ICP (ICP greater than 15 to 20 mm/Hg) should not be delayed because of this anatomic difference, however.
- The intact and open ventricles and cisterns are essential to cerebral integrity. If they are compressed or invisible on a computerized tomography scan, the prognosis is poor.
- The central nervous system has a limited ability for regeneration. Children, though, tend to have better outcomes than adults following severe head injury, although the exact reason for this difference is unclear (Ward, 1995).
- Children have relatively large heads and weak neck musculature; therefore, the head is more likely to sustain impact injuries. Children, unlike adults, may develop hemorrhagic shock from head trauma and subsequent blood loss. Because of the large head size in proportion to the body, it is possible for the child to become hypovolemic from an isolated skull fracture (Sacchetti, Belfer, & Doolin, 2001).

TABLE 31.1 Common Types of Head Injury

Injury	*Description*	*Signs and Symptoms*
Linear skull fracture	Nondepressed fracture of the skull along or perpendicular to a suture line; can be diastatic (separation of sutures), resulting in a "growing" fracture	Fracture site pain and tenderness; swelling; cephalhematoma at fracture site
Basilar skull fracture	Fracture of the bones at the skull base	Headache; altered Glasgow coma scale score; otorrhea (blood or cerebrospinal fluid); hematotympanum; Battle's sign (suggests a mastoid fracture); raccoon's eyes (due to intraorbital bleeding from fracture); agitation; irritability
Depressed skull fracture	Fracture of the skull from a direct blow; can be "ping pong" (indentation in the infant skull)	Altered Glasgow coma scale score (may not always be present); palpable depression at the fracture site; laceration or abrasion of scalp
Concussion	Closed head injury from direct blow or deceleration	Usually no localizing signs; occasionally nausea, vomiting, headache, brief alteration in level of consciousness, amnesia, dizziness
Diffuse axonal injuries	Diffuse white matter damage resulting typically from acceleration-deceleration injuries	Altered level of consciousness
Intracranial bleeding	Vascular injuries resulting in hematoma (intracerebral, subdural, or epidural) or subarachnoid hemorrhage, caused by direct blows to head or violent shaking	Altered level of consciousness, unilateral dilated pupil (sometimes a late sign indicative of herniation); headache; seizures; changes in vital signs; vomiting; irritability. Intracranial bleeding may progress slowly; symptoms may develop hours to days following the injury

Etiology

- Blunt forces—Energy is transmitted to the brain:
  - Bicycle crashes without a helmet
  - Motor vehicle crashes
  - Motorcycle crashes without a helmet
  - Sports (e.g., football, helmet to helmet)
  - Falls from heights to nonyielding surfaces
  - Auto-pedestrian collisions
  - Intentional acts (e.g., shaken-impact syndrome)
  - Acts of violence (e.g., blunt forces to the head)
  - Play activities (e.g., sledding)
- Penetrating forces—Energy is applied directly to the brain:
  - Impalement or other penetrating objects (e.g., lawn darts).
  - Gunshot wounds.
  - Knife wounds.
- Acceleration-deceleration forces:
  - Motor vehicle crashes.
  - Sports activities.
  - Falls.
  - Intentional acts (e.g., shaken-impact syndrome).
- Crushing forces:
  - Pedestrian-motor vehicle crashes.
  - Farm equipment or machinery.
  - Animal bites.

Focused History

Mechanism of Injury

- Bicycle crash:
  - Presence of helmet; condition of helmet post inquiry (e.g., intact or broken)
  - Speed and type of oncoming vehicle.
  - Speed of bicycle.
  - Stationary object struck (e.g., tree or car).

- Motorcycle crash:
  - Presence of helmet.
  - Speed and type of oncoming vehicle.
  - Speed of motorcycle.
  - Stationary object struck (e.g., tree or car).
- Sports-related injury:
  - Use of protective equipment, including helmet.
  - Type of sport.
- Fall from height to nonyielding surface:
  - Height from which the child fell.
  - Surface on which the child fell.
- Pedestrian incident:
  - Speed of vehicle.
  - Child maltreatment (Chapter 46)
- Play activities:
  - Type of activity.
- Gunshot wound:
  - Type of weapon.
  - Caliber of bullet.
  - Distance or range from which bullet was fired.
- Penetrating wound:
  - Type of penetrating object.
  - Impaled or removed prior to emergency medical services arrival.
- Crushing force:
  - Type of farm equipment or machinery.
  - Type of animal (e.g., horse).

Neurologic Symptoms following the Injury

- Loss of consciousness after the injury event.
- Continued loss of consciousness.
- Pupillary changes.
- Visual disturbances.
- Vomiting.
- Seizure activity.
- Headache.
- Decreased activity level.
- Amnesia to the event or ongoing amnesia (short-term).
- Weakness.
- Neck pain.

Injury-related Information

- Witnesses.
- Prehospital treatment.

Focused Assessment

Physical Assessment

1. Assess the airway, respiratory, and cardiovascular systems (Chapter 30).
2. Assess the neurologic system:
   - Assess the level of consciousness with the Glasgow coma scale (GCS), Pediatric Glasgow coma scale (PGCS), or AVPU method:
     - Changes of 2 points in the GCS score indicate potential hypovolemia, hypoxia, or increased ICP. Sudden changes may demand immediate intervention.
     - Score values indicate the following severity of head injury (Dolan, 1997):

       13–15 = mild head injury

       9–12 = moderate head injury

       < 9 = severe head injury
     - Serial documentation of the GCS score and pupillary responses provide ongoing assessment for intracranial hemorrhage, increased intracranial pressure, and brain stem herniation.
     - Each assessment, especially the GCS score, will be useful for the neurosurgeon to determine appropriate treatment guidelines for ICP management.
   - Assess the pupils for:
     - Equality.
     - Size.
     - Reactivity to light and accommodation.
   - Assess neuromuscular activity:
     - Gait.
     - Upper and lower extremity strength.
     - Movement or posturing.
   - Assess the child's activity level and response to the ED environment.
   - Assess for signs of increased intracranial pressure, which can occur very quickly in head trauma:
     - Hypotension and hypoxia related to inadequate airway and breathing or brain stem injury contribute to hypercapnia, hyperemia, and increased ICP.
     - Elevation in ICP from hypoxia can be delayed.
     - Cushing response: a triad of hypertension, bradycardia, and irregular respirations.
     - Decerebrate or decorticate posturing.
     - Seizures (may or may not be related to increased ICP).

- Observe for signs of cerebrospinal fluid leakage (suggestive of a basilar skull fracture):
  - Otorrhea.
  - Rhinorrhea.
- Inspect the face and head for:
  - Surface trauma (lacerations, contusions, and ecchymoses).
  - Battle's sign (ecchymoses in the mastoid area).
  - Raccoon's eyes (periorbial ecchymoses).
- Palpate the head for:
  - Step-offs.
  - Depressions.
  - Elevations.
- Perform (or assist with) an otoscopic evaluation to detect hematotympanum.

3. Assess the remaining body systems (Chapter 30).

Psychosocial Assessment

- Assess the child's and family's coping strategies.
- Assess the child's and family's understanding of the child's head injury.

Nursing Interventions for the Child with a Severe Head Injury

1. Assess and maintain the airway with the jaw thrust maneuver or through insertion of an oral airway while maintaining cervical spine immobilization and stabilization:
   - Prepare for orotracheal intubation with rapid-sequence induction to minimize coughing, agitation, and movement that could increase the ICP. The orotracheal route is preferred due to the possibility of a cribiform plate fracture (Dolan, 1997).
   - Perform a brief neurologic assessment prior to the induction as a guide to future treatment.
2. Administer 100% oxygen by bag-valve-mask ventilation:
   - Although hyperventilation with 100% oxygen has become controversial, it is often initiated in the child with severe head injury:
     - The $PaCO_2$ is maintained at approximately 30–35 mm Hg (Greenes & Madsen, 2000). A lower $PaCO_2$ results in an increased pH and decreased cerebral tissue acidosis; arterioles constrict, decreasing cerebral blood flow, cerebral blood volume, and ICP (Vernon-Levett, 1998). SaO_2 should be maintained at greater than 90%.
     - Caution must be used with hyperventilation, because excessive arteriolar constriction may result, which limits not only cerebral blood flow but also cerebral perfusion, causing hypoxic injury to an already compromised brain.
   - Prepare for mechanical ventilation.
3. Obtain venous access and initiate an intravenous infusion:
   - Administer isotonic intravenous fluids in the child with head injury and signs of hypovolemic shock:
     - Never administer 5% dextrose or 10% dextrose in water.
   - The higher priority in management is maintaining adequate circulation and perfusion. More damage can be done if the patient has a decreased vascular volume and hypotension.
   - Prepare to administer osmotic agents to decrease ICP:
     - These agents remove free water from brain cells within an intact blood brain barrier (McComb & Zlokovic, 1994).
     - Intravenous mannitol may be administered once an indwelling bladder catheter is placed, blood pressure and perfusion are adequate, and there is evidence of increased ICP.
   - Obtain blood specimens for laboratory analysis, such as an ethanol level or toxicology screening, as needed.
4. Measure the child's level of consciousness and neurologic responses.
5. Maintain normothermia during the ED treatment.
6. Perform ongoing assessments of the child's cardiopulmonary, oxygen saturation, and neurologic statuses:
   - These assessments allow early detection of intracranial hemorrhage, increased ICP, and brain stem herniation.
   - A deteriorating neurologic state in any child with an acute brain insult should be considered a life-threatening condition.
7. Insert an orogastric tube to prevent gastric distension.
8. Insert an indwelling bladder catheter to measure urinary output.
9. Prepare for diagnostic testing, such as CT scanning without contrast:

- CT scanning is widely used to identify acute intracranial injury. If the ventricles and cisterns are compressed or invisible on the CT scan, morbidity and mortality are expected.

10. Prepare for operative management:
    - Only 15 to 20% of children with head injury require surgical intervention (Bruce, 1993).
11. Inform the family frequently about the child's condition and results of diagnostic tests.
    - Present the option for family presence (Chapter 28).
12. Provide emotional support to the child and family.
13. Initiate consultations with social services, neurosurgery, and other specialists, as needed.
14. Prepare for transfer or transport to a trauma center (Chapter 10) or admission to the hospital.

Nursing Interventions for the Child with a Mild Head Injury

1. Perform ongoing neurologic assessments. Observe for signs of increased ICP, such as vomiting and changes in level of consciousness.
2. Prepare for diagnostic procedures, such as radiographs and CT scan.
3. Inform the family frequently about the child's condition.
4. Administer an analgesic (e.g., acetaminophen), as prescribed.
5. Provide emotional support to the child and family.
6. Prepare for hospitalization for observation or discharge to home.

Home Care and Prevention

Many head injuries can be prevented through the proper use of protective equipment during play and sports activities. Reinforcement with coaches and adults who supervise sports activities is essential.

Parents should be prepared for changes in their child's usual behavior following a head injury, such as changes in sleep patterns, bad dreams, emotional liability, difficulty staying on task, learning problems, and short-term memory loss (Wright, 1990). Parents of a child with a mild head injury should be instructed to observe their child every 2 hours for the first 24 hours postinjury for changes in the level of consciousness, the child's ability to talk, and movement (Ball, 1998). Parents can be encouraged to provide quiet activities for the child, such as board games, reading, videos, or puzzles (Ball, 1998). Acetaminophen may be prescribed for headache.

Parents should contact the ED or their primary care physician if the child exhibits any of these symptoms in the first few days following a mild head injury (Ball, 1998):

- Severe headaches not relieved with analgesics.
- Persistent vomiting (more than 3 times in 24 hours).
- Projectile vomiting.
- Confusion, restless, excessive sleepiness, or a change in personality.
- Seizure activity.
- Uncoordinated gait or balance; weakness.
- Difficulty eating.
- Rhinorrhea or otorrhea.

Parents should be taught about postconcussive syndrome, which usually lasts 4 to 6 weeks and includes symptoms such as memory loss, headaches, fatigue, mood changes, sleep changes, and difficulty in remembering directions and activities (Wright, 1990). The child needs supervision for safe behaviors (Wright, 1990). Parents can help their child to recover by being patient, taking extra time with the child, giving the child extra help, and providing quiet times for work and school (Wright, 1990). Follow-up visits with the child's primary care physician should be scheduled, and discussions with the child's school nurse and teacher about the child's learning needs should occur before the child reenters school.

Parents whose children sustain a severe head injury may expect a longer rehabilitation process or permanent cognitive and emotional changes. However, the permanent level of function following a head injury is not determined in the ED setting.

Conclusion

Head injuries are a common phenomenon requiring ED treatment. Ongoing assessments and interventions are crucial to detecting early changes in ICP. Home care following a mild head injury is augmented with instructions for the parents and caregivers.

References

Ball, J. (1998). Head injury. In J. Ball (Ed.), *Mosby's pediatric patient teaching guides* (p. I-1). St. Louis: Mosby—Year Book.

Bruce, D. (1993). Head trauma. In M. Eichelberger (Ed.), *Pediatric trauma* (pp. 353-361). St. Louis: Mosby—Year Book.

Dolan, M. (1997). Head trauma. In R. Barkin (Ed.), *Pediatric emergency medicine* (pp. 236-351). St. Louis: Mosby—Year Book.

Greenes, D. & Madsen, J. (2000). Neurotrauma. In G. Fleisher & S. Ludwig (Eds.). *Textbook of pediatric emergency medicine* (4th ed., pp. 1271-1296). Philadelphia: Lippincott, Williams & Wilkins.

McComb, J. G. & Zlokovic, B. (1994). Cerebrospinal fluid and the blood-brain interface. In W. Cheek (Ed.)., *Pediatric neurosurgery* (pp. 167-175). Philadelphia: Saunders.

Sacchetti, A., Belfer, R., & Doolin, E. (2001). Pediatric trauma. In P. Ferrera, S. Colucciello, J. Marx, V. Verdile, & M. Gibbs (Eds.), *Trauma management* (pp. 504-532). St. Louis: Mosby—Yearbook.

Vernon-Levett, P. (1998). Neurologic system. In P. Slota (Ed.), *Core curriculum for pediatric critical care nursing* (pp. 274-359). Philadelphia: Saunders.

Ward, J. (1995). Craniocerebral injuries. In W. Buntain (Ed.), *Management of pediatric trauma* (pp. 177-188). Philadelphia: Saunders.

Wright, C. (1990). Mild head injury: Care of the child at home. Washington, DC: Children's National Medical Center.

32

Spinal Cord Trauma

Kathy Haley, RN, BSN
Christine Nelson, RNC, MS, PNP

Introduction

Spinal column and spinal cord injuries are uncommon in the pediatric population. Unfortunately, half of all children with spinal cord injury die at the scene or within 1 hour of injury (Dickman & Rekate, 1993).

Spinal injury can occur in the cervical, thoracic, lumbar, or sacral spine regions (Table 32.1). Spinal cord injuries include concussions, contusions, lacerations, transections, and hemorrhage; blood vessel injury to the cord itself may also occur (Vernon-Levett, 1998). These injuries result from (Vernon-Levett, 1998):

- *Hyperextension (fracture and dislocation of the posterior elements).*
- *Hyperflexion (fracture or dislocation of the vertebral bodies, discs, or ligaments).*
- *Vertical compression (shattering fractures).*
- *Rotational forces (fractures and rupture of supporting ligaments).*

Younger children tend to have fractures of the upper cervical region, whereas older children and adolescents more often have fractures involving the lower cervical spine area.

Unique to the pediatric age group is the phenomenon of spinal cord injury without radiographic abnormality (SCIWORA). It was first described by Pang & Wilberger (1982). Two thirds of SCIWORA cases occur in children aged 8 years and younger (Dickman & Rekate, 1993), including infants (Kinder, 1991; Lang & Bernardo, 1993).

The phenomenon is more common in the cervical and thoracic spine region and is rarely found in the lumbar spine. The injury is associated with the increased elasticity of the child's immature spine and the greater flexibility from ligamentous laxity:

- During hyperflexion or hyperextension, the spine can elongate without injury.
- The spinal cord stretches beyond its normal range, leading to tears, contusion, or transection.
- The spinal cord and vertebrae return to normal length and alignment, respectively.
- Reversible disk protrusion and transient subluxation are other mechanisms of SCIWORA.
- Symptoms of spinal cord injury may occur immediately or be delayed, in some cases as long as 4 days after injury, and radiographs and computerized tomography studies reveal no bony abnormalities.

Treatment of SCIWORA includes hospitalization, diagnostic tests, such as somatosensory-evoked potentials, spinal radiographs, computerized tomography scans, and immobilization with a Guilford brace or posterior resting splint (Lang & Bernardo, 1993).

Home care of SCIWORA includes wearing the prescribed brace or splint, skin care, bathing with assistance, refraining from organized contact sports, and keeping follow-up appointments with the neurosurgeon (Lang & Bernardo, 1993).

When spinal cord injuries occur, the outcome can be permanent and devastating for the child and their family. Recovery can be maximized by prompt and meticulous assessment, recognition, spinal immobilization, and treatment. The outcome is varied and directly related to the severity of cord injury.

Pediatric Considerations

Spinal injuries in children are related to the following anatomic differences:

- The infant's spine is composed mostly of cartilage, and the intervertebral disk spaces appear wide in relation to the vertebral bodies (Scully & Luerssen, 1995). As the child grows, the vertebral bodies ossify, and the amount of cartilage decreases (Scully & Luerssen, 1995). Children less than 9 years of age are susceptible to cervical spine injuries due to the large head size in proportion to the body, weak neck musculature, and horizontal facets (Eleraky et al., 2000).

TABLE 32.1 Selected Spinal Injuries

Spinal Injury	*Description*
Craniocervical dislocation	Diagnosed in younger children following acceleration-deceleration mechanism of injury. It is usually lethal, because it involves the high spinal cord and brain stem.
"Hangman fracture" (fracture of the posterior arch of the axis)	Occurs in older children; requires immobilization.
Thoracolumbar fractures	Compression fractures—occur with hyperflexion injuries, causing pain with sitting and upon palpation. Treatment includes bed rest. Burst fractures—result from axial loading.

From: Scully & Luerssen, 1995.

- The spine is more elastic and mobile, causing dislocation and spontaneous realignment without bony or ligamental disruption (Lang & Bernardo, 1993). The wedge-shaped vertebrae are prone to forward slipping between adjacent vertebrae (Sullivan, Bruwer, & Harris, 1958).
- The level of maximum flexion in the cervical spine descends as the child grows older. Maximum flexion occurs at C2-C3 in infants and young children; at C3-C4 in children 5 to 6 years of age; and at C5-C6 in adolescents (Baker & Berdon, 1966; Braakman & Penning, 1968; Townsend & Rowe, 1952; Loder, 2001).
- Spinal cord injuries always are suspected in children with multiple injuries.

Etiology

- Blunt forces:
  - Pedestrian incidents.
  - Sports activities (more common in adolescents).
  - Diving. Axial loading occurs when the weight of the body is compressed on the cervical spine.
  - Child maltreatment.
  - Falls.
  - Motor vehicle crashes. Lethal cervical spine injuries caused by passenger-side air bag deployment have been reported in children younger than 8 years of age who were unrestrained front-seat passengers involved in low-speed, front-impact motor vehicle collisions (Murphy, 1999).
  - Acts of violence.
- Penetrating forces:
  - Gunshot wounds.
  - Penetrating wounds.
- Acceleration-deceleration forces:
  - Motor vehicle crashes.
  - Sports activities.
- Crushing forces:
  - Animal bites
  - Machinery
  - Hangings

Focused History

Mechanism of Injury

- Pedestrian incidents:
  - Speed of vehicle
- Sports activity (more common in adolescents):
  - Type of sport
- Diving:
  - Depth of water
  - Type of surface struck (e.g., cement)
- Child maltreatment (Chapter 46)
- Fall:
  - Height from which child fell
  - Yielding or unyielding surface
- Motor vehicle crash:
  - Passenger or driver
  - Type of collision (head-on, T-bone, rear-end, or lateral)
  - Type of safety restraint used
  - Child's position in the car
  - Air bag deployment

- Act of violence:
  - Perpetrator
  - Type of force used
- Gunshot wound:
  - Type of weapon
  - Caliber of bullet
  - Distance from which bullets were fired
- Penetrating wound:
  - Type of penetrating object
  - Impaled or removed
- Crushing wound:
  - Hanging versus autoeroticism
  - Type of biting animal
  - Type of machinery

Neurologic Symptoms following the Injury

- Loss of consciousness after the injury event
- Numbness or tingling in the fingers or toes
- Weakness or paralysis of the upper and/or lower extremities
- Priapism

Injury-related Information

- Witnesses
- Prehospital treatment
- Report of hearing a "crack" or "snap" at the time of injury

Focused Assessment

Physical Assessment

1. Assess the airway and respiratory system.
   - Assess the airway for:
     - Patency.
   - Auscultate the chest for:
     - Respiratory rate. Apnea or bradypnea indicates a high-level spinal cord or brain stem injury.
2. Assess the circulatory system.
   - Auscultate the heart for:
     - Rate. Tachycardia may be present with shock.
3. Assess the neurologic system.
   - Assess the level of consciousness with the Glasgow coma scale, Pediatric Glasgow coma scale, or AVPU (Alert, responds to Verbal stimuli, responds to Painful stimuli, Unresponsive) methods.
   - Assess movement and strength of the extremities:
     - Assess tendon reflexes.
   - Observe for signs of spinal cord injury. The symptoms of spinal cord injury are not easily discerned in young children and are variable depending on the child's age, the injury location, the spinal fracture stability, and other systemic injuries. Generally, signs of spinal cord injury include:
     - Flaccid extremities.
     - Paralysis.
     - Numbness, tingling, and paresthesia.
     - Paresis.
     - Priapism.
4. Assess the abdomen.
   - Inspect the abdomen for ecchymoses or abrasions caused by use of a lap belt in a motor vehicle crash. Chance fracture (posterior transverse fracture through the lumbar vertebral bodies) should be suspected.
     - Assess the rectal tone.
5. Assess the back (performed during the secondary assessment; Chapter 30).
   - Palpate the spinal column for tenderness, leaving the cervical collar intact.
     - Vertebral fractures may be detected.
   - Inspect the back for:
     - Surface trauma.
     - Edema.
     - Deformities.

Psychosocial Assessment

- Assess the child's and family's coping strategies.
- Assess the child's and family's understanding of the spinal cord injury.
  - During emergency department (ED) treatment, the level of function may improve or worsen, and the prognosis usually is not known, causing stress and anxiety for the child and family.

Nursing Interventions

1. Assess and maintain the airway using the jaw thrust maneuver.
   - Prepare for endotracheal intubation in the child with a high cervical spinal cord injury.

- Maintain spinal immobilization to prevent the worsening of an existing spinal cord injury.
  - Assume that any child with a head injury; who is unconscious; or who sustained multiple injuries has a spinal cord injury until proven otherwise.
- Spinal immobilization must remain intact until diagnostic tests and patient assessment findings determine the absence of spinal cord injury.

2. Initiate measures to support respiratory effort.
   - Administer 100% oxygen via face mask or other means, as tolerated by the child.
   - Initiate bag-valve-mask ventilation in the child with apnea or bradypnea.
   - Prepare for mechanical ventilation.
   - Initiate cardiorespiratory and oxygen saturation monitoring.
3. Obtain venous access and initiate an intravenous infusion:
   - Administer medications as prescribed.
     - Administer high-dose methylprednisolone (dosages used vary among institutions) within 6 to 8 hours postinjury. One recommendation is methylprednisolone 30 mg/kg administered over 15 minutes. Then, 5.4 mg/kg/hr is administered for 23 hours if the injury occurred within 8 hours (Woodward, 2000).
4. Perform serial cardiopulmonary and neurologic assessments to detect improvement or worsening in the child's condition.
   - Assess children with lower spinal cord injury for worsening of their respiratory and circulatory statuses, and perform serial neurologic assessments.
   - Neurogenic shock may accompany spinal cord injury (Chapter 40).
   - Perform careful and ongoing assessments for the nonverbal, unconscious, or multiply injured child, to exclude the possibility of spinal cord injury and to measure progression of cord edema.
5. Prepare for diagnostic tests including:
   - Radiographs of the lateral, anterior-posterior, and odontoid views of the cervical spine. In one study of eight children aged 9 to 68 months who fell fewer than 5 feet and sustained cervical spine fractures or cervical spinal cord injury, all had limited range of motion of the neck or neck pain. Therefore, young children who are asymptomatic after sustaining short falls may not require radiographic tests of the cervical spine (Schwartz et al., 1997).
   - Radiographs of the anterior-posterior and lateral views of the thoracic and lumbar spine.
   - Flexion-extension radiographs of the cervical spine. These may be obtained by an experienced physician for the child who does not have vertebral or ligamentous disruption; the child should never move the neck past the range of comfort (Scully & Luerrsen, 1995).
   - Computerized tomography scan.
   - Magnetic resonance imaging.
6. Insert a nasogastric or orogastric tube for gastric decompression.
7. Insert an indwelling bladder catheter for bladder decompression and measurement of urinary output.
8. Provide emotional support to the child and family.
   - The awake child may be very frightened by the ensuing neurologic symptoms and immobilization; continuous consolation by parents and assigned staff is indicated.
   - Use diversion techniques to console the distraught child while observing for facial grimace indicating pain during vertebral palpation.
9. Inform the family frequently of the child's condition.
10. Initiate consultations with social services, neurosurgery, and other specialties, as needed.
11. Prepare for transfer and transport to a trauma center (Chapter 10); prepare for hospitalization.

Home Care and Prevention

Spinal cord injuries can be prevented by teaching children safety measures during sporting and diving activities. It is important to teach parents, coaches, and adults who supervise sports activities how to prevent injuries, including the player's use of proper equipment and the adult's removal of players from action when they complain of numbness, tingling, or electric shock sensations.

Conclusion

Although relatively rare, spinal cord injuries in children evoke feelings of distress in the child, family, and ED staff. Debriefing of the ED staff following the care of such a patient may be needed (Chapter 28). Awareness of the potential for spinal cord injury is imperative, especially in the multiply injured, nonverbal, or unconscious child.

References

Baker, D., & Berdon, W. (1966). Special trauma problems in children. *Radiology Clinics of North America*, *4*, 289-305.

Braakman, R., & Penning, L. (1968). The hyperflexion sprain of the cervical spine. *Radiology Clinics*, *37*, 309-320.

Dickman C., & Rekate, H. (1993). Spinal trauma. In M. Eichelberger (Ed.), *Pediatric trauma* (pp. 362-377). St. Louis: Mosby—Year Book.

Eleraky, M., Theodore, N., Adams, M., Rekate, H., & Sonntrag. V. (2000). Pediatric cervical spine injuries. Report of 102 cases and review of the literature. *Journal of Neurosurgery*, *92*, 12-17.

Kinder, P. (1991). A 6-month-old paraplegic infant with spinal cord injury without radiologic abnormalities (SCIWORA). *Journal of Emergency Nursing*, *17*, 368-369.

Lang, S., & Bernardo, L. (1993). SCIWORA syndrome: Nursing assessment. *Dimensions of Critical Care Nursing*, *12*, 247-254.

Loder, R. (2001). The cervical spine. In *Lovell and Winter Pediatric orthopedics.* R. Morrissy and S. Weinstein (Eds). Philadelphia: Lippincott Williams and Wilkins.

Pang, D., & Wilberger, J. (1982). Spinal cord injury without radiographic abnormalities in children. *Journal of Neurosurgery*, *57*, 114-129.

Schwartz, G., Wright, S., Fein, J., Sugarman, J., Pasternack, J., & Salhanick, S. (1997). Pediatric cervical spine injury sustained in falls from low heights. *Annals of Emergency Medicine*, *30*, 249-252.

Scully, T., & Luerssen, T. (1995). Spinal cord injuries. In W. Buntain (Ed.), *Management of pediatric trauma* (pp. 189-199). Philadelphia: Saunders.

Sullivan, C., Bruwer, A., & Harris, E. (1958). Hypermobility of the cervical spine in children: A pitfall in the diagnosis of cervical dislocation. *American Journal of Surgery*, *95*, 636-640.

Townsend, E., & Rowe, M. (1952). Mobility of the upper cervical spine in health and disease. *Pediatrics*, *10*, 567-573.

Vernon-Levett, P. (1998). Neurologic system. In P. Slota (Ed.), *Core curriculum for pediatric critical care nursing* (pp. 274-359). Philadelphia: Saunders.

Woodward, G. (2000). Neck trauma. In G. Fleisher & S. Ludwig (Eds.). *Textbook of pediatric emergency medicine* (4th ed., pp. 1297-1340). Philadelphia: Lippincott Williams and Wilkins.

33

Oral and Maxillofacial Trauma

Lisa Marie Bernardo, RN, PhD, MPH
Rachael Rosenfield, RN, BSN

Introduction

Injuries to the face and its supporting structures occur with relative frequency in the pediatric population. Because the cranium is disproportionately larger than the face, skull fractures are more common than facial fractures among children younger than 12 years of age (Barkin & Rosen, 1999). Minor injuries, such as corneal abrasions and avulsed teeth, are associated with a rapid recovery and good outcome. Major injuries, such as mandibular and midfacial fractures, require operative management.

Pediatric Considerations

Selected anatomic features are associated with differences in oral and maxillofacial trauma (Haug & Foss, 2000):

- The growing child's primary and secondary dentition affect the use of maxillomandibular fixation because incomplete root formation of the permanent teeth compromises the ability of the dentition to serve as a means for maxillomandibular fixation.
- Rapid bone growth shortens healing time and thus decreases the length of time required for maxillomandibular fixation.
- The growth potential of the septal cartilage of the nose requires early repositioning of the nasal bones and septum to avoid impaired growth.
- Damage to the growing facial bones can result in growth abnormalities, such as ankylosis of the temporomandibular joint or zygomaticomaxillary deficiency.

Etiology

- Blunt forces:
  - Motor vehicle crashes
  - Pedestrian–motor vehicle crashes
  - Falls
  - Sports activities
  - Bicycle crashes
  - Child maltreatment (Chapter 46)
  - Acts of violence
- Penetrating forces:
  - Gunshot wounds
  - Penetrating wounds
  - Machinery
- Acceleration-deceleration forces:
  - Motor vehicle crashes
  - Falls
- Crushing forces:
  - Human bites
  - Animal bites
  - Machinery

Focused History

Mechanism of Injury

- Motor vehicle crash:
  - Child's position in the vehicle
  - Safety restraint usage
  - Type of motor vehicles
  - Speed of vehicle
- Pedestrian–motor vehicle crash:
  - Speed of car
- Fall:
  - Height of fall
  - Surface on which the child fell (yielding or nonyielding)
- Sports activity:
  - Use of protective equipment
  - Type of sport
- Bicycle crash:
  - Helmet use
  - Speed of bicycle
  - Type of crash (moving vehicle or stationary object)
- Child maltreatment (Chapter 46)
- Act of violence:
  - Perpetrator
  - Use of weapons
- Gunshot wound:
  - Caliber of bullet
  - Distance from gun
- Penetrating wound:
  - Type of object
  - Impaled or removed prior to emergency department (ED) arrival
- Human bite:
  - Person involved (family member or other)
- Animal bite:
  - Type of animal
  - Domestic versus wild
  - Rabies status

Symptoms following the Injury

- Ability to maintain a patent airway
- Amount of blood loss
- Loss of consciousness
- Surface trauma to the face or mouth

Injury-related Information

- Witnesses
- Prehospital treatment
- Preservation of avulsed tissue or tooth

Focused Assessment

Physical Assessment

1. Assess the airway and cervical spine:
   - Inspect the airway for:
     - Patency.
     - Presence of foreign bodies.
   - Listen for the child's ability to speak or make age-appropriate sounds.
   - Maintain cervical and spinal alignment.
     - Severe maxillofacial trauma suggests cervical spine involvement.
2. Assess the respiratory system.
   - Auscultate the chest for:
     - Respiratory rate.
     - Adventitious sounds.
3. Assess the cardiovascular system:
   - Auscultate the heart for:
     - Rate.
     - Rhythm.
   - Measure the blood pressure.
   - Palpate central and peripheral pulses for:
     - Presence.
     - Quality.
     - Equality.
   - Assess peripheral perfusion.
     - Observe skin color.
     - Measure core and skin temperature.
     - Measure capillary refill.
4. Assess the neurologic system:
   - Assess the level of consciousness with the Glasgow coma scale or AVPU (Alert, responds to Verbal stimuli, responds to Painful stimuli, Unresponsive) methods.
   - Assess the pupils for:
     - Size.
     - Shape.
     - Reactivity to light.
     - Accommodation.

- Palpate the head for:
  - Depressions.
  - Step-off defects.
  - Pain.
  - Hematomas or swelling.
  - The integrity of the anterior and posterior fontanelle in children younger than 2 years of age.
- Inspect the head for:
  - Surface trauma.
  - Puncture wounds.
  - Gunshot wounds.
  - Foreign bodies, such as glass or metal.
  - Avulsions.

5. Assess the face and oral cavity.
   - Inspect the face for:
     - Deformity.
     - Midfacial fractures are classified with the Le Fort system (Table 33.1). These injuries are rare in children.
     - Surface trauma.
     - Symmetry. Assess for malocclusion by asking the child to smile and grimace and open and close the mouth; inability to perform these tasks is indicative of a mandibular fracture. In a mandibular fracture, the fracture site may be distant from the point of trauma due to the ring structure of the mandible (Barkin & Rosen, 1999). Mandibular fractures occur in any number of combinations.
     - Impaled objects.
     - Raccoon's eyes.
     - Battle's sign.
   - Palpate the forehead, orbits, maxilla, and mandible for:
     - Tenderness.
     - Pain.
     - Step-off deformities.
     - Crepitus.
     - Stability.
   - Test the facial nerves.
     - Test facial nerves by having the child wrinkle the forehead, smile, bare the teeth, and tightly close the eyes (Barkin & Rosen, 1999, p. 426).
6. Inspect the oral cavity and structures (gums, lips, and tongue) for:
   - Lacerations.
   - Loose, chipped, or missing teeth.
     - Tooth avulsion frequently occurs in children 7 to 10 years of age.
     - Missing teeth may be a normal finding unrelated to the trauma. Parents can usually give a reliable dental history.
   - Orthodontic appliances.
     - Damage may be present to orthodontia.
7. Assess the eyes, ears, and nose.
   - Inspect the pupils for:
     - Size.
     - Equality.
     - Reaction to light.

TABLE 33.1 Le Fort Fracture Descriptions

Fracture	*Description*
Le Fort I	Pattern that extends through the zygomaticomaxillary region to the base of the pyriform aperture (Paige, Bartlett, & Whitaker, 2000, p. 1386).
	Horizontal fracture of the maxilla above the alveolar process and horizontal plate of the palatine and palatal processes of the maxilla. Rarely occurs because of the incomplete development of the maxillary sinus.
Le Fort II	Extends superiorly to the infraorbital rims and across the nasofrontal sutures (Paige, Bartlett, & Whitaker, 2000, p. 1386).
	Pyramidal fracture of the orbital floors, lamina papyracea of the ethmoids, and separation of the frontal nasal suture. Rare because of the pliability of the midfacial structures.
Le Fort III	Craniofacial dissociation that extends across the zygomatic arch, zygomaticofrontal region floor of the orbit, and nasofrontal sutures, which ultimately results in separation of the face from the skull base (Paige, Bartlett, & Whitaker, 2000, p. 1386).

- Inspect the eyes for (Table 33.2):
  - Extraocular movements.
  - Visual acuity. Request the younger child to point to a familiar object or family member. Ask the older child about the quality of vision. Perform a visual acuity test.
  - Scleral deformity and hemorrhages.
  - Contact lenses or other foreign bodies.
  - Impaled objects.
- Inspect the external ear canal for:
  - Otorrhea, which may be cerebrospinal fluid.
- Inspect the external ear for:
  - Lacerations.
  - Avulsions.
  - Missing and/or preserved tissue.
- Inspect the mastoid process for ecchymosis (Battle's sign).
- Inspect the nose for:
  - Deformity.
  - Septal deviation or septal hematoma.
  - Rhinorrhea. Clear rhinorrhea may indicate a cerebrospinal fluid leak.
- Palpate the bridge and dorsum of the nose to detect fractures or dislocations.
  - Nasal fractures may be difficult to detect clinically due to swelling (Paige, et al, 2000).

8. Assess the cervical spine while maintaining stabilization.
   - Palpate the cervical spine (posterior neck) for:
     - Tenderness.
     - Pain.
     - Malaligned vertebrae.

Psychosocial Assessment

- Assess the child's and family's coping strategies.
- Assess the child's and family's understanding of the injuries.

Nursing Interventions

1. Assess and maintain airway and cervical spine stabilization.
   - Open and maintain the airway while the cervical spine is manually immobilized in a neutral position.
     - Use the jaw thrust method.
     - Prepare for endotracheal intubation.
   - Suction the mouth and upper airway with a large, rigid tonsilar suction in the presence of debris, blood, or secretions:
     - Avoid deep oral suctioning, because stimulation of the posterior pharynx, larynx, or trachea may cause vagal stimulation with resultant bradycardia.
2. Initiate measures to support respiratory function.
   - Administer supplemental 100% oxygen.
   - Initiate bag-valve-mask ventilation with 100% oxygen in the presence of apnea or ineffective respiratory effort.
   - Prepare for mechanical ventilation.
3. Initiate measures to maintain circulation.
   - Initiate cardiorespiratory and oxygen saturation monitoring.
   - Obtain vascular access and initiate fluid resuscitation.
   - Obtain blood specimens for laboratory analysis:
     - Complete blood count and differential.
     - Prothrombin time and partial thromboplastin time.
     - Type and crossmatching.
     - Toxicology screening (if alcohol or drug use is suspected).
     - Lipase (if parotid gland involvement is extensive).
4. Monitor the neurologic status.
5. Prepare for diagnostic testing, as needed.
   - Radiographs of the face (Barkin & Rosen, 1999).
     - Right and left lateral oblique views.
     - Posteroanterior view of the mandible.
     - Towne view (condylar neck of the mandible).
     - Water's sinus view for midfacial structures, sinuses, and orbits.
     - Panoramic view of the teeth and dentoalveolar structures.
   - Radiograph of the nose (Barkin & Rosen, 1999).
   - Computerized tomography scan.
6. Prepare for interventions.
   - Assist with wound repair with or without conscious sedation for external ear laceration or abrasion.

TABLE 33.2 Comparison of Common Ocular Injuries

Type of Injury	*Description*	*Etiology*	*Physical Assessment*	*Interventions*
Corneal abrasion	Partial or complete removal of the corneal epithelium, which leaves the corneal nerve endings exposed and causes severe pain	■ Introduction of dirt into the eye ■ Exposure to ultraviolet light ■ Infection ■ Contact lenses ■ Foreign objects (e.g., fingers, tree branches)	■ Complaints of pain and a gritty feeling ("piece of sand") in the eye ■ Excessive tearing ■ Pain that worsens with blinking (indicates that the foreign body remains in the eye) ■ Redness, edema, and erythema ■ Photophobia ■ Normal or decreased visual acuity ■ Corneal abrasions from contact lenses appear as an opaque or white area with ill-defined margins	■ Remove contact lenses, if present. ■ Assist with fluorescein staining and ultraviolet light or slit lamp examination. ■ Administer ocular antibiotic drops or ointment. ■ Administer ocular or oral analgesics. ■ Assist with foreign-body removal. ■ Apply an eye patch as prescribed. ■ Avoid eye patching if the abrasion was caused by contact lenses, because of the potential presence of *Pseudomonas* organisms that may worsen a corneal injury. ■ Teach the child and parents methods for eyedrop or ointment installation.
Hyphema	Blood in the anterior chamber of the eye; as the chamber fills with blood, the hyphema becomes half-moon shaped. Risk of rebleeding within 3 to 5 days of the injury Children with sickle cell disease are at greater risk for complications of hyphema.	Blunt force trauma to the eye or head	■ Impaired or normal visual acuity ■ Description of vision as being "blood-tinged" ■ Half-moon appearance of blood at the bottom of the iris	■ Perform visual acuity test. ■ Assist with slit lamp examination. ■ Position the patient upright with the head of the bed elevated 30 to 45 degrees. ■ Patch both eyes, placing a metal shield on the affected eye. ■ Avoid aspirin-containing analgesics. ■ Glaucoma is a long-term complication.
Perforation or rupture of the globe reveals subconjunctival hemorrhage (Paige, et al, 2000)	Rupture of the globe with the potential for protrusion of intraocular contents	Blunt or penetrating forces to the eye or face	■ Decreased vision ■ Intraocular hemorrhage ■ Flat or shallow anterior chamber ■ Irregular pupil or teardrop pupil ■ Presence of a brown-blue spot or line on the conjunctiva, which is intraocular blood	■ Obtain an ophthalmology consultation. ■ Place an eye shield to prevent pressure on the globe. ■ Instruct the child to avoid Valsalva-type maneuvers. ■ Position the child upright.
Orbital blow-out fracture (Paige, et al, 2000).	Fracture to the orbital floor, with the globe absorbing the blow's force and compressing backward into the orbit	Blunt force trauma to the orbit with an object small enough to enter the space between the orbital rims	■ Pain ■ Periorbital edema ■ Ecchymosis ■ Normal or altered vision ■ Subcutaneous emphysema ■ Ipsilateral epistaxis ■ Hyperesthesia of the upper lip and cheek ■ Limited upward gaze with verticle diplopia (entrapped inferior rectus muscle and orbital fat) ■ Enophthalmos	■ Prepare for tomograms. ■ Initiate an ophthalmology consultation. ■ Prepare for possible operative management.

  - Administer local anesthesia.
  - Irrigate with normal saline.
  - Remove devitalized tissue.
  - Realign cartilaginous landmarks.
  - Suture with nonresorbable sutures.
  - Administer oral or intravenous antibiotics as prescribed.
- Assist with wound repair with or without conscious sedation for tooth avulsion:
  - Rinse the avulsed tooth with sterile normal saline (Dale, 2000).
  - If tooth is unable to be reimplanted, the avulsed tissue should be placed in Hank's balanced salt solution, if available, and then in either milk, saline, or saliva if milk or saline is unavailable (Dale, 2000).
- Provide care for avulsed permanent teeth.
  - Thirty minutes is the critical time during which an avulsed tooth may be successfully reimplanted; after 30 minutes, the avulsed tooth has less chance of being successfully implanted, but reimplantation still should be attempted.
  - Hold the avulsed tooth by its crown; gently rinse in a bowl of tap water; do not scrub or scrape; insert into its socket in the right direction (Rudy, 2001).
  - Once the tooth has been placed in socket correctly, have the child apply pressure by biting on a piece of gauze (Rudy, 2001).
  - Alternatively, place the avulsed permanent tooth in a clean container, cover with milk or saline solution, and label the container with the child's name, the date, and the time.
  - Refer the family to a dentist or oral maxillofacial surgeon.
- Assist with septal hematoma drainage or nasal packing, as needed.
- Administer medications, as prescribed.
  - Tetanus prophylaxis.
  - Antibiotics.
- Stabilize impaled objects.
- Assist with tracheostomy, as needed.

7. Insert an orgastric tube for gastric decompression, as needed.
8. Assess for pain; administer analgesics, as prescribed.
9. Inform the family frequently of the child's condition.
10. Provide emotional support to the child and family.
11. Initiate consultations with social services and surgical subspecialists, such as oral maxillofacial surgeons or ophthalmologists.
    - Consult child protective services if child maltreatment is suspected.
    - Contact law enforcement if violence was involved.
12. Prepare for transfer and transport to a trauma center (Chapter 10); prepare for operative management and hospitalization, as needed.

Home Care and Prevention

Following a minor maxillofacial injury, the child returns home with the family. The family will require instructions specific to the rendered ED treatment. Sutures can be removed by the child's primary care physician or by the treating ED physician or specialist. Follow-up with an ophthalmologist may be required for eye injuries.

Major maxillofacial trauma generally requires operative management. The child's facial features may be changed, and reconstructive surgeries may be required. Counseling may be necessary for the family and child to cope with these changes in body image.

Prevention of oral and maxillofacial injuries includes the use of proper protective equipment during sports- and work-related activities, proper positioning and restraint during motor vehicle travel, and conflict resolution measures to prevent violence.

Conclusion

Oral and maxillofacial trauma ranges from minor injuries to major trauma with operative management. Wearing protective equipment while playing sports (e.g., mouth guard, helmets with a face mask) may prevent or ameliorate oral and facial trauma. Children sustaining severe facial trauma may require reconstructive surgeries; psychological interventions and follow-up will be warranted.

References

Barkin, R. & Rosen, P. (1999). Facial trauma. *Emergency Pediatrics: A Guide to Ambulatory Care,* 5th Ed. (pp. 426-433). St. Louis: Mosby—Year Book

Dale, R. (2000). Dentoalveolar trauma. *Emergency Medicine Clinics of North America, 18*(3), 521-538.

Haug, R. & Foss, J. (2000). Maxillofacial injuries in the pediatric patient. *Oral Surgery, Oral Medicine, Oral Pathology, Oral Radiology & Endontics, 90*(2), 126-134.

Paige, K., Bartlett, S. & Whitaker, L. (2000). Facial trauma and plastic surgical emergencies. G. Fleisher & S. Ludwig (Eds.). *Textbook of Pediatric Emergency Medicine* (pp. 1383-1395). Philadelphia: Lippincott Williams & Wilkins.

Rudy, C. (2001). Dental trauma. *School Nurse News, 18*(1), 33-35.

34

Thoracic Trauma

Kathy Haley, RN, BSN
Kathleen Schenkel, RN, BSN, CEN

Introduction

Chest (cardiopulmonary) injuries often occur with multisystem injury and include injuries to the thoracic space, large airways, major thoracic blood vessels, heart, pulmonary parenchyma, and the rib cage (Webster, Grant, Slota, & Kilian, 1998) (Tables 34.1 and 34.2). Blunt chest trauma continues to be more common than penetrating chest trauma in the pediatric population. Emergency thoracotomy is required in fewer than 15% of children with cardiac injury, and 85% can be managed acutely with nonoperative techniques (Haller & Paidas, 1996). Children recover better from chest injury than do adults because of their generally better health status. If the child arrives at the emergency department (ED) in cardiopulmonary arrest after chest injury, the chances of survival are dismal. Emergency department thoractomy is rarely performed; optimal patients for receiving this procedure are those with a single penetrating injury to the left side of the chest who have or had vital signs and pupillary response within 5 minutes before the thoracotomy (Clemence, 2000).

Pediatric Considerations

Several pediatric anatomic features affect thoracic injury patterns.

- The child's ribs are cartilaginous, making rib fractures uncommon.
- When rib fractures are present, a significant force of energy has been sustained.
- Rib fractures can occur with or without flail segments. Although flail chest segments are obvious in adults, they are often less striking in the pediatric patient.
- Children with rib fractures usually present with chest pain and varying degrees of respiratory distress in response to potential intrapleural injury.
- The thoracic cavity is relatively small and affords less protection to the lungs (Soud, Saum, & Pikulski, 1998). There is less ability to dissipate energy throughout the thoracic cavity during the application of blunt forces; this kinetic energy is absorbed by the intrapleural structures, causing injury.
- The child's chest cavity easily can contain a significant volume of blood. Therefore, hypovolemic shock can occur quickly with a hemopneumothorax.
- The mediastinum is mobile, contributing to the low incidence of major vessel and airway injury in the pediatric population (Webster et al., 1998).

Etiology

- Blunt forces:
  - Pedestrian–motor vehicle crashes
  - Motor vehicle crashes
  - Child maltreatment
  - Acts of violence
  - Falls from a height
  - Bicycle crashes
- Penetrating forces:
  - Gunshot wounds
  - Penetrating wounds
- Acceleration-deceleration forces:
  - Motor vehicle crashes
  - Sports activities
- Crushing forces:
  - Animal bites
  - Machinery

TABLE 34.1 Selected Pulmonary Injuries

Injury	*Description*
Pulmonary contusion	Although pulmonary contusion is present on admission, it may not be apparent on radiographs until 24 to 48 hours postinjury. Pulmonary contusion results from blunt force trauma following a motor vehicle crash, bicycle crash, or abusive episode. Signs and symptoms include tachypnea, dyspnea, decreased breath sounds, and general worsening pulmonary status. Specific treatment includes administering high-flow oxygen and initiating cardiorespiratory monitoring. Mechanical ventilation is usually required.
Traumatic asphyxia	An almost exclusively pediatric injury with its own unique pattern. At time of injury, the glottis is closed and the thoracoabdominal muscles are tense. The superficial capillaries of the face, upper chest, and neck are disrupted by the significant, rapid, forceful, backflow up the valveless venous system of the inferior and superior vena cava into the head and neck, resulting in petechiae. Below the injury, no abnormality will be noted. This injury results from blunt force trauma following vehicular and farm equipment runovers. This injury is diagnosed in the unrestrained driver involved in a high-velocity motor vehicle crash; in the unrestrained front-seat passenger held on the lap of a restrained or unrestrained passenger; or in the driver when the child is crushed between the dashboard and the passenger or the steering wheel and the driver. Specific treatment includes high-flow oxygen delivery and cardiorespiratory monitoring.
Tracheobronchial rupture	Tracheobronchial ruptures from blunt thoracic trauma are rare in the pediatric population (Slimane et al., 1999). Death usually occurs within the first hour following tracheobronchial rupture, which is most often the result of blunt force trauma to the neck (Webster et al., 1998). Signs and symptoms include: subcutaneous emphysema, dyspnea, sternal tenderness, and hemoptysis (Webster et al., 1998). Specific treatment includes endotracheal intubation, chest tube insertion, and operative management.

Focused History

Mechanism of Injury

- Motor vehicle crash:
  - Passenger or driver
  - Seating position in vehicle
  - Type of vehicle
  - Type of crash
  - Use of safety restraints
- Bicycle crash:
  - Presence of helmet
  - Speed and type of oncoming vehicle
  - Speed of bicycle
  - Stationary object struck (e.g., tree or car)
- Sports-related injury:
  - Use of protective equipment, including helmet
  - Type of sport
- Fall from height to nonyielding surface:
  - Height from which the child fell
  - Surface on which the child fell
- Pedestrian incident:
  - Speed of vehicle
  - Child maltreatment (Chapter 46)
- Act of violence:
  - Description of the incident
- Gunshot wound:
  - Type of weapon
  - Caliber of bullet
  - Distance or range from which bullet was fired
- Penetrating wound:
  - Type of penetrating object
  - Impaled or removed
- Crushing injury:
  - Type of machinery
  - Type of biting animal

Cardiopulmonary Symptoms following the Injury

- Tachypnea
- Dyspnea
- Hoarse voice
- Facial or truncal petechiae
- Surface trauma to the chest
- Pain

TABLE 34.2 Selected Cardiac and Great-Vessel Injuries

Injury	*Description*
Cardiac contusion	Less common in injured children than in injured adults, it is caused by blunt force trauma to the chest, resulting in myocardial bruising. Presenting signs and symptoms include tachycardia and normal skin color, temperature, and capillary refill. Specific interventions include obtaining a 12-lead electrocardiogram, observation for ectopy, administration of antiarrhythmic therapy or inotropic support, and serial monitoring of creatinine kinase levels.
Cardiac tamponade	This injury is rare in pediatric trauma and is associated with penetrating forces. Once injury occurs, there is an accumulation of blood in the pericardial sac, compressing the heart and causing eventual circulatory collapse. Children may initially appear alert and anxious and rapidly progress to vascular compromise. Signs and symptoms include tachycardia, tachypnea, decreased capillary refill, Beck's triad (distended neck veins [usually not visible in the younger child], muffled heart tones, and a widened pulse pressure). Specific interventions include preparation for a rapid pericardiocentesis and operative management.
Great-vessel injury	Traumatic aortic disruption occurs in the older adolescent population and is the result of acceleration-deceleration or penetrating forces. Signs and symptoms include midscapular back pain, unexplained hypotension, upper extremity hypertension, bilateral femoral pulse deficits, large amounts of initial chest tube drainage, sternal fracture, and widened mediastinum on a chest radiograph (Webster, et al, 1998). Specific treatment is operative management.

Injury-related Information

- Witnesses
- Prehospital treatment

Focused Assessment

Physical Assessment

1. Assess the airway and respiratory system while maintaining cervical spine precautions.
   - Assess the airway for:
     - Patency.
     - Position of the trachea (midline or deviated).
   - Auscultate the chest for:
     - Respiratory rate.
     - Breath sounds may be decreased or absent in a child with a pneumothorax or hemothorax (Table 34.3).
   - Palpate the chest for:
     - Crepitus.
     - Pain/tenderness.
     - Subcutaneous emphysema.
   - Inspect the chest for:
     - Surface trauma.
     - Petechiae (also to the face and neck).
     - Paradoxical movements or flail segments.
2. Assess the cardiovascular system.
   - Auscultate the heart for:
     - Rate. Tachycardia may be present.
     - Rhythm.
   - Measure the blood pressure.
   - Measure capillary refill.
   - Measure skin color and temperature.
3. Assess the face and neck for:
   - Edema.
   - Subcutaneous emphysema.
   - Tracheal deviation.
   - Jugular venous distention.
4. Assess the eyes for subconjunctival hemorrhages.

Psychosocial Assessment

- Assess the child's and family's understanding of the injury.
- Assess the child's and family's coping strategies.

Nursing Interventions

1. Assess and maintain the airway using the jaw thrust maneuver.
   - Prepare for endotracheal intubation.
2. Administer continuous high-flow oxygen.
   - Initiate bag-valve-mask ventilations for the child with apnea or bradypnea.

TABLE 34.3 Comparison of Pneumothoraces

Injury	*Incidence/Mechanism of Injury*	*Signs/Symptoms*	*ED Treatment*
Open pneumothorax (sucking chest wound)	Rare/Penetrating trauma	▪ Respiratory distress. ▪ Decreased/absent breath sounds on the affected side. ▪ "Sucking" sound on inspiration. ▪ Tracheal deviation toward the affected hemithorax.	▪ Initiate positive-pressure ventilation. ▪ Cover the wound with an occlusive dressing. Tape three of the four sides, allowing the fourth to release entrapped air during exhalation. ▪ Prepare for chest tube insertion or operative management.

Simple pneumothrax	Common/Blunt force trauma	▪ Pneumothorax <15% and no other injury:
		  ▪ Commonly asymptomatic.
		▪ Pneumothorax >15% with other injuries:
		  ▪ Respiratory distress.
		  ▪ Absent breath sounds on the affected side.
		  ▪ Pain.
			▪ Prepare for chest tube insertion for lung reexpansion and prevention of tension pneumothorax.

Hemothorax	Rare/Blunt force or penetrating trauma. The source of bleeding is often an intercostal artery lacerated by a fractured rib. Bleeding may also be due to a major vascular injury or pulmonary parenchymal injury.	▪ Signs of hypovolemic shock. ▪ Respiratory distress. ▪ Absent breath sounds on the affected side. ▪ Dullness with percussion.	▪ Prepare for chest tube insertion. ▪ Initiate fluid resuscitation.
Tension pneumothorax (accumulation of air under pressure in the pleural space)	Rare/Blunt or penetrating forces that disrupt the tracheobronchial structures or lung parenchyma. Air enters the pleural space and becomes entrapped. The entrapped air displaces the mediastinum, creating a shift that can interfere with central venous return and lead to decreased cardiac output.	▪ Respiratory distress. ▪ Dyspnea. ▪ Tachypnea. ▪ Decreased breath sounds on the affected side. ▪ Tracheal deviation away from the affected side (difficult to see in the younger child with a short neck). ▪ Distended neck veins (difficult to assess in the younger child). ▪ Profound respiratory distress and failure with eventual circulatory collapse, if unrecognized. ▪ Shock.	▪ Prepare for immediate placement of a needle thoracostomy in the second intercostal space below the second rib at the midclavicular line. ▪ Prepare for chest tube insertion.

- Prepare for mechanical ventilation.
- Initiate cardiorespiratory and oxygen saturation monitoring.
- Prepare for needle decompression, thoracostomy, and chest tube insertion, as needed.

3. Obtain venous access and initiate an intravenous infusion.
   - Obtain blood specimens for laboratory analysis:
     - Creatinine kinase.
     - Complete blood count and differential.
4. Administer analgesics, as prescribed (Chapter 13).
5. Assess the child's neurologic status.
6. Prepare for diagnostic tests.
   - Twelve-lead electrocardiogram.
   - Anterior-posterior and lateral radiographs of the chest.
7. Inform the family frequently about the child's condition.
8. Provide emotional support to the child and family.
9. Initiate consultations with social services, surgery, and other subspecialties, as needed.
10. Prepare for transfer and transport to a trauma center (Chapter 10) or hospitalization.

Home Care and Prevention

Prevention of chest trauma includes routine usage of child safety restraints and other safety measures. Children generally are not discharged from the ED following thoracic trauma, and parents should expect at least one night's hospitalization for observation.

Conclusion

Cardiopulmonary trauma is a potential source of life-threatening injuries in the pediatric population. Although such injuries are rare, emergency nurses must maintain a high index of suspicion for their presence. Attention to cardiorespiratory functioning and worsening of the child's clinical condition are indicators that further interventions are required.

References

Clemence, B. (2000). Emergency department thoracotomy: Nursing implications for pediatric cases. *International Journal of Trauma Nursing*, *6*, 123-127.

Haller, J., & Paidas, C. (1996). Thoracic trauma. In D. Nichols, M. Yaster, D. Lappe, & J. Haller (Eds.), *Golden hour* (2nd ed., pp. 344-371). St. Louis: Mosby—Year Book.

Slimane, M., Becmeur, F., Aubert, D., Bachy, B., Varlet, F., Chavrier, Y., Daoud, S., Fremond, B., Guys, J., deLagausie, P., Aigrain, Y., Reinberg, O., & Sauvage, P. (1999). Tracheobronchial ruptures from blunt thoracic trauma in children. *Journal of Pediatric Surgery*, *34*(12), 1847-1850.

Soud, T., Saum, P., & Pikulski, S. (1998). Trauma-selected systems. In T. Soud & J. Rogers (Eds.), *Manual of pediatric emergency nursing* (pp. 511-539). St. Louis: Mosby—Year Book.

Webster, H., Grant, M., Slota, M., & Kilian, K. (1998). Pulmonary system. In M. Slota (Ed.), *Core curriculum for pediatric critical care nursing* (pp. 33-143). Philadelphia: Saunders.

35

Abdominal Trauma

Kathy Haley, RN, BSN
Nancy L. Mecham, APRN, FNP

Introduction

Potentially life-threatening abdominal injuries are common in the pediatric population (Table 35.1). About 8% of trauma patients admitted to pediatric trauma centers have documented abdominal injuries (Cooper, Barlow, Discala, & String, 1994). Although trauma is considered a surgical disease, fewer than 15% of children with abdominal injury require operative management (Barkin & Marx, 1999). Abdominal trauma is the most commonly unrecognized cause of fatal injuries (Saldino & Lund, 2000). Successful outcome following abdominal trauma is dependent on its prompt recognition, adequate resuscitation, rapid surgical repair when indicated, and severity of additional injuries.

Pediatric Considerations

Anatomic differences place children at greater risk for abdominal trauma than adults because the child's abdomen is less protected from kinetic forces.

- The abdominal wall is thin and protuberant, with less muscle and subcutaneous tissue.
- The abdominal organs are in close proximity, and multiple abdominal organ injuries are possible.
  - The liver and spleen, located below the rib cage, are proportionately larger in children than in adults.
  - When compressed during a trauma event, the compliant ribs do not afford protection to the abdominal organs, leading to liver and splenic damage.
- Large amounts of blood can be lost into the abdominal cavity, masking signs of shock.
  - Children have a remarkable ability to compensate for significant blood losses into the abdominal cavity.
  - Hemorrhagic shock caused by solid-organ injury is a major cause of morbidity and mortality in the injured child.

Etiology

- Blunt forces:
  - Bicycle crashes
  - Child maltreatment (Chapter 46)
  - Pedestrian incidents
  - Falls
  - Sports activities
  - Motor vehicle crashes
  - Acts of violence
- Penetrating forces:
  - Gunshot wounds
  - Penetrating wounds, including impaled objects, such as iron fence posts
- Acceleration-deceleration forces:
  - Motor vehicle crashes
  - Falls
  - Sports activities
- Crushing forces:
  - Animal bites
  - Machinery

TABLE 35.1 Specific Abdominal Injuries

Abdominal Organ	*Frequency of Injury*	*Signs and Symptoms*	*Results of Diagnostic Tests*	*Additional ED Management*
Spleen	Most commonly injured abdominal organ (Wise, Mudd & Wilson, 2002)	■ External left upper quadrant trauma ■ Generalized or localized left upper quadrant pain ■ Kehr's sign ■ Nausea and vomiting ■ Signs of hypovolemic shock	■ Decreased hematocrit ■ Increased white blood cell count ■ CT scan may reveal free fluid in the abdomen	■ Prepare for hospitalization and bedrest. ■ Splenectomy is rarely indicated.
Liver ■ Grade I: subscapular hematoma; capsular tears ■ Grade II: minor parenchymal lacerations ■ Grade III: deep parenchymal lacerations ■ Grade IV: burst liver injuries (Schafermeyer, 1993)	Second most commonly injured abdominal organ (Schafermeyer, 1993); most common source of lethal hemorrhage (Martin & Derengowski, 1998)	■ External right upper quadrant trauma ■ Generalized or localized right upper quadrant pain ■ Diffuse abdominal tenderness or rebound tenderness ■ Abdominal distention ■ Rigidity ■ Kehr's sign ■ Nausea and vomiting ■ Signs of shock	■ Elevated liver enzymes ■ Decreased hematocrit	■ Prepare for hospitalization and observation. ■ Subcapsular hematoma and organ fracture result in hemorrhage, but bleeding often stops spontaneously, allowing a nonoperative approach in most cases.
Duodenum	Duodenal hematoma occurs more often in children, most likely because of lack of rib protection; can result from lap belt injury	Centralized abdominal pain with periumbilical bruising	■ Intraperitoneal air on abdominal radiograph (if hollow viscus is present) ■ Upper gastrointestinal series (as well as computerized tomography scan and ultrasound) locates the injury (Martin & Derengowski, 1998)	Prepare for operative management.
Stomach	Infrequently injured	■ External trauma to the upper abdomen ■ Bloody gastric drainage ■ Boardlike abdomen and severe pain indicate perforation (Martin & Derengowski, 1998)	■ Free air on abdominal radiograph ■ Upper gastrointestinal series locates injured area (Martin & Derengowski, 1998)	Prepare for operative management.
Pancreas	Infrequently injured	■ Diffuse abdominal tenderness ■ Deep epigastric pain radiating to the back ■ Bilious vomiting (Martin & Derengowski, 1998)	Elevated amylase and lipase	Prepare for abdominal computerized tomography scan with contrast; pseudocysts can develop.

Focused History

Mechanism of Injury

- Motor vehicle crash:
  - Passenger or driver
  - Seating position in vehicle
  - Type of vehicle
  - Type of crash
  - Use of safety restraints
  - Vehicular ejection
- Bicycle crash:
  - Presence of helmet
  - Speed and type of oncoming vehicle
  - Speed of bicycle
  - Stationary object struck (e.g., tree or car)
- Sports-related injury:
  - Use of protective equipment, including helmet
  - Type of sport
- Fall from height to nonyielding surface:
  - Height from which the child fell
  - Surface on which the child fell
- Pedestrian incidents:
  - Speed of vehicle
- Child abuse (Chapter 46)
- Act of violence:
  - Description of the incident
- Gunshot wound:
  - Type of weapon
  - Caliber of bullet
  - Distance or range from which bullet was fired
- Penetrating wound:
  - Type of penetrating object
  - Impaled or removed
- Crushing wound:
  - Type of biting animal
  - Type of machinery

Abdominal Signs and Symptoms following the Injury

- Vomiting
- Pain or tenderness
- Surface trauma
- Distention
- Rupture of intra-abdominal contents

Injury-related Information

- Witnesses
- Prehospital treatment

Focused Assessment

Physical Assessment

1. Assess the airway, respiratory, cardiovascular, and neurologic systems (Chapter 30).
2. Inspect the abdomen for:
   - Surface trauma, such as abrasions, ecchymosis, and penetrating objects.
     - A distinctive pattern results from a lap belt injury.
     - Children tend to be at greater risk for lap belt injuries because they frequently ride in the back seat, where the protective restraint devices are commonly lap belts.
     - If the child is too small for a lap belt, the belt tends to ride up on the child's abdomen instead of being correctly positioned at the pelvis.
     - During a motor vehicle crash, deceleration forces pull the child forward against the lap belt. The resulting triad of injuries is: external belt marks (abdominal ecchymosis or actual belt embedment in subcutaneous tissue); hollow viscus injury (duodenum); and lumbar fracture (Chance fracture) (Saldino & Lund, 2000).
3. Observe the child for:
   - Kehr's sign (left shoulder pain). Free blood in the abdomen irritates the diaphragm and the phrenic nerve, referring pain to the left shoulder.
   - Nausea and vomiting.
   - Abdominal distention.
4. Auscultate the abdomen for bowel sounds:
   - The absence of bowel sounds, although nonspecific, is suggestive of an ileus, which typically results after abdominal injury.
5. Palpate the abdomen gently for:
   - Rebound tenderness, pain, and guarding.
     - Peritoneal signs can be obscured by an altered mental status, and abdominal tenderness may be obscured by pain elsewhere.
   - Distention, rigidity, and masses.
6. Assess the remaining body systems.

Psychosocial Assessment

- Assess the child's and family's coping strategies.
- Assess the child's and family's understanding of the injury.

Nursing Interventions

1. Assess and maintain the child's airway and respiratory status.
   - Perform the jaw thrust maneuver.
   - Prepare for endotracheal intubation, as needed, while maintaining cervical spine precautions.
   - Administer continuous high-flow oxygen.
   - Prepare for mechanical ventilation, as needed.
   - Initiate cardiorespiratory and oxygen saturation monitoring.
2. Obtain venous access and initiate an intravenous infusion of lactated Ringer's solution.
   - Obtain blood specimens for laboratory analysis:
     - Complete blood count and differential
     - Liver enzymes
     - Amylase
     - Lipase
     - Type and crossmatch
3. Assess the child's neurologic status.
4. Insert a nasogastric or orogastric tube, because gastric dilatation arising from aerophagia may confound the abdominal assessment, causing abdominal tenderness and simulating peritonitis.
   - Aspirate a sample of stomach contents and evaluate for blood or bile.
   - Reassess the abdomen for distention; if the abdomen remains distended following decompression, suspect intra-abdominal bleeding.
   - Measure the gastric output.
5. Reassess the child's cardiopulmonary, neurologic, and abdominal status frequently.
6. Prepare for diagnostic procedures such as:
   - Ultrasound.
   - Diagnostic peritoneal lavage.
     - The presence of blood in the peritoneal cavity, as determined by ultrasound or diagnostic peritoneal lavage, provides little value other than confirmation of its presence. The child's overall appearance is evidence of ongoing bleeding and is the crux for determining management pathways.
   - Focused abdominal sonography for trauma (FAST).
   - Computerized tomography studies with and without contrast.
7. Inform the family frequently of the child's condition.
8. Provide emotional support to the child and family.
9. Initiate consultations to social services, surgery, and other subspecialities.
10. Prepare for transfer and transport to a trauma center (Chapter 10) or prepare for hospitalization.

Home Care and Prevention

Abdominal injuries can be prevented through the use of car safety restraints and other safety devices during work and play. Parents should be prepared for at least 24-hour hospitalization for observation of the child after an abdominal injury. Analgesics may be withheld to detect changes in the child's condition; therefore, nonpharmacologic measures to relieve pain should be attempted (Chapter 13).

Conclusion

Because of its frequency, emergency nurses should be prepared for abdominal trauma and its sequelae. The emotional support and comfort provided by the nurse during nasogastric or orogastric tube insertion, as well as during frequent abdominal assessments, helps to calm the injured child.

References

Barkin, R. & Marx, J. (1999). Abdominal trauma. In R. Barkin & P. Rosen (Eds.), *Emergency pediatrics* (5th ed.) (pp. 476–487). St. Louis: Mosby—Year Book.

Cooper, A., Barlow, B., Discala, C., & String, D. (1994). Mortality and truncal injury: The pediatric perspective. *Journal of Pediatric Surgery, 29*(1): 33–38.

Martin, S., & Derengowski, S. (1998). Gastrointestinal system. In M. Slota (Ed.), *Core curriculum for pediatric critical care nursing* (pp. 424–460). Philadelphia: Saunders.

Saldino, R., & Lund, D. (2000). Abdominal trauma. In G. Fleisher & S. Ludwig (Eds.), *Textbook of pediatric emergency medicine* (4th ed., pp. 1361–1368). Baltimore: Williams & Wilkins.

Schafermeyer, R. (1993). Pediatric trauma. *Emergency Medicine Clinics of North America, 11*, 187–205.

Wise, B., Mudd, S., & Wilson, M. (2002). Management of blunt abdominal trauma in children. *Journal of Trauma Nursing, 9*(1), 6–13.

36

Genitourinary Trauma

Kathy Haley, RN, BSN
Christine Nelson, RNC, MS, PNP

Introduction

Genitourinary (GU) injury is common in children. Genitourinary injuries occur to the kidney, ureter, bladder, and urethra (Table 36.1). In males, the scrotum, testicles, and penis may be injured, whereas females may sustain injury to the perineal area. Death from GU injury is rare (Lobe, Gore, & Swischuk, 1995). Treatment is specific for the location and extent of injury and may include bed rest, observation, placement of diverting catheters, or surgical exploration.

Pediatric Considerations

The following anatomic differences place children at risk for GU injuries.

- The child's kidney, one of the most frequently injured organs, is larger in relation to abdominal size and is less protected by the lower ribs than is the adult's kidney (Headrick, 1998).
  - The kidney has a greater magnitude of fetal renal lobulation and a lack of perinephric fat (Lobe et al., 1995).
  - The kidney is relatively mobile and can be easily pushed against the ribs or vertebrae, causing crushing or tearing.
  - Rapid deceleration may cause excessive movement of the kidneys and stretching or tearing of the renal vessels.
  - Pre-existing known or unknown renal conditions (e.g., Wilm's tumor, ectopic kidneys, or enlarged kidneys) may be present.
- Although ureteral trauma is rare (Lobe et al., 1995), ureteral elasticity and torso flexibility allow ureteral injuries to occur.
- The bladder essentially is an abdominal organ in small children, making it more vulnerable to injury (Foltin & Cooper, 1997).
  - Full bladders are common in children; while rare, the distended bladder is more likely to rupture in children compared to adults (Foltin & Cooper, 1997).
- Injury to the anterior (distal) urethra is uncommon in boys because of the urethra's mobility; therefore, any injury to this area is most likely iatrogenic (Lobe et al., 1995). Injury to the urethra in females is rare; contusion may result from foreign bodies or self-inflicted trauma (Lobe et al., 1995).
- Although pelvic fractures are often associated with GU injuries in adults, such fractures are less common in children because of the flexible pelvis.

Etiology

- Blunt forces:
  - Motor vehicle crashes or passenger-side air bag deployment (Smith & Klein, 1997)
  - Falls
  - Sports activities (usually associated with a blow to the flank)
  - Kicks to the flank by large animals
  - Child maltreatment (Chapter 46)

TABLE 36.1 Specific GU Injuries and Their Treatment

Organ	*Mechanism of Injury*	*Physical Assessment Findings*	*Additional ED management*

Kidney	▪ Penetrating trauma (gunshot wound, stabbing)
	▪ Blunt trauma
	▪ Rapid deceleration in falls and motor vehicle collision
		▪ Flank tenderness, pain and bruising, hematuria
		▪ Types of injury:
		  ▪ Type 1: renal contusion
		  ▪ Type 2: cortical laceration
		  ▪ Type 3: calyx tear
		  ▪ Type 4: complete tear or rupture
		  ▪ Type 5: vascular pedicle injury
		  ▪ Type 6: ureteropelvic disruption
			▪ Prepare for radiographic tests.
			▪ Prepare for operative management.

Ureter	▪ Acceleration ▪ Deceleration	▪ Flank mass ▪ Leakage of urine from a wound ▪ Oliguria ▪ Enlarging flank mass ▪ Hematuria	▪ Prepare for diagnostic testing, such as ultrasonography, computerized tomography scan, and retrograde pyelography. ▪ Prepare for operative management.
Bladder	▪ Blunt trauma ▪ Penetrating trauma ▪ Self-inflicted trauma (placement of objects into the urethra) ▪ Iatrogenic trauma (e.g., vigorous performance of the Credé maneuver, placement of an abdominal paracentesis catheter, or suprapubic tap)	Four classes: ▪ Contusion: hematuria without renal injury ▪ Extraperitoneal rupture: concommitant pelvic fracture or penetrating injury; extravasation of contrast media ▪ Intraperitoneal rupture: transmission of blunt forces or penetrating forces; assessment findings similar to abdominal trauma ▪ Combined extraperiotoneal and intraperitoneal rupture: pelvic fracture	▪ Prepare for diagnostic testing (retrograde urethrogram). ▪ Prepare for operative management.
Urethra (partial or complete tear)	Blunt trauma	▪ Associated pelvic fracture ▪ Associated straddle injuries	▪ Prepare for retrograde urethrogram to visualize the entire urethra ▪ Avoid placement of an indwelling bladder catheter with the presence of meatal blood.

From: Lobe et al., 1995.

- Straddle mishaps onto the bar of a bicycle or playground equipment
- Industrial mishaps
- Sexual stimulation activities
- Penetrating forces:
  - Gunshot wounds
  - Penetrating injuries
  - Impaled or inserted foreign bodies
- Acceleration-deceleration forces:
  - Motor vehicle crashes
  - Sports activities
- Crushing forces:
  - Animal bites
  - Machinery

Focused History

Mechanism of Injury

- Motor vehicle crash:
  - Passenger or driver
  - Seating position in vehicle
  - Type of vehicle
  - Type of crash
  - Use of safety restraints
- Sports-related injury:
  - Use of protective equipment, including helmet
  - Type of sport
- Kick to the flank by a large animal:
  - Type of animal
  - Size of animal
- Child maltreatment (Chapter 46).
- Act of violence or sexual assault (Chapter 47).
- Gunshot wound:
  - Type of weapon
  - Caliber of bullet
  - Distance or range from which bullet was fired
- Penetrating wound:
  - Type of penetrating object
  - Impaled, inserted, or removed
- Crushing wound:
  - Type of biting animal
  - Type of machinery
  - Falls

Genitourinary Symptoms following the Injury

- Abdominal pain or tenderness
- Flank pain or tenderness
- Surface trauma to the abdomen, flank, or genital area
- Hematuria
- Painful urination or inability to urinate
- Pain with defecation or inability to defecate
- Vaginal bleeding

Injury-related Information

- Witnesses
- Prehospital treatment

Focused Assessment

Physical Assessment

1. Assess the airway, respiratory, cardiovascular, and neurologic systems (Chapter 30).
2. Assess the abdomen.
   - Inspect the abdomen for:
     - Surface trauma, such as abrasions, ecchymosis, and penetrating objects.
   - Observe the child for nausea and vomiting.
   - Auscultate the abdomen for bowel sounds.
   - Palpate the abdomen gently for:
     - Rebound tenderness, pain, and guarding. Peritoneal signs can be obscured by an altered mental status, and abdominal tenderness may be obscured by pain elsewhere.
     - Distention.
     - Rigidity.
   - Inspect the back for surface trauma or penetrating injury.
   - Palpate the back for costovertebral angle tenderness.
3. Assess the GU system.
   - Inspect the genital area for bruising, lacerations, and the presence of a foreign body.
   - Assess for premenarchal or postmenarchal bleeding. Assess for vaginal bleeding; if present, assess the volume of bleeding and the length of time the bleeding has occurred.

- Assess the female genitalia (Chapter 47). In one study of 56 prepubescent girls, hymenal injuries were reported as rarely caused by unintentional trauma; therefore, hymenal injury should suggest sexual abuse (Bond, Dowd, Landsman, & Rimsza, 1995).
- When abuse or assault is suspected, preserve any evidence (e.g., clothing) and proceed with a victim assault assessment (Chapter 47).
- Assess the male genitalia for open wounds, loss of skin, patterns of ecchymosis and constricting objects.
- Penile circumference is assessed for edema and scrotum is assessed for edema and ecchymoses (Engel, 1997).
- Inspect the urinary meatus for the presence of blood. Blood at the urinary meatus is indicative of a urethral tear.
- Inspect the anus for bruising, tears, and for the presence of a foreign body.

4. Assess the remaining systems.

Psychosocial Assessment

- Assess the child's and family's understanding of the injury.
  - Use words that are familiar to the child for describing the genital area.
  - Assure the child's and family's privacy to obtain an accurate history and to protect them from further emotional duress (Bartwik, Goldfarb, & Trachtenberg, 1995).
- Assess the child's and family's coping strategies.
  - GU injuries resulting from assault or abuse can have devastating effects on the child and family.
  - Early assessment with qualified individuals, such as a victim advocate or child abuse team, is beneficial to the child and family (Chapter 47).

Nursing Interventions

1. Initiate measures to maintain airway, breathing, and circulation.
   - Obtain serial assessments to detect signs of hypovolemic shock.
2. Obtain a urine specimen to evaluate for hematuria from a spontaneous voiding in the awake, cooperative child or through urinary bladder catheterization in the unstable child.
   - Do not attempt urinary bladder catheterization in children with blood at the urinary meatus; blood in the scrotum; or an abnormally positioned or abnormally mobile prostate (Lobe et al., 1995).
   - Routine urethral catheter placement should be avoided in boys younger than 5 years of age to avoid the development of future urethral strictures (Lobe et al., 1995).
   - There appears to be no direct correlation between degree of hematuria and severity of injury; therefore, any child who has significant hematuria is suspected of having injury to the kidney or to any other part of the urinary system until proven otherwise (Foltin & Cooper, 1997).
3. Measure urinary output.
4. Administer analgesics to decrease pain and to promote cooperation, if other injuries do not preclude their use (Bartwik et al., 1995).
5. Prepare for wound cleaning and repair.
   - If the child is uncomfortable with or refuses to participate in the assessment and intervention, examination under anesthesia should be performed, especially in cases of sexual assault or abuse.
6. Prepare for diagnostic testing (Barwik et al., 1995; Cline, Mata, Venable, & Eastham, 1998).
   - Computerized tomography scan
   - Radiographs of the kidneys, ureters, and bladder
   - Ultrasonography
   - Intravenous pyleogram
   - Urethrogram
   - Retrograde urethography
7. Inform the family frequently of the child's condition.
8. Provide emotional support to the child and family; maintain the child's modesty and privacy during assessments and treatments.
9. Initiate consultations to social services and medical subspecialties, as needed.
   - Contact child protective services and the police if assault or abuse is suspected.
10. Prepare for transfer and transport to a trauma center if needed (Chapter 10) or prepare for hospitalization and possible operative management.
    - In one study of 22 females with blunt urogenital trauma who experienced examination under anesthesia, 21 were found to have more severe injuries than those demonstrated in the initial ED evaluation (Lynch, Gardner, & Albanese, 1995).
    - Examination under anesthesia should be used in this population to examine and repair the injuries and to accurately determine whether the injury is consistent with its reported mechanism (Lynch et al., 1995).

Home Care and Prevention

Prevention of GU injuries involves the normal safety measures taken for motor vehicles, sports, and other play activities. Preventive measures for child sexual abuse are discussed in Chapter 47. Parents should be prepared for at least a 24-hour hospitalization of the child for observation of worsening symptoms of GU injury.

Conclusion

Emergency nurses should have a high index of suspicion for GU injuries in children with multiple trauma. The nurse must promote the child's modesty and comfort to gain the child's cooperation during a urogenital assessment and treatment.

References

Bartwik, T., Goldfarb, B., & Trachtenberg, J. (1995). Male genital trauma: Diagnosis and management. *International Journal of Trauma Nursing*, *1*, 99-107.

Bond, G., Dowd, M., Landsman, I., & Rimsza, M. (1995). Unintentional perineal injury in prepubescent girls: A multicenter, prospective report of 56 girls. *Pediatrics*, *95*, 628-631.

Cline, K., Mata, J., Venable, D., & Eastham, J. (1998). Penetrating trauma to the male external genitalia, *Journal of Trauma*, *44*(3), 492-494.

Engel, J. (1997). Reproductive system. *Pocket guide to pediatric assessment* (pp. 208-219). St. Louis: Mosby.

Foltin, G., & Cooper, A. (1997). Abdominal trauma. In R. Barkin (Ed.), Pediatric emergency medicine (pp. 335-354). St. Louis: Mosby—Year Book.

Headrick, C. (1998). Renal system. In M. Slota (Ed.), *Core curriculum for pediatric critical care nursing* (pp. 360-386). Philadelphia: Saunders.

Lobe, T., Gore, D., & Swischuk, L. (1995). Urinary tract injuries. In W. Buntain (Ed.), *Management of pediatric trauma* (pp. 371-382). Philadelphia: Saunders.

Lynch, J., Gardner, M., & Albanese, C. (1995). Blunt urogenital trauma in prepubescent female patients: More than meets the eye! *Pediatric Emergency Care*, *11*, 372-375.

Smith, D., & Klein, F. (1997). Renal injury in a child with airbag deployment. *Journal of Trauma*, *42*, 341-342.

37

Submersion Injuries

Jacqueline Jardine, RN, C
Nancy L. Mecham, APRN, FNP

Introduction

Drowning is defined as death occurring within 24 hours of submersion; near-drowning is defined as survival for at least 24 hours after submersion (Dean & Haller, 1995; Baum, 2000). Drowning and near-drowning are the cause of up to 8,000 deaths each year in the United States. The majority of drowning victims are males younger than 20 years of age, and 40% are younger than 4 years of age (Dean & Haller, 1995). One estimate is that the risk of drowning among children 1 or 2 years of age is 10 times higher than the risk for the general population (Dean & Haller, 1995). Among adolescents, alcohol is a risk factor that gives them a sense of false bravado before their coordination is depressed, leading to a drowning episode (Dean & Haller, 1995). School-aged children and adolescents may overestimate their swimming abilities, become fatigued, and then drown.

Ninety percent of drownings are the result of aspiration of water or vomit from struggling, breath holding, and gasping; the remaining 10% of deaths are due to laryngospasm and asphyxia (Ros, 1996). Despite technological advances in pediatric emergency and critical care medicine, the outcomes remain guarded for children sustaining a submersion injury (Nieves, Buttacavoli, Fuller, Clarke, & Schimpf, 1996).

Pediatric Considerations

Children drown in either fresh or salt water.

- Fresh water disrupts surfactant, resulting in alveolar collapse and pulmonary edema (Ros, 1996).
- Salt water causes shunting and edema because of the movement of intravascular fluid into the alveoli (Ros, 1996), resulting in perfusion of nonventilated alveoli, tissue hypoxia and metabolic acidosis, cardiac dysrhythmias, central nervous system changes, or ischemic injury to other organs (Baum, 2000).
- The "diving" response is believed to protect human beings during submersion episodes. Bradycardia and peripheral vasoconstriction occur, preferentially shunting blood to the heart and brain (Rogers, 1998). Rapid brain cooling in cold-water submersions decreases cerebral metabolism and protects the brain from anoxic injury (Rogers, 1998).

Etiology

Younger Children

- Bathtubs:
  - Frequently, an infant is left in a bathtub that is filled with a few inches of water and a younger sibling (usually younger than 4 years of age) is left to supervise while the adult is out of the room, leading to a submersion injury for the infant and/or the toddler, who is unable to recognize or assist a drowning infant (Dean & Haller, 1995). Bathtub drownings in children older than 1 year should arouse suspicion of intentional injury (Chapter 46).
- Hot tubs or spas:
  - Hot tubs, as well as swimming pools or spas, may have uncovered suction devices that trap the child's hair or other body parts, thus forcibly submerging the child (Dean & Haller, 1995).
- Swimming pools.
- Buckets or pails:
  - Young toddlers who are learning to walk pull themselves to a standing position, peer into the bucket filled with chemically treated water, and submarine themselves into the bucket. They are not strong enough to right themselves or to extricate themselves from the bucket, thus leading to a drowning injury associated with a high mortality rate because of the chemical pulmonary injury (Dean & Haller, 1995).
- Toilets.

Older Children and Adolescents

- Swimming pools.
- Large bodies of water, such as lakes, rivers, and oceans.
- Irrigation ditches.

Focused History

- Body of water in which the child was submerged:
  - Bathtub or hot tub
  - Swimming pool
  - Bucket or pail
  - Toilet
  - Large body of water, such as a lake, river, or ocean
- Composition of the water:
  - Fresh
  - Salt
  - Chemically treated (e.g., cleaning chemicals in a bucket or toilet)
- Temperature of the water:
  - Warm
  - Cold
- Length of time the child was left unattended or believed to be submerged; presence of witnesses.
- Events surrounding the submersion:
  - Diving from a height
  - Operating water craft (e.g., jet skis or motorboat)
  - Consumption of alcohol or other substances
- Symptoms following the submersion:
  - Coughing, sputtering
  - Loss of consciousness
  - Loss of cardiopulmonary function
  - Vomiting
- Prehospital treatment:
  - Cardiopulmonary resuscitation
  - Oxygen administration
  - Application of spinal immobilization
  - Intravenous access

Focused Assessment

Physical Assessment

1. Assess the airway and cervical spine.
   - Listen for signs of airway obstruction.
   - Observe for foreign material, such as vomit or water.
   - Assess for signs of spinal cord injury (Chapter 32).
     - The near-drowning may have resulted from a spinal cord injury sustained when the patient dove into shallow water (Chapter 32). Maintain spinal immobilization during the assessment.
2. Assess the respiratory system.
   - Auscultate the chest for:
     - Respiratory rate. Apnea or bradypnea may be present.
     - Adventitious sounds. Rales, rhonchi, or wheezing may be present.
   - Observe the chest for accessory muscle use, such as retractions.
3. Assess the cardiovascular system.
   - Auscultate the heart for:
     - Rate. Asystole or bradycardia may be present.
     - Rhythm.
     - Clarity.
   - Measure the blood pressure.
   - Assess peripheral perfusion.
     - Measure capillary refill. Capillary refill may be more than 2 seconds.
     - Measure core and skin temperature. Hypothermia may be present.
     - Observe skin color. Cyanosis and mottling may be noted.
     - Assess skin texture.
4. Assess the neurologic system.
   - Measure the level of consciousness with the AVPU (Alert, responds to Verbal stimuli, responds to Painful stimuli, Unresponsive) method or Glasgow coma scale method.
   - Measure pupillary response. Pupils may be unresponsive, fixed, and dilated if submersion was prolonged.
   - Observe for posturing.
5. Assess the gastrointestinal and genitourinary systems.
   - Auscultate bowel sounds.
   - Observe for abdominal rigidity.
   - Observe for urinary output.
6. Assess the integumentary system.
   - Observe for surface trauma, especially on the head and face.
7. Assess the musculoskeletal system.
   - Observe for muscle tone and strength.
     - Muscle flaccidity may indicate spinal cord injury.

Psychosocial Assessment

- Assess the family's coping strategies.
  - Finding a submerged sibling or child is devastating for the involved family members. Guilt and fear may be experienced. Early intervention with social services is essential.
- Assess the family's understanding of the injury.
  - Family members may not appreciate the severity of the child's injury. Reports in the popular press about children who survive cold-water submersions may give the family false hope.
  - Presenting the facts as they are available helps the family to make realistic decisions about their child's course of hospitalization and treatment.

Nursing Interventions

1. Assess and maintain the airway and cervical spine.
   - Prepare for endotracheal intubation.
   - Maintain cervical spine precautions until it is determined that a spinal cord injury is not present.
2. Initiate measures to support cardiorespiratory function.
   - Administer 100% oxygen.
   - Prepare for mechanical ventilation.
   - Initiate cardiopulmonary resuscitation as needed.
   - Initiate cardiorespiratory and oxygen saturation monitoring.
   - Evaluate electrocardiogram readings.
     - Nonspecific ST- and T-wave changes may be noted (Rogers, 1998).
3. Obtain venous access and administer intravenous fluids.
   - Administer medications, such as vasopressor agents, as prescribed.
   - Obtain blood specimens for laboratory analysis.
     - Electrolytes. Fresh and salt water rarely have an effect on serum electrolytes because abnormalities occur only when the amount of fluid aspirated exceeds 22 ml/kg, a finding in only 15% of drowning incidents (Ros, 1996).
     - Blood urea nitrogen and creatinine.
     - Creatinine kinase.
     - Complete blood count.
     - Alcohol and toxicology screening, as needed.
     - Anticonvulsant therapy drug levels.
4. Monitor the child's cardiopulmonary and neurologic statuses.
   - Observe for signs of increased intracranial pressure, and titrate the intravenous fluids accordingly.
5. Remove the child's wet clothing and measure the child's temperature.
   - Prepare for active rewarming measures (Chapter 42), such as:
     - Gastric lavage.
     - Peritoneal lavage.
     - Pleural lavage via chest tubes.
     - Warm intravenous fluids.
     - Cardiopulmonary bypass.
   - Observe for electrocardiographic changes, dysrhythmias, and ventricular fibrillation during rewarming.
6. Insert a nasogastric tube to reduce gastric dilation; measure the output.
7. Insert an indwelling bladder catheter to measure urinary output.
8. Prepare for diagnostic tests.
   - Chest radiographs.
   - Cervical spine radiographs.
   - Arterial blood gases.
9. Inform the family frequently of the child's condition.
10. Provide emotional support to the child and family.
11. Initiate consultations with staff from social services, medical subspecialties, and child protective services, as needed.
    - In one study of 21 children sustaining bathtub near-drownings, 67% had a history and physical findings suggestive of child maltreatment or neglect, including incompatible histories or multiple stories of the submersion event as well as severe physical neglect, bruising, fractures, and retinal hemorrhages (Lavelle, Shaw, Seidl & Ludwig, 1995).
12. Prepare for transfer and transport to a tertiary care center (Chapter 10) or hospital admission.

Home Care and Prevention

Children who sustained a witnessed, short submersion and do not lose consciousness or require cardiopulmonary resuscitation generally require 24-hour observation for any complications. Parents should be prepared for this admission. The prognosis for children who arrive at the ED awake and alert is excellent (Dean & Haller, 1995). If cardiopulmonary arrest occurs, the child's chance for survival is poor.

Children must be well supervised when they are in or near water, both in the home and outdoors. Access to swimming pools must be limited by pool barriers, such as fences, that are (Nieves, Buttacavoli, Fuller, Clarke, & Schimpf, 1996):

- Unclimbable.
- Self-closing.
- Self-locking.
- At least 5 ft in height.
- Built to surround the pool on all sides.
- Constructed so that slats or bars are less than 4 inches apart.

Adults who own pools, as well as adolescents, should be trained in cardiopulmonary resuscitation. Water safety training should begin at an early age. As children grow older, these safety rules should be reinforced, and the use of drugs and alcohol during water-related activities should be discouraged. Use of pool covers with motion alarms should be considered.

Conclusion

Drownings and near-drownings may be infrequent occurrences among the pediatric population presenting to the ED, depending on the ED's geographic location. Rapid assessment of the child's condition and prompt interventions may save the child's life. Emergency nurses should be aware of the possible role of child maltreatment or neglect in submersion injuries involving young children. Emergency nurses can become involved in water safety activities in their community to prevent these tragedies from occurring.

References

Baum C. (2000). Environmental emergencies. In G. Fleisher & S. Ludwig (Eds.), *Textbook of pediatric emergency medicine* (4th ed., pp. 943-963). Baltimore: Williams & Wilkins.

Dean, J., & Haller, J. (1995). Submersion injuries. In W. Buntain (Ed.), *Management of pediatric trauma* (pp. 553-568). Philadelphia: Saunders.

Lavelle, J., Shaw, K., Seidl, T., & Ludwig, S. (1995). Ten-year review of pediatric bathtub near-drownings: Evaluation for child abuse and neglect. *Annals of Emergency Medicine*, *25*, 344-348.

Nieves, J. A., Buttacavoli, M., Fuller, L., Clarke, T., & Schimpf, P. C. (1996). Childhood drowning: Review of literature and clinical implications, *Nursing*, *22*(3): 206-210.

Rogers, J. (1998). Respiratory system. In T. Soud & J. Rogers (Eds.), *Manual of pediatric emergency nursing* (pp. 193-232). St. Louis: Mosby—Year Book.

Ros, S. (1996). Near-drowning. In G. Strange, W. Ahrens, S. Lelyveld, & R. Schafermeyer (Eds.), *Pediatric emergency medicine: A comprehensive study guide* (pp. 601-602). New York: McGraw-Hill.

38

Musculoskeletal Trauma

Laurel S. Campbell, RN, MSN, CEN
Donna Ojanen Thomas, RN, MS

Introduction

Musculoskeletal trauma is responsible for 10 to 15% of emergency department visits in urban pediatric hospitals (Bachman & Santora, 2000). Seventy percent of musculoskeletal injuries in young children result from falls; in older children, injuries most often are related to sports activities and motor vehicle or pedestrian-motor vehicle events (Hodge, 1997). In this age group, injuries related to violence are increasingly more common. Emergency care is directed at treatment measures to prevent loss of function, abnormal growth, and deformity (Hodge, 1997). In addition to the costs for medical care of musculoskeletal injuries, incidental costs are attributed to time lost from school and disruption of parents' work schedule.

Pediatric Considerations

Anatomic features affect the child's response to musculoskeletal injury:

- The bones are in a dynamic state of growth and repair that predisposes them to patterns of injury.
  - An increased porosity results in bones that bow, bend, or buckle without complete fracture.
  - Generally, the younger the child, the faster the rate of bone healing (England & Sundberg, 1996). The rate of bone healing is more rapid in children because there is an abundant blood supply to the developing bone.
  - Pediatric bones also have a thick periosteum with a higher bone-forming potential, contributing to faster healing. Nonunion of a fracture is rare in children.
- Abnormal patterns of bone growth associated with diseases such as osteogenesis imperfecta and osteoporosis can result in pathologic fractures.
- Damage to physeal ("growth") centers may lead to acute or chronic disruptions in growth of the affected extremity.
- Joint and ligamental injuries are rare; traumatic forces are more likely to result in physeal injury.
- During periods of rapid growth, bone growth outpaces muscle lengthening ("growing pains"), increasing the adolescent's risk for injury (Overbaugh & Allen, 1994).

Etiology

Blunt Forces

- High-speed or high-impact sports activities:
  - Skiing
  - Snowboarding
  - In-line skating
  - Skateboarding
  - Climbing
  - Bicycling
  - All-terrain vehicle or motor cross
- Traditional sports activities:
  - Soccer
  - Football
  - Softball
  - Basketball
  - Trampolines
  - Gymnastics

- Falls
- Motor vehicle crashes
- Pedestrian-motor vehicle crashes
- Child maltreatment (Chapter 46)

Penetrating Forces

- Gunshot wounds
- Penetrating wounds

Crushing Forces

- Animal bites
- Machinery
- Pedestrian-motor vehicle crashes

Focused History

Mechanism of Injury

- High-speed or high-impact sports activity:
  - Type of activity
  - Use of protective equipment
- Traditional sports activity:
  - Type of activity
  - Use of protective equipment
- Fall:
  - Height from which the child fell
  - Yielding versus nonyielding surface
- Motor vehicle crash:
  - Child's position in the car
  - Use of safety restraints
  - Type of motor vehicle crash
- Pedestrian-motor vehicle crash:
  - Speed of vehicle
  - Type of vehicle
- Child maltreatment (Chapter 46)
- Gunshot wound:
  - Caliber of bullet
  - Range from which bullet was fired
- Penetrating wound:
  - Type of penetrating object
  - Impaled or removed
- Crushing wound:
  - Type of biting animal
  - Type of machinery

Symptoms following the Injury

- Inability to use the extremity:
  - The child may hold or splint affected upper extremity, limp, or refuse to bear weight on affected lower extremity.
- Loss of motor strength
- Loss of neurovascular function
- Open wounds or deformities
- Pain above, below, and at the injury site

Injury-related Information

- Witnesses
- Prehospital treatment rendered
- Time of injury

Focused Assessment

Physical Assessment

1. Assess the airway, respiratory, cardiovascular and neurologic systems (Chapter 30).
2. Assess the musculoskeletal system.
   - Inspect the extremities for:
     - Deformities.
     - Open wounds.
     - Surface trauma.
   - Assess motor strength and movement.
   - Assess neurovascular status for:
     - Pressure sensation.
     - Pain sensation.
     - Skin color and temperature.
   - Assess for pain (Chapter 13).
3. Assess the integumentary system.
   - Observe for surface trauma.

Psychosocial Assessment

1. Assess the child's and family's understanding of the injury.
   - Children who play competitive sports may erroneously believe that they can reenter sports quickly, when a few weeks of treatment and rest may be required. This knowledge may cause distress and anxiety for the child and family.
2. Assess the child's and family's coping strategies.

Nursing Interventions

1. Maintain airway, breathing, and circulation (Chapter 30).
2. Initiate measures to promote musculoskeletal function.
   - Assess sensory, motor, and neurovascular status.
   - Apply a splint or assist with application of a cast.
   - Reassess sensory, motor, and neurovascular statuses frequently and especially after splint application.
3. Assess the child's pain and administer pharmacologic and nonpharmacologic pain relief measures (Chapter 13).
4. Prepare for diagnostic tests.
   - Radiographs of the extremities.
   - Tissue pressure measurements.
5. Inform the family frequently of the child's condition.
6. Provide emotional support to the child and family.
7. Initiate consultations with social services, orthopedists, and medical subspecialtists, as needed. Consult child protective services if child maltreatment is suspected (Chapter 46).
8. Prepare for transfer and transport to a trauma center (Chapter 10), as needed; prepare for hospitalization or discharge to home.

Home Care and Prevention

A number of strategies are helpful to prevent musculoskeletal trauma, especially during sports-related activities:

- Safety equipment is available for a variety of sports-related activities.
  - Emergency nurses should encourage children and adolescents to wear helmets, elbow and knee pads, and wrist guards when the sport involves physical contact or risk of fall at moderate to high speeds.
  - Many musculoskeletal injuries could be prevented through use of protective gear. Nurses should reinforce the importance of safety equipment usage to parents and coaches as well.
- Adult supervision during contact sports is essential, because a lack of adult supervision during sports activities has been correlated with a higher incidence of serious orthopedic injuries (Saperstein & Nicholas, 1996):
  - Parents should encourage their school districts to require qualified adult supervision during and after school hours in sports and recreational activities.
  - Coaches should be familiar with the common injuries associated with their sport (Overbaugh & Allen, 1994).
  - Coaches and adults also should have basic first aid training that includes recognizing an injury and removing the player from the game.
  - Practice sessions place adolescents at a higher risk for injury than does a competitive match because more players are participating and are practicing for longer hours; therefore, for both contact and noncontact sports, medical care from an athletic trainer or coach should be available during these times (Overbaugh & Allen, 1994).
- Young athletes require an adequate recovery time to allow the injury to heal properly.
  - Athletes who sustain injuries may not be willing to rest their injuries and wait for complete recovery to occur, resulting in poor outcomes.
  - Parents, athletes, and coaches should respect the body's need to heal and should identify alternative strategies for keeping the athlete a part of the team (e.g., coaching or mentoring) until the injury heals.
  - Parents and coaches should determine the adolescent athlete's coping abilities related to performance and competition, because increased stress may be associated with increased injuries (Overbaugh & Allen, 1994).
- Encourage young athletes to employ proper training, strengthening, and stretching exercises particular to their sport.
  - Team players should be of the same physical maturation, weight, size, and skill (Overbaugh & Allen, 1994).
  - During the prepubertal years, females' motor strength and skills are equal to or somewhat better than males of the same age; after puberty, however, males' muscle mass increases, and gender separation, even during unstructured games and activities, is advisable (Overbaugh & Allen, 1994).

Specific Injuries

Long Bone Fractures

Fractures are common in children because of their high-speed, high-impact activities. Fractures often occur at the physis (growth plate) in children. Overall, up to 18 to 30% of pediatric fractures involve the physis. Physeal injuries are more common in adolescents than in younger children, with a peak incidence at 11 to 12 years of age (Bachman & Santora, 2000). Most growth plate injuries occur in the upper limbs, particularly in the radius and ulna.

Several classification systems have been described for physeal fractures. The most widely used is that of Salter-Harris who describe five types of growth plate

TABLE 38.1 Salter Harris Classification of Physeal Fractures

Classification	*Description*
Type I	Involves separation of the metaphysis from the epiphysis through the zone of provisional calcification. Type I fractures are generally benign with little chance of growth disturbance if near anatomic reduction is achieved.
Type II	Most common type of physeal fracture. Similar to a type I fracture, except that a portion of metaphyseal bone is displaced with the epiphyseal fragment. The fracture line crosses the germinal growth plate as it courses toward the metaphyis. These fractures usually have a good prognosis.
Types III and IV	Intra-articular injuries that involve the growth plate. Anatomic position must be established to restore normal joint mechanics and prevent growth arrest. Orthopedic consult should be obtained because of an increased risk of functional disability.
Type V	Results from axial compression of the germinal growth plate. Difficult to diagnose and the diagnosis is often made after a growth arrest becomes evident.

Data from: Bachman & Santora, 2000.

TABLE 38.2 Long-Bone Fracture Types

Fracture Type	*Description*
Greenstick	Partial fracture does not completely extend through the bony cortices.
Transverse	Fracture line extends perpendicular to the longitudinal axis of the bone.
Oblique	Fracture line extends at an angle to the longitudinal axis of the bone.
Spiral	Often associated with a twisting force applied as the distal end of the extremity is immobile, the fracture line extends around the longitudinal axis of the bone. The mechanism of injury associated with this type of fracture should raise suspicion of child maltreatment.
Torus fracture ("buckle fracture")	Compression fracture of the bone at the junction of the metaphysis and diaphysis causes "buckling."
Open	Soft tissue and skin are disrupted over the site of the fracture, either from the direct blow to the area or from the jagged edges of the broken bones.
Comminuted	Bone is broken into several pieces.

fractures, each having specific prognostic and treatment implications (Bachman & Santora, 2000). These are described in Table 38.1. Table 38.2 describes types of long bone fractures in children.

Focused Assessment

Physical Assessment

1. Assess the unaffected extremity first and then the affected extremity. Tables 38.3, 38.4, and 38.5 describe upper extremity, lower extremity, and other injuries, respectively.
    - Assess for pain.
        - Gently touch or palpate the extremity; note if point tenderness is present.
        - Ask the child (or parent) to point to the pain.
        - Observe for pain with movement.
        - Ask the child if he or she has pain with movement.
    - Observe for pallor.
    - Test for paresthesias:
        - Lightly touch the fingers or toes and ask the child if he or she can feel the touch.
        - Ask the child if he or she feels "electric shocks" or "pins and needles" in the fingers or toes.
    - Observe for paralysis or ask the child if he or she can move the extremity.
    - Palpate the distal pulses for:
        - Equality.
        - Quality.

TABLE 38.3 Upper Extremity Fractures

Fracture Location	*Etiology*	*Assessment Findings*	*Interventions*
Clavicle	Fall or blow to the shoulder or extended arm	■ Most often occurs between the middle and lateral thirds on radiograph ■ Pain with movement of upper arm and neck ■ Asymmetry of clavicles	■ Immobilize for 3 to 6 weeks with a figure-8 splint. ■ Orthopedic referral if neurovascular compromise.
Proximal humerus	Blunt trauma to the arm or shoulder	■ Epiphyseal fracture (most often Salter-Harris type I or II,) ■ Extreme pain with movement of arm ■ Swelling ■ Rarely displacement	■ Apply a sling and swath dressing or shoulder immobilizer. ■ Prepare for reduction if angulation is great.
Humeral shaft	Direct impact, such as a fall on the elbow or hand; uncommon in children; suspect child maltreatment with a spiral fracture	■ Swelling ■ Localized tenderness ■ Angulation ■ Possible neurovascular compromise	■ Immobilize, possibly with a sugar-tong (long arm) splint with the elbow at 90°. ■ Arrange for evaluation by an orthopedic surgeon.
Supracondylar	■ Fall onto an outstretched arm with the elbow extended, or a fall on the flexed elbow ■ May also occur from a snapping force, as in throwing a baseball too hard	■ Tenderness and deformity of the distal humerus ■ Pain with flexion of the elbow ■ Possible neurovascular compromise—evidenced by pain with extension of the fingers (Volkmann's contracture)	■ Immediately evaluate and immobilize in extension (excessive flexion can compromise perfusion). ■ Orthopedic consultation. ■ Assess neurovascular status before and after immobilization. ■ Prepare for open reduction and internal fixation.
Radial head and neck	Fall onto an outstretched hand. This is relatively uncommon in children.	■ Child often will hold the elbow in flexion ■ Tenderness ■ Ecchymosis ■ Referred pain to wrist	■ Prepare for closed reduction unless displacement is significant. ■ Long arm splint for nondisplaced fracture, including immobilization of wrist and a sling.
Distal radius (Colles' fracture)	Fall on the palm of the hand or a blow to the forearm	■ Pain over fracture side with dorsal angulation and loss of the volar tilt to the distal radial articulating surface ■ Radiographs should include the elbow and wrist	■ Orthopedic consultation. ■ Evaluate for neurovascular compromise. ■ Prepare for closed or open reduction with internal fixation.

Data from: Chetham, 1999.

- Note the skin temperature.
  - The affected extremity may feel cooler than the unaffected extremity.

2. Inspect the affected extremity for:
   - Obvious swelling.
   - Angulation.
   - Crepitus.
   - Soft tissue disruption at the injury site (possible open fracture).
   - Extremity shortening (possible complete fracture).
   - Joint stability above and below the injury.

Psychosocial Assessment

1. Assess the child's understanding of the injury.
   - Often children are injured because they have participated in risky behaviors despite the warnings of "grown-ups." They may not be willing to give details of the mechanism of injury or of the events and circumstances surrounding the injury episode. The child may make up an entirely different history to avoid punishment.
   - Preschool-aged children usually are injured during play or as a result of defiance of parental instruction. They may not give a reliable history if fearful of punishment.

TABLE 38.4 Lower Extremity Fractures

Fracture Location	*Mechanism of Injury*	*Diagnostic Findings*	*Interventions*
Tibia, fibula	Rotational forces and direct impact; most common injuries to the lower extremities in children	▪ May be able to bear weight, usually will limp ▪ Point tenderness ▪ Possible angulation ▪ Possible neurovascular compromise distal to the injury	▪ Orthopedic consultation ▪ Prepare for closed or open reduction. ▪ Observe for compartment syndrome. ▪ Isolated fibular fractures are managed with a short leg walking cast. ▪ Undisplaced tibial fractures can be immobilized in a long leg posterior splint.
Ankle	Inversion or aversion injury; common in children who are in active phases of growth	▪ Usually unable to bear weight ▪ Swelling ▪ Point tenderness ▪ Ecchymosis ▪ Deformity	▪ Be aware of high possibility of epiphyseal fracture. ▪ Prepare for closed reduction if no swelling is present. ▪ Apply a splint until a cast can be applied after swelling is diminished.
Foot	Crushing injuries from heavy objects or fall from height; relatively uncommon	▪ Possible marked swelling, which may compromise neurovascular status	▪ Provide an orthopedic referral, especially if the fracture involves the epiphysis. ▪ Prepare for closed reduction.

Data from: Moon, 1999.

- School-aged children also are injured as a result of play or risk-taking behavior. Older school-aged children may provide a more reliable version of the injury episode.
- Adolescents may fear parental punishment if the injury circumstances included alcohol or risk-taking behaviors; if so, their history may be unreliable. They may give a more detailed history if the parents are not present.

2. Assess the family's understanding of the injury.
   - With child maltreatment, the injury history may be incompatible with the fracture, or there may be a delay in seeking treatment (Chapter 46).
3. Assess the child and family's coping strategies.

Nursing Interventions

1. Assess and maintain airway, breathing, and circulation.
2. Initiate measures to support the musculoskeletal system.
   - Immobilize the affected extremity in the presenting position or position of function unless evidence of neurovascular compromise is present (pallor, pulselessness, paresthesia, cool skin, or paralysis distal to injury). Immobilization can be accomplished with commercially available splints, slings, and swaths.
   - Immobilize the joint above and below the fracture.
     - If a joint injury has occurred, immobilize the bone above and below the affected joint (Hodge, 1997).
   - Assist with manual realignment if neurovascular compromise is present.
   - Apply cold packs to the affected area to decrease swelling and pain (avoid direct contact between cold pack and skin).
   - Elevate the affected extremity.
3. Assess for pain; administer analgesics, as prescribed.
4. Prepare for diagnostic tests.

TABLE 38.5 Description, Assessment, and Interventions of Selected Musculoskeletal Injuries

Injury	*Etiology*	*Physical Assessment*	*Interventions*	*Complications*
Hip fracture	Rare in children, it is usually associated with a high-velocity impact (motor vehicle crash, bicycle crash, fall from significant height).	■ Inability to bear weight ■ Pain with gentle hip movement	■ Immobilize the extremity. ■ Prepare for internal fixation (England & Sundberg, 1996).	Avascular necrosis of the femoral head and growth disturbances: ■ Prognosis is based on the degree of displacement and fracture level. ■ The more proximal the fracture and the greater amount of displacement, the higher the incidence of avascular necrosis (England & Sundberg, 1996).
Femur fracture	Associated with high-velocity impact, it is often included in Waddell's triad (concurrent lower extremity, abdomen/chest, and head injuries following pedestrian-motor vehicle crashes).	■ Inability to bear weight ■ Extremity shortening if fracture is complete ■ Significant angulation and swelling	Interventions depend on the child's age, the amount of displacement, and the psychosocial impact of the treatment: ■ Children younger than 2 years with a nondisplaced fracture with minimal (< 1 to 2 cm) shortening may be treated with spica casting. ■ Older children require longer healing times and would not tolerate prolonged immobilization with casting, so more invasive measures such as external fixation or open reduction with intramedullary fixation are used (England & Sundberg, 1996).	Excessive blood loss: ■ It has been suggested that isolated femur fractures are not associated with as significant blood loss as previously believed. ■ Most children demonstrating hemodynamic instability or need for transfusion had other injuries that contributed to blood loss. Children with isolated femur fractures rarely lose amounts of blood significant enough to require transfusions. (Ciareillo & Fleisher, 1996; Lynch, Gardner, & Gaines, 1996) ■ Serum laboratory values should be monitored as indicators for need for blood transfusion (Ciarallo & Fleisher, 1996; Lynch et al., 1996). ■ Intravenous access and infusion of crystalloid solutions is still appropriate for pediatric patients.
Subluxation of the radial head (nursemaid's elbow)	A common dislocation in young children, it occurs after a traction force (such as a pulling or jerking of the arm by an older child or caregiver) is applied to the extended arm.	■ Symptoms similar to those of fracture ■ Inability or unwillingness to move the arm ■ No point tenderness	■ Reduce the subluxation by supplanting the forearm with the elbow in 90° of flexion (England & Sundberg, 1996) or pronating the forearm with the elbow in extension. Usually a "pop" is felt, and the child will be able to use the arm normally shortly after the manipulation.	None

(continued)

TABLE 38.5 Description, Assessment, and Interventions of Selected Musculoskeletal Injuries (continued)

Injury	*Etiology*	*Physical Assessment*	*Interventions*	*Complications*

Strain	An injury to a muscle-tendon unit, it is relatively uncommon in children.	■ Pain with movement and range of motion
		■ Swelling and ecchymosis
		■ Inability to bear weight on the affected extremity
		■ Often classified as (Saperstein & Nicholas, 1996):
		  ■ *Grade I:* Mild tenderness and pain with passive stretch; usually the child is able to bear weight.
		  ■ *Grade II:* More severe pain with spasm and restricted movement; some swelling and ecchymosis may be present.
		  ■ *Grade III:* A gross defect in the muscle; severe pain with movement; swelling, ecchymosis.
			■ Radiographs may be indicated to rule out tendon avulsion with an attached piece of bone (Hodge, 1997).
			■ Rest the muscle in the lengthened position.
			■ Allow gradual restoration of active motion followed by strengthening exercises until strength is within 90% of that of the contralateral extremity.
				Returning to activity before healing has occurred can result in severe reinjury.

Sprain	This injury to a ligament is more common in children before they experience a growth spurt and in adolescence after the closure of the growth plate (Saperstein & Nicholas, 1996).	■ Often classified as (Hodge, 1997):
		  ■ *Grade I:* Stretched ligament, normal joint stability; child usually can bear weight.
		  ■ *Grade II:* A partial tearing of the ligament with some joint instability, pain with weight bearing, localized soft tissue hemorrhage, and swelling.
		  ■ *Grade III:* A complete ligament tear resulting in an unstable, unusable joint, with ecchymosis, deformity, and swelling. The child will not be able to bear weight on the joint.
		■ Knee ligament sprains occur as a result of contact and noncontact sports activities in which sudden deceleration during running or moving occurs. The force involved in injuring the ligament may also result in an avulsed fracture of the tibia that may require surgery. Knee ligament sprains include (Saperstein & Nicholas, 1996):
		  ■ *Medial collateral ligament (MCL):* Usually associated with an external rotation force such as high-speed impact with another player.
		  ■ *Anterior cruciate ligament (ACL):* Often associated with skiing, basketball, and other sports as a result of hyperextension or combined valgus and external rotation of a flexed knee.
			Depends on the age of the child, the risk of growth disturbance, and whether rupture of the affected ligament has occurred.
			If surgical repair is not necessary or delayed, brace the affected area; have the child avoid sports with jumping or side-to-side motion or rapid deceleration (Saperstein & Nicholas, 1996).
				None

- Obtain radiographs of the extremities:
  - Comparison views of the unaffected extremity may be helpful to confirm suspected elbow fracture or to distinguish a fracture line from a growth plate (England & Sundberg, 1996).

5. Prepare for additional interventions.
   - Closed reduction with conscious sedation
   - Casting
   - Splinting
6. Inform the family frequently of the child's condition.
7. Provide emotional support to the child and family.
8. Initiate consultations with social services, orthopedists, and other medical specialists, as needed. Consult with child protective services if child maltreatment is suspected (Chapter 46).
9. Prepare for transfer and transport to a trauma or tertiary care center (Chapter 10), as needed; prepare for operative management if needed; prepare for discharge to home.

Home Care and Prevention

Depending on the fracture type and location, the child may have to learn proper crutch walking and activity modification on emergency department discharge. The child and family may require instruction in cast care and pain management. A prescription for narcotic analgesics or over-the-counter analgesics should be given to the parent on discharge. If an elastic bandage, sling/swath, or splint is to be used, the child and parent should perform a return demonstration of its application and use, to promote their confidence in doing these applications at home. Finally, parents should be taught about the signs and symptoms of neurovascular compromise and should have the telephone numbers of the emergency department and their primary care physician or other medical specialist to contact if neurovascular compromise is detected.

Quiet play activities, such as board and card games, videos, and other nonstressful games, should be encouraged for a few days until the child grows accustomed to the immobilization. Follow-up for cast removal should be arranged.

Parents must be instructed about proper cast care prior to leaving the emergency department (Ball, 1998):

1. Elevate the extremity higher than the heart level for approximately 2 days or the amount of time prescribed by the physician. Use pillows, towels, or blankets to prop up the extremity.
2. If prescribed by the physician, place a plastic bag of ice on the area of the broken bone.
3. Assess the neurovascular function of the fractured extremity.
   - Have the child wiggle the finger or toes, gently pinch the digits to assess capillary refill, and touch the digits to assess temperature.
     - Increased or decreased skin temperature, tingling without feeling, delayed color return, inability to move the digits, edema, or pain unrelieved by analgesics should be reported to the emergency department or to the primary care physician to prevent compartment syndrome, which is discussed later in this chapter.
4. Keep plaster casts clean and dry.
   - Plaster casts require about 1 to 2 days to dry; therefore, keep the cast uncovered and reposition it frequently to allow for air circulation.
   - If desired, use a portable fan to quicken the drying process; do not use hand-held hair dryers because the heat is too high, resulting in skin burns and mold formation.
   - If tub baths or showers are permitted by the physician, wrap the cast in plastic and keep it out of the tub during bathing.
   - If the cast becomes dirty, rub baking soda on the cast with a damp cloth.
   - If the cast is near the diaper area, change the diaper frequently and tuck the diaper into the cast to avoid soiling of the cast.
5. Dry plastic casts whenever they are wet.
   - If the child is permitted to swim or bathe with the cast, clean it afterward with a mild soap, rinsing well.
6. Apply ice-filled plastic bags to the cast if the child experiences itching.
   - Never apply powder or lotions under the cast.
   - Never place objects, such as a ruler, into the cast to relieve the itching.

Prior to ED discharge, the child with crutches should be taught the basics of crutch walking and should give a return demonstration of the ability to use the crutches while getting up from a chair, to sit down, during three-point gait (weight on one leg), during swing-through gait (weight on both legs), and while walking up and down steps with and without hand rails (Ball, 1998). The child should be instructed that crutches are not to be used as a toy or weapon. Family and friends should not use the crutches, because they are adjusted for the child's height. While the child is using crutches, parents should take the following safety measures (Ball, 1998):

1. Have the child wear a flat, rubber-soled shoe on the uninjured leg to reduce slipping.
2. Remove home hazards, such as scatter rugs, loose carpets, electrical cords, and other household items that may cause a slip and fall.
3. Have a family member assist the child with walking up and down steps to avoid a loss of balance and a fall.

Following a diagnosis of sprains and strains, parents and children should be taught the "RICE" method for home treatment.

1. **R**est the extremity.
2. Apply **I**ce to the injured area every 2 to 3 hours for 30-minute periods during the first 48 hours postinjury.
3. **C**ompress the area with a snug elastic bandage (assess neurovascular status frequently).
4. **E**levate the extremity to decrease edema (Ball, 1998).

The family should contact the ED or their primary care physician if signs of neurovascular compromise, excessive edema, and/or pain unrelieved by analgesics are present (Ball, 1998).

Compartment Syndrome

Compartment syndrome is usually associated with closed trauma to an extremity or circumferential burns. Compartment syndrome is rare in young children unless these injuries are present. Onset of compartment syndrome is rare, but possible, as a result of massive fluid infiltration during resuscitation (Block, Dobo, & Kirton, 1995) or as a result of physical exertion (Bidwell, Gibbons, & Godsiff, 1996).

Each extremity contains several fascial compartments that contain muscle, capillaries, and major sensory nerves. The lower leg has at least five compartments: anterior, lateral, superficial posterior, deep posterior, and posterior tibial. Pressures in compartments can also be affected by casts and circumferential pressure dressings.

Hemorrhage and soft tissue edema associated with trauma or surgery result in increased pressure in the confining fascia of the extremities' muscle compartments. When tissue pressure is near the level of diastolic pressure, capillary flow is diminished. Pressure reduces venous return and results in gradual closure of small arterioles and capillaries. Ischemia can occur even if pulses are present. Eventually, pressures are high enough to occlude arterial supply.

Compartment pressures are measured invasively with commercially available instruments. Pressure is expressed in terms of "absolute" values (normal is less than 10 mm Hg) or in "differential" pressures (diastolic minus compartment pressure) (McQueen & Court-Brown, 1996). Decompression of the compartment is usually recommended if the differential pressure level drops to less than 30 mm Hg or if the absolute pressure rises above 30 to 40 mm Hg (McQueen & Court-Brown, 1996). Absolute compartment pressures may be an unreliable indicator of the need for fasciotomy. Differential pressure measurement may be a better threshold for fasciotomy (McQueen & Court-Brown, 1996).

Etiology

- Circumferential or extensive, deep, partial-thickness, or full-thickness burns to the extremities
- Massive trauma to the extremities (e.g., crushing injury)
- Child maltreatment (tying of a child's leg or arm to a chair or bed to prevent the child from moving)
- Chronic exertional compartment syndrome—pain that decreases with cessation of exercise.
- Acute exertional compartment syndrome—pain that increases after exercise has stopped.
- Recent application of a cast or circumferential dressing

Focused History

Mechanism of injury

- Circumferential or extensive, deep, partial-thickness or full-thickness burns to the extremities:
  - Depth
  - Percent
  - Location
- Crushing or degloving wound:
  - Location
  - Circumstances surrounding the injury
- Child maltreatment (tying of a child's leg or arm to a chair or bed to prevent the child from moving) (see Chapter 46)
- Chronic exertional compartment syndrome—pain that decreases with cessation of exercise:
  - Type of exercise
  - Duration of exercise
  - Duration of symptoms
- Acute exertional compartment syndrome—pain that increases after exercise has stopped:
  - Type of exercise

- Duration of exercise
- Duration of symptoms
- Recent application of a cast or circumferential dressing:
    - Reason for cast or dressing

Symptoms following the injury

- Pain
- Paralysis
- Paresthesia
- Polar (cool skin temperature)
- Pulselessness
- Pallor

Injury-related information

- Onset (sudden versus insidious)
- Prehospital care (e.g., removal of dressing or cast)

Focused Assessment

Physical Assessment

- Assess the musculoskeletal system for pain that:
    - Is out of proportion to the severity of the injury.
    - Occurs with passive stretch.
    - Is located in the muscles near the injury site.
- Palpate the affected muscles.
    - Muscles in the affected compartment are hard.
- Palpate the distal pulses for:
    - Quality.
    - Equality.
- Test for sensation.
    - Sensory deficits may be present distal to the injury.
- Observe and test for paralysis of muscles distal to injury.

Psychosocial Assessment

- Assess the child's response to pain.
    - Young children usually have a predictable response to the pain as well as to the painful procedures involved in diagnosis and treatment.
    - Adolescents may seem stoic during painful diagnostic procedures, but they often experience significant levels of pain.
- Assess the child's and family's understanding of the condition.
- Assess the child's and family's coping strategies.

Nursing Interventions

1. Initiate measures to relieve the pressure.
    - Split an existing cast.
    - Remove any constrictive clothing, dressings, or elastic bandages.
2. Initiate measures to promote peripheral perfusion.
    - Position the extremity at or lower than the level of the heart.
    - Prepare for continuous invasive monitoring of the compartment pressure.
    - Assist with emergency fasciotomy.
    - Monitor peripheral perfusion distal to the injury.
3. Inform the family frequently of the child's condition.
4. Provide emotional support to the child and family.
5. Initiate consultations with social services, orthopedists, and child protective services, as needed.
6. Prepare for transfer and transport to a tertiary care center (see Chapter 10); prepare for operative management.

Home Care and Prevention

Parents should be taught the signs and symptoms of compartment syndrome when their child is discharged from the emergency department with a cast or circumferential dressing. It should be stressed to the parents that a delay in seeking treatment following the onset of symptoms can result in muscle weakness, contractures, and delayed fracture healing. Exertion-induced compartment syndrome can occur in even the most highly trained athletes, so it is difficult to prevent this syndrome in this population. However, these individuals should be taught the signs and symptoms of compartment syndrome and the actions to initiate should they arise.

Conclusion

Although rarely life threatening, musculoskeletal trauma can affect the child's mobility and growth as the child develops. Early recognition of neurovascular compromise may save a child's limb function and improve the functional outcome. Emergency nurses can become involved in teaching coaches, trainers, adults, and adolescents how to recognize and prevent sports injuries.

References

Bachman, D. & Santora, S. (2000). Orthopedic trauma. In G. R. Fleisher and S. Ludwig (Eds.), *Textbook of pediatric emergency medicine* (4th ed., pp. 1435-1478). Philadelphia: Lipincott, Williams and Wilkins.

Ball, J. (Ed.). (1998). Sprains and stains. In J. Ball (Ed.), *Mosby's pediatric patient teaching guidelines* (pp. H-9, H-11, H-12). St. Louis: Mosby—Yearbook.

Bidwell, J., Gibbons, C. & Godsiff, S. (1996). Acute compartment syndrome of the thigh after weight training. *British Journal of Sports Medicine*, *30*,(3), 265-265.

Block, E., Dobo, S., & Kirton, O. (1995). Compartment syndrome in the critically injured following massive resuscitation: Case reports. *Journal of Trauma*, *39*(4), 787-791.

Chetham, M. (1999). Upper extremity injuries. In R. Barkin and P. Rosen (Eds.), *Emergency pediatrics. A guide to ambulatory care* (pp. 524-533). St. Louis: Mosby.

Ciarello, L. & Fleisher, G. (1996). Femoral fractures: Are children at risk for significant blood loss? *Pediatric Emergency Care*, *12*(5), 343-346.

England, S. & Sundberg, S. (1996). Management of common pediatric fractures. *Pediatric Clinics of North America*, *43*(5), 991-1012.

Hodge, D. (1997). Musculoskeletal and soft tissue injuries: Management principles. In R. Barkin (Ed.), *Pediatric emergency medicine: Concepts and clinical practice* (2nd ed., pp. 381-390), St. Louis: Mobsy.

Lynch, J. M., Gardner, M. J., & Gains, B. (1996). Hemodynamic significance of pediatric femur fractures. *Journal of Pediatric Surgery*, *31*(10), 1358-1361.

McQueen, M. & Court-Brown, C. (1996). Compartment monitoring in tibial fractures. The pressure threshold for decompression. *Journal of Bone and Joint Surgery* (British), *78*(1), 99-104.

Moon, S. (1999). Lower extremity injuries, ankle and foot injuries. In R. Barkin and P. Rosen (Eds.), *Emergency pediatrics. A guide to ambulatory care* (pp. 544-555). St. Louis: Mosby.

Overbaugh, K. & Allen, J. (1994). The adolescent athlete: Part II. Injury patterns and prevention. *Journal of Pediatric Healthcare*, *8*(5), 203-211.

Saperstein, A. & Nicholas, S. (1996). Pediatric and adolescent sports medicine. *Pediatric Clinics of North America*, *43*(5), 1013-1033.

39

Burn Trauma

Mary Jo Cerepani, MSN, CRNP, CEN

Introduction

Burns are the second leading cause of death among children aged 0 to 4 years of age and the third leading cause of death in children aged 4 to 9 years (Ray & Yuwiler, 1994). Each year, 2,500 children in the United States die from burns, and nearly 10,000 suffer permanent disability (American Burn Association, 2001). Although most burns are not fatal, they can be disfiguring and disabling.

Children are at greater risk for burn injury because of their inability to recognize a dangerous situation; they also are less likely to respond appropriately when an injury occurs. Table 39.1 outlines risk factors associated with burn injuries in the pediatric population. The purposes of this chapter are to describe the mechanisms of burn trauma and to outline the nursing assessment and intervention of the burn-injured child.

Pediatric Considerations

Children are more likely to sustain a serious burn and more likely to die from it than are adults. This increased likelihood of morbidity and mortality is related to unique physiologic and pathophysiologic changes in children following a burn injury (Bernardo & Sullivan, 1990):

- Children have a larger body surface-area-to-weight ratio than do adults, placing them at increased risk for hypothermia resulting from convective and evaporative heat following a thermal injury.
- Young children have thin, delicate skin and shallow dermal appendages; therefore, a deeper thickness of burn injury occurs at lower temperatures and shorter exposure times and increases children's susceptibility to the effects of thermal injury.
- The child's small airway diameter is easily obstructed by edema and mucus.
  - Inhalation injuries are devastating, because they lead to rapid edema and airway obstruction.
  - Young children rely on the diaphragm for breathing; chest eschar can restrict diaphragmatic movement and impede respiratory effort.
  - Oxygen consumption is high (6–8 ml/kg) in children, and this demand is increased following a burn injury.
- Decreased cardiac output occurs after a burn injury because of decreased preload due to third spacing. Inadequate fluid resuscitation results if this physiologic factor is not recognized early.
- Children have greater metabolic needs because they have less glycogen stored in the liver, resulting in hypoglycemia.
- The ability to concentrate urine increases with age; inadequate fluid resuscitation can impair renal function.

Etiology

Thermal Burns

- Thermal burns result from exposure to hot temperatures. Infants' and children's skin can tolerate exposure to temperatures at or below 111°F (44°C) for extended periods of time. Exposure above that temperature leads to tissue destruction resulting in full-thickness burns.

TABLE 39.1 Risk Factors Associated with Burn Injuries

Age Group	*Developmental Factors and Activities*	*Burn Injury Risk*
Infants	■ Frequently being held by adults during meal times	Scald burn
	■ Crawling infants: pulling tablecloths and hot items onto themselves	Scald burn
	■ Older infants in baby walkers: pulling hot items onto themselves	Scald burn
Toddlers	■ Exploring environment; learning to walk and run; are uncoordinated	Scald burn
	■ Biting on electrical cords; placing fingers into electrical outlets	Electrical burn
	■ Learning to feed self; exploring chemicals kept in the kitchen and bathroom	Chemical burn
Preschoolers	■ Learning to turn on the water for a bath	Scald burn
	■ Imitating parents—grabbing and pulling on pots and pans; striking matches	Flame burn
School-aged children	■ Participating in household cleaning can lead to mixing cleaning agents	Chemical inhalation injury
	■ Experiencing peer pressure and dares to perform potentially dangerous activities	Electrical injury; flame burn
	■ Learning to use matches to light barbecue grills, campfires, candles	Flame burn
	■ Playing with chemistry sets	Chemical and flame injury
Adolescents	■ Working in restaurants	Scald or flame burn
	■ Using gasoline-powered equipment, such as lawnmowers and cars	Flame burn
	■ Using hair dryers or electric radios while standing on a wet bathroom floor	Flame or electrical burn
	■ Being exposed to electricity during home repairs or in the outdoors	Electrical burn
	■ Playing sports outdoors during an electrical storm	Lightning injury
	■ Smoking cigarettes in enclosed spaces where gasoline or flammable agents are stored	Flame or flash burn
	■ Sniffing gasoline or natural gas	Flame or chemical burn
	■ Returning to a burning building to rescue people or pets	Flame burn; inhalation injury

From: Bernardo, L. & Sullivan, K. (1990).

Scalds

- Scald burns are the most common thermal injuries in children younger than 3 years of age.
- The greatest number of scald burns occur in the bathroom and kitchen.
- Contact with hot liquids such as tea, coffee, or water may cause a full-thickness burn in only 1 second.
- Prolonged exposure to tap water heated to 125°F (52°C) or higher may cause a full-thickness burn.
- Immersion in scalding water results in wound demarcation, indicative of child maltreatment (Chapter 46).

Flame

- Flame injuries are more common in older children, yet children aged birth to 5 years are at the greatest risk for fire-related deaths in the home (Benjamin & Heindon, 2002).
- Flame burns are the second most common burns in children 3 years of age and older.
- Flame injuries may be caused by matches or lighters, house fires, faulty electrical wiring, cooking incidents, fireworks, wood stoves, or kerosene heaters.
- The flame burn is often associated with an inhalation injury from the hot air and toxic fumes emanating from the burning substances.
- The combustible material of the surrounding environment may produce toxic fumes (e.g., carbon monoxide), which can significantly compromise the respiratory system. A patient burned outdoors has a lower risk of inhalation injury; however, the absence of a history of entrapment (confinement in a closed space) does not exclude inhalation injury.

Flash burns

- Flash burns are caused by an explosion, ignition of gasoline fumes, or an electrical flash.
- These burns may cause severe facial edema and inhalation injury from increased heat production.

Contact with hot objects

- Contact burns are caused from exposure to hot objects (radiator, iron), hot tar, or hot grease. Many of these burns result in a full-thickness burn.

Chemical Burns

- Chemical burns may be caused by common household cleaners, gasoline, paint removers, disc batteries, and other toxic chemicals stored in the home or garage.

Electrical Injuries

- Electrical injuries are uncommon in the pediatric population:
  - Nonfatal electrical injuries tend to occur in infants and toddlers who bite on electrical cords or place their fingers, tongues, or small objects into electrical outlets.
  - Adolescents may climb on transmission towers, sustaining a fatal high-voltage electrical injury.

Radiation Injuries

- These injuries are rare in the pediatric patient but may result from radiation therapy or from prolonged exposure to ultraviolet light from the sun.

Unintentional vs. Intentional Injuries

- Burn injuries occur at the workplace, home, and in association with vehicular crashes and recreational activity. Most often, these burn injuries are unintentional.
- Intentional burns most often occur to young children; thorough investigation of burn injuries in children is required to detect child maltreatment and to prevent future injuries or death (Chapter 46).

Pathophysiology of Burn Injuries

Burn injuries cause significant changes in local tissue morphology and systemic physiology.

1. Changes in tissue morphology:
   - Tissue destruction following thermal contact is a function of both intensity and duration of exposure (Gaisford, Slater, & Goldfarb, 2002).
   - On the microscopic level, tissue destruction is characterized by a zone effect:
     - The inner zone of coagulation is where irreversible cellular death occurs.
     - The zone of stasis surrounds the zone of coagulation and has the potential for healing if perfusion and moisturization are preserved.
     - The outer zone of hyperemia is characterized by redness and the ability for rapid healing.
2. Changes in systemic physiology, usually found in patients with burns involving more than 20% of total body surface area (TBSA) involvement (Davey, Wallis, Perkins, & Tingay, 1995; Dickerson, Gordon, & Walter, 1998):
   - Cardiovascular system:

- Increased capillary permeability results in fluid shifts from the intravascular space to the interstitial space (third spacing). This fluid and protein shift results in edema, decreased cardiac output, and hemoconcentration.
- The maximum amount of edema occurs 8 to 12 hours postinjury in small burns and up to 24 hours postinjury in large burns. Capillary integrity may be restored 18 to 24 hours postinjury in small burns and up to 30 hours postinjury in large burns.

- Respiratory system:
  - Direct injury to the respiratory tract can occur with the inhalation of smoke and products of combustion. Pulmonary edema results from fluid shifts.
- Neurologic system:
  - Alteration in mental status may result from hypoxia and fluid shifts within the brain tissue.
- Gastrointestinal system:
  - Ileus may occur from peripheral circulatory collapse and is usually found in patients with burns involving 20% of TBSA.
- Genitourinary system:
  - A decreased circulating fluid volume results in a decrease in the renal plasma flow and in the glomerular filtration rate and a subsequent decrease in urinary output. Fluid shifts may cause renal damage, such as tubular necrosis, if intravenous fluid resuscitation is inadequate.
- Metabolic changes:
  - A hypermetabolic state results from a major burn, which increases caloric and nitrogen demands to achieve proper wound healing. Burn wounds are unlike any other disease state that produces such a great demand for glucose, protein, and fat.

Focused History

Mechanism of Burn Injury

- Historical findings for each mechanism of injury are outlined in their respective sections of this chapter.

Injury History

- Time of burn injury:
  - Delays in seeking emergency department (ED) treatment may be indicative of child maltreatment (Chapter 46).
- Duration of contact with the burn agent.
- Location at the time of injury:
  - Establishes an index of suspicion for inhalation injury if the burn occurred in an enclosed space.
- Circumstances surrounding the injury:
  - Presence or absence of adult supervision may be indicative of child maltreatment (Chapter 46).
- Association with another mechanism of injury:
  - Injuries sustained in a motor vehicle crash may be far more significant than that of the thermal burn.
  - Being thrown from an open window or jumping from a significant height during a house fire may result in fractures or internal injuries in addition to thermal and inhalation injuries.

Prehospital Treatment

- Efforts employed to stop the burning process.
- Initial aid to treat the burn wound, including home treatments or remedies (e.g., application of butter).

Focused Assessment

Physical Assessment

The burn wound has the lowest priority; airway, breathing, and circulation are the most important systems to support:

1. Assess the airway.
   - Assess for sounds of airway compromise:
     - Stridor.
     - Hoarseness.
   - Inspect the mouth for burn wounds from chemicals, electricity, or thermal sources.
   - Note the presence of carbonaceous sputum, singed nasal hairs, and lip edema.
2. Assess the respiratory system.
   - Auscultate the chest for:
     - Respiratory rate.
     - Adventitious breath sounds. Adventitious sounds in a patient with a history of entrapment in an enclosed space may indicate an inhalation injury.
   - Inspect the chest for equal expansion and symmetry.
3. Assess the cardiovascular system:
   - Auscultate the heart for:
     - Rate.
     - Rhythm.
     - Quality.
   - Measure the blood pressure.
   - Assess peripheral perfusion:

- Palpate peripheral pulses for equality (circumferential eschar may restrict peripheral perfusion) and quality.
- Measure core and skin temperature.
- Measure capillary refill.
- Inspect the skin color.

4. Assess the neurologic system.
   - Assess the level of consciousness with the AVPU (Alert, responds to Verbal stimuli, responds to Painful stimuli, Unresponsive) method or the Glasgow coma scale (GCS) method.
5. Assess the gastrointestinal and genitourinary systems.
   - Inspect the abdomen for distention or rigidity.
   - Auscultate the abdomen for bowel sounds.
   - Gently palpate the abdomen for pain and tenderness.
   - Observe for vomiting.
   - Note the presence of urinary output.
6. Assess the integumentary system to determine the TBSA burned.
   - Assess the burn wound for
     - Location.
     - Depth. Burns are categorized as superficial, partial-thickness and full-thickness injury on the basis of depth and the ability for regeneration. The differentiation between deep partial-thickness and full-thickness burn injury is often difficult to make at the time of the initial assessment. Table 39.2 summarizes the characteristics of burn wounds.
     - Percentage. Use the Rule of nines or the Lund and Browder chart.
     - Classify the burn injury (Table 39.3).
7. Assess the musculoskeletal system.
   - Observe for circumferential burns of the extremities or digits.
   - Observe for deformities or open fractures.

TABLE 39.2 Summary of Burn Characteristics

Category	*Depth*	*Appearance*	*Pain Level*	*Healing Time*
Superficial	Involves entire epidermis	▪ Red, dry, flaky skin ▪ Similar to a sunburn ▪ Blisters are not present	Painful	3–5 days without scarring
Superficial partial-thickness	Involves only the epidermis and the upper dermal layers	▪ Wet "weeping" areas with or without blister formation ▪ Blanching with pressure ▪ Mild to moderate edema	Very painful	10–21 days, usually without scarring
Deep partial-thickness	Involves the entire epidermis; includes destruction of the dermal papillae but spares sweat glands and hair follicles	▪ Cherry pink or mottled red appearance ▪ May have lost pinprick sensation but retains pressure sensation ▪ Considered a full-thickness burn in children	Very painful	May require excision and grafting
Full-thickness	Involves the epidermis, including destruction of all dermal appendages and epithelial elements	▪ White, charred, and leathery ▪ Firm eschar with thrombosed vessels	No pain	Excision and grafting required, because no spontaneous regeneration is possible

TABLE 39.3 Classification of Burn Injuries

Classification	*Description*
Minor	■ < 10% total body surface area affected by superficial or superficial partial-thickness burns ■ No burns involving the face, hands, feet, joints, or perineum ■ No respiratory involvement ■ No pre-existing diseases
Moderate	■ >10% total body surface area affected by any deep partial thickness or full-thickness burns ■ No burns involving the face, hands, feet, joints, or perineum ■ No respiratory involvement ■ No electrical burn injury ■ No circumferential burn
Major	■ >5% total body surface area affected by full-thickness burns ■ >10% total body surface area affected by deep partial-thickness burns involving the face, hands, feet, joints, or perineum ■ Any chemical burn ■ Any suspicion of inhalation injury ■ Any electrical injury ■ Any preexisting medical condition

- Assess the fingers and toes for color, sensitivity, and motion.

Psychosocial Assessment

- Assess the child's and family's coping strategies:
  - A burn injury is extremely stressful for both the family and the patient.
  - More than one family member may have been involved in the burning episode, including the parents.
  - Other family members may be involved in the ED treatment.
- Assess the child's prior hospital experiences, especially with painful procedures:
  - The pain of burn injuries causes both fear and anxiety in pediatric patients of all ages.
  - Patients and families alike are concerned about the cosmetic appearance following a burn injury; early referral to burn surgeons or plastic surgeons is essential to optimize the patient's cosmetic and functional outcomes.
- Assess the child's and family's dynamics:
  - The child's and family's statements and reactions should be documented precisely as witnessed.
  - In the case of child maltreatment, many stories are changed and children may have a flat affect as a result of the abuse (Chapter 46).
  - Assess for signs of prior abuse by inspecting the child for cigarette burns, burns on the back, signs of demarcation from immersion into hot liquids or bath water, or other scars (Chapter 46).

Table 39.4 lists the nursing diagnoses and expected outcomes.

Triage Decisions

Emergent

- Absence of airway, breathing and circulation
- Shock
- More than 15% of TBSA affected by partial-thickness burns
- More than 10% of TBSA affected by full-thickness burns
- Burns involving the hands, feet, face, or perineum
- Inhalation and chemical injuries

Urgent

- Less than 15% of TBSA affected by partial-thickness burns
- Less than 10% of TBSA affected by full-thickness burns

Nonurgent

- Superficial burns
- No signs of shock
- No suspected child maltreatment

TABLE 39.4 Nursing Diagnoses and Expected Outcomes

Nursing Diagnoses	*Expected Outcomes*
Alteration in fluids, less than body requirements, related to thermal, chemical, electrical, or radiant injury	The patient will have adequate cardiovascular functioning, as evidenced by: ▪ Level of consciousness that is awake and alert. ▪ Verbalizations and vocalizations that are appropriate for age. ▪ Heart rate and blood pressure normal for age. ▪ Capillary refill <2 seconds. ▪ Administration of correctly calculated intravenous fluid resuscitation. ▪ Urinary output normal for age.
Alteration in skin integrity, related to thermal, chemical, electrical, or radiant injury	The patient will have adequate skin covering, as evidenced by: ▪ Application of antimicrobial agents. ▪ Appropriate wound management.
Alteration in thermoregulation, related to major burn wound	The patient will maintain normothermia, as evidenced by: ▪ Normal range of body temperature. ▪ Absence of shivering.
Knowledge deficit, related to burn injury prevention	▪ The family and patient (when appropriate) will learn strategies to prevent burns. ▪ The family will receive counseling and follow-up in the event of suspected or confirmed child maltreatment (Chapter 46).

Nursing Interventions for Moderate and Major Burns

1. Stop the burning process if this has not occurred in the prehospital setting.
   - Extinguish flames by having the child stop, drop, and roll. Alternatively, wrap the patient in a blanket to smother the flames.
   - Apply room temperature water to thermal burns; however, major burn injuries should not be cooled for more than a few minutes because of the child's temperature liability and the risk of hypothermia:
     - Assess for heat dissipation from the skin by holding a hand over the burned area; if heat is felt, the burning process is still in progress.
   - Remove burned clothing; if it has stuck to the tissue, cut around the clothing.
   - Remove any watches, rings, or other objects from injured extremities; because of fluid shifts, a tourniquet-like effect will result in the loss of arterial circulation.
2. Maintain airway patency.
   - Open the airway with the chin lift–jaw thrust technique.
   - Prepare for endotracheal intubation in the patient with a suspected inhalation injury, airway injury, or altered level of consciousness.
3. Initiate measures to support respiratory effort.
   - Administer high-flow oxygen.
   - Initiate assisted ventilations with bag-valve-mask ventilation.
   - Prepare for mechanical ventilation in the patient with suspected inhalation or airway injury.
4. Initiate interventions to support the circulation.
   - Initiate cardiorespiratory and oxygen saturation monitoring:
     - Electrodes can be placed over the burned skin; consider alternative areas, such as unburned shoulders or forehead (Bernardo, 1990).
     - Measure blood pressure, preferably in an unburned extremity. If the extremity is burned, an open gauze pad can be placed over the burn before the cuff is applied. Do not obtain the blood pressure in a circumferentially burned extremity.
   - Obtain venous access with large-bore intravenous catheters, preferably in unburned extremities (burned extremities can be cannulated if the burns are not circumferential).

TABLE 39.5 Calculations for Intravenous Fluid Resuscitation

Percent of the total body surface area burned × child's weight in kilograms × 4 ml = number of ml to be infused in 24 hours, in addition to maintenance.

Administer one half of this amount in the first 8 hours.

Administer one quarter of the original amount in the next 8 hours.

Administer the final one quarter of the solution in the last 8 hours.

Example

25% TBSA burned × 20 kgs × 4 ml = 2,000 ml of lactated Ringer's solution to be infused in 24 hours.

Administer 1,000 ml (1/2 of 2,000 ml) in the first 8 hours (a rate of 125.0 ml/hour).

Administer 500 ml (1/4 of 2,000 ml) in the next 8 hours (a rate of 62.5 ml/hour).

Administer 500 ml (1/4 of 2,000 ml) in the final 8 hours (a rate of 62.5 ml/hour).

- Initiate an intraosseous infusion in an unburned extremity if venous access is not attained within 90 seconds or three attempts. Prepare for a venous cutdown or central line placement, if needed.
- Obtain blood specimens for laboratory analysis:
  - Complete blood count and differential.
  - Electrolytes.
  - Blood urea nitrogen, creatinine, and glucose.
  - Prothrombin time and partial thromboplastin time.
  - Alcohol and toxicology screening, if indicated.
- Initiate intravenous fluid resuscitation in patients with burns involving greater than 10% of TBSA (Davey et al., 1995). Calculate and infuse the correct amount of lactated Ringer's solution for fluid resuscitation based on the calculated TBSA (Table 39.5).

5. Assess the child's neurologic status and assess for pain (Chapter 13).
6. Insert a nasogastric tube for gastric decompression if the burns involve more than 25% TBSA:
   - Measure gastric output:
     - Paralytic ileus can be an early complication of a severe burn injury.
7. Insert an indwelling bladder catheter to measure urinary volume and specific gravity.
   - Urinary output is the best indicator of the adequacy of resuscitation. The formula for calculating urinary output is in Table 39.6.
   - Obtain a urine specimen for:
     - Urinalysis.
     - Urinary chorionic gonadotropin (in postmenarchal females).
     - Toxicology screening, if indicated.
8. Initiate measures to maintain normothermia:
   - Increase the room temperature.
   - Cover the patient with warm blankets or sheets:
     - For wounds covering a large percentage of TBSA, no antimicrobial dressings are needed, because the burn treatment center staff will cleanse and treat the wound on the child's arrival.
   - Administer warmed intravenous fluids.
9. Administer medication, as prescribed:
   - Administer tetanus prophylaxis if the child's immunizations are not current. A burn wound is considered a contaminated tissue that requires tetanus prophylaxis.
   - Administer intravenous narcotic analgesics for pain management. The intravenous route is used because fluid shifts following the burn injury and during fluid resuscitation cause sporadic uptake of medications, leading to inadequate dosing. Suggested intravenous analgesics are:
     - Morphine sulfate, 0.1–0.2 mg/kg/dose, every 2–4 hours, as needed, maximum = 15.0 mg/dose.

TABLE 39.6 Formula for Calculating Urinary Output

Formula	*Example*
Child's weight <30 kg: Urinary output is 1.0–2.0 ml × kg per hour.	1.0–2.0 ml × 25 kg per hour = 25–50 ml per hour minimum urinary output should be maintained.
Child's weight >30 kg: Urinary output is 0.5 ml × kg per hour.	0.5 ml × 40 kg per hour = 20 ml per hour minimum urinary output should be maintained.

- Fentanyl, 1–2 μg/kg/dose, every 30–60 minutes, as needed.

10. Prepare for additional procedures:
    - Prepare for tissue pressure measurements in extremities with circumferential burns.
    - Prepare for escharotomies if tissue pressures are high.
    - Prepare for radiographs, such as chest, extremity, or abdomen, depending on associated injuries.
11. Inform the family frequently of the child's condition; support their presence during ED treatment (Chapter 4).
12. Provide emotional support to the child and family:
    - Explain all procedures and treatments.
    - Encourage the family to touch or hold the child in unburned areas.
    - Be honest about expected outcomes.
    - If child maltreatment is suspected, complete the required reporting forms and photograph the burns; contact social services and child protective services. Explain to the family why this action has been taken (Chapter 46).
13. Initiate consultations with social services personnel, medical subspecialists, and community agencies, as needed.
14. Prepare for transfer and transport to a burn center (Chapter 10).
    - Transfer is initiated for all children with severe burn injuries and, as needed, children with moderate burn injuries.
    - Explain to the patient and family the importance of and need for specialized burn care.
15. Initiate interventions to assist the family whose child has died from burn injuries (Chapter 28); consider a debriefing for the involved staff members.

Nursing Interventions for Minor Burns

1. Stop the burning process.
    - Pour room temperature water over the thermal burn. Never apply ice to the burn, because additional tissue damage may result.
2. Assess the child's level of pain, and initiate pharmacologic and nonpharmacologic interventions prior to performing wound care (Chapter 13):
    - Prepare to administer oral narcotic and nonnarcotic analgesics:
        - Oralet® lollipops (100 μg, 200 μg, 300 μg, or 400 μg).
        - Acetaminophen with codeine.
        - Morphine sulfate concentrated oral solution, 0.2 to 0.5 mg/kg/dose, every 4 to 6 hours.
        - Acetaminophen, 10 to 15 mg/kg/dose, not to exceed 2.6 g over 24 hours.
3. Perform wound care.
    - Wash the burn wound with a mild soap:
        - Leave blisters intact to promote wound healing; debride broken blisters and any necrotic tissue that is present around the wound.
    - Apply an antimicrobial agent to the burn wound:
        - Apply silver sulfadiazine cream if the patient is not allergic to sulfa medications and the burn wound is not on the face (silver sulfadiazine may cause skin discoloration when applied to the face).
        - Apply bacitracin if the child is allergic to sulfa medications and the burn wound is to the face.
        - Encourage the patient to participate in the wound care, if the patient desires to do so. Patients who participate in their wound care may feel a sense of control.
    - Apply a bandage over the burn wound:
        - Facial burns are generally left open to air when ointment is applied.
        - Chest burns can be covered with sterile gauze pads; a cotton t-shirt or stockinette (Hyginette™) dressing can be applied to keep the gauze pads in place.
        - Extremity burns can be covered with gauze pads and a stockinette (Hyginette™).
        - Burned fingers and toes should be separated with small gauze pads to prevent webbing on healing.
        - Perineal burns can be covered with gauze and a diaper; they must be cleaned after each urination or defecation.

Home Care and Prevention

Children with moderate and major burn wounds are hospitalized in burn trauma centers until their wounds are healed. For families whose children have minor burn wounds, home care instructions are reviewed prior to

ED discharge. Parents should be reminded that approximately 10 to 20 days are needed for complete wound healing (Ball, 1998):

- Demonstrate the wound care the family will perform at home; usually, wound care is performed twice a day (Ball, 1998):
  - The parents should wash their hands before changing the burn wound dressing.
  - The child's burn wound should be soaked in warm water for about 10 minutes; The child should be encouraged to play with water toys (Ball, 1998).
- Next, the wound should be gently washed with a clean washcloth and a mild soap to remove all of the antimicrobial agent; if bleeding occurs, gentle pressure should be applied for 30 seconds (Ball, 1998).
  - The wound should be dried with a clean towel.
  - A thin layer of the prescribed antimicrobial ointment should be applied directly onto the gauze pad, and then the pad should be anchored with tape or stockinette (Hyginette™).
  - Provide opportunities for return demonstrations to allay the family's anxieties about performing these procedures at home and to increase their confidence in their ability to comply with the treatment process.
  - Give burn wound supplies to the family on discharge or give the family a prescription for purchase of the supplies.
- Teach the patient and family the signs and symptoms of burn wound infection (fever, redness, swelling, purulent drainage, cloudy fluid, decreased appetite, and decreased activity).
- Assure adequate analgesia with a written prescription or with access to over-the-counter medication:
  - Consider providing an antihistamine, such as diphenhydramine, to allay itching as the wound heals (Ball, 1998).
  - Review with the family strategies for incorporating pharmacologic and nonpharmacologic pain management techniques into their home care.
  - Parents may become very distressed at the wound's appearance as well as their child's crying. Discuss ways for parents to cope with their feelings.
- Have the patient and family return to the emergency department within 24 hours for a wound check and to review the wound care regimen. If an ED return is not possible, make a referral to home care or an appointment with the primary care provider.
- Contact social services and child protective services in cases of suspected child maltreatment; initiate the proper reporting mechanism (Chapter 46).

Specific Burn Injuries

Smoke Inhalation

Pulmonary pathology frequently accompanies major thermal trauma. The presence of an inhalation injury significantly increases the morbidity and mortality associated with a given size of total body surface burn. Three types of inhalation injury are supraglottic, tracheobronchial, and alveolar (Table 39.7). Aggressive diagnostic and therapeutic maneuvers are essential to overall management (Gaisford et al., 2002)

Etiology

Mechanism of burn injury

- Flame
- Chemical

Focused History

Mechanism of burn injury

- Flame. Entrapment in an enclosed space or motor vehicle.
- Chemical. Ingestion or inhalation of a chemical.

Inhalation injury-specific symptoms:

- Rescue from an enclosed space
- Chemical bottle found near the patient
- Respiratory-related symptoms:
  - Drooling, choking
  - Carbonaceous sputum
  - Singed hair
  - Upper airway obstruction

Other historical findings

- Prehospital treatment
- Witnesses
- Involvement of other family members

Focused Assessment

Physical Assessment

1. Assess for signs of potential inhalation injury (Benjamin & Herndon, 2002):
   - Listen for sounds of airway compromise or obstruction:
     - Stridor.
     - Hoarseness.
     - Harsh cough.
   - Inspect the face:

TABLE 39.7 Comparison of Inhalation Injuries and Their Treatment

Injury	*Cause*	*Description*	*Treatment*
Supraglottic injury	▪ Direct heat injury leads to upper airway edema severe enough to cause an obstructive phenomenon. ▪ Heat injury below the vocal cords is uncommon because the child is unable to inhale a large enough volume of air with enough heat-carrying capacity to cause damage.	▪ Obvious edema and associated stridor. ▪ Significant lip and oral edema; the amount of lip edema generally correlates with the amount of vocal cord edema.	▪ Patients with severe lip and vocal cord edema require endotracheal intubation to avert an occlusive phenomenon. ▪ Patients may develop upper airway obstruction secondary to edema during the resuscitative process.
Tracheobronchial injury	▪ Incomplete products of combustion (nitrates, polyvinyls, polyurethane gases) act as toxic agents, damaging the tracheobronchial mucosa and causing a "chemical" injury.	▪ Airway edema; alveolar membrane damage. ▪ Mucosal sloughing and associated tracheobronchitis occur and ultimately lead to a pneumonic process.	▪ Prepare for endotracheal intubation. ▪ Administer intravenous antibiotics, as prescribed.
Alveolar injury	▪ Occurs in a small number of patients (5% of all patients who survive to the emergency department) (Gaisford et al., 2002)	▪ Severe alveolar damage leading to a respiratory distress-type syndrome. ▪ Irreversible hypoxia immediately following extrication from a fire.	▪ These patients generally die rapidly, despite aggressive clinical intervention.

    - Singed facial or nasal hair.
    - Facial burns.
    - Blisters to the lips and face.
    - Soot in the nose and mouth.
    - Carbonaceous sputum.
- Auscultate the chest for:
    - Adventitious sounds.
    - Respiratory rate.
- Observe the chest for:
    - Retractions.
    - Use of accessory muscles.
    - Restricted chest expansion.
- Assess the child's mental status
    - Agitation
    - Stupor

Psychosocial Assessment

- Assess the child's and family's coping strategies.
- Assess the child's and family's understanding of the injury process:
    - Other family members may be affected.
    - The family may not have adequate social or financial resources following a home fire; social services intervention may be needed.

Nursing Interventions

1. Assess and maintain the airway.
    - Prepare for endotracheal intubation.
    - Perform endotracheal lavage and suctioning, as needed.
2. Administer high-flow humidified supplemental oxygen by mask or bag-valve-mask ventilation.
    - Prepare for mechanical ventilation in the child who receives endotracheal intubation.
3. Initiate cardiorespiratory and oxygen saturation monitoring.
4. Obtain venous access and initiate fluid resuscitation:
    - Obtain arterial blood gases and carboxyhemoglobin (CO) levels.
    - CO level >10% indicates potential inhalation injury (Benjamin & Herndon, 2002).
5. Monitor the child's neurologic status.
6. Prepare for diagnostic procedures:

- Chest radiograph.
- Direct visualization of the airway with laryngoscopy or bronchoscopy (Benjamin & Herndon, 2002).

7. Continue with burn wound treatment, as needed.
8. Inform the family frequently of the child's condition.
9. Provide emotional support to the child and family.
10. Prepare for transfer and transport to a burn trauma center (Chapter 10).

Carbon Monoxide Poisoning

Carbon monoxide is a colorless, odorless gas. It affects the brain because carboxyhemoglobin formation hinders systemic oxygen delivery.

Metabolic acidosis and elevation in serum enzymes indicate muscle and liver damage in severe cases. Carboxyhemoglobin levels of 50 to 70% or more are often found in patients who have suffered asphyxiation from a house fire or incomplete products of combustion. When levels of carboxyhemoglobin are 40 to 60%, the patient will have symptoms of confusion, disorientation, or loss of consciousness. Levels of 15 to 40% cause symptoms of headache, nausea, vomiting, or dizziness (American Burn Association, 2001) (Table 39.8).

Etiology

- Poorly ventilated fireplaces
- Space heaters
- Automobile exhaust that leaks into a house from the garage
- Furnaces
- House fires

Focused History

- Rescue from an enclosed space
- Activation of a carbon monoxide detector
- Loss of consciousness

Focused Assessment

Physical Assessment

1. Assess the respiratory system:
   - Auscultate the chest for:
     - Adventitious sounds.
     - Respiratory rate. Tachypnea may be present.
   - Inspect for signs related to inhalation injury in the event of a house fire.
2. Assess the cardiovascular system:
   - Auscultate the heart for:
     - Rate. Tachycardia may be present.
     - Rhythm.
   - Measure the blood pressure.
   - Assess the peripheral circulation.
   - Measure capillary refill.
3. Assess the neurologic system:
   - Measure the level of consciousness with the AVPU method or the GCS.
   - Observe for signs of hypoxia:
     - Agitation.
     - Anxiety.
     - Irritability.
     - Stupor.

TABLE 39.8 Carboxyhemoglobin Levels, Symptoms, and Treatment

Carboxyhemoglobin level	*Symptoms*	*Treatment*
15–40%	Headache, nausea, vomiting, or dizziness	■ Administer 100% oxygen. ■ Obtain arterial blood gas levels and a carboxyhemoglobin level.
40–60%	Confusion, disorientation, or loss of consciousness	■ Administer 100% oxygen. ■ Prepare for endotracheal intubation. ■ Prepare for hyperbaric oxygen therapy. ■ Obtain arterial blood gas levels and a carboxyhemoglobin level.
50–70%	Asphyxiation	■ Administer 100% oxygen. ■ Prepare for endotracheal intubation. ■ Expect a high mortality rate.

Psychosocial Assessment

1. Assess the child's and family's coping strategies.
2. Assess the child's and family's understanding of the injury process:
   - Other family members may be affected.
   - The family may not have adequate social or financial resources to make changes in their home environment; social services intervention may be needed.

Nursing Interventions

1. Assess and maintain the airway:
   - Prepare for endotracheal intubation.
2. Administer high-flow humidified supplemental oxygen:
   - Prepare for mechanical ventilation.
3. Initiate cardiorespiratory monitoring:
   - Avoid oxygen saturation monitoring, because it will read a combination of carboxyhemoglobin plus oxygen-saturated hemoglobin. The monitoring does not differentiate between the two types of hemoglobin, making the readings falsely high.
4. Obtain venous access and initiate fluid resuscitation, as needed.
5. Obtain arterial, venous, or capillary blood gases and carboxyhemoglobin levels.
6. Prepare for a chest radiograph.
7. Continue with burn care treatment, as needed.
8. Inform the family frequently of the child's condition.
9. Provide emotional support to the child and family.
10. Prepare for transfer and transport to a burn treatment center, as needed (Chapter 10).

Chemical Burns

Chemical injuries generally result from the young child's normal curiosity while exploring the kitchen or bathroom and playing with home cleaning agents. The body areas most frequently involved are the head, neck, or extremities because these are most often exposed.

The chemical agents ultimately destroy protein integrity by either a coagulation or denaturation process. This degradation of protein may continue to a depth well below the superficial skin changes that characterize the initial injury presentation. Chemical injuries may be accompanied by significant deep pathology with only minimal cutaneous effect, an important consideration in the resuscitation of children with large chemical injuries. Chemical agents have a prolonged effect after contact with the skin and go on to cause progressive damage if immediate intervention is not accomplished.

Chapter 45 outlines the treatment of chemically-exposed patients.

Electrical Injuries

Electrical injuries occur from contact with high or low electrical voltage (Table 39.10). When electrical current is involved, there is always a chance of ventricular fibrillation and other dysrhythmias. Tissue injury results from electricity because the energy is converted to heat. Cutaneous injury generally results from the relationship that exists between the passage of current and body resistance. Electric current has a propensity to cause necrosis of tissue as a result of thrombosis of major vascular systems. The electrical current injures the endothelial cells of small and medium blood vessels, resulting in the deposition of fibrin and platelets, which may ultimately occlude the vessel.

TABLE 39.9 Comparison of Electrical Burn Injuries

Characteristic	*Low-Voltage Injuries*	*High-Voltage Injuries*
Voltage	120–1000 volts	>1000 volts
Current	Alternating (household electrical outlets, fuse boxes)	Direct (power lines)
Where injuries occur	Home	■ Outdoors ■ Workplace
Effect on body systems: neurologic cardiovascular musculoskeletal skin	■ Loss of consciousness ■ Ventricular fibrillation ■ Possible compartment syndrome ■ Full thickness burns	■ Coexisting injuries from falls ■ Renal failure from myoglobinuria ■ Muscle necrosis ■ Full thickness burns

Unlike thermal injury, an electrical injury may be a progressive and dynamic lesion that evolves over many days. Children who sustain high-voltage electrical injuries may present with a multitude of problems that are significantly different from those exhibited by children who present with thermal cutaneous injuries. Aggressive intervention is essential to manage the many potential facets of pathology that can occur in high-voltage electrical injuries.

Etiology

- Alternating current sources:
  - Fuse boxes in the home
  - Electrical outlets in the home
  - Home appliances
- Direct current sources:
  - Power lines
  - Defibrillators

Focused History

- Source of the electrical current
- Voltage of the electrical current
- Amount of time the child was in contact with the electrical source
- Path of the electricity

Focused Assessment

Physical Assessment

1. Assess the respiratory system.
   - Auscultate the chest for:
     - Respiratory rate.
     - Adventitious sounds.
2. Assess the cardiovascular system.
   - Auscultate the heart for:
     - Rate.
     - Rhythm.
     - Quality.
   - Measure the blood pressure.
   - Assess the peripheral circulation:
     - Palpate the peripheral pulses for quality; equality.
     - Assess core and peripheral temperature.
     - Measure capillary refill.
     - Assess skin color and texture.
3. Assess the neurologic system.
   - Assess the level of consciousness with the AVPU method or the GCS.
4. Assess the integumentary system.
   - Inspect the skin for thermal wounds, entrance and exit wounds.
5. Assess the musculoskeletal system:
   - Observe for deformities or dislocations.
   - Observe for impaired mobility.
   - Assess for the presence of the six P's
     - Assess for *pain*.
     - Test for *paresthesia*.
     - Palpate for *pulselessness*.
     - Observe for *pallor*.
     - Test for *paralysis*.
     - Palpate for *polar*

Nursing Interventions for Major Electrical Injuries

1. Assess and maintain the airway and cervical spine.
   - Prepare for endotracheal intubation.
   - Initiate spinal immobilization as needed.
2. Maintain respiratory function.
   - Administer 100% oxygen.
   - Prepare for mechanical ventilation.
   - Initiate cardiorespiratory and oxygen saturation monitoring:
   - Monitor the child for electrocardiogram changes.
3. Obtain venous access and initiate fluid resuscitation.
   - Fluid administration flushes myoglobin and hemoglobin from the kidneys. These proteins precipitate in the renal tubules and can result in acute tubular necrosis if urinary output is not maintained.
   - Obtain blood specimens for laboratory analysis:
     - Creatine kinase.
     - Creatine kinase-MB.
   - Administer analgesics as prescribed.
4. Monitor the neurologic status.
   - Observe for seizure activity.
   - Administer medications, as prescribed, for seizure activity.
   - Assess for pain.
   - Administer analgesics as prescribed.
5. Insert a nasogastric tube and indwelling bladder catheter.
   - Obtain a urine specimen for:
     - Urinalysis.
     - Myoglobin.
   - Measure urinary output.
     - Note the color of urine (tea-colored or black urine indicates the presence of myoglobin).

6. Inspect the electrical injury for its location; calculate the TBSA affected and the severity:
   - Remove any jewelry from the injured extremity to decrease the tourniquet-like effect, which may cause vascular ischemia.
7. Assess the injured extremities for fascial compartment compression, because of the propensity for vessel thrombosis and associated muscle nonviability.
   - Prepare for tissue pressure measurement and subsequent fasciotomy in the operating room.
   - Monitor peripheral pulses and peripheral perfusion continuously so that impaired circulation may be recognized and appropriate decompression procedures may be quickly instituted.
8. Inform the family frequently of the child's condition.
9. Provide emotional support to the child and family.
10. Initiate consultations with social services personnel and medical subspecialists.
11. Prepare for transfer and transport to a burn treatment center (Chapter 10).

Nursing Interventions for Minor (Localized) Electrical Injuries

1. Inspect the electrical injury for its location; calculate the TBSA affected and the severity.
2. Obtain an electrocardiogram.
3. Obtain blood specimens for laboratory analysis:
   - Creatine kinase.
   - Creatine kinase–MB.
4. Obtain a urine specimen for myoglobin.
5. Initiate consultation with a burn treatment center, plastic surgeon, or pediatric surgeon.
6. Provide follow-up for subsequent treatment:
   - Patients must be examined regularly (i.e., daily) to detect the presence of underlying nonviable tissue in the areas of entrance and exit wounds and over the intervening areas. This inspection detects evolving nonviable tissue and allows for the initiation of appropriate interventions, such as debridement.
7. Prepare for hospitalization, because patients with electrical injuries should be observed for a minimum of 24 hours.

Lightning Injuries

Lightning kills between 80 and 100 people a year in the United States alone. Lightning is direct current of 100,000,000 volts, and up to 200,000 amps (American Burn Association, 2001). Multiple strikes can occur on the same location.

Etiology (American Burn Association, 2001)

- Direct strike:
  - The lightning directly contacts the patient.
- Side flash:
  - Current flows between a person and a nearby object struck by lightning.
  - Current travels on the surface of the body and not through it, resulting in superficial cutaneous burns (splashed on spidery and arborescent pattern).

Focused History

- Nature of the injury:
  - How and where the injury occurred.
  - Witnesses to the event.
- Symptoms following the lightning strike:
  - Loss of consciousness; seizure.
  - Cardiopulmonary arrest.
  - Amnesia.
  - Additional systemic injuries (e.g., if the child was thrown into the air).
- Treatment initiated:
  - Cardiopulmonary resuscitation

Focused Assessment

Physical Assessment

1. Assess the respiratory system:
   - Auscultate the chest for:
     - Respiratory rate.
     - Adventitious sounds.
2. Assess the cardiovascular system:
   - Auscultate the heart for:
     - Rate.
     - Rhythm.
     - Quality.
   - Measure the blood pressure.
   - Assess peripheral perfusion.
   - Measure capillary refill.

3. Assess the neurologic system.
   - Assess the level of consciousness with the AVPU method or the CGS method.
   - Observe for seizure activity.
   - Assess for signs of a spinal cord injury (Chapter 32).
4. Assess the integumentary system.
   - Inspect the skin for thermal wounds.
   - Inspect the skin for lightning spots.
5. Assess the musculoskeletal system.
   - Observe for deformities or dislocations.
   - Palpate the peripheral pulses for intensity and equality.
   - Observe for impaired mobility.

Psychosocial Assessment

- Assess the child's and family's coping strategies.
  - Additional family members or friends may have been involved in the lightning strike.
  - Parents may blame each other or may blame coaches or other adults if outdoor sports activities were in progress during the lightning strike.
- Assess the child's and family's understanding of the lightning injury.

Nursing Interventions

1. Assess and maintain airway and cervical spine immobilization.
   - Prepare for endotracheal intubation as needed.
   - Maintain spinal precautions.
2. Initiate measures to promote respiratory function.
   - Administer supplemental oxygen.
   - Prepare for mechanical ventilation.
   - Administer cardiopulmonary resuscitation if needed.
   - Initiate cardiorespiratory and oxygen saturation monitoring:
     - Monitor the patient for electrocardiogram changes.
3. Obtain venous access and initiate fluid resuscitation to flush myoglobin and hemoglobin from the kidneys.
   - These proteins precipitate in the renal tubules and can result in acute tubular necrosis if urinary output is not maintained.
   - Obtain blood specimens for laboratory analysis:
     - Creatine kinase.
     - Creatine kinase–MB.
4. Monitor the neurologic system.
   - Observe for seizure activity:
     - Administer anticonvulsant therapy, as prescribed.
   - Assess for pain (Chapter 13):
     - Administer analgesics, as prescribed.
5. Remove any watches, rings, belts, clothing, or anything that may cause a tourniquet-like effect.
6. Insert an indwelling bladder catheter:
   - Monitor urinary output.
     - Obtain urine for myoglobin.
7. Assess peripheral pulses for vascular compromise, which may necessitate escharotomy.
8. Inform the family frequently of the child's condition.
9. Provide emotional support to the child and family.
10. Initiate consultations with social services personnel and medical subspecialists as needed.
11. Prepare for transfer and transport to a burn treatment center (Chapter 10) or trauma center; prepare for hospitalization.

Radiation Therapy Injuries

Radiation therapy may cause skin reactions in the treated area (Table 39.10).

Patients and caregivers should be given the following instructions:

- Wash the treated area with tepid water and soft washcloth.
- Do not use any soaps, lotions, deodorants, medicines, cosmetics, talcum powder, or other substances in the treated area.
- Protect the area from the sun. If possible, cover treated skin with light clothing before going outside. Apply a PABA-free sunscreen or a sunblocking product with a protection factor of a least 15.

TABLE 39.10 Acute Radiation Morbidity Scoring Criteria

Score	*Criteria*
0	No change over baseline
1	Follicular, faint or dull erythema; epilation; dry desquamation; decreased sweating
2	Tender or bright erythema; patchy, moist desquamation; moderate edema
3	Confluent, moist desquamation other than skin folds; pitting edema
4	Ulceration; hemorrhage necrosis

Burn Prevention

Children of all ages are at risk for burn injuries, especially in the home setting. Simple everyday acts of bathing, cooking, using gasoline or kerosene-powered equipment, storing paint and household chemicals, using a fireplace, having a gas or electric furnace, and even using electricity place everyone at risk for a burn injury.

Because of the severity of the injuries that can result, fire and burn prevention should be an ongoing concern for every individual and family.

Kitchen Safety

The kitchen is the single most dangerous room in the home for burns. Extra care must be taken when food is being cooked, especially if there are children in the house. A fire extinguisher and box of baking soda should be kept readily available to quell a fire. Guidelines for kitchen safety are given in Table 39.11.

Bathroom Safety

The bathroom is the second most dangerous room for thermal and electrical burns. Guidelines for bathroom safety are listed in Table 39.12.

General Home Fire Prevention

House fires are a leading cause of death in infants and children. Guidelines to prevent fires in the home include those listed in Table 39.13.

Burn Safety Outdoors

See Table 39.14 for a list of burn safety measures during outdoor activities.

Teaching Children Burn Safety

Children as young as preschoolers can be taught the basic principles of burn safety. They can also be taught how to respond should a fire or other emergency occur in the home setting. Emergency nurses can teach basic burn prevention strategies to children and families:

Before fire occurs

- Identify two escape routes from every room in the house, in the event that a room is blocked by flames or smoke.
- Obtain escape ladders to provide a safe exit from second or third floor bedrooms and ensure that they are easily accessible and in good condition.

TABLE 39.11 Guidelines for Kitchen Safety

Safety Measure	*Rationale*
Turn pot handles inward while cooking.	Avoids unintentional contact with a curious child's hand or an adult's hand or body.
Avoid lifting and carrying boiling or hot liquids.	Decreases risk of spilling or splashing.
Avoid wearing loose-fitting clothes, especially loose housedresses or full sleeves; keep potholders, dish towels, and curtains away from the stove.	Prevents the fabric from hanging too close to hot burners and igniting.
Keep electrical cords away from crawling infants and young children; avoid overloading electrical circuits with small kitchen appliances; consider unplugging small appliances after each use.	Deters children from biting on them and helps family members avoid tripping over them; avoids electrical fires.
Store detergents, cleaning fluids, drain cleaners, and other dangerous substances where curious children cannot get to them.	Prevents burn and poisoning injuries.
Contain grease fires with a lid and turn off the burner. Do not throw water on the fire.	Water may cause the grease to splash out of the pan, spreading the flames.
Set a timer while cooking.	Serves as a reminder to turn off the oven or any burners after use.
Remove any metal or aluminum foil before heating foods in a microwave oven.	Avoids a potential fire or spark.
Carefully test the temperature of foods and beverages heated in a microwave before feeding them to infants and young children.	Microwaves can heat liquids very quickly, without necessarily warming the container.

TABLE 39.12 Guidelines for Bathroom Safety

Safety Measure	*Rationale*
Always test the temperature of bath water before placing an infant or child into the tub.	Avoids scald burns.
Keep electrical appliances and cords away from the tub.	Avoids electrical injuries.
Set the water heater temperature at or below 125°F (52°C)	Prevents scald injuries.
Never leave children alone while they are in the bathtub.	Children may slip or bump the hot water faucet, causing a scald injury; drowning may occur.
Teach children to turn on the cold water first, and then the hot water.	Avoids scalding injuries.

TABLE 39.13 General Home Fire Prevention

Safety Measure	*Rationale*
Always make sure matches and lighters are out of children's reach.	Avoids flame burns; the most frequent cause of fatal home fires is carelessly discarded cigarettes.
Install smoke detectors outside of each bedroom and on every floor.	Alerts family members to the presence of fire regardless of their location in the home.
Check smoke detectors and carbon monoxide regularly; a recognized time for checking them is at the end of daylight savings time.	Ensures that the batteries are functioning.
Extinguish all cigarettes and ashes completely prior to their disposal.	Prevents fires.
Unplug any appliance when the electrical cord begins smoking or gives off a strange odor.	Prevents electrical fires.
Check the plugs and cords on all lights and appliances regularly to make sure that they are not damaged or frayed. Replace them when damage appears.	Prevents electrical fires.
Do not overload outlets or extension cords.	Prevents electrical fires.
Do not run extension cords under rugs.	Cord damage or breakage may go undetected.
Replace blown fuses with ones of the correct amperage.	Avoids overloading the electrical circuit.
If an odor of gas is noted, go to a neighbor's to call for help; do not turn on electrical lights or strike a match to see where the gas fumes are originating.	Electrical sparks created inside the telephone could be enough to ignite the gas.
Have furnaces checked each fall before using them; have chimneys cleaned periodically.	Prevents carbon monoxide poisoning; prevents flame injuries.
Close bedroom doors at night.	The barrier between the family member and the smoke may provide critical, lifesaving minutes.
Place "tot finders" stickers in bedroom windows.	May alert firefighters to the presence of children in the home.

TABLE 39.14 Burn Safety Measures for Outdoor Activities

Safety Measure	*Rationale*
Avoid smoking cigarettes while filling the lawn mower or other tools with gasoline.	Prevents a possible spark that would ignite the gasoline.
Turn gas- or kerosene-powered tools off before adding more fuel.	A spill could be ignited by a spark from the engine.
Store gasoline and other flammable liquids in metal safety containers outside of the house.	Prevents ignition and fire.
When starting a charcoal grill, use an electric starter, solid fuel, or specialized charcoal starter fuel. Never add more liquid fuel once the fire has started.	Prevents a flash-type burn.
When starting a propane gas grill, always have the match lit before turning on the gas. Keep the grill and propane tank stored outside, away from the house.	Prevents an explosion and burn injury.
Keep children away from outdoor grills; keep starter fuels, matches, and lighters out of their reach.	Prevents flame and chemical burns.
Leave fireworks to the professionals; attend community-sponsored fireworks events.	Fireworks cause thousands of burns and fires each year.
When camping, clear the campfire area of leaves and brush; soak the campfire with water and ensure that it is completely out before going to bed or leaving the campsite.	Prevents an uncontrolled fire; prevents inhalation and flame burns.
Never build a fire inside a tent.	Prevents home and inhalation injuries
Seek shelter in a lightening storm	Prevents lightening injuries

- Establish a meeting place outside the house so family members will know immediately if anyone is left inside. Teach children never to return to the burning home to retrieve pets, toys, or other family members.
- Practice family fire drills so that all family members are familiar with what they should do and where they should go.
- Teach children how to call for help (911 or other emergency number). Consider placing the emergency number on a speed dial or having the number posted on the telephone.

When fire occurs

- Teach children to get out of the house or building as quickly as possible and stay out.
- Call 911 or other emergency number immediately.
- Teach children that if they have to go through smoke to crawl on their hands and knees out of the house; smoke rises toward the ceiling, so traveling low to the floor prevents inhalation of smoke.
- If trapped in a room, close the door and try to keep as much smoke from entering as possible. Cover all of the cracks around the door and air vents. Hold a cloth, wet, if possible, over the mouth and nose and try to signal from a window for help. If there is a telephone in the room, call 911 or other emergency number immediately and advise them about the entrapment and its location.

When clothing catches fire

- Teach children to stop, drop, and roll in the event that their clothes catch fire. Running fans the flames and worsens the situation:
  - Stop what you are doing.
  - Drop to the floor and cover your face with your hands.
  - Roll until the flames are smothered.
- Teach young children to get an adult right away if someone else's clothes catch on fire; teach school-aged children and adolescents to smother the flames by wrapping the person in a blanket, sheet, or rug.

Conclusion

Burn injuries cause needless death and disability in the pediatric population. Emergency nurses can become involved in preventing burn injuries by teaching burn safety courses to children and parents. Practicing burn safety with children identifies adults as role models and reinforces burn safety behaviors.

References

American Burn Association. (2001). *American Burn Association life support manual.* Chicago, IL: Author.

Ball, J. (1998). Home care of burns. In J. Ball (Ed.), *Mosby's pediatric patient teaching guides* (pp. B-16). St. Louis: Mosby—Year Book.

Benjamin, D. & Herndon, D. (2002). Special considerations of age: The pediatric burned patient. In D. Heindon (Ed.), *Total burn care* (2nd ed., pp. 427-438). Philadelphia: Saunders.

Bernardo, L. (1990). Emergency department treatment of burns. In R. Trofino (Ed.), *Care of the burn-injured patient* (pp. 351-380). Philadelphia: Davis.

Bernardo, L., & Sullivan, K. (1990). Care of the pediatric patient with burns. In R. Trofino (Ed.), *Care of the burn-injured patient* (pp. 249-276). Philadelphia: Davis.

Davey, R., Wallis, K., Perkins, K., & Tingay, M. (1995). Thermal and electrical injuries. In W. Buntain (Ed.), *Management of pediatric trauma* (pp. 431-449). Philadelphia: Saunders.

Dickerson, P., Gordon, M., & Walter, P. (1998). Burns. In M. Slota (Ed.), *Core curriculum for pediatric critical care nursing* (pp. 652-675). Philadelphia: Saunders.

Gaisford, J., Slater, H., & Goldfarb, I. (2002). *The management of burn trauma: A unified approach.* Pittsburgh: Synapse Publications.

Ray, L., & Yuwiler, J. (1994). *Child and adolescent fatal injury databook.* San Diego: Children's Safety Network.

40

Shock

Sarah Martin, RN, MS, PCCNP, CPNP, CCRN
Michelle R. Morfin, RN, MS, CNP, CS, CCRN

Introduction

Shock is categorized as hypovolemic, cardiogenic, or maldistributive (anaphylactic, neurogenic, or septic). The common pathway of all types of shock is inadequate tissue perfusion and oxygen supply to meet the metabolic needs of the tissues. Inadequate tissue perfusion results in anaerobic metabolism, with the accumulation of lactic acid and a metabolic acidosis. As the shock state progresses, microvascular perfusion is impaired, resulting in cellular damage and the release of vasoactive substances, and eventual individual organ dysfunction. Death results if treatment does not stop the cascade of these events.

Etiology

Tables 40.1 and 40.2 describe the etiology of each shock state.

Focused History

Patient History

- Antecedent illness that could cause hypovolemia:
  - Fever (Chapter 12).
  - Gastroenteritis (Chapter 19).
  - Burn injury (Chapter 39).
- Recent infection
- History of cardiac disease, surgery, or syncopal episodes:
  - Cardiogenic shock may be a sequela of closure of the patent ductus arteriolus in a neonate with a ductal-dependent lesion (Chapter 17).
- Exposure to allergens:
  - Insect bites.
  - Nuts.
  - Eggs.
  - Shellfish.
  - Certain antibiotics (e.g., penicillin and sulfonamides).

Focused Assessment

Physical Assessment

1. Assess the airway and respiratory systems.
   - Assess the airway for patency.
   - Auscultate the chest for:
     - Respiratory rate. May be increased or decreased dependent on the type of shock and the stage of illness.
     - Adventitious sounds.
   - Inspect the chest for:
     - Accessory muscle use.
2. Assess the cardiovascular system.
   - Auscultate the heart for:
     - Rate. An increased heart rate may reflect a compensatory measure to increase cardiac output.
     - Rhythm.

TABLE 40.1 Comparison of Hypovolemic and Cardiogenic Shock States

Parameter	*Hypovolemic*	*Cardiogenic*
Etiology	Abnormal loss of circulating volume: ▪ Blood: Hemorrhage (e.g., trauma and gastrointestinal blood loss), inadequate replacement ▪ Water: Diarrhea, vomiting, hyperglycemia, diabetes insipidus; redistribution of intravascular volume: vasodilator therapy, sepsis ▪ Plasma: Capillary leak syndrome, peritonitis, burns, nephrotic syndrome, and hypoproteinemia	▪ Congenital heart disease ▪ Acquired heart disease ▪ Acidosis ▪ Electrolyte imbalances ▪ Drug toxicities ▪ Cardiac tamponade ▪ Dysrhythmias
Pathophysiology	▪ Excessive volume loss, resulting in decreased venous return, decreased ventricular filling, and decreased stroke volume, with eventual decreased cardiac output	▪ Impaired myocardial muscle function, leading to decreased cardiac output
Physical assessment	▪ Tachycardia ▪ Hypotension (late sign) ▪ Decreased peripheral pulses ▪ Cool, mottled skin ▪ Oliguria ▪ Altered mental status	▪ Tachycardia ▪ Hypotension (late sign) ▪ Decreased peripheral pulses ▪ Cool, mottled skin ▪ Oliguria ▪ Altered mental status
Treatment	▪ Assess and maintain airway patency and respiratory function. ▪ Obtain venous access with two large-bore intravenous catheters; initiate fluid resuscitation with colloid and crystalloid fluids. ▪ Measure intake and output. ▪ Correct the source of hypovolemia.	▪ Assess and maintain airway patency and respiratory function. ▪ Obtain venous access. ▪ Initiate fluid restriction as prescribed. ▪ Administer inotropic and vasoactive therapy as prescribed. ▪ Administer diuretic therapy as prescribed. ▪ Measure intake and output.

From: Taketomo, Hodding & Kraus, 2001; Tuite, 1997.

- Palpate the peripheral pulses for:
  - Equality.
  - Quality.
- Measure capillary refill time:
  - Capillary refill greater than 3 seconds indicates poor peripheral perfusion.
- Observe skin color and temperature.
- Measure the blood pressure.

3. Assess the neurologic system.
   - Assess the child's level of consciousness with the AVPU (Alert, responds to Verbal stimuli, responds to Painful stimuli, Unresponsive) method or Glasgow coma scale.
   - Observe the child's response to the environment and procedures.
   - Inspect the pupils for:
     - Size.
     - Reactivity.
     - Equality.

Psychosocial Assessment

- Assess the child's and family's understanding of the current health condition.
- Assess the child's and family's coping strategies and social support system:
  - Children in shock can be near death on emergency department (ED) presentation. Consider the family members' emotional needs (Chapter 28).

TABLE 40.2 Comparison of Maldistributive Shock States

Parameter	*Anaphylactic*	*Neurogenic*	*Septic*
Etiology	■ Allergen	■ Spinal cord injury ■ High levels of spinal anesthesia ■ Nervous system damage ■ Ganglionic and adrenergic blocking agents	■ Infectious organisms
Pathophysiology: vascular abnormality (vasodilation) that precedes a maldistribution of blood flow	■ Hypersensitivity reaction, causing vasodilation and capillary leakage	■ Vasodilation caused by loss of sympathetic nervous system tone ■ Spinal shock occurs with transection above T1, where trauma to the cervical or high thoracic spinal cord often injures the descending sympathetic pathways.	■ Following an insult with an infectious agent, a series of events is produced by chemical mediators and cascades, resulting in endothelial cell destruction, massive vasodilation, increased capillary permeability, microemboli formation, and resultant vasoconstriction of organ beds and depressed myocardial contractility.
Physical assessment	■ Hives ■ Dyspnea ■ Wheezing ■ Chest tightness ■ Hypotension	■ Bradycardia ■ Hypotension ■ Initially, warm extremities, low diastolic blood pressure, and a wide pulse pressure are found, which are related to the interruption of sympathetic outflow from the cervicothoracic region of the spinal cord. ■ Vasomotor tone vanishes, resulting in pooling of blood in the extremities and inadequate venous return. ■ Altered mental status ■ Oliguria	■ Tachycardia ■ Hypotension ■ Delayed capillary refill ■ Cool extremities
Treatment	■ Assess and maintain airway patency and cardiopulmonary function. ■ Administer epinephrine 1:1,000 subcutaneous (0.01 ml/kg, maximum dose of 0.5 ml). ■ Avoid re-exposure to allergen.	■ Assess and maintain airway patency and cardiopulmonary function. ■ Obtain venous access and initiate intravenous fluids at normal maintenance infusion rates. ■ Administer vasopressor therapy as prescribed.	■ Assess and maintain airway patency and cardiopulmonary function. ■ Obtain venous access and administer intravenous fluids. ■ Administer vasopressor and antibiotic therapy, as prescribed.

From: Taketomo et al, 2001; Tuite, 1997.

Nursing Interventions for all Types of Shock

1. Maintain airway patency:
   - Prepare for endotracheal intubation.
2. Administer supplemental oxygen:
   - Provide 100% oxygen through a nonrebreather mask for the child with adequate respiratory function.
   - Provide bag-valve-mask ventilation to the child requiring assisted ventilation.
   - Prepare for mechanical ventilation.
3. Initiate continuous cardiopulmonary and oxygen saturation monitoring.
4. Initiate cardiopulmonary resuscitation if needed.
5. Obtain venous access and initiate intravenous infusions with large-bore catheters:
   - Administer medications as prescribed:
     - Initiate fluid bolus and fluid replacement therapy for hypotension.
     - Initiate vasopressor therapy for hypotension.
     - Initiate antibiotic therapy for suspected infection.
   - Obtain blood for laboratory studies:
     - Arterial blood gas.

- Electrolytes.
- Complete blood count with differential and platelet count.
- Cultures.

6. Insert a nasogastric tube as needed for gastric decompression; measure its output.
7. Insert an indwelling bladder catheter as needed; measure urinary output.
8. Measure intake and output.
9. Provide frequent updates on the child's condition to the family; consider having the family present during procedures and treatment (Chapter 4).
10. Initiate social support through social services, clergy, or other consultation.
11. Prepare for transfer and transport to a tertiary care facility as needed (Chapter 10).
12. Initiate debriefing for the staff if the child dies in the ED (Chapter 28).

Home Care and Prevention

A high index of suspicion and early recognition of shock states prevent subsequent decompensation and mortality. Children who are allergic to foods, bee stings, and other allergens should wear a Medic Alert bracelet and carry an Epi-pen Jr® with them at all times. Family members must be prepared for possible allergen exposure.

Conclusion

A high index of suspicion is indicated for potential shock states among children who present for ED treatment. Early recognition of shock and intervention with these children may enhance their outcomes.

References

Taketomo, C. K., Hodding, J. H., & Kraus, D. M. (2001). *Pediatric dosage handbook* (8th ed.). Hudson, OH: Lexi-Comp., Inc.

Tuite, P. (1997). Recognition and management of shock in the pediatric patient. *Critical Care Nursing Quarterly*, *20*(1), 52-61.

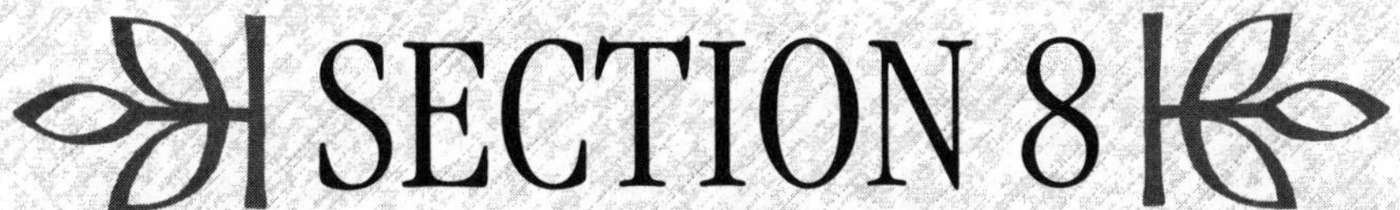

Environmental-Related Emergencies

41

Heat-related Emergencies

Jeanette H. Walker, RN, BSN

Introduction

Heat-related emergencies are a common occurrence in the United States. They can be mild events that respond readily to simple management techniques or life-threatening events that require immediate intervention. To provide appropriate care, the emergency department (ED) nurse must understand normal and abnormal thermoregulation and be able to identify children at risk for heat injuries.

Heat-related deaths occur most commonly in adults, particularly the elderly, but children are also vulnerable to serious injury or death. Children are at high risk if left in an intense heat environment, such as a closed car. Temperatures in a car parked in the sun can rise to 60°C (140°F) in 15 minutes (Mellor, 1997). Death in a heated car is more common in children younger than 12 months but has occurred in older children. In 1998, four preschool-aged children died in Utah when they climbed into a trunk of a car and were undetected for a long time. Similar deaths have resulted in children who climb into trunks of cars and cannot safely get out. Legislation is being proposed to have trunks equipped with a latch that allows them to be opened from the inside. The purpose of this chapter is to discuss common heat-related emergencies, their assessment, and nursing interventions.

Pathophysiology

Thermoregulation, the maintenance of normal body temperature, is accomplished by balancing heat load and heat dissipation:

- *Heat load* is determined by metabolic, kinetic, and environmental conditions. Metabolism produces about 100 kcal of heat per hour. Muscle activity during exercise produces 300 to 600 kcal or more of heat per hour. The body also absorbs heat from the environment (Waters, 2001).
- *Heat dissipation* occurs primarily through evaporation of sweat. If the ambient humidity is 75% or higher, evaporation slows. At 90% to 95% humidity, evaporation ceases altogether (Mellor, 1997). *Radiation*, the transfer of heat through electromagnetic waves, and *conduction*, the transfer of heat through direct contact, also play a role in heat dissipation.
- *Convection* is heat loss by the transfer of heat through air currents. Excess clothing, low wind velocity, and an air temperature that is near body temperature can impede convection.

The hypothalamus acts as a thermostat. When heat begins to build, the hypothalamus signals the autonomic nervous system to reduce sympathetic vasoconstrictor tone. Cardiac output rises, increasing circulation to the skin. Heat from the core is lost as the blood circulates to the periphery and sweating begins (Mellor, 1997).

When the body reaches the point that dissipation can no longer keep up with heat accumulation, the body temperature begins to rise. Cellular enzyme systems fail above 42.0°C (107.6°F). Further heat insult denatures proteins and results in organ and system failure (Mellor, 1997).

Pediatric Considerations

Several physiological factors increase the risk of heat-related emergencies in children (Mellor, 1997; Barkin & Rosen, 1999):

- Children have a greater surface area to mass ratio, allowing for greater transfer of heat from the environment to the body.
- Children have an increased production of metabolic heat per kilogram of body weight when moving and a poor ability to acclimate to hot conditions because of immature thermoregulatory control mechanisms.
- Children have a lesser ability to convey heat through the blood from the body core to the body surface.

Several developmental, behavioral, and health risk factors predispose children to heat-related emergencies:

- Young children do not instinctively think to replace fluid losses and may ignore thirst or be unable to interpret thirst as a need for fluids. They are dependent on adults to meet these needs.

- Teenaged and preadolescent athletes account for more than 1,000 cases of heat exhaustion reported annually among athletes in the United States. (Mellor, 1997). They push themselves harder and are less likely to replace fluid losses.
- Vapor-impermeable uniforms, helmets, and shoulder pads worn when children participate in organized sports limit heat dissipation by decreasing evaporation of sweat and convection of heat.
- Chronic childhood diseases, such as cystic fibrosis, quadriplegia, and congenital anhidrosis, decrease the ability to sweat or cause excess losses of sodium.
- Acute febrile illnesses, which are common in young children, also increase the risk for heat injury.
- Drugs such as antihistamines, phenothiazines, anticholinergics, beta-blockers, and alcohol, as well as street drugs, including phencyclidine (PCP) and D-lysergic acid diethylamide (LSD), impair normal sweating. Amphetamines and cocaine increase muscle activity and heat production. Any of these agents may increase the risk of heat injury.

Focused History

- Length of exposure to heat
- Temperature and humidity level during exposure
- Activities preceding onset of symptoms
- Pre-existing illnesses or drug use
- Treatment prior to arrival in the emergency department

Focused Assessment

Physical Assessment

The standard pediatric assessment is done (Chapter 6). Signs and symptoms of heat-related injuries are discussed under specific conditions later in this chapter.

Psychosocial Assessment

- Was the child properly supervised prior to the illness?
- Is the child's condition the result of caregiver neglect or ignorance of the child's needs?
- Was housing on upper floors without air conditioning a factor?

A list of nursing diagnoses and expected outcomes is shown in Table 41.1.

Triage Decisions

Emergent

- Child is experiencing respiratory or cardiac arrest.
- Child has a temperature greater than 40.0°C (104.0°F).
- Child has a decreased level of consciousness.

Urgent

- Child has a temperature between 38.0 and 40.0°C (100.4 and 104.0°F) with mild changes in mental status.

Nonurgent

- Child is alert with a temperature less than 38.0°C (100.4°F).

Specific Heat-related Emergencies

There are three common heat-related emergencies: heat cramps, heat exhaustion, and heat stroke. Table 41.2 compares the signs and symptoms and interventions for each condition.

Heat Cramps

Heat cramps are painful spasms that result from profuse sweating and loss of electrolytes during prolonged peri-

TABLE 41.1
Nursing Diagnoses and Expected Outcomes

Nursing Diagnoses	*Expected Outcomes*
Hyperthermia, associated with increased body temperature and decreased heat loss	Temperature will return to normal level through interventions to increase heat loss.
Risk for fluid volume deficit, related to electrolyte losses and inadequate fluid replacement	Hydration status will return to normal through interventions to replace fluid and electrolytes and decrease losses.
Knowledge deficit, related to risks of illness from heat exposure	Parent will have an understanding of factors that may lead to hypothermia on discharge from the ED by discharge teaching.

TABLE 41.2 A Comparison of Heat Cramps, Heat Exhaustion, and Heat Stroke

Type	*Assessment Findings*	*Nursing Interventions*
Heat cramps	■ Sudden, painful, and brief muscle spasms during or following exercise ■ Normal or slightly elevated body temperature ■ Normal mental status	■ Move the child into a cool environment to rest. ■ Treat mild dehydration with oral fluid and electrolyte replacement. A mixture of 1 teaspoon of sodium chloride (table salt) to 500 ml of water given over 1 to 2 hours is usually sufficient. ■ Treat severe dehydration intravenously with a 20 ml/kg of 0.9% normal saline given over 1 to 2 h.
Heat exhaustion	■ Fatigue ■ Headache ■ Nausea and vomiting ■ Diarrhea ■ Muscle cramps ■ Tachypnea ■ Hypotension ■ Mild changes in mental status ■ Moist skin, patient may be sweating profusely	■ Move the child into a cool environment; use fans in the emergency department if necessary. ■ Treat mild dehydration and sodium depletion with oral fluid and electrolyte replacement (see the interventions for heat cramps). ■ Treat severe isotonic or hypotonic dehydration with 0.9% normal saline, 20 ml/kg over 30 to 60 minutes. ■ Spray water over the child's body to increase evaporative losses. ■ Use a fan to increase convective heat loss.
Heat stroke	■ Nausea and vomiting ■ Headache ■ Neurologic changes progressing from ataxia, confusion, and disorientation to coma. ■ Flushed skin, hot, and dry. ■ Tachycardia ■ Hypotension	■ Secure airway. ■ Assist with intubation, if necessary. ■ Establish intravenous access and start 0.9% normal saline, 20 ml/kg over 30 to 60 minutes. ■ Continuously monitor temperature, pulse, respirations, blood pressure, and level of consciousness. ■ Insert an indwelling urinary catheter and monitor urinary output. ■ Give diazepam 0.2 to 0.3 mg/kg intravenously to prevent shivering. ■ Initiate rapid cooling until the temperature is less than 39.0°C (102.2°F). ■ Give ice baths. ■ Spray the child with water and cool with fan; apply ice bags to groin, axilla, and neck if an ice bath is not available.

Data from: Mellor, 1997; Barkin and Rosen, 1999; Baum, 2000.

ods of exercise in hot conditions. Sodium depletion can potentiate the effect of calcium on skeletal muscle. Cramping usually affects the large muscle groups being used, most commonly the legs. Heat cramps may occur during activity or several hours later. Drinking hypotonic fluids (water) to replace fluid losses contributes to the cramping, because it worsens the hyponatremia by diluting the circulating sodium.

Heat Exhaustion

Heat exhaustion is a condition resulting from exposure to high temperatures, excessive sweating and insufficient fluid and/or salt replacement. The core temperature ranges from 38.0 to 40.0°C (100.4 to 104.0°F) (Lee-Chiong & Stitt, 1995). There are two types of heat exhaustion:

1. *Hyponatremic* heat exhaustion results from replacement of fluid and electrolyte losses with water only.
2. *Hypernatremic* heat exhaustion results from loss of fluid and electrolytes without replacement of any kind.

If not treated promptly, heat exhaustion may progress to heat stroke which can be fatal.

Heat Stroke

Heat stroke is a life-threatening emergency. Heat stroke can result from direct exposure to the sun's rays or from high environmental temperatures without exposure to the sun. It is characterized by a temperature greater than 41.0°C (106.0°F). The body's ability to dissipate heat is overwhelmed and sweating is impaired. The brain is particularly sensitive to heat; therefore, neurologic symptoms occur early. Profound volume depletion occurs. Respiratory alkalosis and metabolic acidosis are common. Without immediate intervention, widespread organ injury and death can occur (Yarbrough & Bradham, 1998).

Heat stroke can be divided into two categories (Mellor, 1997):

1. *Classic* or *nonexertional* heat stroke usually affects infants and small children with predisposing illness and is likely to occur during heat waves. It develops over a period of days.
2. *Exertional* heat stroke develops rapidly and occurs most commonly in vigorously active individuals who are not acclimated to a hot environment.

Home Care and Prevention

Instruct parents to:

- Never leave a child alone in a car, especially in warm temperatures. Keep car windows open in the driveway at home to prevent children from becoming locked in the car.
- Be aware of and educate other supervising adults (parents, babysitters, and coaches) of the dangers involved with strenuous exercise in a hot environment.
- Provide children participating in strenuous exercise with adequate fluid and electrolytes and allow plenty of rest.
- Schedule athletic practices for early morning or in the evening.
- Be especially careful to take precautions if the child has a preexisting health condition that increases the risk of heat illness.

Conclusion

Children, because of various physiological and developmental factors, are at risk for hyperthermia. Emergency department nurses must be aware of the different types of heat-related injury and intervene to prevent a mild case of heat exhaustion from progressing into life-threatening heat stroke. Parents and children must be given information about prevention of these conditions.

References

Barkin, R. M., & Rosen, P. (1999). *Emergency Pediatrics* (5th ed., pp. 330–335). St. Louis: Mosby—Year Book..

Baum, C. R. (2000). Environmental and exertional heat illness. In G. R. Fleisher & S. Ludwig (Eds.), *Textbook of pediatric emergency medicine* (4th ed., pp. 951-955). Philadelphia: Lippincott, Williams & Wilkins.

Lee-Chiong, T. L., & Stitt, J. T. (1995). Heatstroke and other heat-related illnesses. *Postgraduate Medicine, 98*(1), 26–36.

Mellor, M. F. (1997). Heat-induced illnesses. In R. M. Barkin (Ed.), *Pediatric emergency medicine: Concepts and clinical practice* (2nd ed., pp. 496–499). St. Louis: Mosby.

Waters, T. A. (2001). Heat illness: Tips for recognition and treatment. *Cleveland Clinic Journal of Medicine, 68*(8), 685–687.

Yarbrough, B. & Bradham (1998). Heat illness. In Rosen, P. & Barkin, R. (Eds.), *Vol. I, Emergency medicine concepts and clinical practice* (4th ed., pp. 986–1002). St. Louis: Mosby.

42

Cold-related Emergencies

Jeanette H. Walker RN, BSN

Introduction

Cold injuries in children result from immersion in cold water or prolonged exposure to a cold environment. Injury occurs when the body is unable to produce sufficient heat to balance heat losses. Children are at high risk of developing hypothermia as a result of other illnesses or injuries. An infant undressed and left uncovered in a cool environment can become hypothermic during examination and therapeutic procedures. It is essential that emergency nurses be aware of the factors that increase the risk and be able to provide immediate, effective treatment. The purpose of this chapter is to discuss selected conditions related to exposure to cold temperatures and nursing interventions to treat and prevent these conditions.

Pathophysiology

Hypothermia exists when the core body temperature falls below 35.0°C (95.0°F). It is usually caused by accidental exposure to cold temperatures.

Human core temperature is normally maintained within 0.6°C (1.0°F). This represents a fine balance between heat production and heat loss. When core temperature begins to fall below 37.0°C (98.6°F), physiologic mechanisms that produce and conserve heat are activated (Baum, 2000):

- Cooled blood stimulates the hypothalamus to increase muscle tone and metabolism (oxidative phosphorylation and high energy phosphate production) and to augment heat production by 50% during non-shivering thermogenesis.
- When muscle tone reaches a critical level, shivering begins, and heat production increases two to four times basal levels.

Although surface temperature of the body, especially the extremities, may drop nearly to environmental temperatures, several mechanisms work to conserve heat and to protect blood and core structures from ambient air temperature, humidity, and wind (Baum, 2000). Sweating ceases, decreasing heat loss by evaporation, and vasoconstriction of cutaneous and subcutaneous vessels reduce losses further. Table 42.1 describes other responses to decreasing body temperature.

There is a misconception that cold penetrates. However, in reality, heat flows from hot to cold. The speed of the movement depends on the temperature difference. The greater the difference, the faster the heat flows from the warm body to the cold environment.

The thermal conductivity of water is approximately 30 times greater than that of air (Bessen, 1996). Thus, immersion in cold water produces a more rapid decline in body temperature than does exposure to cold air. Death occurs in 15 minutes in water at 0°C (32.0°F) (Baum, 2000). Heat is also lost by the following methods:

- *Evaporation*—Most commonly, evaporation of sweat
- *Convection*—The transfer of heat through air currents
- *Radiation*—The transfer of heat through electromagnetic waves
- *Conduction*—The transfer of heat through direct contact

Pediatric Considerations

Infants and young children are at significantly high risk for hypothermia, particularly in cold water immersions. Physiologic, health, and behavioral factors may increase the risk:

- Physiologic factors:
  - Large body-to-surface-area ratio
  - Minimal subcutaneous fat
  - Thin skin with increased permeability
  - Delayed shivering and inefficient ability to produce heat

- Health and behavioral factors:
  - Malnutrition
  - Drug or alcohol intoxication, which can impair the ability to feel the cold and the body's ability to react normally to the cold stimulus (Ciorciari & Hodge, 1997).
  - Incapacitating illnesses such as severe infection or diabetic ketoacidosis, and immobilizing injuries such as paralysis
  - Hypothyroidism and Addison's disease
  - Trauma

Focused History

- Type of exposure (such as submersion in cold water or exposure to cold outdoor environment)
- Temperature of the environment; wind chill and humidity factors
- Length of exposure
- Preexisting medical conditions that might increase the risk for hypothermia
- Drug or alcohol use

Focused Assessment

Physical Assessment

The signs and symptoms of hypothermia depend on the degree of hypothermia and are listed in Table 42.1.

Any child with cold skin, altered mental status, and bradycardia should be considered to be hypothermic until proven otherwise (Ciorciari & Hodge, 1997). The standard pediatric assessment is done (see Chapter 6).

A low-reading thermometer is essential. Ordinary thermometers do not record less than 34.0°C (93.2°F). Rectal or indwelling urinary catheter probes are designed to measure low temperatures. An esophageal probe will most accurately measure core temperature.

1. Assess heart rate and rhythm, and blood pressure.
2. Assess for other injuries.
3. Grade the hypothermia as mild, moderate, or profound (Ciorciari & Hodge, 1997):
   - *Mild*—32.2–35.0°C (90.0–95.0°F).
   - *Moderate*—26.2–32.0°C (79.2–89.6°F)
   - *Profound*—less than 26.2°C (79.2°F)

TABLE 42.1 Signs and Symptoms of Cold Injury

Body Temperature and Pathophysiology	***Signs and Symptoms***
32.0–35.0°C (89.6–95.0°F) Sympathetic response causes peripheral vasoconstriction	▪ Shivering ▪ Chattering teeth ▪ Dysarthria ▪ Clumsiness ▪ Poor capillary refill
28.0–32.0°C (82.0–89.6°F) Body function slows down progressively. The metabolism slows approximately 6% for each degree decrease in body temperature. At 28.0°C the basal metabolic rate falls by half. Oxygen consumption and carbon dioxide production decrease. Compensatory mechanisms fail.	▪ Decreases in shivering ▪ Decrease in heart rate and blood pressure ▪ Apathy ▪ Disorientation
25.0–28.0°C (77.0–82.0°F) Cardiac conduction decreases and cardiac irritability increases. Circulatory collapse begins as stroke volume, filling pressure, contractility, and heart rate decrease.	▪ Dysrhythmias, ranging from bradycardia to ventricular fibrillation ▪ Coma ▪ Cardiopulmonary arrest
<25.0°C (77.0°F) The body's physiologic needs may still be met.	▪ Apnea ▪ Asystole

Data from: Ciorciari & Hodge, 1997; Bessen, 1996; Barkin, 1999.

TABLE 42.2 Nursing Diagnoses and Expected Outcomes

Nursing Diagnoses	*Expected Outcomes*
Hypothermia related to cold exposure	Temperature will be increased after warming measures.
Decreased tissue perfusion (cerebral, cardiopulmonary, renal)	Tissue perfusion will be improved or return to normal, as evidenced by vital signs and the child's level of consciousness.
Inability to maintain spontaneous respirations	Respirations will be spontaneous and nonlabored.

Psychosocial Assessment

- Children are at risk for cold injuries because they are likely to become absorbed in outdoor play and sporting activities, often not realizing that an injury is occurring. Also, they are more likely to wear clothing that restricts circulation or to continue playing in wet clothing.
- Homelessness places children at special risk for cold injuries.
- The child should always be assessed for evidence that abuse or neglect may have contributed to the injury. For example, was the child improperly clothed for the conditions or left outside for an extended period of time without supervision?

Nursing diagnoses and expected outcomes are shown in Table 42.2.

Triage Decision

Emergent

- History of cold exposure if a child is experiencing respiratory or cardiac arrest or altered mental status.

Urgent

- History of cold exposure, child's temperature is above 35.0°C (95.0°F) and child is experiencing mild to moderate respiratory distress and minimal changes in mental status.

Nonurgent

- History of cold exposure, child has normal or slightly subnormal temperature and no respiratory distress or change in mental status.

Nursing Interventions

1. Maintain airway, breathing, and circulation.
   - Assist with cardiopulmonary resuscitation as necessary.
   - Handle the child gently, because rough handling may precipitate ventricular fibrillation.
2. Assist with intubation as necessary.
   - Administer warmed, humidified 100% oxygen.
3. Continuously monitor oxygen saturation.
4. Establish intravenous access.
   - Administer intravenous fluid warmed to 36.0 to 40.0°C (96.8 to 104.0°F) (Barkin, 1999).
5. Monitor heart rate and rhythm continuously.
   - Be prepared to treat dysrhythmias.
6. Gently remove all wet or cold clothing.
7. Assist with rewarming techniques (Table 42.3).

Specific Cold-related Emergencies

Frostbite

Localized cold injuries result from failure to provide or maintain adequate protection from the environment. Children who live in colder climates and participate in winter sports are at risk for these injuries.

Frostbite occurs when ice crystals form within the soft tissues as a consequence of exposure to the cold (Ciociari & Hodge, 1997). The incidence and severity of frostbite in children is directly influenced by environmental factors, including wind chill, humidity, and contact with good thermal conductors, such as water or metal. Severe injury can occur at temperatures above freezing if these factors are present (Rabold, 1996). Exposed areas of the body most often affected are the hands, feet, cheeks, chin, and nose. Early cold injury is referred to as *frost nip*. Frost nip will quickly progress to frostbite if treatment is not initiated promptly. Health care workers must be able to recognize and differentiate signs of frostbite and initiate the proper treatment immediately.

The initial body response to prolonged exposure to cold temperatures is peripheral vasoconstriction, which

TABLE 42.3 Rewarming Techniques

Mild Hypothermia	*Moderate Hypothermia*	*Profound Hypothermia*
Passive Rewarming ▪ Layered blankets ▪ Warm room	**Active Rewarming** ▪ Intravenous access prior to warming in case dysrhythmias occur ▪ Electric warming blankets or pads; hot water bottles ▪ Radiant warming ▪ Forced air ▪ Blanket warming	**Core Rewarming** ▪ Warmed intravenous fluids ▪ Warmed, humidified oxygen ▪ Warmed nasogastric, peritoneal, bladder, or pleural lavage ▪ Extracorporeal circulation on heart-lung machine

Data from: Ciorciari & Hodge, 1997; Barkin, 1999.

compromises blood flow to the area. The blood becomes more viscous, decreasing capillary perfusion and causing sludging and thrombosis. The surrounding tissue becomes ischemic, with an increase in vascular permeability, resulting in swelling. When the tissue temperature drops below 0°C (32.0°F), freezing ice crystals begin to form in the extracellular compartment. Intracellular fluid is drawn out by osmosis, resulting in cellular dehydration, denatured proteins, enzyme destruction, and altered cellular membranes. The end result is irreversible tissue damage (Danzi, 1998).

Focused History

The history is the same as was discussed earlier in this chapter.

Focused Assessment

The clinical findings of frostbite depend on the severity of the exposure. Frostbite is classified as superficial or deep (Table 42.4) or by degrees (Table 42.5). The standard pediatric assessment is done:

1. Airway and breathing.
   - Frostbite often occurs simultaneously with hypothermia. Stabilization and prevention of life-threatening events always take priority over the treatment of local cold injury (See the discussion of hypothermia.)
2. Circulation and skin integrity of the affected area:
   - Swelling.
   - Pliability of tissue.

TABLE 42.4 Clinical Findings in Frostbite

Description	*Signs and Symptoms*
Superficial ▪ Involves the skin and subcutaneous tissue	▪ Burning, tingling, and numbness may be present. ▪ Tissue will not reperfuse after blanching. ▪ A grayish cast to the skin may be present while the underlying tissue remains soft. ▪ Skin may become painful and flushed with rewarming. ▪ Fluid-filled blisters may develop over the next 24 hours.
Deep ▪ Involves the muscles, nerves, blood vessels, and bone	▪ Tissue will appear pale or gray, is hard, and cannot be depressed. ▪ There is a lack of sensation in the involved area. ▪ After warming, the area will become grossly swollen. ▪ Tissue will eventually turn purple-black and dry with small hemorrhagic blebs.

TABLE 42.5 Classification of Frostbite

Degree	*Signs and Symptoms*
First	Mottled skin; edema; erythema; white or yellowish plaque at injured area; burning and tingling; no tissue loss
Second	Blister formation (clear or milky fluid); paresthesia and anesthesia of area
Third	Deeper blisters (purple, blood-containing fluid); necrosis of skin with ulceration and edema; involvement of subcutaneous tissue
Fourth	Necrosis with gangrene; injury through the dermis; possible muscle and bone involvement

From: Tucker and Schauben, 1998, p. 665.

- Skin color.
- Sensation.
- Peripheral pulses.
- Capillary refill.
- Presence of blistering, necrosis, or gangrene.

Nursing Interventions

1. Remove wet or constrictive clothing.
2. Establish intravenous access with two large-bore intravenous catheters.
3. Prepare to treat life-threatening emergencies.
4. Elevate and immobilize the affected limb.
5. Avoid any mechanical friction, because this will increase tissue injury.
6. In severe cases, keep the injured area away from sources of heat until rapid rewarming can be done.
   - Warming and refreezing can markedly increase the injury.
7. Give analgesics prior to rewarming.
8. Initiate rapid rewarming measures.
   - Apply warm packs to the face and ears:
   - Submerge extremities in a warm water bath:
     - Use a warm water bath of 40.0 to 42.0°C (104.0 to 107.6°F) measured with a thermometer (Rabold, 1996).
     - If desired, add chlorhexidine gluconate (Hibiclens) for cleansing.
     - Carefully suspend the affected part in the bath; do not allow it to touch the sides or bottom.
     - Maintain the water temperature. Always remove the body part before adding hot water.
     - Continue rewarming until the area is completely thawed. The part will feel pliable, and erythema will be present distal to the injury.
     - Rewarming may take up to an hour in cases of severe freezing.
9. Provide postwarming care.
   - Elevate the extremity.
   - Separate the fingers or toes with sterile gauze to prevent tissue-to-tissue contact.
   - Reevaluate the injury frequently for changes in color, increased edema, increased or decreased sensation, and formation of blisters.
10. Provide wound care.
    - Blister management is controversial. Some practitioners advocate debridement; others feel that all blisters should be left intact. Most agree that hemorrhagic blisters should not be debrided because desiccation of deep dermal layers will worsen the outcome.
    - Apply topical silver sulfadiazine (Silvadene, SSD, Thermazene) cream to open wounds, if desired.
    - Topical aloe vera has been shown to improve the microcirculation (Danzi, 1998).
    - Consider administration of prophylactic systemic antibiotics.
    - Update tetanus immunity, as needed.

Home Care and Prevention

- Avoid lengthy exposure to cold.
- Wear layered, loose-fitting clothing.
- Avoid wearing tight-fitting footwear that may impair circulation.
- Keep dry.
- Be aware that wind chill, humidity, or contact with water or metal can increase the risk of sustaining a cold injury.
- Keep small children away from potential hazards such as frozen lakes or streams.

Conclusion

Children are at risk for cold injuries because of physiologic, health, and behavioral factors. Infants can experience hypothermia simply from being examined in a cold room. Nurses must understand the conditions that place infants and children at risk for cold injuries and be familiar with rewarming techniques for any condition, from mild frostbite to severe hypothermia.

References

Barkin, R. M. (1999). Hypothermia and frostbite. In R. M. Barkin & P. Rosen (Eds.), *Emergency pediatrics* (5th ed., pp. 335-341). St. Louis: Mosby—Year Book.

Baum, C. R. (2000). Accidental hypothermia. In G. L. Fleisher & S. Ludwig (Eds.), *Textbook of pediatric emergency medicine* (4th ed., pp. 955-959). Philadelphia: Lippincott Williams & Wilkins.

Bessen, H. A. (1996). Hypothermia. In J. E. Tintinalli, E. Ruiz, & R. L. Krome (Eds.), *Emergency medicine: A comprehensive study guide* (4th ed., pp. 846-849). New York: McGraw-Hill.

Ciorciari, A. J., & Hodge, D., III. (1997). Environmental emergencies. In E. Crain & J. Gershel (Eds.), *Clinical manual of emergency pediatrics* (3rd ed., pp. 180-182). New York: McGraw-Hill.

Danzi, D. F. (1998). Frostbite. In P. Rosen & R. Barkin (Eds.), *Vol. I, Emergency medicine concepts and clinical practice* (4th ed., pp. 953-962). St. Louis: Mosby.

Hofstrand, H. J. (1997). Accidental hypothermia and frostbite. In R. M. Barkin (ed.), Pediatric emergency medicine (2nd ed., pp. 500-508). St. Louis: Mosby.

Rabold, M. (1996). Bite and other localized injuries. In J. E. Tintinalli, E. Ruiz, & R. L. Krome, (Eds.), *Emergency medicine: A comprehensive study guide* (4th ed., pp. 843-846). New York: McGraw-Hill.

Tucker, C. and Schauben, J. (1998). Environmental and toxicologic emergencies. In T. E. Soud and J. S. Rogers (Eds.), *Manual of pediatric emergency nursing* (pp. 622-659). St. Louis: Mosby.

43

Bites and Stings

Jeanette H. Walker, RN, BSN

Introduction

Bites and stings are responsible for thousands of pediatric visits to the emergency department (ED) each year. Most present few problems to the child other than transient swelling and discomfort. They are easily managed with over-the-counter antihistamines and analgesics. However, the ED nurse must be prepared to recognize and treat the child who presents with a toxic envenomation from a number of sources, including spiders, scorpions, and snakes. Animal and human bites account for 1% of all ED visits (Ciociari, 1997) and pose a risk for disfigurement, rabies, and infection. Emergency nurses must be aware of the types of bites that might occur in their area of practice. The purpose of this chapter is to discuss common bites and stings that may occur in the pediatric patient and specific nursing interventions.

Pediatric Considerations

Bites that may not present a threat to an adult will be much more severe in a child because the child receives a larger dose of venom per kilogram of body weight than does an adult. The smaller the child, the greater the threat to the child's health.

Focused History

- Type of bite (spider, snake, animal).
- Time the bite occurred.
- Location of the bite on the child's body.
- Activities that might have placed the child at risk for getting bitten (e.g., playing outdoors in tall grass, around woodpiles, in sheds, garages, and barns).
- Allergies.
- Past medical history.
- Immunization status.
- First aid rendered at the scene. Prehospital interventions may include the following:
  1. Reassure and calm the victim.
  2. Immobilize the extremity in a neutral position at a level just below the heart.
  3. Remove constricting clothing and jewelry from the affected area.
  4. Do not attempt incision and suction. No animal studies have demonstrated increased survival rates when these techniques were used. Incision can result in damage to deeper structures. Oral suction increases the risk of infection (Herman & Skokan, 1999).
  5. Place a constricting band at least 2 cm wide, 5 to 10 cm proximal to the wound, loose enough to allow one finger beneath and preserve normal distal arterial pulses if the transport time to a hospital is more than 1 hour (Hodge & Tecklenburg, 2000).
  6. Transport the child to a medical facility as quickly as possible.

Focused Assessment

The standard pediatric assessment is done (Chapter 6). The following information must also be obtained:

- Location and number of bite marks, punctures, and scratches.
- Appearance of the bite (redness, swelling, drainage, discoloration).

A list of nursing diagnoses and their expected outcomes is given in Table 43.1.

TABLE 43.1 Nursing Diagnoses and Expected Outcomes

Nursing Diagnoses	*Expected Outcomes*
Pain, related to tissue injury and effects of venom	The child will be pain free through the use of medications and nonpharmacologic approaches, and lessening of the effects of the venom.
Altered tissue perfusion, renal, cerebral, cardiopulmonary, peripheral, related to the effects of the venom	The child will be well perfused, as evidenced by normotension, capillary refill <3 seconds, strong peripheral pulses, good sensation in all extremities, adequate urinary output, and alert and oriented mental status.
Risk for infection, related to loss of skin barrier	The risk for infection will be minimized by wound debridement, administration of tetanus prophylaxis, and appropriate use of antibiotics.

Triage Decisions

Emergent

- Any child who has been bitten by a poisonous snake or spider
- Any child who is exhibiting signs of respiratory distress or altered level of consciousness or signs of shock
- Any child bitten by a marine animal

Urgent

- Child experiencing local signs without circulatory impairment

Nonurgent

- None

Specific Conditions

Snake Bites

Snakes inflict around 45,000 bites each year in the United States and approximately 8 thousand are poisonous (Cohen, 1998). Fifty percent of the bite victims are children (Herman & Skokan, 1999). Most bites occur in adolescents and young adults while they are trying to handle or provoke the snake. Bites usually occur during the summer months and involve the upper extremities. Males are far more likely to be bitten than females (Hodge & Tecklenburg, 2000). Younger children are most likely to be bitten on the lower extremities (Herman & Skokan, 1999; Hodge & Tecklenburg, 2000).

The majority of venomous snakes in this country are pit vipers from the Crotalidae family, including rattlesnakes, cottonmouths, water moccasin, and copperheads. They are found in most areas of the country and are responsible for 99% of venomous snake bites. Coral snakes of the Elapidae family, found in the Southeast and Southwest and "exotic" nonindigenous snakes account for the other 1% (Hodge & Tecklenburg, 2000).

Pathophysiology

The severity of the bite depends on:

1. The type of snake:
   - *Pit viper venom* contains a combination of toxins (primarily hemotoxins). The venom is injected by the snake's fangs and is more dangerous than that of a coral snake because a large amount can be injected. The venom can cause the following signs and symptoms:
     - Local tissue necrosis.
     - Hemolysis of red blood cells.
     - Defects in coagulation with disseminated intravascular clotting.
     - Increased prothrombin times and decreased platelet counts with active bleeding.
     - Hypovolemic shock.
     - Renal failure secondary to prolonged hypotension and rhabdomyolysis.
     - Massive pulmonary edema.
   - *Coral snake venom* contains mainly neurotoxic components that produce mild local signs even in the case of major envenomations. The coral snake has teeth and must chew the victim to inject the venom. Systemic signs are delayed. However, once they begin, they are severe and progress rapidly. They include:
     - Nausea and vomiting.
     - Mental status changes.
     - Bulbar palsy, the destruction of the nerve centers of the medulla oblongata, characterized by an inability to speak and swallow.
     - Ptosis, drooping of the upper eyelids resulting from paralysis of the oculomotor nerve.

- Visual changes.
- Descending muscle paralysis leading to respiratory distress and respiratory failure.

2. The age, health, and size of the victim.
3. The site and number of bites.
4. The time lapse before the victim receives definitive treatment.
5. The amount of venom injected. Snake bites vary from a "dry" bite with little or no envenomation (as many as 30% of all bites) (Schexnayder & Schexnayder, 2000) to multiple bites causing marked tissue necrosis and/or severe systemic signs and symptoms.

Nursing Interventions

1. Ensure adequate airway.
2. Establish two large-bore intravenous catheters, one for crystalloid resuscitation and one for administration of antivenom, if necessary.
3. Obtain laboratory studies to include:
   - Urinalysis.
   - Complete blood count.
   - Platelets.
   - Creatinine.
   - Prothrombin time.
   - Partial prothrombin time.
   - Blood urea nitrogen.
4. Monitor vital signs.
5. Perform sequential circumferential measurements of the affected area every 15 to 30 minutes to assess the rate of spread and effectiveness of treatment.
6. Consider administration of vasopressors and monitoring of central venous pressure if the patient is exhibiting signs of shock.
7. Grade the envenomation of pit viper bites to determine the need for antivenom (Table 43.2).
8. Administer other therapy as necessary, including:
   - Pain medications.
   - Broad-spectrum antibiotics (not routinely needed).
   - Tetanus toxoid or tetanus immune globulin, depending on the patient's immunization status.
   - Wound debridement.

TABLE 43.2 Grading of Pit Viper Envenomation

Severity	*Findings*	*Laboratory Changes*
Minimal	■ Fang marks with mild local swelling and redness ■ Minimal or no systemic signs	■ No significant laboratory changes
Moderate	■ Fang marks with slowly progressing swelling and redness ■ Systemic signs including: ■ Nausea ■ Vomiting ■ Perioral paresthesia ■ Metallic taste ■ Weakness ■ Tachycardia	■ Decreased fibrinogen ■ Decreased platelet count ■ Hemoconcentration
Severe	■ All bites to the head and neck ■ Fang marks with rapidly progressing swelling and redness affecting the entire extremity ■ Systemic signs including: ■ Changes in mental status ■ Hypotension ■ Shock ■ Respiratory distress ■ Spontaneous bleeding ■ Convulsions	■ Increased clotting times ■ Anemia ■ Disseminated intravascular coagulation ■ Coagulopathy ■ Metabolic acidosis

TABLE 43.3 Antivenom Information

Antivenom Information and Supply	*Precautions/Nursing Implications*
1. Contact the local poison control center in your area. 2. Call the Antivenom Index at: 520-626-6016. 3. Contact the local zoo in the area. Zoos are required to keep adequate antivenom stores for any venomous snake in the possession of the zoo.	1. Snake antivenom consists of hyperimmune horse serum that can cause anaphylactic or delayed serum sickness reactions. A skin test should be performed for sensitivity. If the test result is positive, consult a toxicologist. 2. Be prepared to treat anaphylaxis even in patients with negative results to a skin test. 3. For best results, administer antivenom within 6 hours to patients with moderate to severe envenomation. In severe envenomation, antitoxin may be given up to 24 hours after the bite. 4. Instruct the parent or patient to watch for signs of serum sickness, which may occur within 1 to 3 weeks. Symptoms include fever, malaise, edema, headache, arthralgia, myalgia, and lymphadenopathy.

Data compiled from: Primm, 1997, and Hodge & Tecklenburg, 2000.

9. Administer antivenom (Hodge & Tecklenburg, 2000). Table 43.3 lists information and precautions concerning antivenom.
   - Dilute 5 vials in 250 ml of normal saline (125 ml of normal saline for infants weighing less than 10 kilograms) and administer slowly (1 to 2 ml/hr) for the first 10 to 20 minutes. If no adverse reaction is noted, the rate can be increased to complete the total volume in 2 hrs.
   - Continue to administer the antivenom in 5-vial aliquots until there is no further progression of swelling. As many as 75 vials may be necessary.
10. Monitor the patient for adverse reactions.
11. Treat anaphylaxis related to antivenom, as necessary:
    - Secure airway as necessary.
    - Establish intravenous access.
    - Administer epinephrine:
      - .01 ml/kg, 1:1,000 subcutaneously.
      - 0.1 ml/kg, 1:10,000 intravenously or endotracheally.
    - Administer antihistamines. The child can be premedicated to prevent or minimize allergic reactions:
      - H_2 blockers (cimetidine, ranitidine).
      - H_1 blockers (diphenhydramine).
      - B_2 agonists and/or aminophylline to ease bronchospasm.
      - Corticosteroids for anti-inflammatory effects and possible prevention of late-phase allergic response (Herman, Erickson, & Bowman, 1996).

Spider and Insect Bites

Fifty species of spiders found in the United States have fangs capable of penetrating human skin. Only two species, the black widow and the brown recluse, can cause fatalities (Ciorciari, 1997).

Pathophysiology and Nursing Interventions

Table 43.4 lists signs, symptoms, and treatment of various spider bites.

1. The *black widow* is found in every state except Alaska. The female is responsible for all human envenomation because the male is not big enough to inflict bites. The female black widow is shiny black and has a characteristic red or orange hourglass marking on the abdomen. She is typically found in sheltered corners of fields, gardens, outbuildings, barns, and garages. In areas where outdoor toilets are used, the bite is likely to involve the buttocks or genital area.
2. The *brown recluse* is most commonly found in the Mississippi, Ohio, and Missouri river basins. It prefers warm, dry areas such as abandoned buildings, woodpiles, and cellars (Otten, 1998). It may be dark or light brown and has a dark, violin-shaped spot centered so that the violin neck extends backward across the cephalothorax.

Several species of scorpion are found in the United States. The only medically significant stings occur in the

TABLE 43.4 Spider and Insect Bites

Spider/Insect	*Local Signs*	*Systemic Signs*	*Treatment*
Black widow spider	■ May or may not have initial pain ■ Mild redness and swelling ■ Two tiny puncture marks may be noted	■ Painful spasms of large muscles of abdomen, back, and extremities ■ Abdominal rigidity mimicking peritonitis or appendicitis ■ Weakness, hypertension ■ Respiratory arrest in young children ■ Rarely, death	■ Provide oral analgesics and reassurance in most cases. ■ Provide parenteral narcotics and benzodiazepines in more significant cases. ■ Administer antivenom in severe cases. Be prepared to treat anaphylaxis; watch for signs of serum sickness.
Brown recluse spider	■ May or may not have initial pain ■ Mildly reddened macule or papule that progresses to a hemorrhagic lesion with central necrosis	■ Rash, fever, chills, headache, myalgias, nausea, vomiting ■ Hemolysis resulting in hemoglobinuria ■ Thrombocytopenia ■ Renal failure ■ Disseminated intravascular clotting ■ Rarely, death	■ Provide wound care. ■ Dapsone may prevent necrosis by inhibiting infiltration of polymorphonuclear leukocytes. ■ Prepare for cosmetic repair of large necrotic areas by a plastic surgeon.
Hobo spider (northern brown spider)	■ May cause necrotic lesion similar to a brown spider bite	■ Headache ■ Visual disturbances ■ Weakness ■ Hallucinations	■ Same as for brown spider
Bark scorpion	■ Immediate burning and tingling	■ Tachycardia ■ Increased secretions ■ Muscle fasciculations ■ Opisthotonos ■ Roving eye movements ■ Delirium ■ Pulmonary edema	■ Administer beta-blockers. ■ Administer benzodiazapines. ■ Administer antivenom (available in Arizona).
Hymenoptera (bees, wasps, hornets, ants)	■ Local swelling, pain, redness, itching	■ Usually none ■ Possibility of anaphylactic reaction	■ Remove the stinger, if present, by carefully scraping it off. Avoid compressing the sting sack and injecting more venom (Banner, 1988). ■ Provide wound care.

Southwest, by the bark scorpion. The scorpion may be straw-colored, yellow, or light brown and is approximately 5 cm in length (Herman & Skokan, 1999).

Animal Bites

Children experience bites from a variety of animals and even each other during childhood. The majority of animal bites involve dogs, cats, humans, and rodents. Although parents are concerned about cosmetics, excessive bleeding, or rabies, the most common complication is infection (Ciociari, 1997).

Infection is a concern because of the variety of organisms found in the human mouth. Dog bites are associated with a lower incidence of infection than human bites, but cat bites or scratches have a higher risk for infection (Hodge & Tecklenburg, 2000). Rabies is the most serious concern. Rabies is commonly carried by raccoons, foxes, skunks, undomesticated dogs and cats, and bats (Chapter 26).

Pathophysiology

Skin and soft tissue injuries are the first concern in evaluating animal or human bites. The two major types of bite wounds are (Ciociari, 1997):

1. *Puncture*—This small break in the skin carries a significant risk of infection.
2. *Lacerations*—Controversies exist concerning suturing lacerations, but generally those on the face are sutured because the risk of infection is lower on the face.

Nursing Interventions

1. Clean the wound, irrigate under pressure: Clean with benzalkonium chloride, which kills rabies.
2. Anticipate the need for an X-ray to identify underlying fractures.
3. Obtain a wound culture if the wound is infected.
4. Assist with suturing, as necessary.
5. Administer tetanus toxoid.
6. Administer antibiotics, if appropriate, to prevent infection (may be intramuscular, intravenous, or oral).
7. Report bites to animal control department, per protocol.
8. Give follow-up information to family regarding signs and symptoms of infection, need to return to the emergency department, and wound care.

Marine Animal Bites and Stings

Marine animal (aquatic organisms) bites and stings occur in areas of the country near the ocean. These organisms usually do not prey on people but cause injuries when they are disturbed . These bites can result in a secondary infection from contaminated fresh and salt water. The three groups of aquatic organisms include (Emergency Nurses Association, 1994):

- Creatures that bite and may transmit a neurotoxic venom (sharks, barracudas, octopi, sea snakes).
- Creatures that sting by means of nematocysts or stinging capsules and produce an acid wound, such as jellyfish, hydrozoans anemones, and corals.
- Creatures that have spines, producing traumatic puncture wounds, and release toxins from venom sacs, producing cardiovascular, respiratory, or neurologic complications (stingray, scorpion fish, and sea urchin).

Pathophysiology and Nursing Interventions

Emergency department staff must be familiar with the types of marine bites and stings that occur in their area of practice and the proper treatment. Tables 43.5 and 43.6 list signs, symptoms, and treatment of invertebrate and vertebrate stings and bites.

Home Care and Prevention

- Avoid areas inhabited by snakes.
- Do not attempt to tease, play with, or capture snakes.
- Wear high-top boots and long pants when working, playing, or hiking in areas inhabited by snakes, spiders, or other insects.
- Become familiar with the insects and spiders in the area.
- When possible, avoid areas where there is an increased risk of encountering insects and spiders.
- Shake out clothing, sleeping bags, and shoes when camping.
- Do not allow children to play barefoot in the grass.
- Avoid wearing brightly colored or flowered clothing, which is more likely to attract stinging insects.
- Teach children about pets and how to approach them.
- Teach children to avoid unfamiliar animals or pets and what to do if approached by one.
- Be aware of types of marine animals capable of inflicting a toxic envenomation.
- Avoid contact with marine animals that can be harmful.

TABLE 43.5 Clinical Features and Treatment of Some Common Invertebrate Stings and Bites

Animal	*Injury*	*Treatment*
Portuguese man-of-war (nematocyst)	Electric shock-like sensation; multiple linear welts; headache; muscle cramps; nausea; vomiting; shock; cardiovascular collapse	Avoid fresh water:* rinse in sea water. Apply alcohol or vinegar. Apply baking soda and seawater paste to tentacles. Scrape tentacles off. Take nematocyst precautions.**
Fire coral (nematoycyst)	Redness; urticaria; hemorrhage; zosteriform rash; abdominal pain	Same as above.
Jellyfish (nematocyst)	Painful welts with characteristic pattern; muscle spasms; respiratory distress with sea wasp and sea nettle	Same as above. Administer antivenom for sea wasp.
Elkhorn coral	Intense stinging; weeping ulcers; septic sloughing; ulcer, if untreated	Same as above. Debride wound. Administer antibiotics.
Sea urchin	Intense pain; redness; swelling; partial motor paralysis; irregular pulse; delayed granulomas	Promptly remove spine, surgically, if necessary. Immerse in hot water (45°C) for 30 to 90 minutes to reduce pain.
Sea cucumber	Contact dermatitis; corneal injury	Take nematocyst precautions. Conduct a thorough eye exam.
Coneshell	Local reaction; pain; paresthesia; respiratory paralysis; death	Apply a loose tourniquet. Apply direct pressure. Administer naloxone. Administer neostigmine (use with caution).
Octopus	Minimal local reaction; occasionally neurotoxic symptoms	Symptomatic. Apply direct compression with gauze and bandage.

Adapted from: Prasad, 1993, pp. 791–792. Used with permission.
*Fresh water will cause nematocytes to activate.
**Nematocyst precautions include wearing gloves and using tweezers to remove the nematocytes to prevent poison injection into the caregiver.

TABLE 43.6 Clinical Features and Treatment of Some Common Vertebrate Stings and Bites

Animal	*Injury*	*Treatment*
Stingray	Intense pain; edema; syncope; paralysis; muscle spasms; seizures; vomiting; diarrhea	Provide thorough wound irrigation and wound care. Apply local suction. Administer antibiotics.
Catfish	Local pain; edema leading to gangrene; occasional systemic signs	Immerse in hot water; provide wound care.
Weeverfish	Pain; swelling; ischemia; gangrene	Immerse in hot water. Explore the wound. Administer antibiotics.
Scorpionfish	Intense pain; rash vesicles; severe gastrointestinal symptoms; respiratory distress; seizure; cardiac dysrhythmias	Immerse in hot water. Irrigate wound. Explore wound. Administer antivenom.

Adapted from: Prasad, 1993, pp. 791–792. Used with permission.

Conclusion

A variety of bites and stings may result in emergency department visits. Nurses should be familiar with the types of bites that are common in their area of practice and how to obtain the necessary antivenom. Bites and stings can be more serious in pediatric patients because of their small size. Prevention is the key to avoiding bites and stings.

References

Banner, W. Jr. (1988). Bites and stings in the pediatric patient. *Current problems in pediatrics, 18*(1), 5-69.

Ciorciari, A. J. (1997). Wound care and minor trauma. In E. F. Crain & J. C. Gershel (Eds.), *Clinical manual of emergency pediatrics* (3rd ed., pp. 643-655). New York: McGraw-Hill.

Emergency Nurses Association. (1994). *Emergency nursing core curriculum*, 5th ed. Park Ridge, IL: Author.

Herman, B. E. & Skokan, E. G. (1999). Bites that poison: A tale of spiders, snakes, and scorpions. *Contemporary Pediatrics, 8*, 41-65.

Herman, B. E., Erickson, T., & Bowman, M. J. (1996). Spider bites. In G. R. Strange, W. R. Ahrens, S. Lelyveld, & R. W. Schafermeyer (Eds.), *Pediatric emergency medicine: A comprehensive study guide.* (pp. 593-598). New York: McGraw-Hill.

Hodge, D. & Tecklenburg, F. W. (2000). Bites and Stings. In G. R. Fleisher & S. Ludwig (Eds.), *Textbook of pediatric emergency medicine* (4th ed., pp. 979-998). Philadelphia: Lippincott Williams & Wilkins.

Otten, E. J. (1998). Venomous animal injuries. In P. Rosen & G. Barkin (Eds.), *Volume I, Emergency medicine concepts and clinical practice* (4th ed., pp. 924-940. St. Louis: Mosby.

Prasad, N. H. (1993). Marine animal envenomation. In E. J. Reisdorff, M. R. Roberts, & J. G. Wiegenstein. *Pediatric emergency medicine* (pp. 789-793). Philadelphia: Saunders.

Schexnayder, S. M. & Schexnayder, R. E. (2000). Bites, stings and other painful things. *Pediatric Annals, 29*(6), 354-358.

44

Toxicologic Emergencies

Rose Ann Soloway, RN, BSN, MSEd, DABAT

Introduction

There are hundreds of thousands of drugs and chemicals in use, any of which may be involved in a poisoning or poison exposure. A poison exposure *is an inappropriate contact with or use of a chemical, drug, or natural toxin, by any route of exposure.* Poisoning *means that symptoms actually resulted from a drug, toxin, or chemical poison exposure. Most poison exposures are managed at home with the assistance of a poison center, but seriously poisoned children are referred or transported to the emergency department (ED) for treatment.*

Perhaps more than any other common pediatric emergency, poisoning elicits multisystemic responses in its victims. Proper assessment and treatment of a poisoned child require knowledge of normal growth and development plus astute history-taking and physical assessment skills. The purpose of this chapter is to discuss poison exposures that are common and potentially dangerous and for which accurate and effective ED assessment and treatment can have a significant impact on patient outcome.

Epidemiology

In 2000, the American Association of Poison Control Centers Toxic Exposure Surveillance System reported 2,168,248 human poison exposures (Litovitz, Klein-Schwartz, & White et al., 2001). The majority of exposures in young children are unintentional; intentional exposures (e.g., suicide and abuse of drugs and chemicals) predominate after the age of 13 years. Therefore, as the age of poisoning victims increases, the number of fatalities increases (Table 44.1).

Pediatric poison exposures reflect the availability of potentially poisonous substances (Table 44.2). More than 90% of all exposures occur in a residence (Litovitz et al., 2001), but the substances most commonly involved are not necessarily the most dangerous. The leading causes of fatalities from poison exposures among all ages are listed in Table 44.3.

Following a poisoning or poison exposure, the patient may be asymptomatic or symptomatic. In the *asymptomatic patient*, no obvious life-threatening effects are observed. The poison center is contacted to determine if any treatment is required. (The poison center may have been contacted by the family before an asymptomatic patient arrives in the ED, to determine if evaluation is necessary). In the *symptomatic patient*, the obvious effects are observed. The patient's condition is stabilized in the ED, and the poison center is contacted to determine if a specific antidote, treatment, or clinical or laboratory assessment is required.

Pediatric Considerations

Pediatric considerations in poison exposures relate to children's physiologic immaturity and developmental maturation. Infants' small size, immature organ systems, and high metabolic needs place them at great risk of dangerous medical consequences from many poison exposures. Toddlers' immature taste buds allow them to swallow items that seem noxious to adults. Their small size and immature organ systems place them at greater risk than adults of dangerous medical consequences of poison exposures.

Normal curiosity and imitation lead to unintentional poisonings in children of almost any age. Toddlers learn by imitating adults and climb to reach and ingest a medicine or product used by adults. They are unable to associate cause and effect, making them susceptible to repeated poison exposures. Older children desire self-sufficiency, which may lead to inappropriate medication use. Although school-aged children can read labels, they may not understand them completely. They also may have an imperfect grasp of cause and effect, leading to possible problems with the use of household products and school

TABLE 44.1 Number of Pediatric Poison Exposures and Fatalities, 2000

Age (yr)	*Number of Exposures*	*Percent of All Exposures*	*Number of Fatalities*	*Percent of All Fatalities in Database (All Ages)*
Under 6	1,142,796	52.7	20	2.2
6-12	151,221	7.0	6	.7
13-19	160,505	7.4	66	7.2

From Litovitz et al., 2001.

TABLE 44.2 Most Common Pediatric Poison Exposures, 2000

Less than 6 Years of Age	*6–19 Years of Age*
Cosmetics and personal care products	Analgesics
Cleaning substances	Bites and envenomations
Analgesics	Cleaning substances
Plants	Cough and cold preparations
Cough and cold preparations	Cosmetics and personal care products
Foreign bodies	Plants
Topical medicines	Foreign bodies
Antimicrobials	Stimulants and street drugs
Vitamins	Antidepressants
Gastrointestinal preparations	Food products and food poisoning

From: Litovitz et al., 2001.

chemicals. Preadolescents and adolescents experiment with drugs and alcohol, including inhalants. Adolescents may be exposed to poisons in the workplace.

Etiology

Pediatric poison exposures occur unintentionally or intentionally:

- Unintentional poison exposures:
  - A change in family routine may precipitate poison exposures, either because routinely locked medications and chemicals are left within reach or because less attention is paid to children and their activities. Environmental factors (e.g., a carbon monoxide leak or chemical spill) may affect all family members.
  - Infants may be poisoned as a result of therapeutic errors (Ellenhorn, 1997, p. 13; Litovitz, 2001). The wrong drug may be dispensed or administered. Parents may administer a drug intended for older children, mistakenly thinking that a smaller dose will be safe for younger children. They may misread the label or administer extra doses because of confusion about who is administering the medicine. Infants and toddlers may be poisoned by older siblings who want to "help" while parents aren't looking, and toddlers may pick up containers left within their reach by family members.

TABLE 44.3 Most Common Causes of Poison-Related Fatalities, All Ages, 2000

Analgesics
Antidepressants
Sedatives/hypnotics/antipsychotics
Stimulants and street drugs (Most, but not all, deaths were associated with illegal drugs.)
Cardiovascular drugs
Alcohols
Anticonvulsants
Muscle relaxants
Gases & fumes
Chemicals

From: Litovitz et al., 2001

- Intentional poison exposures
  - Parents or caregivers may intentionally administer a poison or medication that results in a poison exposure to either harm the child or to create symptoms in the child so emergency care can be rendered (e.g., factitious disorder by proxy; Chapter 46).
  - Preadolescents and adolescents may deliberately incur a poisoning (e.g., alcohol, illicit drugs, or medications) as a suicide gesture or suicide attempt (Chapter 27).

Focused History

Historical information about both asymptomatic and symptomatic patients following a poison exposure or poisoning is obtained as applicable from the patient, the parents or caregivers, and witnesses.

Family History

- Recent visitors at the home
- A change in the home environment, including home improvement projects or restoration
- Medicines used by family members (prescription, nonprescription, foreign, herbal, homeopathic, veterinary, and dietary supplements)
- Witnesses to the event
- Involvement or exposure of other children or adults
- History of psychiatric illness in the patient, family members, or others with whom the child spends time

Patient History

- Concurrent intentional or unintentional trauma, which may be precipitated by exposure to drugs or chemicals
- Time recently spent outside of the home, and the length of time
- Agent to which the child was exposed:
  - Time of the exposure.
  - Route of the exposure (Table 44.4).
  - Symptoms after the exposure, their time of onset, and the sequence of their appearance.
  - First aid measures employed, by whom, and when. The effects of inappropriate first aid treatment may need to be reversed prior to the initiation of appropriate treatment.

Focused Assessment

Physical Assessment

Children with suspected poison exposure require a physical assessment (Table 44.5).

TABLE 44.4 Route-specific History Findings

Route	*Historical Data*
Ingestions	Availability of the medication or product container. Sometimes the actual contents of the product are different from what the parent thinks.
	The number of pills or amount of fluid in the container prior to and after the exposure.
Inhalations	Availability of the chemical container or product.
	Exposure to a fire while in an enclosed space (risk of carbon monoxide and cyanide poisoning).
Cutaneous or ocular exposures	Availability of the product container. Sometimes the actual contents of the product are different from what the parent thinks (e.g., a lawn care product that seems like fertilizer may also contain an insecticide).
	The amount of the substance in the container prior to and after the exposure.

1. Assess the respiratory system.
   - Auscultate the chest for:
     - Respiratory rate. Tachypnea or bradypnea may be present, depending on the poison exposure.
     - Adventitious sounds. Wheezing may be heard with aspirated substances.
2. Assess the cardiovascular system.
   - Auscultate the heart for:
     - Rate. Tachycardia or bradycardia may be present, depending on the poison exposure.
     - Rhythm. Irregular heart rhythms may occur with selected poison exposures.
   - Measure the blood pressure.
   - Assess peripheral perfusion.
     - Palpate peripheral pulses for quality and equality.
   - Measure core and skin temperature.
   - Inspect the skin for:
     - Color.
   - Measure capillary refill.
3. Assess the neurological system.
   - Measure the level of consciousness with the AVPU (Alert, responds to Verbal stimuli, responds to Painful stimuli, Unresponsive) method or the GCS method.

TABLE 44.5 Symptomatology, Poison Exposure, Assessment, and Interventions

Symptomatology	*Poison Exposure*	*Assessment and Interventions*

Symptomatic	No history of poison exposure	■ Maintain a high index of suspicion that a poisoning may have occurred.
		■ Consider poisoning in children with:
		  ■ Multiple symptoms.
		  ■ Abnormal assessment findings (e.g., abnormal electrocardiograph).
		  ■ Abnormal laboratory findings with no obvious cause.
		■ Immediately consult the poison center.

Symptomatic	History of poison exposure	■ Initiate further evaluation and treatment. ■ Symptoms (toxidromes) vary among the toxic agents (Table 44.6). ■ Consult the poison center.
Asymptomatic	History of poison exposure	■ Initiate a complete physical and psychosocial assessment and appropriate interventions. ■ Consult the poison center.

TABLE 44.6 Toxicologic Syndromes (Toxidromes)

Toxin	*Vital Signs*	*Mental Status*	*Symptoms*	*Clinical Findings*	*Laboratory Findings*
Acetaminophen	Normal (early)	Normal	Anorexia, nausea, vomiting	RUQ tenderness, jaundice (late)	Abnormal LFTs
Amphetamines	Hypertension, tachycardia, tachypnea, hyperthermia	Hyperactive, agitated, toxic psychosis	Hyperalertness	Mydriasis, hyperactive bowel sounds, flush, diaphoresis	Increased CPK
Anticholinergics	Hypotension, hypertension, tachycardia, hyperthermia	Altered (agitation, lethargy to coma), hallucinations	Blurred vision	Dry mucous membranes, mydriasis, diminished bowel sounds, urinary retention	ECG abnormalities
Arsenic (acute)	Hypotension, tachycardia	Alert to coma	Abdominal pain, vomiting, diarrhea, dysphagia	Dehydration	Renal failure, abnormal abdominal radiograph; dysrhythmias
Arsenic (chronic)	Normal	Normal to encephalopathy	Abdominal pain, diarrhea	Melanosis, hyperkeratosis, sensory motor neuropathy, hair loss, Mees' lines, skin cancer	Pancytopenia, proteinuria, hematuria, abnormal LFTs
Barbiturates	Hypotension, bradypnea, hypothermia	Altered (lethargy to coma)	Slurred speech, ataxia	Dysconjugate gaze, bullae, hyporeflexia	Abnormal ABGs
Beta-adrenergic antagonists	Hypotension, bradycardia	Altered (lethargy to coma)	Dizziness	Cyanosis, seizures	Hypoglycemia, ECG abnormalities
Botulism	Bradypnea	Normal unless hypoxic	Blurred vision, dysphagia, sore throat, diarrhea	Ophthalmoplegia, mydriasis, ptosis, cranial nerve abnormalities	Normal
Carbamazepine	Hypotension, tachycardia, bradypnea, hypothermia	Altered (lethargy to coma)	Hallucinations, extrapyramidal movements, seizures	Mydriasis, nystagmus	ECG abnormalities
Carbon monoxide	Often normal	Altered (lethargy to coma)	Headache, dizziness, nausea, vomiting	Seizures	Elevated carboxyhemoglobin, ECG abnormalities, metabolic acidosis

(continued)

TABLE 44.6 Toxicologic Syndromes (Toxidromes) (continued)

Toxin	*Vital Signs*	*Mental Status*	*Symptoms*	*Clinical Findings*	*Laboratory Findings*
Clonidine	Hypotension, hypertension, bradycardia, bradypnea	Altered (lethargy to coma)	Dizziness, confusion	Miosis	Normal
Cocaine	Hypertension, tachycardia, hyperthermia	Altered (anxiety, agitation, delirium)	Hallucinations, paranoia	Mydriasis, tremor, perforated nasal septum, diaphoresis, seizures, active bowel sounds	ECG abnormalities, increased CPK
Cyclic antidepressants	Hypotension, tachycardia, hyperthermia	Altered (lethargy to coma)	Confusion, dizziness	Mydriasis, dry mucous membranes, distended bladder, flush, seizures	Prolonged QRS complex, cardiac dysrhythmias
Digitalis	Hypotension, bradycardia	Normal to altered, visual hallucinations	Nausea, vomiting, anorexia, visual disturbances	None	Hyperkalemia, ECG abnormalities, increased digoxin level
Disulfiram/ethanol	Hypotension, tachycardia	Normal	Nausea, vomiting, headache, vertigo	Flushed, diaphoresis, tender abdomen	ECG abnormalities (ventricular dysrhythmias)
Ethylene glycol	Tachypnea	Altered (lethargy to coma)	Abdominal pain	Slurred speech, ataxia	Anion gap metabolic acidosis, osmolal gap, crystalluria, hypocalcemia, renal failure
Iron	Hypotension (late), tachycardia (late)	Normal unless hypotensive, lethargy	Nausea, vomiting, diarrhea, abdominal pain, hematemesis	Abdominal tenderness	Hyperglycemia (child), leukocytosis (child), heme-positive stool/vomitus, metabolic acidosis, radiopaque material on abdominal radiograph
Isoniazid	Often normal	Normal or altered (lethargy to coma)	Nausea, vomiting	Seizures	Anion gap metabolic acidosis
Isopropyl alcohol	Hypotension, bradypnea	Altered (irritability, lethargy to coma)	Nausea, vomiting	Hyporeflexia, breath odor of acetone	Ketonemia, ketonuria, no glycosuria or acidosis
Lead	Hypertension	Altered (lethargy to coma)	Irritability, abdominal pain (colic), nausea, vomiting, constipation	Peripheral neuropathy, seizures, gingival pigmentation	Anemia, basophilic stippling, radiopaque material on abdominal radiograph, proteinuria
Lithium	Hypotension (late)	Altered (lethargy to coma)	Diarrhea, tremor	Weakness, tremor, ataxia, myoclonus, seizures	Leukocytosis, ECG abnormalities, renal abnormalities (diabetes insipidus)
Mercury	Hypotension (late)	Altered (psychiatric disturbances)	Salivation, diarrhea, abdominal pain	Stomatitis, ataxia, tremor	Proteinuria, renal failure
Methanol	Hypotension, tachypnea	Altered (lethargy to coma)	Blurred vision, blindness, abdominal pain	Hyperemic disks	Anion gap metabolic acidosis, increased osmolal gap
Opioids	Hypotension, bradycardia, bradypnea, hypothermia	Altered (lethargy to coma)	Slurred speech, ataxia	Miosis, absent bowel sounds	Abnormal ABGs
Organophosphates/ carbamates	Hypotension, bradycardia/tachycardia, bradypnea/tachypnea	Altered (lethargy to coma)	Diarrhea, abdominal pain, blurred vision, vomiting	Salivation, diaphoresis, lacrimation, urination, defecation, miosis, fasciculations, seizures	Depressed red blood cells and plasma cholinesterase activity

(continued)

RUQ = right upper quadrant; LFT = liver function tests; CPK = creatinine phosphokinase; ECG = electrocardiogram; ABGs = arterial blood gases.

From: Goldfrank et al., 1994.

TABLE 44.6 Toxicologic Syndromes (Toxidromes) (continued)

Toxin	*Vital Signs*	*Mental Status*	*Symptoms*	*Clinical Findings*	*Laboratory Findings*
Phencyclidine	Hypertension, tachycardia, hyperthermia	Altered (lethargy to coma)	Hallucinations	Miosis, diaphoresis, myoclonus, blank stare, nystagmus, seizures	Myoglobinuria, leukocytosis, increased CPK
Salicylates	Hyperthermia, tachypnea	Altered (lethargy to coma)	Tinnitus, nausea, vomiting	Diaphoresis, abdominal tenderness	Anion gap metabolic acidosis, respiratory alkalosis, abnormal LFTs and prothrombin time/partial prothrombin time, positive iron chloride
Sedative-hypnotics	Hypotension, bradypnea, hypothermia	Altered (lethargy to coma)	Slurred speech, ataxia	Hyporeflexia, bullae	Abnormal ABGs
Theophylline	Hypotension, tachycardia, tachypnea, hyperthermia	Altered (agitation)	Nausea, vomiting, diaphoresis	Diaphoresis, tremor, seizures, dysrhythmias	Hypokalemia, hyperglycemia, metabolic acidosis, ECG abnormalities

RUQ = right upper quadrant; LFT = liver function tests; CPK = creatinine phosphokinase; ECG = electrocardiogram; ABGs = arterial blood gases.

From: Goldfrank et al., 1994.

- Observe the child's:
  - Gait.
  - Motor function.
  - Sensory function.
  - Reflexes.

4. Assess the gastrointestinal and genitourinary systems.
   - Assess the abdomen for:
     - Distention.
     - Bowel sounds.
   - Note the presence of vomiting.
   - Measure urinary output.
5. Assess the integumentary system.
   - Assess for topical contamination (Chapter 45).
   - Assess for burns, wounds, or other signs of trauma or neglect (Chapter 46).
6. Assess the child's overall appearance.
   - Note the child's hygiene and level of nourishment.
   - Weigh the child; compare to established norms.

Psychosocial Assessment

- Assess the quality of the child's and family's interaction patterns.
  - Intentional poisoning or unintentional poisoning from neglect in the young child may have occurred (Chapter 46).
  - Intentional poisoning as a plea for attention may have occurred in the older child.
- Assess the child's and family's coping strategies.
- Assess the parents' response to the poison exposure (e.g., extreme guilt versus nonchalance).
- Assess parental familiarity with age-specific growth, development, and behavior; assess whether the poison exposure is typical of the child's age and developmental level.

Table 44.7 outlines selected nursing diagnoses and expected outcomes.

Triage Decisions

Emergent

- Known or suspected poison exposure with:
  - Inability to maintain a spontaneous patent airway.
  - Respiratory distress or insufficiency.
  - Cardiovascular compromise.
  - Altered level of consciousness.

Urgent

- Known or suspected poison exposure to a toxic substance.

Nonurgent

- None

TABLE 44.7 Nursing Diagnoses and Expected Outcomes

Nursing Diagnoses	*Expected Outcomes*
Ineffective airway and breathing patterns, related to poison exposure	■ The child will have a patent airway. ■ The child will have adequate respiratory efforts, as evidenced by adequate oxygen saturation measurements and effective respiratory rate and rhythm.
Potential for injury, related to poison exposure	The child will be free from further injury as evidenced by: ■ Adequate airway, breathing, and circulation. ■ Adequate neurological functioning. ■ Serum electrolytes and other components within normal limits. ■ Effective removal of the poison.
Knowledge deficit, related to anticipatory guidance of poison prevention	■ Parent or caregiver will verbalize methods for poison prevention, such as locking poisonous household chemicals. ■ Parent or caregiver will verbalize age-appropriate expectations and developmental considerations. ■ Parent or caregiver will receive the telephone number for the local poison center: 1-800-222-1222.

Nursing Interventions

1. Assess and maintain airway, breathing, and circulation (Chapter 30).
   - Initiate maneuvers to maintain airway patency, such as positioning, suctioning, and insertion of an oral airway.
   - Prepare for endotracheal intubation in the child who cannot maintain spontaneous airway patency.
   - Administer 100% oxygen through a nonrebreather mask; initiate assisted ventilations in the child who is not maintaining adequate respiratory effort.
   - Initiate cardiorespiratory, blood pressure, and oxygen saturation monitoring.
     - Observe and analyze cardiac rhythm.
     - Obtain a 12-lead ECG, if indicated.
2. Obtain venous access and initiate an intravenous infusion, as needed:
   - Obtain blood for toxicology screening.
     - Toxicology screening is initiated to identify the presence or absence of some suspected drugs or chemicals. The terms *drug screen*, *negative drug screen*, and *comprehensive toxicology screen* are meaningless unless it is known exactly which substances are being screened for. The drugs included in a drug screen vary among institutions.
     - Ask the laboratory what bodily fluid is preferred; depending on the drug and the test to be used, blood or urine may be required. In some circumstances (e.g., for unknown drugs or mushroom spores), gastric fluid can be tested.
     - Provide the laboratory with as much information as possible about the patient's history and condition to help the laboratory narrow down the testing procedures.
     - Become familiar with the laboratory's procedures and definitions. For example, serum levels of therapeutic drugs may be performed only on specified days, and *stat* may be defined in hours, not minutes.
3. Initiate decontamination procedures (Table 44.8).
4. Prepare to administer antidotes, as prescribed.
   - Antidotes are available for relatively few substances, although they can be lifesaving in some poisonings (Table 44.10)

TABLE 44.8 Route of Exposure and Decontamination Procedures

Route of Exposure	*Decontamination Procedure*
Ocular	Irrigation with tap water or normal saline through intravenous tubing or a Morgan lens for at least 20 minutes after exposure to an acid and 30 minutes after exposure to an alkaline substance. Irrigation has been sufficient when a pH strip, touched gently to the cul de sac, registers a neutral pH.
Dermal	Irrigation with running water for the same length of time as ocular exposures. With older children and adolescents, effective irrigation can be achieved in a shower. Emergency nurses may need to initiate hazardous materials decontamination procedures to protect themselves and the patient (Chapter 45). Depending on the poison, local and/or systemic effects may be expected.
Inhalation	Removal of the child to fresh air, then other measures as indicated by the nature of the poison, including oxygen administration, respiratory support, observation for pulmonary effects (which are delayed for some poisons), and assessment and treatment of systemic effects.
Ingestion	May require gastrointestinal decontamination (Table 44.9). The use of specific measures depends on the poison, its physical form, the amount, and the time between exposure and presentation.

TABLE 44.9 Methods of Gastrointestinal Decontamination

Gastrointestinal Decontamination Method	*Indications*	*Contraindications*	*Procedure*	*Specific Considerations*
Ipecac syrup-induced emesis Mechanism: Induces emesis through local gastric irritation and systemically by stimulation of the chemoreceptor trigger zone	Drugs and chemicals that are: ■ Ingested in potentially dangerous amounts ■ Not adsorbed to activated charcoal (e.g., iron, lithium) ■ Too large to be retrieved by gastric lavage ■ Best treated quickly, at the site and time of the poison exposure, to prevent absorption	■ Inability to protect the airway ■ Current or anticipated depressed level of consciousness ■ Current or anticipated seizures ■ Ingestion of caustic substances ■ Third trimester of pregnancy ■ History of recent myocardial infarction	■ Administer with 4–8 oz of any fluid patient will drink (need not be water). ■ Repeat dose once if there is no emesis within 30 minutes. ■ If second dose is ineffective, the need for additional gastrointestinal decontamination measures depends on expected absorption time of ingested substance and the patient's clinical condition. ■ Dose: ■ 6–11 months: 10 ml ■ 12 months to approximately 10–12 years [100 pounds]: 15 ml ■ Over 100 lb: 30 ml	■ Recommended by poison centers for home use in selected circumstances. ■ Infrequently used in emergency departments. Most children poisoned seriously enough to need emergency department care require activated charcoal, which may be administered after gastric lavage and is sometimes used without first performing a gastric evacuation procedure.

(continued)

TABLE 44.9 Methods of Gastrointestinal Decontamination (continued)

Gastrointestinal Decontamination Method	*Indications*	*Contraindications*	*Procedure*	*Specific Considerations*
Activated charcoal ■ Mechanism: Specially processed form of charcoal possesses multiple binding sites; adsorbs to most substances, thereby preventing their absorption into the bloodstream ■ Available suspended in sorbitol, in an aqueous solution, and as a powder to be measured and mixed with water.	Ingestion of potentially dangerous or life-threatening quantities of most drugs and poisons	■ Substances not adsorbed to activated charcoal (e.g., iron, lithium, ethanol, caustic chemicals)	■ Single doses are indicated for most serious ingestions. ■ Administer orally or via gastric tube. ■ Dose: ■ Infants and toddlers: 0.5–1.0 g/kg of body weight, 25 g minimum/dose ■ Older children: 25–50 g/dose ■ Adolescents and adults: 50–100 g/dose	■ Multiple doses of activated charcoal, every 2 to 6 hours, will enhance the elimination of some drugs, including carbamazepine, cyclic antidepressants, digitalis, phenobarbital, and theophylline. ■ If multiple doses of charcoal are indicated, the presence of bowel sounds must be verified prior to administration of each dose. ■ If multiple doses of charcoal are indicated, a cathartic must *not* be administered more than once per day, to avoid fluid and electrolyte disturbances. ■ Warn parents of the passage of black stools, which is normal and expected but may be alarming. ■ Commercial suspensions are much easier to administer. Charcoal powder is difficult to measure and mix properly.
Cathartics: ■ Sorbitol, alone or in suspension with activated charcoal ■ Magnesium citrate ■ Mechanism: Promotes elimination of charcoal-poison complex	Ingestions for which activated charcoal is administered		Administer with or after activated charcoal. ■ Dose for sorbitol: ■ Young children: 0.5 g/kg ■ Adolescents: 1 g/kg ■ Dose for magnesium citrate: ■ 4 ml/kg	In children receiving multiple doses of activated charcoal, administer no more than once a day. Do not administer with each charcoal dose.
■ Whole bowel irrigation ■ Mechanism: Removes ingested substances before absorption by flushing through the gastrointestinal tract (Tenenbaum, 1987)	Ingestions in which above methods are insufficient to prevent life-threatening effects, e.g., from enteric-coated drugs, sustained release preparations, and substances not adsorbed to activated charcoal. ■ Indicated if standard gastric emptying procedures have failed or if substance has entered the intestinal tract	■ Gastrointestinal bleeding ■ Gastrointestinal tract abnormalities	■ Dose for polyethylene-glycol: ■ Administer with or after activated charcoal. ■ Young children: 0.5 l/h orally or by nasogastric tube until rectal effluent is clear or drug removal is documented. ■ Adolescents: 1 l/h orally or by nasogastric tube until rectal effluent is clear or drug removal is documented.	Procedure is similar to preparations used before gastrointestinal procedures and surgery. There is a slight risk of fluid and electrolyte imbalance (Kaczorowski & Wax, 1996). Intact pills can be identified in rectal effluent. Observe for vomiting and electrolyte imbalance. An antiemetic may be required.

TABLE 44.10 Selected Substances with Specific Antidotes

Substance	*Antidote*
Acetaminophen	*N*-acetyl-L-cysteine (NAC)
Benzodiazepines	Flumazenil (Romazicon)
Carbon monoxide	Oxygen, including hyperbaric oxygen
Cyanide	Taylor cyanide antidote treatment kit: ▪ Amyl nitrite ▪ Sodium nitrite ▪ Sodium thiosulfate
Digitalis	Digitalis Fab fragments (Digibind)
Envenomations ▪ Pit viper (Crotalidae) ▪ Coral snake (Elapidae) ▪ Black widow spider (Lactrodectus)	Antivenom
Ethylene glycol	Fomepizole, ethanol
Iron	Deferoxamine
Isoniazid (INH)	Pyridoxine
Methanol	Fomepizole, ethanol
Opioids	Naloxone
Organophosphate insecticides	Atropine Pralidoxime (2-PAM)

5. Prepare the patient for specific diagnostic tests.
   - Radiographs:
     - Radiographs may be useful in some conditions, such as button battery ingestions.
     - If a button battery has been swallowed, it is a medical emergency if the battery is retained in the esophagus, but the patient is in no danger if the battery has passed at least to the stomach (Litovitz & Schmitz, 1992).
     - Radiopaque drugs and chemicals (Table 44.11) can be visualized on abdominal films, indicating their placement and amount.
     - Some swallowed packets of illegal drugs may also be visualized with radiographs.
6. Prepare for possible enhanced elimination modalities.
   - Forced diuresis:
     - It is occasionally indicated for substances that are eliminated renally (e.g., lithium).
     - It is used less often in children than adults because of the risk of fluid and electrolyte disturbances.
   - Ion-trapping:

TABLE 44.11 Radiopaque Substances

C	Chloral hydrate, Calcium Carbonate, Crack vials
H	Heavy metals, Health foods (bone meal)
I	Iron, Iodides
P	Psychotropics (phenothiazines and other neuroleptics, cyclic antidepressants), Potassium (enteric-coated), Phosphates, Packages (cocaine, heroin)
E	Enteric-coated preparations (e.g., aspirin, potassium chloride, sodium chloride)
S	Slow-release preparations (sustained-release), Solvents (CCL_4, $CHCl_3$)

From: Schwartz & Goldfrank (1994).

- This occurs by administration of sodium bicarbonate, which alkalinizes the urine, promoting elimination of salicylates and phenobarbital.
- Extracorporeal elimination (hemodialysis or hemoperfusion):
    - This is indicated for serious poisoning by ethylene glycol, methanol, salicylates, lithium, and theophylline, among others.
    - Dangerously poisoned children who are too young for hemodialysis or hemoperfusion may be candidates for exchange transfusion.

7. Initiate consultations, as needed.
    - Poison center:
        - Early consultation with the poison center is the best way of assuring that a child's condition does not worsen unnecessarily and assuring that appropriate treatment options are considered as the child's condition changes. Call 1-800-222-1222 to be automatically connected to the closest poison center.
    - Social services.
    - Child protective services, if child neglect is suspected (Chapter 46).
    - Pediatric medical subspecialists.
    - Hazardous materials personnel (Chapter 45).
8. Inform the family frequently of their child's condition; provide psychosocial and emotional support to the child and family (Chapter 4).
9. Reassess the child's cardiorespiratory and neurological status.
10. Prepare for transfer and transport to a tertiary care facility (Chapter 10), hospital admission, or discharge to home.

Home Care and Prevention

Discharge to home after an unintentional poisoning requires anticipatory guidance to prevent future poison exposures (Table 44.12). Emergency nurses should provide the parents with the poison center telephone number, 1-800-222-1222, to keep by the telephone. The parents should be reminded that the poison center will call the family to be sure that the child is recovering as expected, to refer the child for additional care if indicated, and to answer any questions about the poisoning episode. The poison center will take this opportunity to send poison prevention information to the home; the local poison center may provide the emergency department with poison prevention materials for distribution at their discretion. Parents may not be receptive to poison prevention education following the emergency treatment. Once their anxiety has diminished somewhat, they may be more receptive than ever.

Parents should receive discharge instructions specific to the poison and the treatment. Parents may need to observe their child for specific effects following the treatment, such as dark stools following charcoal administration.

TABLE 44.12 Anticipatory Guidance for Poison Prevention

- Identify the most dangerous poisons at home and where they are stored: medicines, caustic cleaning products, pesticides, antifreeze, windshield washer solution, alcoholic beverages, hydrocarbons.
- Purchase medicines and household products in child-resistant packaging. Replace caps securely after use.
- Lock dangerous poisons out of sight and reach of children.
- Store products in their original containers.
- Do not take medicines in front of children. Children learn by imitation!
- Do not call medicine "candy."
- Before taking or giving a drug, read the label. If necessary, put on your eyeglasses and turn on the light.
- Give prescription medicines only to the person for whom they were prescribed. Give over-the-counter medicines only as recommended on the label, unless your pediatrician advises otherwise.
- Discard old medicines.
- Call your poison center before a poisoning occurs. The poison center will send you information about poisons specific to your area, information about teaching poison prevention to children, and telephone stickers with the poison center's emergency phone number.
- Be prepared for a possible poisoning emergency. Keep syrup of ipecac on hand, to use only if directed by the poison center.
- Keep activated charcoal on hand, if recommended by the poison center. Use only if directed by the poison center.
- Keep the telephone number of the poison center on or near the telephone (1-800-222-1222).
- Call the poison center immediately in case of a possible poisoning.

Selected Toxicological Emergencies—Poisoning by Pharmaceutical Agents

Acetaminophen

Sources

- Hundreds of brand-name and generic prescription and nonprescription medicines, including single- and multiple-ingredient analgesics and combination drugs for allergies, colds, and insomnia.

Routes of Exposure

- Oral tablets (regular and sustained-release)
- Liquids
- Rectal suppositories

Mechanism of Toxicity

- For children over the age of 10 years, metabolism of acetaminophen results in the production of small amounts of *N*-acetyl-*P*-benzoquinoneimine (NAPQI), a toxic metabolite that is usually detoxified by the enzyme glutathione.
  - In an overdose, larger amounts of NAPQI are generated; the resulting accumulation depletes glutathione and damages hepatocytes.
  - A different metabolic pathway in young children provides some protection from liver damage, but this protection is not complete in all cases.
- Because hepatotoxic effects are due to metabolites, the onset of toxicity is delayed.
  - The earliest symptoms are gastrointestinal, occurring 6 to 14 hours after exposure. Over 24 to 72 hours, liver enzymes rise, gastrointestinal symptoms increase, and right upper quadrant pain may develop.
  - If antidotal treatment with *N*-acetyl-*L*-cysteine (NAC) is begun within eight hours, recovery is expected without toxic sequelae. If not, progressive liver injury is possible and may be fatal unless a liver transplant is performed.

Focused History

- Exact product ingested (brand name, strength, regular or sustained-release).
- Time of ingestion.
- Acute or chronic exposure.
- Intentional or unintentional exposure.
- If this information is not available, or if the history may not be reliable, a toxic exposure must be presumed to have occurred unless ruled out by laboratory evaluation. The presence or absence of symptoms and their time and sequence of onset may help confirm or refute the history.

Focused Physical Assessment

- Gastrointestinal system
  - Gastrointestinal symptoms (nausea and vomiting).
  - Right upper quadrant pain.

Laboratory Tests

- A blood sample for acetaminophen levels must be drawn *no sooner than* 4 hours after exposure, to allow time for peak absorption.
- Obtain a repeat level four hours after the first if:
  - The history is uncertain.
  - The ingestion is chronic.
  - Sustained-release dosage forms are involved.
- Toxicity is predicted by plotting the level of acetaminophen in the blood and time of ingestion on the Rumack-Matthew nomogram (Figure 44.13).
- Other laboratory studies include baseline hepatic and renal function studies.

Nursing Interventions

- Support airway, breathing, and circulation (Chapter 30).
- Perform gastrointestinal decontamination with gastric lavage and administer activated charcoal with a cathartic in patients with a toxic dose confirmed by history or laboratory analysis.
- Administer NAC (Table 44.13) if a toxic level is found at any time after four hours postingestion.
  - Once the need for NAC has been established, further acetaminophen levels are no longer necessary.
  - The full course of therapy must be completed even if acetaminophen levels subsequently decline, because the antidote is used to treat the effects of the metabolite, which is not being measured.

Special Considerations

- A child may ingest a fatal dose of acetaminophen, yet experience no symptoms of consequence for a day or more; however, the ideal time to administer the antidote, which is highly effective in preventing fatalities, is within 8 hours of the overdose, before significant metabolism of the drug and symptoms occur; however, later administration is

Figure 44.1 Nomogram for assessment of acetaminophen toxicity.

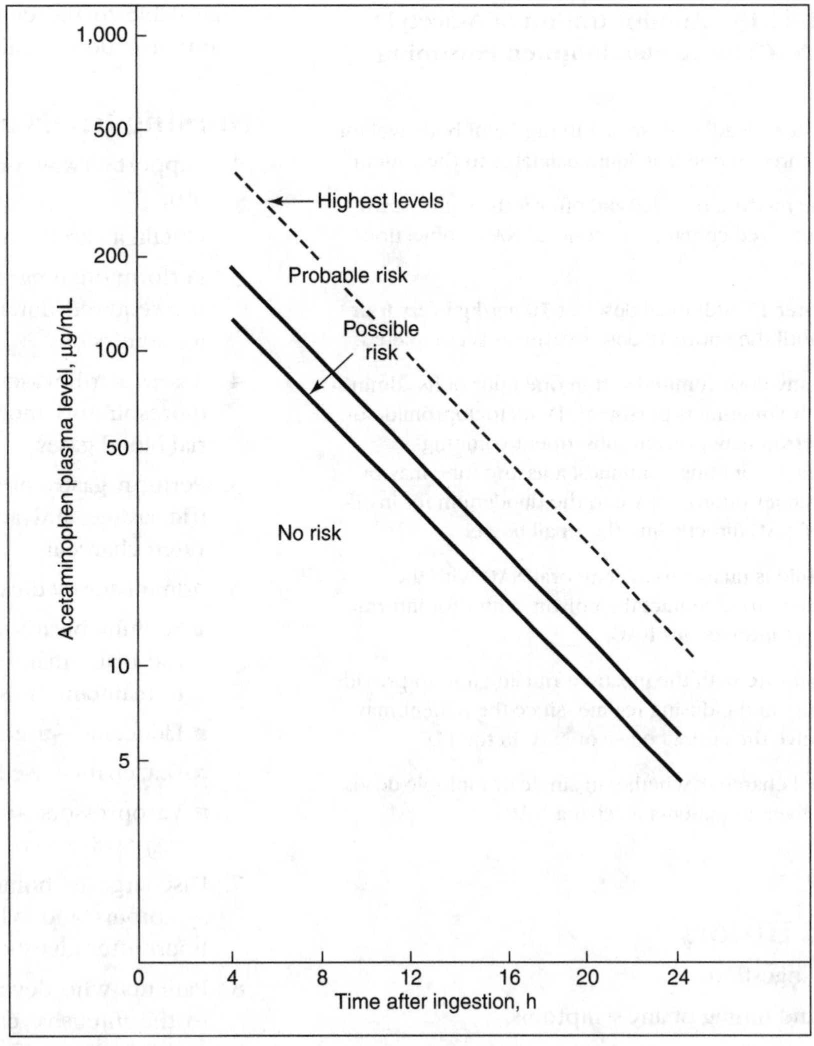

From: Rumack, Peterson, Koch, & Amara. (1981). Used with permission.

still useful. Therefore, the emergency nurse must have a high index of suspicion for acetaminophen poisoning.

- Consider the possibility of acetaminophen poisoning in virtually any patient who presents with an intentional drug overdose: it is widely available, frequently involved in drug overdoses, causes no early symptoms, is readily treated, yet may cause death if the diagnosis is not made.
- Also consider acetaminophen poisoning in children who present with gastrointestinal complaints as well as those with evidence of hepatic abnormalities.

Tricyclic Antidepressants

Sources

- Numerous oral preparations, including amitriptyline, clomipramine, desipramine, doxepin, imipramine, nortriptyline, protriptyline, and trimipramine. None of these drugs is intended for use in very young children.
- Imipramine is sometimes prescribed for nocturnal enuresis in children aged 5 years and older.
- Preteens and adolescents may receive these drugs for treatment of depression.

Route of Exposure

- Oral tablets

Mechanism of Toxicity

- Anticholinergic effects, alpha-adrenergic blocking effects, decreased reuptake of norepinephrine, and cardiac membrane depressant effects occur to a greater or lesser extent, depending on the exact agent involved.
- Any ingestion of tricyclic antidepressants is potentially dangerous in a young child.

TABLE 44.13 Administration of *N*-acetyl-L-cysteine (NAC) for Acetaminophen Poisoning

1. Administer a loading dose of 140 mg/kg of body weight, diluted three to one in a liquid palatable to the patient.
2. Pour the mixture over ice and offer it through a straw from a covered container to conceal NAC's objectionable odor.
3. Administer 17 additional doses of 70 mg/kg every four hours until the entire 18-dose treatment is completed.
4. Repeat any dose vomited within one hour of its administration. If vomiting is persistent, IV metoclopromide or ondansetron may prevent subsequent vomiting episodes. If vomiting continues, a gastric tube may be placed under fluoroscopy into the duodenum for instillation of NAC directly into the small bowel.
5. If the child is unable to tolerate oral NAC with the above measures, contact the poison center for information about intravenous NAC.
6. Communicate with the inpatient nursing unit to provide continuity in the dosing regime, since the patient may not receive the entire course of NAC in the ED.
7. Activated charcoal, whether in single or multiple doses, can be given to patients receiving NAC.

Focused History

- Time of ingestion.
- Nature and timing of any symptoms.

Focused Physical Assessment

- Cardiovascular system:
  - Significant dysrhythmias, with ECG changes including sinus tachycardia and prolonged PR, QRS, and QT intervals.
  - Hypotension.
- Neurologic system:
  - Seizures. Severe toxicity presents as the sudden onset of seizures and coma within 30 minutes of ingestion, though not all children present so dramatically.
  - Hallucinations.
  - Coma.
- Gastrointestinal system:
  - Decreased bowel sounds.

Laboratory Tests

- Laboratory measures of the drugs themselves correlate generally with expected toxicity, but will not be available to the emergency department staff and, in any case, do not guide treatment.

Nursing Interventions

1. Support airway, breathing, and circulation (Chapter 30).
2. Obtain a careful history.
3. Perform ongoing physical assessments to determine the required duration of observation and the need for admission.
4. Assess cardiovascular status, with continuous cardiorespiratory monitoring and measurement of arterial blood gases.
5. Perform gastrointestinal decontamination with gastric lavage and administer multiple doses of activated charcoal.
6. Administer medications:
   - Sodium bicarbonate—the first-line drug to treat the many manifestations of this overdose. Titrate to maintain the serum pH between 7.45 and 7.55.
   - Lidocaine—used to treat ventricular dysrhythmias.
   - Diazepam—used to treat seizures.
   - Vasopressors—used to treat hypotension not responsive to positioning or intravenous fluids.
7. Discharge to home children who present without symptoms and who remain asymptomatic for six hours after ingestion.
8. Patients who develop symptoms must be admitted to the intensive care unit for at least 24 hours for multiple doses of activated charcoal and continuous ECG monitoring.

Special Considerations

- Amoxapine is an antidepressant without the significant cardiac toxicity of other cyclic antidepressants; in overdose, it causes status epilepticus. Aggressive treatment of seizures (Chapter 18) is necessary to prevent hypoxic brain injury and significant hyperthermia.

Calcium Channel Blockers

Sources

- Drugs used to treat hypertension, angina, and arrhythmias, including bepridil, diltiazem, felodipine, isradipine, nicardipine, nifedipine, nimodipine, and verapamil.

Routes of Exposure

- Oral
- Intravenous

Mechanism of Toxicity

- In overdose, side effects are extensions of therapeutic effects.
- By slowing calcium influx into myocardial and nodal cells and vascular tissue, these agents cause conduction delays, decreased peripheral resistance, and decreased myocardial contractility.
- Ingestion of any amount of these drugs is dangerous and potentially lethal in children. Because many preparations are sustained-release, the onset of toxicity may be delayed and the duration of symptoms may be prolonged.

Focused History

- Time of ingestion
- Number of pills ingested, regular or sustained-release
- Onset of symptoms

Physical Assessment

- Cardiovascular system:
  - Hypotension, decreased cardiac output, conduction delays, heart block and other dysrhythmias.
- Neurologic system:
  - Depressed CNS function, hypoxia, seizures, and metabolic acidosis.
- Metabolic system:
  - Hyperglycemia, because calcium is required for insulin release.

Laboratory Tests

- None specific to the drug; levels not generally available.

Nursing Interventions

1. Support airway, breathing and circulation (Chapter 30).
2. Perform careful ongoing assessments of respiratory, cardiovascular, neurological, and metabolic status in every child who may have ingested or even sucked on these preparations.
3. Perform vigorous gastrointestinal decontamination with gastric lavage if the ingestion is recent.
   - Syrup of ipecac is contraindicated because of the risk of bradycardia.
   - Administration of activated charcoal and a cathartic are indicated.
   - Consider whole bowel irrigation if it is possible that pills have moved into the intestinal tract and for sustained-release preparations.
4. Administer intravenous calcium supplementation (preferably calcium chloride) in symptomatic children, although this is not always effective in reversing hypotension and other cardiovascular effects.
   - Glucagon may increase heart rate, though this, too, is not always effective.

Special Considerations

- As calcium channel blockers become more widely prescribed, they account for an increasing number of serious poisonings and fatalities (Litovitz et al., 2001).
- There is no antidote for overdose, and there are no universally effective treatments. It is essential that every possibility of ingestion of these drugs in children be considered a potentially fatal event. Rapid action to decontaminate the gastrointestinal tract and treat early manifestations of toxicity may present the best chance a child has of surviving ingestion of a calcium-channel-blocking drug.

Digitalis

Sources

- Pills, liquids, and intravenous preparations.
- Plants including *Digitalis purpurea* (foxglove) and *Nerium oleander* (oleander).
- Toad toxins (bufotoxins).

Routes of Exposure

- Oral:
  - Intentional or unintentional overdose of medication.
  - Ingestion of plant material or teas brewed from plant material.
  - Compounds containing bufotoxins found in topical aphrodisiacs or nonwestern medicines (Kwan, Paiusco, & Kohl, 1992; Centers for Disease Control and Prevention, 1995).
  - Chronic toxicity in patients taking digitalis.
- Intravenous preparations—intentional or unintentional overdose.

Mechanism of Toxicity

- Digitalis binds to and inhibits the action of Na^+-K^{++}-ATPase at receptors on cardiac and smooth muscle, resulting in increased intracellular sodium and calcium, depleted intracellular potassium, and markedly increased extracellular potassium.

Focused History

- Determine if the overdose is:
  - Acute.
  - Chronic.
  - Acute in a child undergoing chronic therapy. A child prescribed digitalis will be seriously (acutely) poisoned at a lower serum level than a patient with an acute overdose only, because receptor sites are already saturated.

Focused Physical Assessment

- Cardiovascular system:
  - Bradycardia and numerous other dysrhythmias, including heart block, and hypotension due to a decrease in nodal conduction and cellular contraction.
- Neurologic system:
  - Lethargy.
  - Visual changes, including yellow or greenish "halos" in chronic overdoses.
- Gastrointestinal system:
  - Elevated serum potassium levels, unless the patient is on concomitant diuretic therapy.
  - Gastrointestinal effects (nausea and vomiting).
  - Signs of dehydration (Chapter 19)

Laboratory Tests

- Serum digitalis level
- Serum hepatic studies (Digitalis is metabolized by the liver.)
- Serum renal studies (Digitalis is excreted by the kidneys.)

Nursing Interventions

1. Support airway, breathing, and circulation (Chapter 30).
2. Initiate continuous ECG and blood pressure monitoring.
3. Administer digoxin immune Fab fragments (Digibind) to the child with severe or life-threatening ECG abnormalities (Table 44.14).
4. Perform gastrointestinal decontamination with gastric lavage and activated charcoal.
5. Initiate intravenous hydration, if needed.

TABLE 44.14 Administration of Digoxin Immune Fab Fragments (Digibind)

1. Notify the pharmacy that Digibind is required. Too commonly, hospital pharmacies stock insufficient amounts of Digibind (Dart et al., 1996) and it may be necessary to obtain additional supplies from other facilities. A delay in procuring and administering the antidote could cost the child's life.
2. Dosing depends on the amount of digitalis ingested; each vial of 40-mg Digibind will bind 0.6 mg of digitalis.
3. If the ingested amount of digitalis is unknown, contact the local poison center to calculate the Digibind dose; the calculation includes the digitalis level, its volume of distribution, and patient characteristics.
4. Determine whether the laboratory is measuring *total* or *free* digitalis levels.
   - *Free* digitalis level (unbound digitalis): This level determines if the child is at risk for continued toxicity and if a child who requires therapeutic levels of digitalis remains adequately digitalized.
   - *Total* digitalis level (digitalis already bound to the antidote plus free digitalis): This is not useful for determining management of an overdose.

Special Considerations

- Although a therapeutic digitalis level is 0.5 to 2.0 ng/ml, toxicity is possible within that range.

Diphenoxylate/Atropine

Sources

- Oral prescription drug used to treat diarrhea, such as Lomotil® or generic preparations

Route of Exposure

- Oral

Mechanism of Toxicity

- The combination of an opioid and atropine (an anticholinergic) slows peristalsis, the desired therapeutic effect.
- Children can experience significant opioid toxicity from diphenoxylate, yet delayed absorption may mean delayed toxicity.
- The opioid effects may occur as long as 24 hours after ingestion (McCarron, Challoner, & Thompson, 1991).

- *In young children, the ingestion of even one tablet is significant.*

History

- Number of pills ingested
- Time of ingestion
- Symptoms since ingestion

Focused Physical Assessment

- Respiratory system:
  - Respiratory depression, bradypnea.
- Neurologic system:
  - Pinpoint pupils.
  - Decreased level of consciousness.

Laboratory Tests

- None

Nursing Interventions

1. Support airway, breathing, and circulation (Chapter 30)
2. Perform gastrointestinal decontamination with gastric lavage and administer activated charcoal and a cathartic, depending on the time of postingestion.
3. Administer naloxone to treat symptoms of opioid overdose.
4. Hospitalize and initiate 24-hour cardiorespiratory monitoring for young children with a history of any ingestion of this drug.

Special Considerations

- Because the onset of symptoms is delayed, it can be difficult to convince parents and healthcare professionals that an apparently healthy child is at risk for significant opioid toxicity.

Iron

Sources

- Numerous types of vitamin and mineral supplements, both pediatric and adult, in solid and liquid formulations.
- Prenatal vitamins with iron and adult-strength iron supplements are a significant cause of poisoning death in young children. Serious iron poisoning also occurs in pregnant teens who deliberately take overdoses of their own prenatal vitamins.

Route of Exposure

- Oral

Mechanism of Toxicity

- Initially, iron has a corrosive effect on the gastrointestinal mucosa, causing significant bleeding which contributes to cardiovascular shock.
- The damaged gastrointestinal mucosa allows increased absorption of iron, which damages hepatocytes and blood vessels.
- As iron is metabolized, generation of hydrogen ions contributes to metabolic acidosis.
- The ultimate effects of iron poisoning depend on the amount ingested and the rapidity with which the child receives adequate medical care.
- Mild toxicity is predicted with ingestions of 20 to 40 mg/kg of elemental iron, and significant toxicity with ingestions of ≥60 mg/kg.
- As few as 10 adult-strength iron supplements are potentially lethal to a 10-kg child.
- Iron poisoning is described in stages, although poisoning events in individual children may occur differently (Table 44.15).

Focused History

- Type of iron preparation.
- Amount of iron preparation.
- Time of ingestion.
  - If a patient with a history of iron ingestion seems asymptomatic, assess for the occurrence of any gastrointestinal symptoms in the last 12 to 24 hours.

Focused Physical Assessment

- Cardiovascular system:
  - Hypotension may occur.
- Gastrointestinal system:
  - Dehydration may occur.

Laboratory Tests

- Immediate serum iron level
- Total iron-binding capacity (although the total iron-binding capacity may be misleading if iron levels are high):
  - Draw both at the time absorption probably will have occurred (about 1 to 2 hours after ingestion of a liquid preparation, 2 to 4 hours after ingestion of a solid). Draw immediately if the time since ingestion is longer than that or if the time of ingestion is unknown.

TABLE 44.15 Phases of Iron Poisoning

Phases	*Onset of Symptoms Postingestion*	*Symptoms*
Phase I	30 minutes to 2 hours	■ Nausea ■ Vomiting ■ Diarrhea (may be bloody) ■ Abdominal discomfort
Phase II	2 to 12 hours	■ "Latent phase": children become asymptomatic and appear to have recovered. However, significant toxicity is developing.
Phase III	12 to 48 hours	■ Sudden cardiovascular collapse. ■ Metabolic abnormalities and hepatic injury (acidosis and coagulopathies). ■ Decreased level of consciousness, coma, pulmonary edema, and hepatorenal failure. ■ Children who survive this phase may recover fully or may develop complications such as intestinal necrosis, causing their death days or weeks later.
Phase IV	2 to 4 days	■ This phase may occur in seriously poisoned children who survive their poisoning episode; this includes pyloric stenosis, secondary to corrosive injury, that requires corrective surgery.

- Immediate complete blood count
- Electrolytes
- Hepatic studies
- Renal studies
- Arterial blood gases
- Immediate stool guiac
- Blood for typing and crossmatching if the stool is guiac-positive

Nursing Interventions

1. Support airway, breathing, and circulation (Chapter 30).
2. Perform gastrointestinal decontamination if the ingestion was recent (about 1 hour for a liquid preparation or a few hours for solid dosage forms). Activated charcoal is not effective and is not indicated, unless other substances that do adsorb to charcoal were also ingested.
3. Obtain an abdominal radiograph if adult-strength tablets were involved, to aid in documenting the position and number of the ingested iron pills. A negative radiograph does not negate the possibility of ingestion of an iron-containing preparation.
   - Liquids and pediatric chewable vitamins with iron will not be visible on a radiograph.
4. If a potentially dangerous number of iron pills have reached the intestinal tract, initiate whole-bowel irrigation until all pills have been counted in the rectal effluent or a subsequent radiograph documents their passage.

5. Administer deferoxamine, the antidote for iron poisoning. Deferoxamine complexes with iron, forming ferrioxamine, which is water soluble and excreted renally.
   - The usual intravenous dose of deferoxamine is 15 mg/kg per hour.
   - Deferoxamine is indicated for symptomatic children with a serum iron level of 350 μg/dl and for all children with a level greater than 500 μg/dl.
   - Large doses of deferoxamine can cause significant hypotension, usually when given too quickly or at greater than 15 mg/kg per hr, thereby limiting its use in dangerously poisoned children.
   - Deferoxamine should not be administered intramuscularly to an iron-poisoned child, because there may be insufficient or erratic absorption in hypotensive children.

Special Considerations

- The potential dangers of iron overdose are underestimated by parents and health care professionals alike, who recognize that iron is an essential dietary element and may believe it to be innocuous. For this reason, early signs of iron toxicity are sometimes not recognized as serious; children progress through the asymptomatic phase and then are brought to the emergency department after becoming seriously ill.
- Iron is prescribed regularly for pregnant women who are likely to have young children at home. If a child has ingested iron, determine if other siblings may have done the same.

Isoniazid (INH)

Sources

- Oral drug used to treat tuberculosis

Route of exposure

- Oral

Mechanism of Toxicity

- An overdose of isoniazid rapidly depletes the body's stores of pyridoxine (vitamin B_6).
  - Pyridoxine is necessary for synthesis of gamma-aminobutyric acid (GABA), an inhibitory neurotransmitter.

Focused History

- Family or patient treatment for tuberculosis
- Refractory seizures prior to presentation

Focused Physical Assessment

- Neurologic system:
  - Seizures or a postictal state.

Laboratory Tests

- Arterial blood gases

Nursing Interventions

1. Support airway, breathing, and circulation (Chapter 30).
2. Initiate measures to control seizure activity (Chapter 18).
3. Administer intravenous pyridoxine:
   - Known dose of ingested INH: Administer an equal amount of pyridoxine.
   - Unknown dose of ingested INH: Administer 5 g of pyridoxine.
4. Administer diazepam:
   - Diazepam enhances the effects of GABA, but it is not a substitute for pyridoxine.
5. Treat acidosis.
6. Perform gastrointestinal decontamination with gastric lavage, activated charcoal, and a cathartic.

Special Considerations

- The incidence of tuberculosis in the United States has risen in recent years. There is increased prevalence among some immigrant groups and patients infected with the human immunodeficiency virus. Consider medical, social, and environmental factors when assessing the likelihood of INH as a cause of recalcitrant seizures.

Oral Hypoglycemic Agents

Sources

- Oral agents taken by adults with Type 2 diabetes, including chlorpropamide, glipizide, glyburide, and tolbutamide

Route of Exposure

- Oral

Mechanism of Toxicity

- Hypoglycemia is the failure to maintain normal glucose homeostasis (Goldfrank, Flomenbaum, Lewin, et al., 1994, p. 579). When serum glucose levels fall below 45 mg/dl, symptoms occur.

- Delayed onset of hypoglycemia, which may be persistent, especially with the second-generation sulfonylureas such as glipizide and glyburide, may be appreciated.
- Any amount of these drugs is dangerous in children, who may not manifest significant hypoglycemia until nearly 24 hours after ingestion.

Focused History

- Suspected or witnessed ingestion
- Neurologic changes indicative of hypoglycemia such as tremulousness; irritability; cool, clammy skin; unconsciousness; and seizures

Focused Physical Assessment

- Neurologic system:
    - Altered level of consciousness
    - Signs of hypoglycemia

Laboratory Tests

- Immediate serum glucose level
- Serum glucose levels repeated at least every 2 hours

Nursing Interventions

1. Support airway, breathing, and circulation (Chapter 30)
2. Initiate measures to control seizure activity (Chapter 18).
3. Obtain an immediate serum glucose level and administer intravenous glucose, if needed.
    - Because of small glycogen stores, children may not respond sufficiently to glucagon. In these cases, consider octreotide acetate.
4. Perform gastrointestinal decontamination with gastric lavage, activated charcoal, and a cathartic.
5. Monitor serum glucose levels closely.

Special Considerations

- Following the ingestion of oral hypoglycemic agents, the child should be hospitalized for 24 hours of observation.

Salicylates

Sources

- Aspirin (acetylsalicylic acid), in regular, sustained-release, and enteric-coated formulations, alone or in combination with prescription and nonprescription drugs.
- Bismuth subsalicylate, in over-the-counter gastrointestinal preparations.
- Oil of wintergreen (methyl salicylate), sold alone as a liquid, and found in over-the-counter topical preparations to relieve muscle and joint pains and green rubbing alcohol.

Routes of Exposure

- Oral
    - Poisonings may occur from acute or chronic ingestion of aspirin and aspirin-containing drugs or from ingestion of oil of wintergreen, which is intended for external use only.
- Rectal suppositories
- Topical

Mechanism of Toxicity

- Stimulation of the CNS respiratory center leads to metabolic abnormalities.
- Disruption of carbohydrate and lipid metabolism leads to additional metabolic abnormalities and disruption of thermal regulation. If a child is acidotic, salicylate moves more easily into the central nervous system.
- Other manifestations of salicylate toxicity include gastrointestinal irritation and altered platelet function.
- Acute, chronic, and acute poisonings in someone taking the drug chronically are all possible.
- Acute ingestion of salicylates can lead to rapid deterioration, even in children who do not appear acutely ill on presentation.
- Depending on the time since ingestion, children may present with no metabolic abnormalities, respiratory alkalosis, or metabolic acidosis.

Focused History

- Suspected or known salicylate ingestion:
    - Determine the exact preparation, how much is missing, over what period of time the drug was taken, and the nature of the illness for which it was taken.
    - Because aspirin is metabolized hepatically and excreted renally, the child's health history is important to ascertain renal or hepatic abnormalities.
- Unknown salicylate ingestion:
    - Ascertain concurrent or recent illnesses in the child and if aspirin was administered during the illness.
    - Aspirin may be given initially to treat a fever but actually causes a fever if chronic toxicity develops.

- Chronic salicylate intoxication can mimic a number of viral or flu-like presentations.
- Ascertain if salicylate preparations are in the home.

Focused Physical Assessment

- Respiratory system:
  - Tachypnea, signs of pulmonary edema
- Cardiovascular system:
  - Fever
  - Diaphoresis
- Neurologic system:
  - Lethargy, seizures, and coma may occur.
  - Tinnitus is common.
  - Hyperthermia.
- Gastrointestinal system:
  - Signs of dehydration (Chapter 19)
  - Gastrointestinal bleeding
- Metabolic system:
  - Electrolyte imbalance
  - Coagulopathies

Laboratory Tests

- Obtain serum electrolyte levels, glucose levels, renal and hepatic function tests, and arterial blood gases.
- Ingestion of liquid preparation:
  - Obtain a salicylate level 1 to 2 hours after ingestion.
- Ingestion of a solid (tablet) preparation:
  - Obtain a salicylate level 6 hours after ingestion and then serial levels to confirm that the level is declining.
- Ingestion of a solid preparation in a chronic ingestion or a large acute ingestion in a chronic user:
  - Obtain a salicylate level immediately and 6 hours later. Then obtain serial levels to confirm that the level is declining.

Nursing Interventions

1. Support airway, breathing, and circulation (Chapter 30).
2. Perform gastrointestinal decontamination and administer activated charcoal.
3. Obtain a serum salicylate level and correct fluid and electrolyte imbalances:
   - Administer intravenous sodium bicarbonate to achieve a urine pH of approximately 8.0, because salicylates are eliminated more quickly in alkaline urine.
4. Hydrate with intravenous fluids containing supplemental potassium.
5. Predict toxicity by plotting the salicylate level and time of ingestion on the Done nomogram (Figure 44.2). A subsequent serum salicylate level is often necessary to rule out continued absorption from sustained-release or enteric-coated preparations, or from a concretion of aspirin tablets in the stomach.
6. Prepare for hemodialysis in children with significant symptoms, salicylate levels greater than 100 mg/dl after acute poisoning or lower salicylate levels after chronic ingestion.
7. Initiate supportive care:
   - Continue ongoing cardiorespiratory monitoring.
   - Obtain serial salicylate levels to assure that serum salicylate levels are decreasing.

Special Considerations

- At one time, aspirin was a leading cause of poisoning death in children. Because of passive measures to prevent salicylate poisoning (child-resistant containers, limited number of baby aspirin tablets per bottle), many healthcare providers are unfamiliar with its disastrous history. Consequently, emergency professionals may not appreciate the rapidly fatal effects of salicylate poisoning. Many parents do not think of aspirin as particularly dangerous and may not call a poison center until their children are symptomatic. Teenagers will attempt suicide with aspirin simply because it is so widely available.
- A high index of suspicion, careful history, vigorous gastrointestinal decontamination, and careful attention to salicylate levels and the child's response to treatment are imperative to prevent unnecessary fatalities from this common drug.

Sympathomimetic Drugs

Sources

- Legal drugs:
  - Decongestants, including phenylpropanolamine and ephedrine. Although phenylpropanolame was recently removed from the market, the product remains in homes.
  - Stimulants, including caffeine.
  - Methylphenidate (Ritalin™), a prescription drug used to treat hyperactivity and attention-deficit disorders.
  - Weight control agents, including amphetamines and related drugs. (Fenfluramine and dexfenfluramine were removed from the market, but remain available in some homes.)

Figure 44.2 Nomogram relating serum salicylate concentration and expected severity of intoxication at varying intervals following the ingestion of a single dose of salicylate.

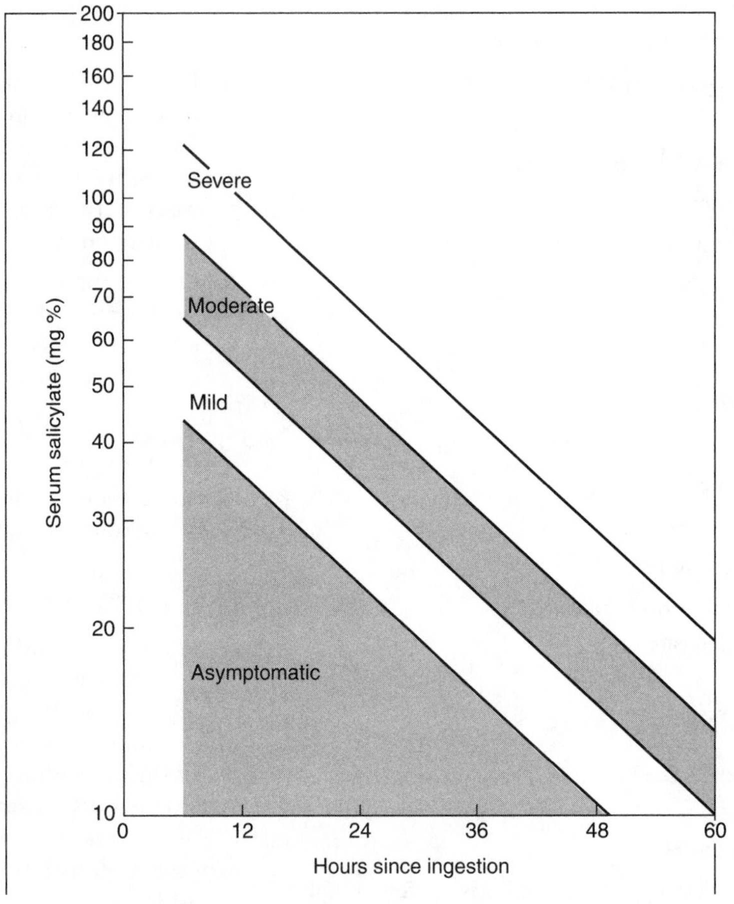

From: Done, 1960. Used with permission.

- "Street speed" (or any number of other rapidly changing names), including legal drugs packaged and sold illegally, often as stimulants.
- Herbal drugs and dietary supplements containing ephedrine, derived from the plants of the genus *Ephedra* (ma huang).

- Illegal drugs:
  - Cocaine—injection, inhalation ("snorting"), and smoking of "crack"; ingested by children who find it or teens and adults attempting to avoid arrest for drug possession.
  - Illicit amphetamines ("speed")—injection, ingestion, and smoking "ice."
  - MDMA ("Ecstasy") and other hallucinogenic amphetamines—ingestion.

Routes of Exposure

- Oral
- Injection
- Inhalation

Mechanism of Toxicity

- Uncontrolled stimulation of the sympathetic nervous system ("fight or flight" response) causes tachycardia, tachypnea, hypertension, miosis, and CNS stimulation.
- The half-life of cocaine is about 4 to 6 hours, and of amphetamines about 18 to 24 hours. Clinically, poisonings by these agents cannot be differentiated, and the treatment is the same.

Focused History

- Often difficult to obtain when the poisonings involve illicit substances or legal substances diverted for illicit sale:
  - Determine whether ingested illegal drugs were contained in some type of vial, condom, balloon, or package; leakage of the drug from containers can cause continuing effects, and sudden breakage could have catastrophic consequences.
- Central nervous system effects (seizures, agitation, tremors, or hallucinations)

- Cardiac effects (chest pain, hypertension, or tachycardia)

Focused Physical Assessment

- Respiratory system:
  - Tachypnea
- Cardiovascular system:
  - Chest pain from myocardial ischemia
  - Tachydysrhythmias
  - Hypertension
  - Peripheral vasodilation with central vasoconstriction
- Neurologic system:
  - Headache from extreme hypertension
  - Agitation
  - Tremors
  - Seizures
  - Hyperthermia

Laboratory Tests

- Laboratory identification of the agent involved can help predict the duration of effects.
- Other studies will be dictated by the child's physical condition, such as whether the child has evidence of cardiac or CNS involvement.

Nursing Interventions

1. Support airway, breathing, and circulation (Chapter 30):
   - Initiate measures to control ventricular dysrhythmias and hypertension.
2. Support neurologic function:
   - Initiate measures to control hyperthermia and seizures.
3. Provide gastrointestinal decontamination with gastric lavage and activated charcoal in oral ingestions. (Ipecac syrup is contraindicated because of the risk of seizures.)
4. Consider abdominal radiographs, because ingested packets of drugs may be visible.

Special Considerations

- Although substance abusers will often smoke or inject drugs to obtain the most rapid effects, these substances also are absorbed from the gastrointestinal tract. This poses a hazard to children who swallow legal or illegal stimulants and to those under arrest who presumably swallowed drugs and are released to jail sooner than is medically wise. If the child has used illegal drugs, the presentation and clinical course may be affected by adulterants such as quinine, lidocaine, strychnine, and a host of other substances.
  - Idiosyncratic reactions may occur from usual doses of these drugs; overdose is not necessary for a patient to present with the sudden onset of significant symptoms.

Theophylline

Sources

- Regular and sustained release preparations used to treat asthma. Indications are declining as other, less toxic drugs have become available, but theophylline is sometimes still prescribed.

Route of Exposure

- Oral

Mechanism of Toxicity

- The mechanisms of toxicity are not well described, although the consequences of therapeutic and intentional theophylline overdose are well known.
- Gastrointestinal symptoms, seizures and dysrhythmias are signs of early toxicity.

Focused History

- Determine if the drug is taken therapeutically. An acute ingestion in someone already taking the drug is more dangerous than the same ingestion in someone who is not.

Focused Physical Assessment

- Cardiovascular system:
  - Tachycardia
  - Dysrhythmias
- Neurologic system:
  - CNS stimulation, including tremors and seizures
- Gastrointestinal system:
  - Nausea and vomiting
- Metabolic system:
  - Electrolyte abnormalities, especially hypokalemia

Laboratory Tests

- Immediate theophylline level
- Immediate electrolyte levels
- Immediate arterial blood gases

Nursing Interventions

1. Support airway, breathing, and circulation (Chapter 30).
   - Initiate ECG monitoring
2. Perform thorough gastrointestinal decontamination with gastric lavage and activated charcoal administration. Multiple doses of activated charcoal are indicated.
   - Ipecac syrup is contraindicated because of the risk of seizures.
   - Consider whole-bowel irrigation in children who have swallowed sustained-release drugs.
3. Monitor serum theophylline and electrolyte levels.
4. Maintain fluid and electrolyte balance; administer potassium supplementation, as needed.
5. Prepare for charcoal hemoperfusion (preferred) or hemodialysis in children with theophylline levels greater than 80 μg/ml after an acute ingestion and at lower levels for children with chronic ingestions or life-threatening symptoms.

Special Considerations

- Children with a theophylline overdose can deteriorate rapidly, so it is essential that they be evaluated and treated expeditiously. Even children who have been maintained on a stable dose of theophylline for some time can develop toxicity; the therapeutic range is narrow and can be affected by numerous drug interactions and concurrent acute illnesses.
- Seriously poisoned children may present with the sudden onset of seizures and dysrhythmias, without prodromal symptoms.

Selected Toxicological Emergencies—Poisoning by Nonpharmaceutical Agents

Caustic Substances

Sources

- Acids (e.g., hydrochloric or sulfuric acid often found in household products):
  - Toilet bowl cleaners, some bathroom cleaning products, swimming pool chemicals, automobile batteries, and products used to clean concrete and bricks.
- Alkaline chemicals (e.g., sodium hydroxide, potassium hydroxide, calcium hydroxide, or sodium carbonate, often found in household products):
  - Drain openers, laundry detergent, electric dishwasher detergent, oven cleaner, industrial-strength cleaners, wet and powdered cement, and liquid from damaged dry cell batteries.
- Hydrofluoric acid has a different toxicity from other caustics and will be considered separately.

Routes of Exposure

- Ingestion
- Inhalation
- Ocular
- Dermal

Mechanism of Toxicity

- *Acids* dehydrate tissue and precipitate surface proteins, resulting in coagulation necrosis. A hard eschar develops, which inhibits penetration of the acid into deeper tissue.
- *Alkalines* cause a liquifaction necrosis; disrupted cell membranes provide no barrier to deeper penetration of the chemical with continuing injury. Saponification, a result of alkaline action on lipids in cell membranes, causes the soapy appearance of the tissue.
- For all tissues affected, injury can range from mild irritation to full thickness chemical burns; the degree of severity can be compared to first, second, and third degree thermal burns (Chapter 39). The extent of injury after ingestion, dermal, or ocular exposure to a caustic substance is determined by:
  - The pH of the product, with the most severe injury expected with products with a pH of ≤2 or ≥12.
  - The duration of contact with tissue. Even substances that usually are mildly irritating at worst, such as household bleach, can cause more significant injury with prolonged contact.
  - The product formulation. Liquid substances quickly transit the oropharynx and esophagus, so the greatest injury is typically seen in the stomach. Granular substances may adhere to tissues in the mouth and oropharynx, causing a greater likelihood of burns to the lips, tongue, oropharynx, and esophagus.
  - The adequacy of irrigation, for ocular and dermal exposures.
- Pulmonary edema may occur after inhalation of caustic substances. It is usually delayed for at least several hours, during which time cellular membrane destruction occurs, with subsequent leakage of capillary fluid into the lungs and disruption of gas exchange across alveolar membranes.

Focused History

- Treatment must be initiated prior to or concurrent with the history and assessment.

- Identify the *exact* product, so that the poison center can advise about the pH, or check the pH of the product itself.
- Determine if the exposure was unintentional or intentional.
- Suicidal ingestions in teenagers and adults usually involve larger amounts of product and more significant injury (Chapter 27).

Focused Physical Assessment

- Ingestion:
  - Examine for visible burns.
  - Evaluate respiratory function. Oral edema may compromise the airway. Product may have been aspirated.
  - Ascertain presence or absence of oral, chest, or epigastric pain.
  - Assess for abdominal distention.
- Ocular exposure:
  - Examine the cornea and affected skin.
- Dermal exposure:
  - Determine depth, percent, and extent of injury (Chapter 39).

Laboratory Tests

- Oral exposures: serum electrolytes
- Dermal exposures: as for thermal injuries (Chapter 39)
- Inhalation exposures: arterial blood gases

Nursing Interventions

1. For all exposures, support airway, breathing, and circulation (Chapter 30)
2. Oral exposures:
   - Administer a small amount of water if the child is able to swallow.
   - Assess for visible burns to the lips, face, and oropharynx.
   - Evaluate respiratory function, because oral edema may compromise the airway and some product may have been aspirated. Maintain the airway and prepare for a tracheostomy, if necessary.
   - Assess for chest or epigastric pain, although absence of such pain does not rule out esophageal or gastric burns.
   - Assess for abdominal distention, which may indicate perforation.
   - Obtain a thorough laboratory evaluation and monitor for acid-base imbalances.
   - Anticipate gastrointestinal bleeding and consult a gastroenterologist. Esophagoscopy may be performed soon after ingestion or may be delayed for 24 or 48 hours.
   - Anticipate the administration of antibiotics if infection develops. The use of steroids is controversial and steroids are generally not used in the management of these patients.
3. Inhalation exposures:
   - Assess respiratory function.
     - The delayed onset of pulmonary edema may be anticipated with such common inhalants as chlorine gas.
     - When ignited, a number of products and chemicals generate phosgene gas, a severe respiratory irritant.
   - Assess for carbon monoxide and cyanide poisoning if exposure was a result of fire.
4. Ocular exposures:
   - Irrigate the eye immediately if it has not already been done in the prehospital setting. Prolonged irrigation is needed until the ocular pH returns to neutral, a minimum of 20 minutes for acids and 30 minutes to 1 hour for alkaline chemicals.
   - Check ocular pH by gently touching a pH strip to the cul de sac.
   - Examine the cornea for injury.
   - Treat the corneal injury.
   - Consult an ophthalmologist.
5. Dermal exposures:
   - Irrigate the skin immediately if it has not already been done in the prehospital setting (Chapter 45).
   - Determine the extent of injury as for a thermal burn of similar degree (Chapter 39). The child with a severe chemical burn is at risk of the same systemic effects as a child with a thermal burn of similar degree; fluid loss, electrolyte imbalance, and risk of infection must all be considered.

Special Considerations

- Caustic burns can be devastating, painful injuries that require long-term treatment. Ocular exposures may lead to permanent blindness. Dermal exposures may cause scarring. Survivors of caustic ingestions may face decades of repeated surgeries to maintain esophageal patency.
- Emergency staff must protect themselves from the same consequences by careful handling of the patient, any contaminated clothing, and the caustic material itself (Chapter 45).

Hydrofluoric Acid

Sources

- Rust removers for home and commercial use, air conditioning coil cleaners, wire wheel cleaners, and industrial products to etch glass and computer chips

Routes of Exposure

- Oral
- Ocular
- Dermal (most common, from using the product without gloves or with damaged gloves)
- Inhalation

Mechanism of Toxicity

- Unlike other acids, hydrofluoric acid can penetrate intact skin and complex with magnesium and calcium.
- With hydrofluoric acid concentrations of greater than 50%, tissue burns are immediately evident, as they would be with other acids.
- With hydrofluoric acid concentrations of less than 50%, skin effects are delayed and may be minimal.
- The absorption of hydrofluoric acid causes the delayed onset of deep pain at the site of exposure and may cause hypomagnesemia and fatal systemic hypocalcemia.
- Severe toxicity has been reported with small body surface area exposures (Bertolini, 1992), with pediatric ingestions (Klasner, Scalzo, Blume, et al., 1996), and with inhalation.

Focused History

- Product name, to determine the hydrofluoric acid concentration
- Time of exposure
- Nature and timing of symptoms
- Time and type of decontamination procedures. (Often, decontamination has not been initiated because skin exposures initially may be painless.)

Focused Physical Assessment

- Integumentary system:
  - Assess for ocular, dermal, and oral burns (Chapter 39)

Laboratory Tests

- Serial calcium levels for exposures greater than the most trivial skin contact, inhalation, and ingestion, to determine the risk of hypocalcemia and subsequent ventricular fibrillation

Nursing Interventions

1. For all exposures:
   - Support airway, breathing, and circulation (Chapter 30).
   - Initiate continuous cardiorespiratory monitoring.
   - Monitor electrolyte, calcium, and magnesium levels.
   - Treat decreased calcium levels with intravenous calcium chloride or calcium gluconate.
2. Decontaminate ocular exposures.
   - Immediate consultation with ophthalmology is essential; opinions differ as to the best therapy, but as is often the case, such disagreement simply highlights the fact that there are no universally effective treatments.
3. Decontaminate dermal exposures.
   - Treat by irrigating for at least 20 minutes.
   - Closely monitor calcium levels.
   - Treat pain:
     - The delayed pain that develops at the site of exposure is deep, severe, and often not controlled by narcotics. The key to treatment is replacement of tissue calcium. This can sometimes be accomplished by application of a calcium gel, which is rubbed in until the pain subsides; application is repeated as pain recurs.
     - Often, fingers are the site of exposure, with intense pain and blanching.
     - Intra-arterial calcium infusion is often the treatment of choice, not only to relieve pain but to prevent destruction of soft tissue and bone.
4. Treat inhalation exposures:
   - Initiate treatment as in respiratory injury from other causes.
   - Monitor serial calcium levels.
5. Treat ingestion exposures:
   - Perform dilution; then initiate a gastrointestinal consultation. The child is at risk for complications of caustic ingestion as well as the potentially fatal effects of hypocalcemia.

Special Considerations

- Parents are astounded to learn that agents of such extreme toxicity may be in the garage or laundry room. Because toxicity is unexpected, parents may not seek advice until a child is ill. Unfortunately, healthcare providers not familiar with this poisoning may underestimate the extreme toxicity of seemingly minimal exposures.

Ethanol

Source

- Alcoholic beverages
- Mouthwash
- Cosmetics (facial toners, astringents, or hair spray)
- Antidote for ethylene glycol and methanol poisoning

Routes of Exposure

- Oral
- Dermal
- Intravenous (for therapeutic administration)

Mechanism of Toxicity

- Ethanol is a central nervous system depressant.
- In children, ethanol commonly causes hypoglycemia (Ellenhorn, 1997, p. 1133).
- Acute poisoning causes CNS depression, respiratory depression, and ataxia; hypoglycemic effects include seizures and coma.
- Extremely high ethanol levels, coma, and death can result from ingestion of household products containing ethanol and from binge drinking.
- Preteens and teenagers may be chronic ethanol abusers who develop a tolerance for CNS depressant effects.

Focused History

- Time of ingestion (determines the usefulness of gastrointestinal decontamination)
- Ingestion of other drugs (potential for enhanced CNS depressant effects)
- Type of product ingested
- Amount of ethanol ingested

Focused Physical Assessment

- Respiratory system:
  - Respiratory depression occurs with acute poisoning.
- Neurologic system:
  - CNS depression and ataxia occur with acute poisoning.
  - Seizures and coma can result from hypoglycemia.

Laboratory Tests

- Serum ethanol level
- Serum glucose level
- Electrolytes
- Arterial blood gases

Nursing Interventions

1. Support airway, breathing, and circulation (Chapter 30).
2. Obtain blood for laboratory tests.
3. Initiate gastric decontamination with gastric lavage if the ingestion has been within the past hour, because lavage may retrieve some unabsorbed ethanol.
   - Activated charcoal is ineffective.
4. Maintain fluid and electrolyte status.
5. Monitor arterial blood gases and ethanol and glucose levels; monitor acid-base balance.
6. Prepare for hemodialysis in severely symptomatic patients.

Special Considerations

- Because of their small size, young children are especially susceptible to the CNS depressant effects of ethanol, something that parents may not realize when giving a children "just a taste" of an alcoholic beverage or some beer to "help them sleep."
- Teenagers who are inexperienced drinkers overestimate their capacity for alcohol or drink on a dare. Some preteens and teenagers will be ethanol dependent, and so must be monitored for withdrawal symptoms when being treated for other conditions (Chapter 27).

Ethylene Glycol

Sources

- Automobile antifreeze (nearly 100% ethylene glycol).
- Related chemicals such as diethylene glycol and ethylene glycol monobutyl ether, found in some solvents and cleaning products.
  - Although the degree of toxicity may differ from ethylene glycol, effects and treatment are the same.

Routes of Exposure

- Oral
  - Unintentional ingestions in children (The chemical has a sweet taste.)
  - Used as an ethanol surrogate or in suicide attempts by adolescents and adults

Mechanism of Toxicity

- Toxicity occurs as a result of metabolism by alcohol dehydrogenase.

- Production of several organic acids causes significant acidosis.
- One metabolite is oxalic acid, which precipitates with calcium to form calcium oxalate crystals; these are deposited in soft tissue and in the kidneys, where they may cause renal failure.
- Because toxicity results from the action of metabolites and not that of the ethylene glycol itself, the onset of symptoms is delayed for approximately 12 to 24 hours.
- Beginning about 8 to 10 hours after ingestion, calcium oxalate crystals may be identified in the urine.
- Effects similar to those of alcoholic inebriation may occur initially. They are accompanied or followed by lethargy, abdominal pain, ataxia, seizures, coma, and renal failure; death may occur.
- An anion gap metabolic acidosis will be pronounced, and there will be a widened osmolal gap.
- Ethylene glycol poisoning should be suspected in any child with CNS depression accompanied by metabolic acidosis.

Focused History

- Identify potential sources:
  - Child playing near someone working on a car.
  - Use of ethylene glycol as an ethanol surrogate, intentionally or otherwise.
  - Have someone examine the home or other locations where the patient spent time within the previous 24 hours.
- Time of symptom onset

Focused Physical Assessment

- Neurologic system
  - Lethargy
  - Ataxia
  - Seizures
  - Coma
- Gastrointestinal system
  - Abdominal pain

Laboratory Tests

- Ethylene glycol levels
- Ethanol levels
- Arterial blood gases
- Baseline renal function studies
- Examination of urine for oxalate crystals

Nursing Interactions

1. Support airway, breathing, and circulation (Chapter 30).
2. Initiate gastrointestinal decontamination if the ingestion was within the previous hour.
3. Obtain serum laboratory tests to determine if there are anion and osmolar gaps.
4. Administer an antidote, either fomepizole (Antizol™) or ethanol. These drugs are competitive inhibitors of alcohol dehydrogenase, which is necessary for ethylene glycol metabolism:
   - Fomepizole:
     - Loading dose: 15 mg/kg, administered intravenously.
     - Subsequent doses: 10 mg/kg every 12 hours for 4 doses. Then, 15 mg/kg every 12 hours until ethylene glycol level is <20 mg/dl.
   - Ethanol:
     - Titrate an intravenous ethanol drip to achieve and maintain a blood ethanol level of 100 mg/dl.
     - Monitor serum glucose levels to prevent ethanol-induced hypoglycemia.
   - Administer pyridoxine, which may enhance the conversion of toxic metabolites to carbon dioxide and water.
   - Administer sodium bicarbonate to correct acidosis, which may be refractory.
5. Prepare for hemodialysis.
   - Hemodialysis is required if the ethylene glycol level is greater than 50 mg/dl.

Special Considerations

- Small amounts of ethylene glycol can cause significant toxicity and death. Parents and others may underestimate the danger from small ingestions, because the child is typically asymptomatic for many hours.
- The best time to recognize and treat ethylene glycol poisoning is before any symptoms occur. Onset of symptoms indicates the presence of toxic metabolites, with the likelihood of significant CNS and renal consequences, including permanent renal damage and peripheral neuropathies in children who survive.

Methanol

Sources

- Windshield washer fluid (nearly 100% methanol)
- Some gasoline additives

- Chafing dish fuel
- Model airplane fuel

Route of Exposure

- Oral

Mechanism of Toxicity

- Methanol is metabolized briefly to formaldehyde, then to formic acid and other organic acids.
- Formic acid is responsible for optic nerve changes, leading to permanent blindness.
- Significant acidosis also is characteristic of this poisoning.
- Symptoms are caused by metabolites; therefore, no symptoms or vague symptoms occur for 10 to 12 hours or longer after ingestion. Then, children will complain of such ocular symptoms as dim, blurred, or double vision.
- Symptoms of inebriation, abdominal pain, and lethargy also may occur, followed by seizures and coma.
- Anion gap metabolic acidosis will be pronounced, and there will be a widened osmolar gap.

Focused History

- A high index of suspicion is essential.
- Time of symptom onset.
- Access to methanol-containing fluids.

Focused Physical Assessment

- Neurologic system:
  - Ocular symptoms such as dim, blurred, or double vision.
- Metabolic system:
  - Metabolic acidosis.

Laboratory Tests

- Serum methanol levels
- Serum ethanol levels
- Arterial blood gases

Nursing Interventions

1. Support airway, breathing, and circulation (Chapter 30).
2. Obtain blood for laboratory tests; determine if anion and osmolar gaps are present.
3. Perform gastrointestinal decontamination if the ingestion was within the previous hour.
4. Administer an antidote, either fomepizole (Antizol) or ethanol. These drugs are competitive inhibitors of alcohol dehydrogenase, which is necessary for methanol metabolism.
   - Fomepizole:
     - Loading dose: 15 mg/kg, administered intravenously.
     - Subsequent doses: 10 mg/kg every 12 hours for 4 doses. Then, 15 mg/kg every 12 hours until methanol level is <20 mg/dl.
   - Ethanol:
     - Titrate an intravenous ethanol drip to achieve and maintain a serum ethanol level of 100 mg/dl.
     - Monitor serum glucose levels to prevent ethanol-induced hypoglycemia.
     - Both ethanol and methanol are metabolized by alcohol dehydrogenase; when both agents are present, alcohol dehydrogenase will preferentially metabolize ethanol. Maintenance of serum ethanol level of 100 mg/dl prevents generation of toxic metabolites of methanol.
5. Administer folic acid:
   - It enhances the conversion of toxic metabolites to nontoxic compounds; leucovorin may be given instead if the child is still asymptomatic.
6. Administer sodium bicarbonate to correct acidosis, which may be refractory.
7. Prepare for hemodialysis:
   - Hemodialysis is required if the methanol level is greater than 50 mg/dl.
8. Continuously assess the child's neurological status.
9. Obtain ophthalmologic consultation; hyperemic discs are characteristic of early methanol poisoning.

Special Considerations

- Methanol is toxic in small amounts, and symptoms are delayed. Parents may underestimate the danger to children who are playing nearby when someone is working on a car.
- The best time to institute treatment is before symptoms occur. Otherwise, permanent blindness and permanent peripheral neuropathies are possible in patients who survive.

Hydrocarbons

Sources

- Gasoline
- Kerosene
- Turpentine

- Lighter fluid
- Charcoal lighter fluid
- Furniture polish
- Lamp oil
- All hydrocarbons of low or relatively low viscosity

Routes of Exposure

- Oral
- Dermal
- Ocular
- Inhalation

Mechanism of Toxicity

The toxicity of hydrocarbons differs, depending on the route of exposure:

Ingestion exposure

- Sources (see above)
- Mechanism of toxicity
  - Toxicity occurs from aspiration into the lungs, not actual ingestion.
  - Aspiration of even small amounts of hydrocarbons may result in disruption of surfactant with alveolar collapse, respiratory irritation, and pneumonitis.
  - Hypoxia produces cyanosis and CNS depression.
  - Initial respiratory findings include coughing, wheezing, and rales.
  - Pneumonitis produces typical systemic effects of infection, including fever.
- Focused History
  - Ascertain if the child coughed or choked. If either occurred when the child attempted to swallow the product, the risk of aspiration is great.
  - Time of ingestion.
- Focused physical assessment
  - Respiratory system. Assess signs of respiratory distress, such as coughing, wheezing, rales.
- Laboratory tests
  - Arterial blood gases
- Nursing interventions
  - *For all ingestions*, support airway, breathing, and circulation
  - *For ingestion without evidence of aspiration*, dilute the hydrocarbon. Observe at home for 24 hours for the development of respiratory effects.
  - *For ingestion with evidence of aspiration*—asymptomatic child—support respiratory function. Obtain a chest radiograph, no sooner than 2 hours after the event, to assess pulmonary changes. If, at 2 hours, the chest radiograph is negative and the child shows no signs of pulmonary damage, the child may be discharged home. The poison center will follow-up for 24 hours for the unlikely development of delayed pulmonary effects. If the child has symptoms and/or the chest radiography shows signs of pulmonary damage, admit the child for observation.
  - *For ingestion with evidence of aspiration*—symptomatic child—support respiratory function, obtain a chest radiograph immediately, and admit for symptomatic and supportive care.
- Special considerations
  - Parents are often unaware that tiny amounts of these products can be dangerous or even fatal to their children; products such as charcoal lighter fluid, lamp oils, and furniture polish are often within children's reach. On the other hand, parents are alarmed by labels advising that "Ingestion can be fatal." In fact, ingestion is not fatal, but aspiration can be.

Ocular and dermal exposures

- Sources (see above)
- Routes of exposure
  - Eye
  - Skin
- Mechanism of toxicity
  - These products have a defatting action on both skin and ocular tissue.
  - Depending on the duration of exposure, effects may range from mild irritation or corneal abrasion to corneal burns.
  - Likewise, effects on the skin range from mild irritation to full-thickness burns after lengthy contact, such as might occur if someone is trapped under a vehicle in a pool of spilled gasoline.
- Focused History
  - Time of exposure
  - Duration of exposure
- Nursing interventions
  - Eye: ocular pain, tearing, redness.
  - Integumentary system: partial, deep-partial, and full-thickness burns.
- Laboratory tests
  - For significant dermal injury, as for thermal burns (Chapter 39).

- Nursing interventions
  - Support airway, breathing, and circulation (Chapter 30).
  - For ocular exposures, initiate irrigation of the eye. If there is evidence of ocular pain or irritation after irrigation, obtain ophthalmologic consultation for possible corneal injury.
  - For dermal exposure, initiate irrigation. Remove the patient's contaminated clothing.
  - Initiate burn wound care (Chapter 39).

Inhalation exposure

- Sources
  - All of the aforementioned sources plus butane, propane, toluene, and other hydrocarbons used as aerosol propellants and solvents; helium; nitrous oxide
- Routes of exposure
  - Workplace use in areas with insufficient ventilation
  - Deliberate abuse ("huffing," "bagging," or "sniffing")
- Mechanism of toxicity
  - In most cases, the mechanism of toxicity is displacement of oxygen and asphyxiation. Hypoxia leads to euphoria (the desired effect for inhalant abusers), sensitization of the myocardium, and an increase in circulating catecholamines, resulting in the sudden onset of ventricular fibrillation and death.
- Focused history
  - Workplace exposure: Determine if other victims were exposed, as one or more workers along with unprotected rescuers may become unconscious.
  - Suspected abuse exposure: Determine the product name, because some hydrocarbons are associated with toxicities other than the consequences of hypoxia, especially with long-term use.
- Focused physical assessment
  - Respiratory system: respiratory distress.
  - Cardiovascular system: dysrhythmias
  - Neurologic system: altered level of consciousness
- Laboratory tests
  - Although many hydrocarbons can be evaluated in the laboratory, these tests are not available and not helpful to emergency department personnel, and are often used for forensic purposes instead.
- Nursing interventions
  - Support airway, breathing, and circulation (Chapter 30).
  - Initiate measures to control seizures and treat dysrhythmias.
  - Follow up with the involved workplace management; consider reporting to OSHA (the Occupational Safety and Health Administration).
  - Follow up with counseling for intentional abuse.
- Special considerations
  - *Sudden sniffing death syndrome* describes the outcome of concentrating and inhaling hydrocarbons and some other substances such as nitrous oxide: a sudden shout, running for several yards, then collapsing in ventricular fibrillation. Parents are usually unaware of inhalant abuse by their children, because the products abused are legal and readily available.

Organophosphate Insecticides

Sources

- Numerous products intended for indoor and outdoor residential applications, by homeowners and professional pest control applicators, and agricultural pesticides (diazinon, dursban, fenthion, malathion, and many others).

Routes of exposure

- Ingestion
- Inhalation
- Dermal
- Toxicity is the same by all routes of exposure.

Mechanism of Toxicity

- Organophosphate insecticides are acetylcholinesterase inhibitors.
- By binding to acetylcholinesterase, they allow continued action of acetylcholine at receptor sites throughout the nervous system.
- They also prevent the hydrolysis of acetylcholine and the reuptake of choline into presynaptic nerve cells.
- If not disrupted, this acetylcholinesterase-organophosphate bond becomes permanent in about 24 hours.
- The initial result is excessive cholinergic stimulation, eventually followed by depletion of acetylcholine and decreased cholinergic stimulation.
- Muscarinic effects can be remembered by the mnemonic "SLUDGE": Salivation, Lacrimation, Urination, Defecation, GI (nausea, diarrhea), Eyes (pinpoint pupils)/Emesis.

- Nicotinic effects can be remembered by the mnemonic "MTWtHF": Mydriasis, muscle twitching, and muscle cramps; Tachycardia; Weakness; Hypertension; Fasciculations. Central nervous system effects include lethargy, seizure, and coma. What the mnemonic doesn't describe is significant bronchorrhea, which may present the biggest challenge in early ED management.

Focused History

- Product name
- Amount of product involved in the exposure
- Routes of exposure
- Time of exposure

Focused Physical Assessment

- Respiratory system: bronchorrhea.
- Cardiovascular system: tachycardia and hypertension.
- Neurologic status: lethargy, seizures, and coma.

Laboratory Tests

- Red blood cell cholinesterase level.
- The more easily obtained plasma cholinesterase level is less useful because it can be affected by many things besides actual acetylcholinesterase inhibition.

Nursing Interventions

1. For all exposures:
   - Support airway, breathing, and circulation (Chapter 30).
2. Ingestion exposure:
   - Initiate gastrointestinal decontamination.
   - Administer an intravenous infusion of atropine.
     - Atropine occupies muscarinic acetylcholine receptor sites and terminates symptoms of cholinergic excess.
     - Titrate atropine to the production of bronchial secretions.
     - Repeat the dose as needed to keep the bronchial tree clear.
     - The pediatric dose is 0.05 mg/kg, repeated every 10 to 30 minutes as necessary. The endpoint is not a specific total dose, but drying of pulmonary secretions.
     - Auscultate for the disappearance of rales and observe for lessening of bronchorrhea.
     - Monitor for tachycardia. (If administration of atropine results in significant tachycardia, organophosphate poisoning is unlikely to be the cause of the patient's symptoms.)
   - Administer an intravenous infusion of pralidoxime (2-PAM):
     - 2-PAM cleaves the organophosphate-acetylcholinesterase bond before it becomes permanent.
     - Administration of pralidoxime can begin concurrently with atropine, but must begin within 24 hours of exposure, before the organophospate-acetylcholinesterase bond becomes permanent. The dose is 25 to 50 mg/kg. This dose may be repeated in one hour and then every 6 to 12 hours as needed. The goal is not a specific amount but relief of muscle weakness, especially diaphragmatic weakness. Both drugs may be needed for days, depending on the half-life of the pesticide and its degree of fat-solubility.
3. Dermal exposure:
   - Initiate decontamination procedures (Chapter 45).
   - Discard any contaminated leather garments, belts, shoes, etc.; leather is skin and absorbs these chemicals.

Special Considerations

- The amounts of atropine and 2-PAM needed may seem excessive to the emergency nurse unfamiliar with organophosphate insecticide poisoning. Fearful of tachycardia or other effects of atropine "overdose," the emergency nurse may be reluctant to administer the large amounts needed. In fact, a seriously poisoned child can tolerate the huge amounts needed, up to several grams of atropine over the course of treatment. It cannot be overemphasized that sufficient amounts of these drugs are the mainstays of treatment of this life-threatening poisoning.

Conclusion

Children experiencing poison exposures or poisonings benefit greatly from the advice rendered by poison centers. Poison centers offer expert advice about recognizing and treating poison exposures 24 hours a day, 7 days a week. Regional poison centers are staffed by board-certified medical toxicologists, board-certified clinical toxicologists, and registered nurses and pharmacists who are nationally certified as specialists in poison information. These resources should be used, because nonspecialist sources of toxicology information are likely to provide incorrect or misleading advice (Mullen,

Anderson, & Kim, 1997; Wigder, Erickson, Morse, & Saporta, 1995).

Emergency nurses who contact their local poison center gain the obvious immediate benefit of expert, individualized treatment advice. Other benefits of contacting the poison center include:

- Follow-up by the poison center, whether the child is discharged home or admitted to an inpatient unit, assuring continuity of care.
- Anonymous entry of the child's case into the only national database of human poison exposures. The American Association of Poison Control Centers Toxic Exposure Surveillance System records poison exposures and their associated medical outcomes, identifies trends in poisonings, and identifies previously unsuspected hazards amenable to regulatory action or educational intervention. These data also guide research to improve the recognition and treatment of poisoning.
- Every poison center in the United States may be reached by calling 1-800-222-1222. Callers are automatically connected to the correct poison center.

References

Bertolini, J. (1992). Hydrofluoric acid: A review of toxicity. *Journal of Emergency Medicine*, *10*, 163-168.

Centers for Disease Control and Prevention. (1995). Deaths associated with a purported aphrodisiac—New York City, February 1993-1995. *MMWR*, *44*, 853-855, 861.

Dart, R., Start, Y., Fulton, et. al. (1996). Insufficient stocking of poisoning antidotes in hospital pharmacies. *JAMA*, *276*, 1508-1510.

Done, A. (1960). Salicylate intoxication: significance of measurements of salicylate in blood in cases of acute ingestion. *Pediatrics*, *26*, 800-807.

Ellenhorn, (1997). *Ellenhorn's medical toxicology: Diagnosis and treatment of human poisoning* (2nd ed). Baltimore: Williams & Wilkins.

Goldfrank, L. Flomenbaum, N., Lewin, N., Weisman, R., Howland, M., & Hoffman, R. (Eds.). (1994). *Goldfrank's toxicologic emergencies* (5th ed, pp. 577-588). Norwalk CT: Appleton & Lange.

Goldfrank, L., Flomenbaum, N., Lewin, N., Weisman, B., Howland, M., & Hoffman, R., (Eds.). (1998). Vital signs and toxic syndromes. In *Goldfrank's Toxicologic Emergencies* (6th ed.). Stamford, CT: Appleton & Lange.

Kaczorowski, J. & Wax, P. (1996). Five days of whole-bowel irrigation: A case of pediatric iron ingestion. *Annals of Emergency Medicine*, *27*(2), 258-263.

Klasner, A., Scalzo, A., Blume, C., Johnson, P., & Thompson, M. W. (1996). Marked hypocalcemia and ventricular fibrillation in two pediatric patients exposed to a fluoride-containing wheel cleaner. *Annals of Emergency Medicine*, *28*(6), 713-18.

Kwan, T., Paiusco, A. & Kohl, L. (1992). Digitalis toxicity caused by toad venom. *Chest*, *102*, 949-50.

Litovitz, T. & Schmitz, B. (1992). Ingestion of cylindrical and button batteries: An analysis of 2382 cases. *Pediatrics*, *89*, 747-757.

Litovitz,T. L., Klein-Schwartz, W., White, S., Cobaugh, D., Youniss, J., Omslaer, A., & Benson, B. (2001). 2000 Annual Report of the American Association of Poison Control Centers Toxic Exposure Surveillance System. *American Journal of Emergency Medicine*, *19*, 337-395.

McCarron, M., Challoner, K., & Thompson, G. (1991). Diphenoxylate-atropine (Lomotil) overdose in children: An update (report of eight cases and review of the literature). *Pediatrics*, *87*, 694-700.

Mullen, W., Anderson, I., & Kim, S. (1997). Incorrect overdose management advice in the Physician's Desk Reference. *Annals of Emergency Medicine*, *29*, 255-261.

Rumack, B., Peterson, R., Koch, G., & Amara, I. (1981). Acetaminophen overdose: 662 cases with evaluation of oral acetylcysteine treatment. *Archives of Internal Medicine*, *141*, 380-385.

Tenenbaum, M. (1987). Whole-bowel irrigation in iron poisoning. *Journal of Pediatrics*, *111*(1), 142-145.

Wigder, H., Erickson, T., Morse, T., & Saporta, V. (1995). Emergency department poison advice telephone calls. *Annals of Emergency Medicine*, *25*, 349-542.

45

Hazardous Material and Biochemical Emergencies

Roger K. Keddington, APRN, MSN, CEN, CCRN

Introduction

Hazardous material (HAZMAT) and biochemical exposures are real risks for children. These emergencies are increasingly a concern in patient care, and all emergency department (ED) personnel must be properly prepared for these situations. A child who is contaminated may be especially challenging to treat; not only does the child suffer from the effects of the exposure, but also any residual hazardous material may pose significant risk to emergency personnel and other patients. The purpose of this chapter is to discuss hazardous material and biochemical exposures, their effects, and how to treat specific exposures.

A hazardous material is defined as any substance, chemical, material, or waste that poses a risk to life, health, safety, property, or the environment if improperly handled. (Kirk, Cisek, & Rose, 1994; Burgess, Keifer, Barnhart, Richardson, & Robertson, 1997). The Federal Emergency Management Agency identifies five types of hazardous incidents with the "B-NICE" acronym. Biological, Nuclear (radiation), Incendiary, Chemical, and Explosive. (Federal Emergency Management Agency, 2000). Poisindex lists nearly 600,000 substances that can be hazardous (Leonard, 1993).

Biohazard risk refers to the use of biological agents used to kill or injure others. Agents like this used by terrorists are also referred to as weapons of mass destruction (Henretig et al., 2000). Examples of weapons of mass destruction include anthrax, small pox, bubonic plague, and nerve gas (Noeller, 2001).

Pediatric Considerations

Developmental Factors

Infants

Typically, young infants do not initiate hazardous material or biochemical contact. They may be exposed unintentionally by being in the vicinity where an adult is somehow exposed. Infants may also be exposed in a public area where agents may be present. Some hazardous materials may even be brought home on parent's clothing or other work materials.

Toddlers and Preschoolers

These children are more mobile and, as their curiosity increases, they may have access to a variety of serious agents without recognition of the hazards. Toddlers and preschoolers experience much of their environment through oral exploration, which can lead to exposure. With their increased independence, they can find many products stored around the house.

School-aged Children and Adolescents

School-aged children are increasingly independent and spend more time away from home. This independence can lead to exposure to a variety of chemicals. Older children are often curious about the effects of various chemicals, experimenting by mixing household agents without regard to chemical interactions. The release of defense sprays in school has also become somewhat common (Claman & Patterson, 1995).

Household Factors

Most hazardous material exposures in children occur at home. According to the American Association of Poison Control Centers, in 2000 there were more than 117,000 exposures of children under 6 years of age to household cleaning substances. Of these, more than 18,800 were exposures involving household chloride bleach. It is estimated that 47% of homes with a child under the age of 5 had at least one pesticide stored in an unlocked cabinet within reach of the child (U.S. Environmental Protection Agency, 2001).

Environmental Factors

In addition to households, industries, businesses, and schools contain hazardous materials that can pose serious risk to children. Examples include cleaners, organic solvents, paints, rat or mouse poisons, disinfectants, and automobile products.

Physiologic Factors

Pediatric physiologic factors that can influence the absorption of the substance and its systemic effects are listed in Table 45.1.

Etiology

A HAZMAT incident can occur anywhere. The likelihood of children being involved in some of these incidents is high (Lamminpaa & Riihimaki, 1992; Lipscomb, Kramer, & Leikin, 1992; Cyr, 1988). In the 1980s, the majority of serious hazardous material incidents occurred in rural areas without the assistance of highly trained personnel (Plante & Walker, 1989).

Billions of tons of chemicals are transported across the United States yearly, creating situations in which multiple patients could be exposed. In 2000 there were 17,454 transportation incidents involving hazardous materials with 227 injuries (United States Department of Transportation, 2001).

Four main routes of exposure to hazardous material exist (Emergency Management Institute, 1992):

- *Inhalation.* Inhalation allows the hazardous material to quickly gain access into the blood through the lungs, producing dangerous systemic effects and direct effects on the pulmonary system. *Aerosol exposure* is the inhalation of droplets or fumes of a hazardous material. Examples of aerosol exposures include gases such as chlorine, vapors from pesticides, fumes from petroleum-based products, and self-defense chemical sprays.
- *Absorption.* Usually substances that are in direct contact with the skin do not pass into the bloodstream. However, certain chemicals may pass through the skin very easily, producing systemic effects. Contact exposures may cause only minor erythema and irritation of the body's surface or can result in severe local or systemic reactions. The amount of area exposed and the condition of the patient's skin, including temperature and hydration, can affect the body's reaction to a hazardous material (Emergency Management Institute, 1992). Once a hazardous material is on the skin or clothing, it can give off hazardous fumes even though there is no direct contact on the caregiver's body.
- *Ingestion.* Hazardous materials in contact with mucosal membranes of the mouth or nose can cause

TABLE 45.1 Physiologic Considerations in Pediatric HAZMAT and Biohazard Exposures

Physiologic Differences in Children	*Nursing Considerations*
Smaller body mass and larger body surface area affect absorption and severity of effects.	More rapid absorption of hazardous materials and more serious systemic effects can occur.
	Children's larger body surface area makes temperature control difficult, and copious amounts of water used in decontamination may lead to hypothermia.
Smaller airways that can easily obstruct with minimal swelling.	Pediatric inhalation exposures can quickly lead to respiratory distress.
Skin is thinner and more fragile.	Children have an increased risk of absorption of chemicals and toxicity from skin exposure.
Higher metabolic rate contributes to an alveolar ventilation that can be as great or greater than in an adult.	Any respiratory contact with hazardous materials can lead to more significant effects in a child than in an adult in the same situation. Even with low levels of contaminants in the air, a child's high respiratory rate and rapid pulmonary air exchange can lead to a significant exposure over time.
A child's vascular and gastrointestinal system can absorb materials quickly.	Hazardous materials can be transported rapidly into the circulatory system and reach lethal levels.
A child's immune system is immature.	Children are more susceptible to infections or illness for which they have not been immunized.

local or systemic effects. Common examples of hazardous material ingestions include gasoline, antifreeze, household cleaning products, and acids. Hazardous materials may be ingested in suicide attempts. Once ingested, certain substances may saturate the body, releasing hazardous fumes ("off gassing") from the body. Examples include pesticides and fertilizers. This off-gassing of a hazardous material from a patient can put emergency caregivers at risk when they have not been properly prepared or protected. (Merritt & Anderson, 1989).

- *Injection.* This exposure is due to a puncture injury, wounds, or other surface trauma. Once a hazardous material is introduced under the dermal layer, systemic absorption or tissue injury can occur.

The effect of the substance on the patient is determined by the type of exposure as well as the chemical makeup, pH, concentration, amount, and the length of time the substance is in contact with the patient.

Focused History

In situations where the history is vague or unclear, or the substance remains unknown, assume that full treatment is needed and that the patient is a potential risk to caregivers until proven otherwise (Burgess et al., 1997). The following are important components of the history:

- Type of substance and its potential effects on the child or others. (Some methods and resources for hazardous material identification are listed in Tables 45.2 and 45.3.)
- Time involved. The length of time of exposure and how long since the exposure.
- The concentration of the substance.
- The location of exposure. Determine if the area had adequate ventilation or was enclosed.
- The potential for multiple types of exposure.
- Other areas the child has been to that may now be contaminated.
- The risk that the substance may pose to others.
- The history or identification of others who may be exposed.
- Unusual or suspicious illnesses or complaints.

Focused Assessment

In many hazardous material exposures, decontamination takes place before an in-depth assessment is done. Appropriate personal protective gear should be used if it will be necessary to have contact with the patient prior to decontamination. Protective gear should continue to be worn if the patient can potentially contaminate others after decontamination. Protective gear is described later in this chapter. However, an evaluation of the following

TABLE 45.2 Resources for Hazardous Material Identification

Resource	*Description/Comments*
United States Department of Transportation Identification Standards	This agency establishes identification standards for transporting hazardous materials. This system has been designed as a national standard to help reduce confusion in chemical transport and can be cross-referenced for more information. Transportation vehicles are required to have several placards visible that list the following: ■ The hazardous properties of the material. ■ A four-digit number for identification of the material. ■ United Nations hazardous reference number (Plante & Walker, 1989).
Material Safety Data Sheets (MSDS)	Government regulations require businesses to maintain a MSDS for every chemical used. Each data sheet describes the exposure risks of the material, serious dosage levels, treatment, and chemicals contained in the substance. Information can be found on the MSDS web site: http://www.chem.utah.edu/MSDS/msds.html. However, information on the chemicals' physiologic effects may be incomplete or inaccurate. Ingredients listed as inert on MSDS may actually be toxic (Kirk et al. 1994).
Local and national governmental agencies	These agencies provide 24-hour support and up-to-date information. They include the Chemical Transportation Emergency Center, local fire departments, and regional poison control centers (Table 45.3).

TABLE 45.3 Hazardous Material Incident Information Resources

Agency	*Description, Phone Number, and Web Site (If Applicable)*	
Chemical Transportation Emergency Center (CHEMTREC)	24-hour information on all hazardous products with an emphasis on transportation emergencies	1-800-424-9300 International: 703-527-3887
National Response Center and Terrorist Hotline	24-hour identification of hazardous material and incident control	1-800-424-8802 or 1-202-267-2675
Agency for Toxic Substance and Disease Registry	24-hour assistance for health-related effects	1-404-725-5754
National Pesticide Telecommunications	Information regarding pesticide exposures	1-800-858-7378
Radiation Emergency Assistance Center/Training Site (REACTS)	Emergency consultation for radioactive incidents	1-865-576-3131 1-865-576-1005
Regional poison control center	Lists poison control centers that offer 24-hour identification of hazardous materials and their treatment	http://www.medicinenet.com
CDCP—Centers for Disease Control and Prevention	Information on biohazards and diseases	1-770-488-7100
National Antimicrobial Information Network	Information on biohazards	1-800-447-6349
Federal Emergency Management Agency	Emergency response to terrorism; job aid. Helpful plastic reference book	http://www.usfa.fema.gov/usfapubs/
Local fire department	Support in decontamination and caring for hazardous material and contamination incidents	
Chemical Emergency Preparedness and Prevention office (CEPP)	http://www.epa.gov/swercepp/ Information on prevention, risk management, planning and emergency response. Also has information about international programs and counterterrorism	
Agency for Toxic Substances and Disease Registry (ATSDR)	http://www.atsdr.cdc.gov Provides toxicology facts, summaries of hazardous materials and their emergency response	
National Pesticide Tele-network	http://www.nptn.orst.edu Accesses online poisoning handbook	

should be done immediately, and critical interventions should be performed:

- Airway
- Breathing
- Circulation
- Disability

A thorough head-to-toe assessment should be completed after proper decontamination.

Triage Decisions

Emergent

Any hazardous material exposure posing a risk to the child's life or the lives of others should be classified as emergent. A child with hazardous material exposure requires attention not only to the immediate condition but also to the risk the exposure might pose to others.

- Rapidly identify situations in which an exposure involves hazardous material that gives off fumes or gases, or in which a child might be grossly contaminated. Also watch for unknown or suspicious substances being brought to the ED. If any of these situations occur, the child and those with them should be removed from the triage area. Place the child in a location where initial decontamination can begin and where gases and hazardous materials will not increase the risks to others.
- Any area where the child has been should be sealed off until it is clear that no residual contamination is present and the area has been decontaminated. Emer-

gency department staff may need to use protective gear if immediate risks are identified.

- It is imperative that hazardous materials do not spread within the hospital system. If there is a risk that hazardous or biohazardous materials have been brought to the emergency department, the ED staff should not only protect themselves but involve the hospital engineers and local health department to ensure that nothing is spread in the ventilation system or to other hospital areas.

Urgent

All hazardous material injuries other than emergent ones should be classified as urgent because of the unpredictable nature of chemical exposures. Frequent reassessment is needed to recognize the effects of delayed toxicity (Kirk et al., 1994).

Nonurgent

Nonurgent classification should not be used for patients with hazardous material contamination.

Nursing Interventions

Preparation for Decontamination

By law, each state is required to establish a state emergency response commission (SERC) and local emergency planning committees (LEPC) (Ferazani, Fucaloro, Hayes, & Schroeder, 1995). The emergency department should work with these agencies as well as local fire and emergency agencies to establish a coordinated plan that is practical and useful (American Health Consultants, 2001). Not only does this type of plan improve communication but it can maximize the efficient use of resources and establish important roles in a contamination emergency before it occurs.

- Provide personal protective gear for staff involved with the child. The U.S. Environmental Protection Agency has identified and defined four levels of protection for working with hazardous materials (Cox, 1994). These four levels were originally determined for those who work with hazardous materials but have been widely adopted in rescue work and hazardous material decontamination (Table 45.4). Decontamination in a hospital setting generally requires level B or C (Table 45.4). Level B protection uses a positive pressure device along with protective clothing. Level C protection can be achieved with a full-face air-purifying respirator with a multichemical filter cartridge; disposable chemical-resistant coveralls of a protective material such as tyvek; and double-gloving with nitrile gloves, rubber overboots, and duct tape for sealing all seams and openings. The Occupational Safety and Health Administration (OSHA) has strict guidelines about the training required for those who use this equipment (Lynch, 2001).

Prehospital Decontamination

Initiate prehospital decontamination if possible. Ideally, decontamination should be performed by special HAZMAT teams in the field prior to the child's transport to a hospital. This reduces the risk to both prehospital

TABLE 45.4 U.S. Environmental Protection Agency HAZMAT Protection Levels

Level	*Indications*	*Respiratory Protection*	*Clothing*	*Gloves*
Level A	HAZMAT workers dealing in areas of very high concentration of toxic materials need Level A protection.	Self-contained, positive-pressure breathing device	Fully encapsulated chemical-resistant suit	Double layers of attached chemical-resistant gloves
Level B	Full respiratory protection is needed; low concentrations of hazardous materials are expected.	Positive-pressure respiratory protection, self-contained or attached to hose	Chemical-resistant overalls with head and foot protection.	Double layers of chemical-resistant gloves, taped to sleeve
Level C	There are low levels of hazardous material; air contamination is expected to be minimal.	Face mask with canister filter	Chemical-resistant suit	Chemical-resistant gloves and boots
Level D	There is no danger of hazardous material exposure.	None; simple face mask, if desired	Standard work clothes	Gloves, if desired

personnel and the emergency department staff (Cox, 1994). However, HAZMAT teams are expensive and may not be available in all communities. Even when HAZMAT teams are available, the seriousness of child's exposure to a hazardous material contamination may not be fully appreciated, and the child may be transported to an emergency department before proper decontamination has occurred (Cox, 1994).

Emergency Department Decontamination

During a hazardous material or biohazard incident it is likely that contaminated patients will be brought directly to the emergency department by family or friends without any prior decontamination. This is especially true if the contamination occurred in the home. For this reason it is important that each emergency department has a well-thought-out plan of what actions will be taken when patients present to the ED without warning (Kohlmeier, 1985). Biologic incidents pose a special problem. Victims may present to an ED following an incubation period. There may not be any incident or history to alert medical personnel to the exposure. Primary caregivers may put themselves at risk unknowingly (McLaughlin, 2001).

- Emergency personnel should be sufficiently trained to identify a potential exposure as quickly as possible. This will help reduce the risk of hazardous or communicable materials getting spread through the department or rest of the hospital. Establish a decontamination area near the ED to receive contaminated patients. This area should be designed and prepared for water run off and for the collection and disposal of contaminated materials. Resuscitation supplies should be available. Other considerations for establishing a decontamination area are listed in Table 45.5. Three clearly marked and secured areas or zones should be established.

  1. *Hot Zone*—This is the initial area where gross decontamination takes place. The risk of exposure to the hazardous material is higher in this area.
  2. *Warm Zone*—The risk of exposure to hazardous materials is lower. Specific cleaning of wounds or detailed decontamination can be done.
  3. *Cold Zone*—The patient is fully decontaminated. No protection is needed and further treatment can proceed as indicated. (U. S. Environmental Protection Agency, 1997a).

- Be aware of toxic odors. Most exposures will not pose a serious risk to emergency department staff if rapidly identified and properly decontaminated. However, a small percentage of patients may still pose significant risk to healthcare workers because of off-gassing

TABLE 45.5 Setting Up an ED Decontamination Area

Set-Up Needs	*Outdoor Set-Up*	*Indoor Set-Up*
Ventilation system	Ventilation is not generally required outdoors. Keep the decontamination area away from hospital air intakes.	A ventilation system is required to provide a negative pressure flow of air. All air from the area has to be vented to the outside. Charcoal filters are recommended in air systems.
Collection of drainage	Drainage collection can be established with plastic wading pools or commercial collection tanks. In some cases it may be possible to allow some hazardous materials to go down the sewer system. Check with your local authorities.	Plastic wading pools or commercial collection tanks can be used for drainage collection. It must be designed for easy access, cleaning, and hazardous material disposal.
Water source	Water for bathing and irrigation must be available. Temperature control of the water is needed for pediatrics.	It is easier to establish a water source with temperature control inside the hospital.
Privacy	A curtain system or a commercial decontamination tent is needed to maintain privacy.	Individual rooms and curtains to provide privacy are easily established.
Environmental	A decontamination tent with heaters and lights may be needed. There must be a safe way to provide outdoor decontamination during bad weather or cold conditions.	Temperature control and lighting are usually easily designed in an internal decontamination area.
Cost and care	An outside decontamination area can usually be established relatively inexpensively. Time is needed for setup and preparation before patient decontamination can start.	The cost of establishing an area indoors can be expensive. Set-up time in preparation for a hazardous material incident is usually less than for an outdoor system.

(Shultz, Cisek, & Wabeke, 1995), as for example, in those patients exposed to an organophosphate or pesticides. If chemical odors from the patient are detected, or if there is a history of an exposure involving a substance that could pose continued risk, the patient should be treated in a negative pressure area where fumes cannot expose the rest of the hospital. Staff should continue to use adequate respiratory protection and appropriate protective clothing until it is clear that there is no more risk. If indoor resources do not exist to safely care for this patient, it may be necessary to continue care in an outdoor decontamination area with adequate outdoor ventilation.

Specific Interventions in Decontamination

1. *Care of the child in the hot zone:* Medical care in the decontamination area is mostly symptomatic and supportive. The major goals of decontamination are to remove the hazardous material from the patient, if possible; to stop the toxic effects of the substance; and to keep the child from contaminating those caring for him or her. Because contact with hazardous materials is probable, respiratory and contact protection using protection levels B or C is recommended (Levitin & Siegelson, 1996). During decontamination, consider the privacy needs of the child and recognize that help may be needed to thoroughly decontaminate all areas of the body.

   Assessment and treatment of the child should focus on only the most basic concerns: airway, breathing, circulation, and disability. All other treatments should be delayed until after decontamination. If respiratory distress is likely or present, oxygen should be administered immediately. Any medical devices applied before the patient is decontaminated should be replaced with clean devices after decontamination so that hazardous materials are not transported from the hot zone to other areas.

   Nursing diagnoses to consider when treating patients exposed to hazardous materials are shown in Table 45.6.

   The steps in the process of decontaminating pediatric patients include:

   - Remove contaminated clothing immediately. This can eliminate 70 to 80% of the contaminant (Cox, 1994).
   - Place contaminated clothing or waste in plastic bags for proper disposal. Place patient infomation tag on bag as it may be necessary for forensic evidence. It may be necessary to store this waste in the hot zone until those qualified to remove hazardous wastes can arrive.
   - Remove large pieces of the contaminant with forceps prior to the shower. Some contaminants, such as elemental metals (sodium, lithium) may explode on contact with water. These types of contamination should be covered with mineral oil and removed completely before water irrigation. (Kirk et al., 1994).
   - Wash the child with copious amounts of water for at least 15 minutes. A mild soap may be helpful in removing contaminants (Emergency Management Institute, 1992; Kirk et al., 1994). Vigorous scrubbing of the skin should be avoided, especially in children because skin damage can occur easily. If hot water is used, the risk of chemical reactivity is increased. Cool water showers are recommended for decontamination. However, cool water showers can be very uncomfortable and may result in hypothermia in pediatric patients. A warm shower will be better tolerated and will decrease the risk of hypothermia. It is important to control the water temperature for decontamination. The decision to use warm versus cool water should be

TABLE 45.6 Nursing Diagnoses and Expected Outcomes

Nursing Diagnoses	*Expected Outcomes*
Ineffective airway clearance related to hazardous material inhalation	Airway will be open and respirations will be unobstructed.
Risk (to patient and staff) for poisoning related to hazardous material effects	Risk will be minimized by proper decontamination techniques.
Altered tissue perfusion; renal, cerebral, or cardiopulmonary effects related to hazardous material	Tissue perfusion will be normal, as evidenced by capillary refill, blood pressure, level of consciousness, and urinary output.
Infection and risk of infection	Infection will be controlled so as to minimize the spread of illness and risk to others.

based on the type and extent of the contamination and the needs of the patient.

- The decontamination process should start with any contaminated wounds, followed by the eyes, mucous membranes, skin, nail beds, and hair. Patients exposed to aerosol contamination should have the mouth, nose, and ears carefully cleaned. Ocular exposures require prompt removal of contact lenses and irrigation of the eyes. The folds of the skin as well as all body openings should be carefully cleaned (Emergency Management Institute, 1992). Irrigation runoff should flow away from cleaned areas and down so that previously washed places are not recontaminated (Kirk et al., 1994; Leonard, 1993).

2. *Care of the child in the warm zone.* After the child is decontaminated, he or she can move to the warm zone, an area where emergency department staff provide further treatment and verify that the patient has received adequate decontamination. There is less risk to emergency department staff in the warm zone, and level C or D protection should be adequate. (Table 45.4.) A more thorough assessment can be conducted and attention can be given to wounds or injuries that might require special irrigation and decontamination. When dealing with any type of a biohazard incident the healthcare professional should maintain communication with local public health agencies and civil authorities. Epidemiology studies may be part of continuing care (McLaughlin, 2001). The early involvement of a specialist in infectious disease is also important.
3. *Care of the child in the cold zone.* When it is verified that the child is fully decontaminated, the child is moved to the cold zone, where definitive treatment is given. The cold zone can be located in any area of the emergency department. HAZMAT protection is not needed in this area. Each decontamination area should be clearly marked so that people and supplies do not cross over from a contaminated area to a clean area.
4. *Cleanup.* After any decontamination process there should be a plan for decontamination of involved staff, equipment, and rooms. Proper cleanup will include the disposal of any hazardous materials or collected waste.

Specific HAZMAT Emergencies

Because of the vast number and types of hazardous materials, a comprehensive explanation of all types of exposures is beyond the scope of this chapter. But in all cases of hazardous material or biohazard exposure, the following actions should be included as part of any treatment guidelines:

1. Evacuate the patient from the exposure area.
2. Remove contaminated clothing.
3. Wash contaminated surfaces thoroughly with mild soap (no oils) and water.
4. Provide oxygen therapy for patients with respiratory involvement.

Additionally, attention must be given to the airway, breathing, circulation, disability, and any other injury or specific problem.

Chemical Hazards

Some of the specific types of materials likely to be encountered in the pediatric population are listed. The focus of these specific guidelines is to address the hazardous material exposure; attention to other medical needs of the patient is assumed.

Chlorine Gas

Chlorine gas is used as a disinfectant and for water purification.

Pathophysiology

Commonly, chlorine is used in association with residential swimming pools and spas. Chlorine gas has a strong, pungent odor and may be seen as a greenish-yellow vapor cloud. It is heavier than air and can move out easily from its source. Chlorine gas can cause sloughing of airway epithelium and intense inflammation of the respiratory system (Segal & Lang, 2001).

Signs and Symptoms

- *Mild exposure:* Burning sensation of the nose, mouth, and throat associated with irritation of the eyes.
- *Increased exposure:* Paroxysmal cough. In some cases, the cough will be associated with hematemesis. Headache, weakness, wheezing, nausea, nasal drainage, hoarseness, tachypnea, chest pains, and palpitations may also occur.
- *Severe exposure:* Productive cough and difficulty breathing, cyanosis, worsening respiratory status, and rales because of pulmonary edema and congestion. Severe hematemesis and death can occur because of progressive respiratory failure.

Nursing Interventions

Chlorine gas usually dissipates quickly, so these patients generally pose little risk for contaminating other healthcare workers. Unless there is gross chlorine contamination, these patients do not have to be decontaminated before coming to the emergency department.

1. Remove clothing to reduce the risk of off-gassing. Any exposure residue on the clothing or skin can cause trapped gasses to be released.
2. Provide 100% oxygen for respiratory exposure.
3. Treat bronchoconstriction with inhaled bronchodilators. Intubation may be necessary in severe cases.
4. Rinse eyes with tepid water.
5. Thoroughly wash the mouth and face if chlorine generating compounds have been ingested.
6. Do not induce vomiting because of the risk of aspiration.

Hydrocarbons

Hydrocarbons include gasoline, kerosene, and their constituents. These products may be found in glues, propellants, lighter fluids, and other products.

Pathophysiology

Hydrocarbons can defat the skin and mucous membranes, causing irritation and chemical burns. They can be absorbed though the lungs, skin, or gastrointestinal tract. Inhalation injuries are common with exposure to these products. Ingestion and surface exposure may also be seen (Maffeo, 1996).

Signs and Symptoms

- Respiratory exposure: Nausea, vomiting, light headedness, and dizziness. Chronic inhalation can lead to irreversible central nervous system injury.
- Systemic exposure: Cardiac dysrhythmias and liver and renal abnormalities.
- Severe exposure: Unconsciousness and respiratory depression.

Nursing Interventions

1. Wash any solvents from the skin with large amounts of a mild soap and water.
2. Provide oxygen therapy for inhalation exposures.
3. Irrigate eyes with copious amounts of water if they have been exposed.
4. Do not induce vomiting in patients with ingestion exposures because of the risk of aspiration. If the substance must be removed from the stomach, it should be done by gastric lavage while there is appropriate airway control with a cuffed endotracheal tube to prevent aspiration.

Methanol (Methyl Alcohol)

Methanol can be found in many household products including paint removers, glass cleaners, brake fluid, antifreeze, and windshield washer and deicer.

Pathophysiology

- Methanol ingestion may be identified by the presence of an increased anion and osmolar gap. Treatment focuses on life-support measures.

When metabolized by the liver, methanol forms formic acid, which inhibits mitochondrial respiration. This results in tissue hypoxia and metabolic acidosis, which can lead to optic nerve damage and blindness (Likosky, 2001).

Signs and Symptoms

Signs and symptoms can be delayed for many hours, making contamination more difficult to successfully treat. Symptoms include:

- Visual disturbances.
- Nausea, vomiting, and abdominal pain.
- Headache, weakness, and dizziness.
- In severe cases, coma and seizures associated with cerebral edema. Death results from myocardial depression, bradycardia, hypotension, shock, and respiratory arrest.

Nursing Interventions

1. Contaminated clothing should be removed, and the child should be washed with water if the skin or eyes are involved. After 30 to 60 minutes of ingestion, the methanol is usually already absorbed into the system, so gastric lavage may not be helpful.
2. Treat inhalation exposures with oxygen.
3. Ethanol infusion and dialysis may be indicated, depending on the severity of contamination.
4. Do not induce vomiting because of the risk of central nervous system depression.

Self-Defense Sprays

These products are commonly available in many stores. There has been a 40% increase in sales yearly in the last several years. Various chemicals may be used in self-defense sprays; the most common are oleoresin capsicum (cayenne pepper) and chloroacetophenone (Mace) (Claman & Patterson, 1995).

Pathophysiology

Self-defense sprays are classified as irritants and cause direct irritation to nerve endings of the eyes, mucous membranes, respiratory system, and skin.

Signs and Symptoms

Most symptoms are self-limiting and will resolve after 20 minutes.

- Contact dermatitis, erythema, edema, vesication, purpura, difficulty breathing, pulmonary edema, and lacrimation are among the symptoms.
- Conjunctivitis may persist for 1 to 2 days.
- Bronchopneumonia may develop if prolonged exposure in an enclosed space has occurred.
- Laryngospasm can occur. Asthmatics may be more sensitive to bronchoconstriction and at greater risk for respiratory arrest (Ross & Siddle, 1998).

Nursing Interventions

Treatment focuses on removal of the agent and irrigation.

1. Provide fresh air or oxygen to alleviate respiratory complaints.
2. Irrigate the eyes for up to 30 minutes.
3. Provide a cool shower for 10 minutes. Avoid scrubbing and soap initially. During the initial part of the shower additional chemicals may be released from the hair, temporarily worsening eye and skin irritation.
4. Add mild soap (no oils in soap) after the first 10 minutes. Oils in the soap decrease the effectiveness of breaking up and removing some of the sprays.
5. Blot dry with a towel. Avoid vigorous scrubbing.

Organophosphates

Organophosphates are found in many insecticides.

Pathophysiology

Organophosphates interfere with the normal degradation of cholinesterases of acetylcholines and function as a nerve agent. They inhibit nerve fibers from resetting after activation, so that nerves remain in a constant state of excitement. Initially, the interference of organophosphates is reversible if treated; however, after approximately 48 hours, the blockade of the enzyme is not reversible, and normal nervous function can return only after the synthesis of new enzymes, a process that takes weeks to months (Noeller, 2001).

Signs and Symptoms

- Immediately after exposure, headache, nausea, dizziness, anxiety, and restlessness may occur.
- With continued exposure, muscle fasciculation, weakness, abdominal cramps, pulmonary edema, and respiratory failure may occur.
- Continued interference with acetylcholine also leads to a glandular hypersecretion. The resulting signs and symptoms are known by the acronym SLUDGE: Salivation, Lacrimation, Urination, Defecation and Gastrointestinal upset, and Emesis (Rothrock, 1999).

Nursing Interventions

The use of protective clothing and respiratory protection is very important for hospital staff involved in the decontamination. Off-gassing is a risk with these patients.

1. Remove all clothing and wash exposed surfaces several times with soap and water.
2. Initiate life support measures and seizure precautions.
3. Administer medications as ordered. Atropine and pralidoxime may be required for severe cases (Chapter 44).
   - Atropine antagonizes the hypersecretion effects of organophosphates and can be given as a dose of 0.02 mg/kg up to a total dose of 1 mg. If this dose shows some positive effect, it should be administered in large enough doses to keep SLUDGE effects reversed. Atropine may not help in reversing respiratory muscle weakness.
   - Pralidoxime can be used in early stages of organophosphate contamination to restore some enzyme function, and may help to restore some respiratory function.
4. Consider gastric lavage or administration of activated charcoal if the child has ingested organophosphates.

Biohazards

Anthrax (*Bacillus anthracis*)

Pathophysiology

Anthrax is an aerobic, gram-positive bacteria. It is spore forming and nonmotile. It is naturally occurring in soil throughout the world. Spores can be cultured and developed to spread very easily. The anthrax outbreak of October 2001 demonstrated a virulence of this disease that had not been previously appreciated. Anthrax is associated with three types of infections.

- *Cutaneous* infections are the most common. If the bacteria gets into broken or open skin, an infection can develop about 12 days after exposure. Patients present with puritic macula or papule, then vesicles appear. After one to two weeks a painless depressed black eschaar dries, loosens, and falls off.
- *Gastrointestinal* infections are rare and associated with eating contaminated meat. Patients present with an oropharyngeal infection or abdominal infection.
- *Inhalation-caused* infections are rare, but can be fatal. Spores inhaled into the alveoli are ingested by macrophages and transported to the mediastinal lymphatic system. The bacteria can then germinate and reproduce. The course of the illness is worsened by the toxins the bacteria produces. Initial presentation may include fever, dyspnea, cough, headache, nausea and vomiting, abdominal pain, and chest pain (Inglesby et al., 1999; Broussard, 2001).

Signs and Symptoms

- Inhalational anthrax initially presents with fever, dyspnea, cough, headache, nausea and vomiting, abdominal pain, and chest pain.
- With a worsening inhalational anthrax the patient will develop worsening shortness of breath, diaphoresis, shock, hemorrhagic meningitis, delirium, and coma.

Nursing Interventions

1. Remove any contaminated clothing and thoroughly shower with soap.
2. Prevent any material with anthrax spores from coming into the hospital.
3. Anthrax is not contagious from one person to another; however, the spores can move about easily in the air.
4. Anthrax usually responds well to appropriate antibiotics if started early enough. Ciproflaxin is the antibiotic of choice.

Botulism

Botulinum toxin occurs from *Clostridium botulism*. It is considered to be the most poisonous substance known to man.

Pathophysiology

Clostridium botulism is usually found in unprocessed or poorly processed foods. It can also be found in improperly cared for or cooked food. Once ingested, the clostricium toxin, Botulinum, spreads into the body and binds in the neuromuscular junction, blocking acetycholine. This leads to a rapid paralysis. Botulism is not easily spread (Arnon et al., 2001; Broussard, 2001).

Signs and Symptoms

- A sudden and rapidly spreading descending flaccid paralysis occurs. This can be confused with Guillian Barre syndrome.

Nursing Interventions

1. Prepare for intubation and airway management.
2. Treat symptomatically. The patient may require weeks or months of intubation before neurologic function begins to return.
3. Although the patient may be paralyzed, botulism has no effect on cerebral function and the patient may be completely aware of his/her surroundings.

Plague

Yersinia pestis bacilli are naturally occurring bacteria that spread from the fleas of rats to humans. Plague can also be mechanically aerosolized.

Pathophysiology

- Usually the bacteria enter the body through a flea bite and migrate to the lymph nodes where the bacteria reside in the lymph (Inglesby, 2000; Broussard, 2001).

Signs and Symptoms

- Tender lump (bubo) develops in the lymph 2–8 days after exposure.
- Fever, nausea, and vomiting may develop.

Nursing Interventions

- Treat symptomatically and with antibiotics.

Tularemia

Francisella tularensis is a bacteria that has caused plague-like outbreaks throughout the world.

Pathophysiology

- Usually tularemia is a waterborne infection.

- Tularemia has also caused pneumonia (Dennis et al., 2001; Broussard, 2001).

Signs and Symptoms

- Pharyngitis, pneumonitis.
- Pleuritis.
- Sepsis.

Nursing Interventions

- Treat with antibiotics.
- With treatment, 2% fatality.

Smallpox

Pathophysiology

Smallpox (variola major) is an easily spread virus with a 30% fatality rate. Since the last outbreak in the 1960s, vaccination has eliminated these infections. Smallpox spreads slower than does chicken pox, but the virus can last up to 24 hours on surfaces. There is no transmission until a rash appears. The patient is infectious at the onset of the rash for 7–10 days until the rash becomes scaly (Henderson et al., 1999; Broussard, 2001).

Signs and Symptoms

- High fever, malaise, severe headache, and backache.
- Maculopapular rash that starts in the mouth, pharynx, face, and forearms, then spreads to trunk and legs. Rash becomes vesicular and then pustular.
- Death is thought to result from the toxemia associated with immune complexes and antigens. Encephalitis can also develop.

Nursing Interventions

A key to treating smallpox is preventing its spread to others.

- Initiate strict isolation. These patients should avoid being in the hospital, or a special hospital designated for smallpox patients should be established.
- Administer vaccination to all those exposed.
- Treat the patient symptomatically.

Prevention of HAZMAT Exposure

Complete prevention of HAZMAT exposure is difficult because of the large number of chemicals used daily. The potential risk of exposure increases each day. However, some steps can be taken to reduce this risk.

- Make sure that all chemical substances are kept out of reach and sight of children, preferably in a cupboard that can be locked.
- Lock all substances and keep them in their original containers. Use child-resistant caps.
- Dispose of unneeded chemicals rather than keeping products that have little or no use.
- Be familiar with the product warnings and the way to use each product properly.
- Look for alternatives to hazardous products that may be just as effective but less dangerous. Some alternatives to chemicals are listed in Appendix A.
- Emergency department staff must be sufficiently trained to work in any hazardous situation they may encounter (Gough & Markus, 1989; O'Neil, 1994).
- An education plan should exist to train the staff not only about the proper use of equipment and personal protection devices but also about the effects of various hazardous materials and what to expect during a contamination incident.

Summary

Children who have been exposed to hazardous materials or biohazards are at risk to have rapid and serious complications. These children can pose a significant risk to all those who come in contact with them, including emergency department staff and other emergency patients. Proper planning and preparation are essential to providing safe and effective care. Every emergency department should have a clear protocol and guidelines established to successfully care for the pediatric patient exposed to hazardous materials.

A

Products, Their Effects, and Safer Alternatives

Products	*Hazardous Ingredients*	*Dangers*	*Alternatives*
Aerosol sprays	Butanol; butane; propanol	Flammable; irritating; explosive	Pump-type sprays; potpourri
Ammonia-based cleaners	Ammonia; ethanol	Irritating; toxic; corrosive. (Forms poison gas when mixed with bleach.)	Vinegar; salt and water for surfaces; baking soda and water for the bathroom
Antifreeze	Ethylene glycol	Toxic. Sweet smell and taste leads to frequent poisoning.	Unknown. (Use caution; take to a collection center.)
Batteries	Sulfuric acid; lead	Corrosive; toxic	Unknown. (Use caution; recycle.)
Brake fluids	Glycol ethers; heavy metals	Flammable; toxic	Unknown. (Take to a collection center.)
Disinfectants	Diethylene glycol; sodium; hypochlorite; phenols	Corrosive; toxic	One-half cup borax in 1 gallon of water
Drain openers	Sodium hypochlorite; sodium or potassium hydroxide	Corrosive; toxic	Plunger; flush with boiling water and one-quarter cup baking soda
Flea repellants	Carbamates; organophosphate; pyrethrins	Toxic	Eucalyptus leaves where pet sleeps; brewer's yeast in diet
Floor and furniture polishes	Diethylene glycol; petroleum distillates; nitrobenzene	Flammable; toxic	One part lemon juice with two parts olive or vegetable oil
Furniture strippers	Acetone; methyl ethyl ketone; toluene; xylenes	Flammable; toxic	Sandpaper
Latex paints	Resins; glycol; ethers; esters	Flammable	Limestone-based white wash or casein-based paint
Oil-based paints	Ethylene; aliphathydrocarbons; petroleum distillates	Flammable; toxic	Latex- or water-based paints
Oven cleaners	Potassium or sodium hydroxide; ammonia; lye	Corrosive; toxic	Baking soda and water; salt on spills that are still warm
Photographic chemicals	Silver; acetic acid; ferrocyanide; hydro quinone	Corrosive; toxic; irritating	Unknown. (Use caution; take to collection center.)
Pool chemicals	Muriatic acid; sodium hypochlorite algicide	Corrosive; toxic	Unknown. (Use caution; use until gone and take container to a collection center.)
Rat and mouse killers	Lead arsenate; coumarin (warfarin); strychnine	Toxic	Remove food and water sources; clear garbage; cover holes and drains where rats may enter; use mechanical traps; get a cat.
Roach and ant killers	Organophosphates; carbamates	Toxic	Roaches: traps; boric acid; ants: chili pepper and cream of tartar in ants' path
Rug and upholstery cleaners	Naphthalene; oxalic acid; diethylene glycol	Irritating; toxic; corrosive	Dry cornstarch sprinkled on rug and then vacuumed up
Toilet bowl cleaners	Muriatic or oxalic paradichlorobenzene; calcium hypochlorite	Irritating; toxic; corrosive	Toilet brush and baking soda; mild detergent
Thinners and turpentines	N-butyl alcohol; isobutyl ketone; petroleum distillates	Flammable	Use water with water-based paints
Transmission fluids	Hydrocarbons; mineral spirits	Flammable; toxic	Unknown. (Take to a collection center.)
Used oils	Hydrocarbons (e.g. benzene); heavy metals	Flammable; toxic	Unknown; recycle. *Note:* It is illegal to dispose of oil on or in the ground.

From: Phoenix Arizona, Phoenix at Your Fingertips, 1997.

References

American Health Consultants. (2001). JCAHO president calls for bioterror preparedness. *Hospital Peer Review, 26*(12), 165-166.

Arnon, S. S., Schechter, R., Inglesby, T. V., et al. (2001). Botulinum toxin as a biological weapon. *JAMA, 285*(8), 1059-1070.

Broussard, L. A. (2001). Biological agents: Weapons of warfare and bioterrorism. *Molecular Diagnosis, 6*(4), 323-333.

Burgess, J. L., Keifer, M. C., Barnhart, S., Richardson, M., & Robertson, W. O. (1997). Hazardous materials exposure information service: Development, analysis, and medical implications. *Annals of Emergency Medicine, 29*(2), 248-254.

Claman, F. L. & Patterson, D. L. (1995). Personal aerosol protection devices. Caring for the victims of exposure. *Nurse Practitioner, 20*(11), 52-58.

Cox, R. D. (1994). Decontamination and management of hazardous materials exposure victims in the emergency department. *Annals of Emergency Medicine, 23*(4), 761-770.

Cyr, J. C. (1988). Case review: Multivictim emergency care: A case study of organophosphate poisoning in sixty-seven children. *Journal of Emergency Nursing, 14*(5), 277-279.

Dennis, D. T., Inglesby, T. V., Henderson, D. A., et al. (2001). Tularemia as a biological weapon. *JAMA, 285*(21) 2763-2773.

Emergency Management Institute. (1992). Hazardous materials workshop for EMS providers. Washington, DC: U.S. Government Publication.

Federal Emergency Management Agency. (2000). *Emergency responses to terrorism, Job aid.* Available: http://www.usfa.fema.gov/usfapubs.

Ferazani, L., Fucaloro. A, Hayes, N., & Schroeder, W. (1995). Preparing for a hazardous materials accident. *Journal of Healthcare Protection Management, 12*(1), 111-115.

Gough, A. R. & Markus, K. (1989). Hazardous materials protections in ED practice: Laws and logistics. *Journal of Emergency Nursing, 15*(6), 447-480.

Henderson, D. A., Inglesby, T. V., Bartlett, J. C., et al. (1999). Smallpox as a biological weapon. *JAMA, 281*(22), 2127-2137.

Henretig, F. M., Cieslak, T. J., Madsen, J. M., Eitzen, E. M., & Fleisher, G. R. (2000). The emergency department response to incidents of biological and chemical terrorism. In: *Textbook of Pediatric Emergency Medicine* (4th ed., pp. 1763-1784), Lippincott Williams & Wilkins, Philadelphia, 2000.

Inglesby, T. V, Henderson, D. A., Bartlett, J. G., et al. (1999). Anthrax as a biological weapon. *JAMA, 281*(18), 1735-1745.

Inglesby, T. V., Dennis, D. T., Henderson, D. A., et al. (2000). Plague as a biological weapon. *JAMA, 238*(17), 2281-2290.

Kirk, M. A., Cisek, J., & Rose, S. R. (1994). Emergency department response to hazardous materials incidents. *Emergency Medicine Clinics of North America, 12*(2), 461-481.

Kohlmeier, C. A. (1985). Protocols: Acute hazardous material exposure. *Journal of Emergency Nursing, 11*(6), 249-254.

Lamminpaa, A. & Riihimaki, V. (1992). Pesticide-related incidents treated in Finnish hospitals—A review of cases registered over a 5-year period. *Human and Experimental Toxicology, 11*, 473-479.

Leonard, R. B. (1993). Hazardous materials accidents: Initial scene assessment and patient care. *Aviation, Space, and Environmental Medicine*, June 1993, 546-551.

Levitin H. W. & Siegelson, H. J. (1996). Hazardous materials, disaster medical planning and response. *Emergency Medicine Clinics of North America, 14*(2), 317-348.

Likosky, D. (2001). Methanol. *Medicine Journal, 2*(1). Available: http://www.emedicine.com/neuro/topic217.htm.

Lipscomb, J. W., Kramer, J. E., & Leikin, J. B., (1992). Seizure following brief exposure to the insect repellent N, N-Diethyl-m-Toluamide. *Annals of Emergency Medicine, 21*(3), 315-317.

Lynch, A. C. (2001). A chemical decontamination plan for an emergency department. *Journal of Healthcare Protection Management, 17*(2), 55-61.

Maffeo, R. (1996). Gasoline exposure. *American Journal of Nursing, 96*(8), 47.

McLaughlin, S. (2001). Thinking about the unthinkable. *Health Facilities Management*, July 2001, 26-32.

Merritt, N. L. & Anderson, M. J. (1989). Malathion overdose: When one patient creates a departmental hazard. *Journal of Emergency Nursing, 15*(6), 463-465.

Noeller, T. P. (2001). Biological and chemical terrorism: Recognition and management. *Cleveland Clinic Journal of Medicine, 68*(12), 1001-1013.

O'Neil, K. (1994). Emergency department planning for hazardous materials victims: Getting started. *Journal of Emergency Nursing, 20*, 41-44.

Phoenix Arizona, Phoenix at your fingertips. (1997). *Household hazardous materials.* [Online]. Available: http://www.ci.phoenix.az.us/fire/hsehazrd.html.

Plante, D. M. & Walker, J. S. (1989). EMS response at a hazardous material incident: Some basic guidelines. *Journal of Emergency Medicine, 7*, 55-66.

Ross, D. & Siddle, B. (1998). Use of force, policies and training recommendations: Based on the medical implications of oleoresin capsicum. Millstadt, Ill: PPCT Management Systems, Inc.

Rothrock, S. C. (1999). *The Pediatric Emergency Pocketbook* (3rd ed.). Winterpark, Florida: Mako Publishing.

Schultz, M, Cisek, J., & Wabeke, R. (1995). Simulated exposure of hospital emergency personnel to solvent vapors and respirable dust during decontamination of chemically exposed patients. *Annals of Emergency Medicine, 26*(3), 324-329.

Segal, E. & Lang, E. (2001). Toxicity, chlorine gas. *Emedicine Journal, 2*(5). Available: http://www.emedicine.com/emerg/topic851.htm.

U.S. Department of Transportation. (2001). *Department of Transportation Office of Hazardous Materials.* [Online]. Available: http://hazmat.dot.gov

U.S. Environmental Protection Agency. (1997a). *Pesticides and child safety.* [Online]. Available: http://www.epa.gov/opp00001/citizens/childsaf.html.

U.S. Environmental Protection Agency. (2001). *Pesticides and child safety.* [Online] 12/2001. http://www.epa.gov/pesticides/citizens/childsaf.htm.

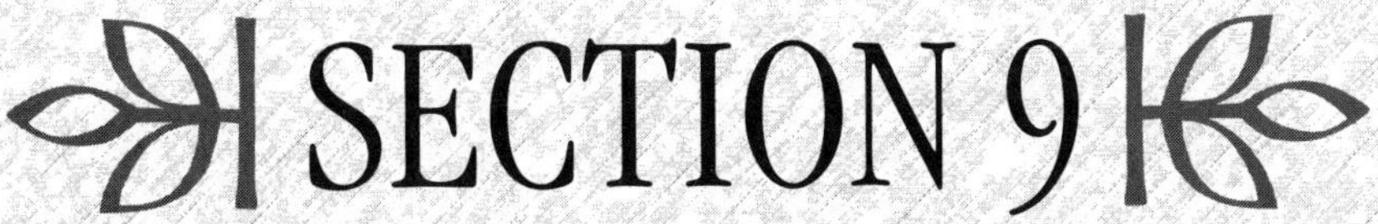

Psychosocial Emergencies

46

Child Abuse and Neglect

Susan J. Kelley, RN, PhD, FAAN

Introduction

Child maltreatment (CM), a serious social and public health problem, is frequently encountered by emergency nurses. The severity of CM ranges from emotional neglect to child fatalities. Emergency nurses play a critical role in the identification, treatment, and prevention of CM.

Child maltreatment generally is grouped into four major categories: neglect, physical abuse, sexual abuse, and psychological maltreatment (Table 46.1). Although the behaviors that characterize these forms of maltreatment are distinct from each other, it is important to note that these different types of abuse often co-occur. The purpose of this chapter is to discuss the recognition and treatment of children suffering from child neglect and physical abuse; Chapter 47 discusses child sexual abuse.

Etiology and Epidemiology

According to the *Fifty-State Survey* conducted by Prevent Child Abuse America, 3,244,000 children were reported to child protective services (CPS) in 1999 as alleged victims of child maltreatment, a rate of 46 of every 1,000 in the population (Peddle & Wang, 2001). Approximately 1,070,000 were substantiated as victims of child maltreatment, a rate of 15 per 1,000 children. Almost half (46%) of all cases of substantiated child maltreatment involved children who were victims of neglect, while 18% experienced physical abuse, 9% were sexually abused, and 4% were victims of emotional abuse and domestic violence. Almost one-quarter (23%) of the children were reported to be victims of multiple forms of child maltreatment.

In 1999, an estimated 1,396 children died as a result of child maltreatment, nearly four children per day. Children under five years account for 80% of child fatalities, with children under one year accounting for 40% of those deaths.

Focused History

The child and parent are interviewed separately to determine if there are any discrepancies between the parents' and the child's accounts of the injury or the living conditions. When interviewed alone, the child is more likely to accurately report the cause of the injury and the identity of the abuser. If more than one caretaker is present, interviewing each separately may reveal discrepancies in offered explanations.

- Family risk factors and history associated with child abuse and neglect:
  - Social isolation; lack of family support
  - Loneliness
  - Maternal history of experiencing domestic violence
  - Substance abuse (Kelley, 2002).
  - Poverty (major single risk factor for failure to thrive)
  - Economic pressures and other stressors
  - Crowded or inadequate housing
- Parental risk factors or history associated with child abuse and neglect:
  - Low self-esteem
  - Social isolation
  - Reliance on physical punishment for discipline
  - Lack of knowledge of normal growth and development, leading to unrealistic expectations of children
  - Role reversal
  - Childhood history of abuse
  - Depression

TABLE 46.1 Categories of Child Maltreatment

Category	*Definition*	*Description*
Neglect	Failure to meet a child's basic needs, including food, shelter, clothing, health care, education, and a safe environment	Includes acts of omission rather than commission, as in the case of physical abuse May or may not be intentional Also includes failure-to-thrive syndrome, where an infant or child is inadequately nourished, leading to poor growth and development
Physical abuse	Physical injury to a child inflicted by a parent or caretaker through excessive and inappropriate physical force	Typically episodic and often the result of "corporal punishment" Factitious disorder by proxy (Munchausen syndrome by proxy) is an unusual yet very serious form of physical abuse in which a caregiver, typically a mother, induces illness in a child
Sexual abuse	Any sexual contact between a child and adult (or considerably older child) whether by physical force, persuasion, or coercion Includes noncontact acts, such as exhibitionism, sexually explicit language, showing children sexually explicit materials, and voyeurism	(Chapter 47)
Psychological maltreatment	Parental or caregiver behaviors that are cruel, degrading, terrorizing, isolating, or rejecting	Can occur independently and is almost always embedded within or accompanying other forms of maltreatment (Hart, Binggeli, & Brassard, 1998) One of the most difficult types of CM to document and particularly difficult to determine in an emergency department setting where contacts with families are generally brief

  - Substance abuse
- Child risk factors and history associated with child abuse and neglect (Kelley, 2002):
  - Prematurity
  - Prenatal drug exposure
  - Developmental disability
  - Physical disability
  - Chronic illness
  - Product of a multiple birth

Focused Assessment

Physical Assessment

1. Assess the respiratory system.
   - Auscultate the chest for:
     - Respiratory rate. Tachypnea may be present in the child with respiratory distress; bradypnea may be present in the child with shock.
   - Observe the chest for:
     - Bruises.
     - Paradoxical movement. Blunt force trauma to the chest may have occurred.
2. Assess the cardiovascular system.
   - Auscultate the heart for:
     - Rate. Tachycardia may be present in early shock or dehydration; bradycardia may be present with late shock.
   - Measure the blood pressure:
     - Hypotension may be seen in late shock.
   - Palpate peripheral pulses for:
     - Equality.

- Quality.

3. Assess the neurological system.
   - Assess the child's level of consciousness with the AVPU method (Alert, responds to Verbal stimuli, responds to Painful stimuli, Unresponsive) or GCS (Glasgow coma scale) method.
     - A decreased level of consciousness may indicate shock, head injury, or ingestion of toxins.
4. Assess the integumentary system.
   - Assess for alterations in skin integrity.
   - Note the presence of:
     - Bruises—location, age.
     - Scars—location, pattern. Any geometric pattern is unlikely to be unintentional.
5. Assess the child's overall hygiene and appearance.
   - Assess for appropriate clothing according to season.
   - Note personal and dental hygiene.
     - Lack of personal and oral hygiene may be an indicator of neglect.

Psychosocial Assessment

- Assess the child's and family's interaction patterns.
- Assess the family's involvement with CPS.
  - Parents may volunteer this history.
  - The local CPS office may be contacted.
- Assess the family's socioeconomic status:
  - Level of income.
  - Source of income.
  - Level of education.
  - Housing.
- Assess the family's composition:
  - Availability of social support.
  - Family strengths and weaknesses.
  - History of parental substance abuse.

A list of nursing diagnoses and expected outcomes is in Table 46.2.

Triage Decisions

Emergent

- Severe dehydration or malnutrition leading to shock
- Life-threatening injury
- Unstable vital signs
- Impaired airway, breathing, or circulation

Urgent

- Dehydration requiring fluid replacement
- Skeletal fractures without circulatory impairment
- Minor burns
- Parents or caregivers who are likely to leave the emergency department prior to treatment

Nonurgent

- Absence of life-threatening health conditions
- Parents or caregivers who are reliable and not likely to leave the emergency department

TABLE 46.2 Nursing Diagnoses and Expected Outcomes

Nursing Diagnoses	*Expected Outcomes*
Ineffective individual coping (parent)	▪ Parent identifies available social support. ▪ Parent verbalizes willingness to attend parenting support group. ▪ Parent verbalizes frustrations regarding parenting.
Altered growth and development	▪ Parent verbalizes understanding of strategies to promote physical and emotional growth. ▪ Parent is referred to primary care provided for follow-up.
Altered parenting	▪ Parent verbalizes understanding of risk of harm to child through use of corporal punishment. ▪ Parent verbalizes alternatives for discipline. ▪ Parent verbalizes understanding of behaviors needed to eliminate neglect.

Nursing Interventions

1. Assess and maintain airway, breathing and circulation as needed in cases of life-threatening trauma (Chapter 30).
2. Initiate measures to diagnose and treat injuries, as outlined in the trauma-specific chapters (Chapters 31–40).
3. Prepare for diagnostic procedures.
4. Provide psychosocial support.
   - Establish a rapport with the family.
   - Convey genuine concern and understanding.
   - Use a nonjudgmental, noncritical approach.
     - Judgmental attitudes hinder communication and limit information.
     - Acknowledge the demands of parenting.
     - Discuss alternatives to corporal punishment.
     - Focus on the health and well-being of the child.
     - Encourage parents to discuss their feelings about the child's maltreatment; such feelings may include anger, grief, or guilt.
5. Document the history and observed injuries.
   - All statements made by the child and parents are written in quotation marks.
   - The time of all statements is documented, in case the history changes over time.
   - The injuries are documented for their size, shape, color, and location.
6. Photodocument all injuries.
   - Use a hospital photographer for reliable and professional photographs.
   - If a photographer is not available, use a high-quality 35-mm camera or an instant camera that is kept in the emergency department.
   - Document the child's name, birthdate, and medical record number; include a ruler in the photo, as well as a standard color chart.
7. Report suspected child abuse and neglect to CPS and hospital protection team (if available).
   - Every state has a law requiring the reporting of suspected child maltreatment to designated child protection or law enforcement authorities. Although anyone in any state may report a suspicion of child abuse, reporting laws usually mandate reporting only for professionals who have regular contact with children (Myers, 2002). In each of the 50 states, nurses are mandated reporters.
   - Mandated reporters do *not* need to have actual knowledge of child abuse or neglect.
   - Reporting requirements provide that a report must be made if the mandated reporter suspects or has reason to believe that a child has been abused or neglected (Myers, 2002); the nurse does not need to "know for sure" that abuse or neglect occurred. A professional who postpones reporting until all doubt is eliminated probably violates the reporting law (Myers, 2002).
   - Reporting laws deliberately leave the ultimate decision about whether abuse or neglect occurred to investigating officials, not to mandated reporters (Myers, 2002).
   - Emergency nurses reporting CM in good faith are typically immune from civil or criminal liability, while nurses who knowingly or intentionally fail to report suspected abuse or neglect are subject to civil or criminal liability. Some states impose criminal liability even if the mandated reporter did not realize the child was abused when a reasonable professional would have suspected abuse (Meyers, 2002). Deliberate failure to report suspected abuse is a crime (Myers, 2002).
   - An emergency nurse, physician, or social worker should inform the parents of this report. It should be stressed that the report is a legal requirement and is not vindictive towards the parents.
   - Parents should be alerted to the possibility they will be contacted by CPS and that a home visit is likely to occur. They should also be informed that this is a referral for services, and not a criminal complaint.
   - Arrangements should be made with hospital security or local law enforcement agencies should the ED staff suspect that a parent will elope from the ED with the child.
8. Prepare for the child's transfer and transport to a tertiary care center, hospitalization, or discharge to CPS.
   - Immediate removal of the child from the abusive home is necessary when there is imminent danger to the child's safety.
9. Refer the family to other health care professionals, as necessary.
   - Primary care provider for follow-up assessment and services.
   - Social worker for information on community resources.
   - Support groups for parenting and child care.
   - Public health or community health nursing services.
   - Public assistance programs, such as WIC (Women, Infants, and Children).

Specific Child Maltreatment Emergencies

Child Neglect

Neglect, the most prevalent form of child maltreatment, receives considerably less attention than other forms of child maltreatment (Erickson & Egeland, 2002). Physical neglect tends to be chronic, while physical abuse is typically episodic. In addition to physical neglect, a child may be subjected to emotional, medical, or educational neglect.

Parents suspected of neglect often have inadequate financial resources, lower educational attainment, lack of parenting skills, and poor problem-solving skills. Neglect may also be manifested in failure-to-thrive (FTT) syndrome, a diagnostic term used to describe a lack of growth according to expected norms for age and gender, which typically occurs in the first 2 years of life (Frank, Drotar, Cook, Bleiker, & Kasper, 2001).

Focused History

Family and social history

- Unsafe or unsanitary housing conditions
- Poverty
- Lack of supervision of child, resulting in unintentional injuries or poisonings

Patient history

- Inadequate immunization status
- Abandonment
- Educational neglect, such as frequent school absences or truancy
- Unattended medical problems
- Inadequate dietary intake

Focused Assessment

Physical Assessment

1. Specific growth parameters are evaluated.
   - Assess the child's anthropometric measures (weight, height, and head circumference):
     - A child's weight falling below the fifth percentile for age on an anthropometric or growth chart may be at risk for failure-to-thrive syndrome. Underlying medical causes for poor weight gain have to be explored.
   - Assess the child's nutritional status:
     - Children with neglect may be malnourished.
   - Assess the child's hygiene:
     - Inappropriate clothing for the season and poor personal and oral hygiene (such as unattended dental caries) may be observed.
2. Assess for age-appropriate interactions.
   - Note the infant's and child's attentiveness to the environment:
     - Children with a dull, inactive, and excessively passive and fatigued appearance may be neglected. Also, children who are detached or excessively fearful may be neglected.
   - Observe for bald spots on an infant's head:
     - Bald spots may result if the infant is left in a crib for long periods of time.
   - Observe for developmental delays (Chapter 4)
     - A Denver Development Screening Test may be performed to chart the child's development progress.

Psychosocial Assessment

- Assess the child's and family's interaction patterns.
- Assess the family's prior involvement with CPS.
- Assess the family's socioeconomic status.
- Assess the family's composition.

Nursing Interventions

1. Prepare for diagnostic procedures.
2. Provide psychosocial support to the child and family.
3. Utilize careful written and photodocumentation of the child's history and observed neglect.
4. Report cases of suspected neglect to CPS and the hospital child protection team (if available).
5. Refer the family to other health care professionals, as necessary.
6. Provide discharge instructions related to proper child care and community resources.

Home Care and Prevention

Parents may need guidance in exploring community resources available to them for assistance with housing, food, and other basic necessities. Referrals to such agencies may be initiated in the emergency department or at a later date. Educating parents on proper nutritional choices and dental care (Chapter 5) and providing resources to accomplish these recommendations requires patience and the support of other hospital and community resources. Emergency nurses may choose to teach parenting classes to community groups or may choose to be involved in local shelters or homeless clinics to provide counseling to these families.

Physical Abuse

Many cases of child physical abuse are identified in the emergency department when a caregiver seeks treatment for the inflicted injury; however, in some instances, the inflicted injury is identified when the child is being treated for an unrelated illness or injury. For example, an infant's inflicted rib fracture may be diagnosed when a chest radiograph is obtained to rule out pneumonia.

The injuries related to physical abuse may range from a cutaneous lesion to death. In addition to physical injury, a body of literature has documented the psychological damage associated with physical abuse, such as (Kolko, 2002):

- Medical or health problems and psychobiological problems
- Intellectual or academic problems
- Cognitive or perceptual and attributional problems
- Aggression or behavioral dysfunction
- Psychiatric disturbances and posttraumatic stress disorder
- Interpersonal problems

Factitious disorder by proxy (FDBP), also known as Munchausen syndrome by proxy (MSBP), is a rather rare form of physical abuse in which a parent falsifies a child's illness through fabrication or creation of symptoms and then seeks medical care (Rosenberg, 2001) (Table 46.3). Although less common, FDBP may also involve falsification of psychological or developmental symptoms (Ayoub, Deutsch, & Kinscherff, 2000).

Focused History

Family and social history

- Denial of any knowledge of cause or mechanism of injury:
  - Parent reluctant to give information
  - Parent blames sibling for injury
- Delay in seeking medical attention:
  - Abusive parents ignore the seriousness of an injury in the hope that the injury will heal without medical attention, thereby avoiding detection and legal action.
- Inappropriate emotional response to severity of injury.
- Previous placement of a child in foster care.
- Previous involvement with CPS.
- Presence of "crisis" factors at home (e.g., drug or alcohol use).
- Previous history of abuse in the caregiver.
- Family history of sudden infant death syndrome or unexplained deaths.
- Family history of bleeding or bone disorders.

Patient history

- Past health history, including a history of repeated injuries or hospitalizations:
  - Abusive parents often seek medical care at many different treatment facilities to avoid being identified.
  - The child's medical record, when available, may provide documentation of previous suspicious injuries.
- History inconsistent with existing injury or inconsistencies in the provided history—a cardinal finding.
- Child developmentally incapable of specified self injury:
  - Determine if the child is developmentally able to have injured himself or herself in such a manner; suspect child abuse if the child's developmental capabilities do not coincide with the mechanism or severity of injury.
- Acute change in the child's behavior or activity without any provided history (e.g., sudden limp, fussy, swollen arm).

Focused Assessment

Physical Assessment

1. Assess the neurological system.
   - Assess the child's level of consciousness using the AVPU (Alert, responds to Verbal stimuli, responds to Painful stimuli, Unresponsive) method or GCS (Glasgow coma scale) method.
     - Children with an altered level of consciousness may have craniocerebral trauma, most likely a subdural hematoma.
   - Observe the head for swelling or edema of the scalp, lacerations, and other signs of trauma.
     - Inflicted head injuries are the leading cause of death from child abuse. The majority of deaths from head trauma among children younger than two years are the result of maltreatment (Alexander, Levitt, & Smith, 2001).
     - Inflicted head injuries may result from direct trauma, from vigorous shaking or a combination of direct trauma and shaking. Resultant injuries are diagnosed as shaken impact syndrome. Shaken impact syndrome is a unique and prevalent form of intracranial injury that may have no external evidence of head trauma.
     - Shaken impact syndrome results from acceleration-deceleration injuries due to vigorous shak-

TABLE 46.3 Factitious Disorder by Proxy

- Most victims are infants and toddlers (Rosenberg, 2001).
  - School-aged children may be abused in this manner.
  - Older children may aid in the parents' deceptions to protect them or because of an intense fear of retribution by the FDBP parents.
- Mothers are the perpetrators in the vast majority of identified cases of FDBP (Rosenberg, 2001).
  - Frequently, the mother has chronic, poorly defined medical problems.
  - In many instances the mother has trained in one of the healthcare professions and is adept at making falsified information appear credible (Ayoub, Deutsch & Kinscherff, 2000).
  - The mother often appears genuinely and sometimes overconcerned over her child's illness and when the child is hospitalized, rarely leaves the child's bedside.
  - Perpetrator typically continues victimizing the child in the hospital (Rosenberg, 2001).
- Parents may induce physical findings in their children by:
  - Manual suffocation.
  - Administration of drugs or toxic substances or contaminating central lines.
  - Placing their own blood in the child's urine, vomitus, or stool specimens.
- Drugs often used in FDBP include:
  - Laxatives to induce severe diarrhea.
  - Insulin to induce hypoglycemia and seizures.
  - Ipecac to induce vomiting.
  - Drugs or alcohol to cause an alteration in level of consciousness.
  - Salt may be added to an infant's formula to induce hypernatremia.
- Clinical indicators of FDBP are:
  - Recurrent illnesses for which no cause is identified.
  - Unusual symptoms that do not make clinical sense.
  - Symptoms that are observed only by the parent.
  - Frequent visits to various hospitals that result in normal findings.
  - The presence of drugs that induced the symptoms in a toxicology screen.
  - Discrepancies between the history and physical findings.
  - Numerous hospitalizations at many different hospitals.
- Clinical presentations often include (Rosenberg, 2001):
  - Seizures.
  - Apnea.
  - Diarrhea.
  - Vomiting.
  - Bleeding rash.
  - Fever.
  - CNS depression.

ing, which may or may not involve blunt trauma to the head.

- Physical findings in shaken impact syndrome include: retinal hemorrhages, subdural or subarachnoid hemorrhages, cerebral edema, grip marks to chest and upper arms, and fractures of the humeri or ribs.

2. Assess the abdomen.

- Observe the abdomen for bruising or other signs of external trauma:
  - Abdominal injuries are the second leading cause of fatal child abuse.
  - Blunt abdominal trauma, the most common type of inflicted abdominal trauma in children, is usually the result of a child's being punched or kicked in the abdomen (Ludwig, 2001). It

may result in intra abdominal hemorrhage with few external signs of trauma.

- Visceral injuries rarely produce immediately specific signs or symptoms that lead to prompt identification (Ludwig, 2001).
- The high mortality resulting from these injuries may be due to: exsanguinating intra-abdominal hemorrhage, delay in seeking medical attention, or failure of emergency personnel to make the correct diagnosis when lifesaving surgery is needed.
- Severe internal injuries may not be immediately detected because of the parent's failure to give an accurate history of trauma and because there may be little or no external evidence of abdominal trauma at the time of examination.

- Observe for vomiting, guarding, abdominal pain, and signs of cardiovascular failure.
  - Bilious vomiting may be present, suggesting an obstruction.

3. Assess the integumentary system for signs of trauma.
   - Observe for cutaneous lesions:
     - Cutaneous lesions are the most common manifestation of physical abuse and are the most easily recognized sign of abuse.
     - The pattern of a bruise typically reflects the method or instrument used to injure a child.
     - A comparison of intentional versus unintentional bruises is described in Table 46.4.
     - Cutaneous lesions resulting from blunt forces and instruments are described in Table 46.5.
   - Observe for burns.
     - Inflicted burns are involved in approximately 10% of substantiated cases of child abuse and are the third leading cause of death related to child abuse.
     - Ten to 25% of burns in children are deliberately inflicted by adults and are more common in younger children (Jenny, 2001).
     - Children who repeatedly suffer burns should be carefully evaluated for abuse.
     - Suspicion should be raised when treatment for burns is delayed more than 24 hours or when the parent who was not home at the time of the burning seeks health care.
     - Table 46.6 compares unintentional and intentional burn patterns from scalds, contact with hot objects, and cigarettes.
4. Assess the musculoskeletal system.
   - Observe for deformed extremities, indicating long bone fractures:
     - Injuries to bones are more common in abused children younger than 2 years, whereas unintentional fractures occur more commonly among school-aged children.
     - Fractures and dislocations that are inconsistent with the mechanism of injury are highly suspect.
     - Table 46.7 compares fracture types with their probable cause.
   - Observe for pain, tenderness, edema, and inability to use the extremity:
     - In cases of inflicted injury, caretakers often delay seeking medical treatment; therefore, manifestations typically seen in the acute phase of skeletal injury, such as swelling and tenderness, may not be present.
5. Assess the eyes and ocular ability:
   - Perform simple vision screening by having the verbal child count fingers or objects; have the preverbal child or infant follow/track an object.
   - Inflicted eye injuries may leave no external evidence of trauma. Thus, an ophthalmologic exami-

TABLE 46.4 Comparison of Intentional and Unintentional Bruising

Characteristic	*Unintentional*	*Intentional*
Location	Bony prominences (forehead, elbows, knees, and shins) or anterior surfaces	Unusual places or areas usually protected by clothing; multiple bruises; bruises over noncontiguous areas
Color	Uniform color, indicating a singular time of injury	Multiple colors, indicating varying stages of healing with multiple episodes of injury
Shape	Uniform shape, such as a skinned knee or a scratch on the arm	Varying configurations and shapes

Data from: Elvik, 1998.

TABLE 46.5 Cutaneous Lesions Resulting from Intentional Injury

Method of Injury	*Resulting Cutaneous Lesions*
Doubled-over extension or lamp cords	Characteristic loop-shaped marks are typically found on the back, buttocks, upper arms, and thighs.
Belt, strap, buckle, or stick	These result in linear marks often found over curved body surfaces.
	An imprint of the belt buckle may be noted.
Spoon, paddle, spatula, or hairbrush	These implements result in oval or other shaped marks.
Hand	Characteristic parallel linear marks may be noted, representing the spaces between the fingers.
Coat hanger	Hangers leave a wider loop mark caused by the hanger's flat base.
Cords or ropes	Rope "ligature" marks on the ankles, wrist, or torso indicate that a child has been bound.
	Cords or rope used to bind ankles, wrists, and neck leave thin, circumferential bruises; thicker marks may indicate that the child has been tied with sheets.
Clothes or objects to gag infants and young children to stop their crying.	Gag marks leave down-turned lesions at the corners of the mouth.
Human forces:	
▪ Grabbing	▪ Circular or oval marks on the upper arm may be the result of a caregiver forcibly grasping a child and applying pressure to the site.
▪ Hair pulling	▪ Areas of irregular hair loss characterized by broken, uneven hair may result from a child's being pulled by the hair (traction or traumatic alopecia).
▪ Force-feeding	▪ Bleeding under the scalp also may result from hair pulling.
▪ Physical forces:	▪ Injuries to the labial frenulum and lingual frenulum may result from a bottle or spoon being forced into the child's mouth.
▪ Blunt	▪ Teeth may be loosened or knocked out from blunt trauma to the face.
	▪ Oral lacerations also may occur from a direct blow to the face.
Human bites	Marks may resemble a double horseshoe or are an irregular doughnut-shaped mark.
	Bite marks are measured to determine if they were inflicted by an adult or child. (Adult bite marks have a 3-cm or greater distance between the canines.)
	Human bites typically do not leave puncture marks.

nation by indirect light is essential in suspected cases of child abuse.

- Eye injuries that can result from physical abuse include:
  - Periorbital hematomas.
  - Fractures of the orbital or facial bones.
  - Subconjunctival hemorrhage.
  - Dislocated lens.
  - Retinal detachment.
  - Retinal hemorrhage (almost pathognomonic).
  - Hyphema.
  - Corneal abrasion.
  - Optic atrophy.

6. Assess the ears.
   - Observe for evidence of inflicted injuries:
     - Contusions about the external ear.
     - Ecchymoses on the internal surface of the pinna may be the result of boxing the ear and crushing it against the skull or pinching the ear.
     - Battle's sign (the presence of discoloration behind the ear), indicative of a basilar skull fracture (Chapter 31).
   - Perform or assist with an otoscopic examination to detect hemotympanum and perforation of the tympanic membrane, resulting from a direct blow to the ear.

TABLE 46.6 Comparisons of Intentional and Unintentional Burn Injuries

Burn Etiology	*Intentional*	*Unintentional*
Scalds: ■ Immersion injuries—occur when the child is forcibly held in the hot water for a prolonged period of time, such as a few minutes	■ Tend to be full thickness. The presence of clothing tends to cause more severe burns because there is longer contact between the hot water and the skin. Initially the clothing is protective; the extent of the burn depends on the duration of exposure to the hot liquid.	Tend to be partial thickness
	■ Typically uniform in depth	Uneven in depth
	■ Symmetrical	Asymmetrical
	■ Have sharp lines of demarcation	Usually not as clearly demarcated on the edges
	■ Often involve bilateral burns of the feet, hands, and buttocks	May be unilateral; if bilateral, burn depth is not deep
	■ Usually spare flexion creases because the child flexes the extremities in the hot water	May not be deep or extensive
	■ Often appear "sock-shaped" on the feet, "glove-shaped" on the hands, and "doughnut-shaped" on the buttocks ■ Doughnut-shaped burns occur when a child is forcibly held down in water with the buttocks flat against the bathtub. The unburned area ("donut-hole") is the result of the buttocks being forcibly held down against the bottom of the tub and thus, that area, being spared prolonged contact with the hot water.	Are not extensive or severe and do not depict the configuration of the hot object
Oral burns	May occur from excessively hot food or fluids placed in the child's mouth	
Intentional pour burns	Usually on the back; usually don't have a splash pattern	
Contact burns	Depict the patterned configuration of a heating object including: ■ Steam irons ■ Electric stove burners ■ Hot plates ■ Forks ■ Knives ■ Radiators (Toddlers being toilet trained may be placed on radiators to dry their wet diapers, resulting in burns to the buttocks.) ■ Hair dryers ■ Candles ■ Curling irons ■ Car cigarette lighters ■ Cigarette lighters	
Cigarette burns	Occur from deliberate attempts to burn the child	May occur when sudden movement causes momentary contact with a lighted cigarette
	Found on the soles of the feet, palms of the hands, buttocks, or back	Typically occur about the face when a child walks into a lighted cigarette held by an adult at waist height
	Well circumscribed; typically 6 to 8 mm in diameter and indurated at the margins	Usually shallower, more irregular, and less circumscribed than deliberately inflicted ones

TABLE 46.7 Comparison of Fracture Type and Probable Cause

Type of Fracture	*Probable Cause*
Spiral fracture of long bones	Intentional twisting of the extremity; spiral fractures of the humerus are particularly suspicious; femoral fractures in infants and toddlers are often a result of abuse
Rib fractures	Frequently multiple, bilateral, and posterior, often reflecting a squeezing of the chest.
Skull, nose, or facial fractures	Frequently the result of abuse
Fractures to the sternum, spinous processes, scapulae; humeral fractures in children less than 3 years of age	Result of intense blunt forces
Femur fractures in children younger than 1 year of age (nonambulatory)	Frequently the result of abuse
Fractures of the epiphyseal-metaphyseal junction; transverse fractures	Result of abuse
Multiple fractures of different ages	Result of abuse

Psychosocial Assessment

- Assess the child's and family's interaction patterns.
- Assess the family's prior involvement with CPS.
- Assess the family's composition.
- Consult with the child's primary care provider to determine if there have been prior episodes of suspicious behaviors or injuries.
- Evaluate the risk for subsequent injury if the child is discharged home from the emergency department.
- Ascertain the availability of social support systems.

Nursing Interventions

1. Assess and maintain airway, breathing, and circulation (Chapter 30)
2. Obtain specific diagnostic tests to determine the extent of the injuries, to find a medical cause for the injury, and to determine if prior injuries have occurred.
    - Obtain radiographs of the injured extremity to identify previous fractures:
        - Multiple fractures, especially bilateral, in various stages of healing indicate repeated abuse.
        - The possibility that multiple fractures are related to an underlying disease, such as osteogenesis imperfecta, scurvy, syphilis, rickets, neoplasia, or osteomyelitis should be considered. The presence of these rare disorders can be ruled out by appropriate diagnostic procedures.
    - Obtain a skeletal survey in children younger than 2 years of age in whom abuse is suspected (Elvik, 1998).
    - Obtain coagulation studies to rule out blood dyscrasias for multiple bruises (Elvik, 1998).
    - Obtain skull radiographs and computerized tomography scans to determine the presence of bilateral skull fractures, multiple skull fractures, skull fractures with widths greater than 5 mm, subdural hematomas, separation of sutures arising from chronic subdural hematoma.
    - Obtain cervical spine radiographs to detect subluxation or dislocation; anticipate SCIWORA injury (Chapter 32).
3. Provide psychosocial support.
4. Utilize careful written and photodocumentation of the child's history and observed injuries.
5. Report cases of suspected abuse to CPS and the hospital child protection team (if available).
6. Refer the family to other health care professionals as necessary.
7. Prepare for transfer or transport to a tertiary care center, hospitalization, or discharge to CPS.

Home Care and Prevention

Emergency nurses should make opportunities to provide information related to prevention of child abuse and neglect to all families. This can be accomplished by providing printed materials and information on seeking support on parenting issues. Nurses can locate local chapters of Parents Anonymous, a self-help organization for abusive and neglectful parents, and identify parental stress telephone hotlines. In addition, ED nurses routinely can provide information to parents on normal child growth and development.

Nurses may also help to prevent abuse and neglect by helping families to identify sources of social support, home health nurses, parenting classes, and home visitation programs (e.g., Healthy Families America, an initiative of the National Committee to Prevent Child Abuse). Families should be referred to community resources.

Conclusion

Child maltreatment is a disease that can be prevented. Astute observations of child and family dynamics, understanding of the causes of intentional and unintentional injury, and prompt recognition of serious injury help emergency nurses to decrease this disease's associated morbidity. Emergency nurses are mandated by law to report suspected abuse and neglect. Collaborating with the hospital's child protection team is one strategy that emergency nurses can use to facilitate the care of children in their hospital.

References

Alexander, R. C., Levitt, C. J., & Smith, W. L. (2001). Abusive head trauma. In R. M. Reece & S. Ludwig (Eds.), *Child abuse: Medical diagnosis and management* (2nd ed., pp. 47–80). Philadelphia: Lippincott Williams & Wilkins.

Ayoub, C. C., Deutsch, R. M., & Kinscherff, R. (2000). Muschausen by proxy: Definitions, identification, and evaluation. In R. M. Reece (Ed.), *Treatment of child abuse: Common ground for mental health, medical, and legal practitioners* (pp. 213–225). Baltimore: The John Hopkins University Press.

Elvik, S. (1998). Child maltreatment. In T. Soud & J. Rogers (Eds.), *Manual of pediatric emergency nursing* (p. 486–605). St. Louis: Mosby—Year Book.

Erickson, M. F., & Egeland, B. (2002). Child neglect. In J. E. B. Myers, L. Berliner, J. Briere, C. T. Hendrix, C. Jenny, & T. A. Reid (Eds.), *The ASPAC handbook on child maltreatment* (2nd ed., pp. 3–20). Thousand Oaks, CA: Sage Publications.

Fountain, K. & Pierce, B. (1998). Child abuse and neglect. In L. Newberry (Ed.), *Sheehy's Emergency nursing principles and practice* (4th ed., pp. 743–753). St. Louis: Mosby—Year Book.

Frank, D. A., Drotar, D., Cook, J., Bleiker, J., & Kasper, D. (2001). Failure to thrive. In R. M. Reece & S. Ludwig (Eds.), *Child abuse: Medical diagnosis and management* (2nd ed., pp. 307–337). Philadelphia: Lippincott Williams & Wilkins.

Hart, S. N., Binggeli, N., & Brassard, M. (1998). Evidence for the effects of psychological maltreatment. *Journal of Emotional Abuse*, 1, 27–58.

Jenny, C. (2001). Cutaneous manifestations of child abuse. In R. M. Reece & S. Ludwig (Eds.), *Child abuse: Medical diagnosis and management* (2nd ed., pp. 23–45). Philadelphia: Lippincott Williams & Wilkins.

Kelley, S. J. (2002). Child maltreatment in the context of substance abuse. In J. E. B. Myers, L. Berliner, J. Briere, C. T. Hendrix, C. Jenny, & T. A. Reid (Eds.). *The APSAC handbook on child maltreatment* (2nd ed., pp. 105-117). Thousand Oaks, CA: Sage Publications.

Kolko, D. J. (2002). Child physical abuse. In J. E. B. Myers, L. Berliner, J. Briere, C. T. Hendrix, C. Jenny, & T. A. Reid (Eds.), *The APSAC handbook on child maltreatment* (2nd ed., pp. 21–54). Thousand Oaks, CA: Sage Publications.

Ludwig, S. (2001). Visceral injury manifestations of child abuse. In R. M. Reece & S. Ludwig (Eds.), *Child abuse: Medical diagnosis and management* (2nd ed., pp. 157–175). Philadelphia: Lippincott Williams & Wilkins.

Myers, J. E. B. (2002). The legal system and child protections. In J. E. B. Myers, L. Berliner, J. Briere, C. T. Hendrix, C. Jenny, & T. A. Reid (Eds.), *The APSAC handbook on child maltreatment* (2nd ed., pp. 305–327). Thousand Oaks, CA: Sage Publications.

Peddle, N. & Wang, C. (2001). *Current trends in child abuse prevention, reporting, and fatalities: The 1999 fifty-state survey.* Chicago: Prevent Child Abuse America.

Rosenberg, D. A. (2001). Munchausen syndrome by proxy. In R. M. Reece & S. Ludwig (Eds.), *Child abuse: Medical diagnosis and management* (2nd ed., pp. 363–383). Philadelphia: Lippincott Williams & Wilkins.

47

Child Sexual Abuse

Marilyn K. Johnson, RN

Introduction

Child sexual abuse was first recognized as a common problem in the 1980s. As public awareness and reporting of suspected abuse has increased, so have requests to evaluate children for possible sexual abuse (Finkel & DeJong, 2001). There is no universal definition for child sexual abuse. Most definitions cover a wide range of sexual activities including situations in which there is no physical contact. Child sexual abuse is often defined as the involvement of children or adolescents in sexual activities they do not understand, to which they cannot give informed consent, or that violate social taboos (Finkel & DeJong, 2001). The legal definition can vary slightly from state to state.

In 1997, 3.1 million children were reported for child abuse and neglect to child protective services in the United States. Of these, 1,054,000 (8%) were confirmed for sexual abuse (Wang & Daro, 1998). Approximately 20% of girls and 9% of boys experience sexual abuse before reaching 18 years of age. Girls were sexually abused three times more often than boys, according to the 1996 National Incidence Study (NIS) conducted by the federal government (Sedlak & Broadhurst, 1996).

The true incidence of sexual abuse is unknown. There is a recent documented upward trend in number of reports. The National Center on Child Abuse/Neglect estimates that the current annual incidence of sexual abuse is between 75,000 and 250,000 cases per year (Ludwig, 2000). Most estimates do not include child prostitution and those children who are victims of pornographic exploitation.

Child sexual abuse is complex and not merely the act of sexual intercourse. Sexual abuse describes a range of behaviors including (Reece, 2000):

- Sexual touching.
- Forced masturbation.
- Digital or object penetration.
- Exposing a child to exhibitionism or other forms of sexual behavior.
- Using a child in the production of pornography.

Adults are not the only perpetrators of sexual abuse. Adolescents are perpetrators in at least 20% of all sexual abuse cases (some surveys state up to 50%). Preadolescents make up an additional 5 to 10%. Many abusers are successfully employed, active in community affairs, and do not have prior criminal records (Finkel & DeJong, 2001). Child abuse is often generational unless discovered and stopped. Many perpetrators are adults who were molested as children. An incident of abuse will most likely have an impact on not just that particular victim but on a multitude of others. Perpetrators often commit many crimes against multiple victims before being caught. The incest perpetrator may have fewer victims but more incidents of abuse, while the out-of-home perpetrator has more victims but fewer instances with each victim (Becker, 1994).

Small children may imitate behaviors they have seen (or had perpetrated on themselves). This should not be confused with normal age-related sexual curiosity and self-stimulating behaviors. Typically children do not act out explicit details of the sexual act or perform intrusive acts on others unless they have sexual knowledge beyond their normal age-related development. When a concern exists about these behaviors, a physical examination should be done by a pediatric healthcare provider with expertise in this area.

Sexual abuse of children is a crime in every state in the United States, although specific laws pertaining to sexual abuse vary from one jurisdiction to another (Kelley, 1994). Emergency department (ED) nurses need to be knowledgeable as to the laws of their own jurisdiction pertaining to sexual abuse. If sexual abuse is suspected, the nurse is required by law to report to the appropriate agency.

Focused History

Children can be groomed by a perpetrator for increasing sexual involvement over a period of time. It is a secret between the perpetrator and the child, accompanied with threats of harm or coercion for a special favor. The child is confused because the activity may "feel good." Children don't know the exact physical act of intercourse unless they have been taught. They may state that "he put it inside" even though only intra labial intercourse may have occurred without any penetration into the vaginal opening. The child may report getting "peed on" or that they "got wet with sticky stuff."

Getting a history from an adult is standard procedure. It is equally as important to obtain a history from any child capable of talking (Finkel & DeJong, 2001). Guidelines when obtaining a history include:

- Interview the caregiver and the child separately. Allowing the child to hear the caregiver may influence the child's response and affect the legal process. The child may not be comfortable sharing details of the abuse with the caregiver in the room.
- Direct communication to the child on his or her developmental and emotional level. This develops trust and cooperation between the child and the healthcare professional. If the examiner is unhurried, nonjudgmental, and empathetic, the child will be more likely to view the clinician as understanding and will therefore be more likely to share both the details of the events and the accompanying affective associations. While talking, the child also observes the interviewer's reaction to what he or she says. If the interviewer appears uncomfortable listening or insensitive to the child's needs, the child may stop talking. It is critical that the interviewer be nonjudgmental and facilitating without being leading (Finkel & DeJong, 2001).
- Use only open-ended questions such as: "Can you tell me why you are here?" (It is vital for the legal case that no ideas are placed into the child's mind.)
- Document all statements by the child about the abuse with quotations preceded by the question that elicited response.
- Document all explanations of the incident given by caregivers. A complete medical history from caregivers is imperative for the medical staff to understand findings on the physical exam.
- Document any syndromes or medical conditions (e.g., Crohn's disease, lichen et atrophicus) plus any surgical interventions, especially in the genital or anal areas (e.g., female circumcision).
- Reassure the child that what happened is not his or her fault.

Focused Assessment

Physical Assessment

The examination includes a standard head-to-toe assessment with all parts of the body being examined. Very young children may do best being examined in the caregiver's lap. Two positions are recommended when examining the genitalia of young girls. One is the frog-leg position and the other is the knee-chest position. (The child lies prone on the exam table with knees tucked under the thorax) (Ludwig, 2000).

Examination findings may be categorized as (Finkel, 2000):

- Medical findings that confirm the allegations with medical certainty.
- Nonspecific findings that can be related to specific events by history or other investigative details.
- Findings that are nonspecific and are seen in both abused and nonabused children.
- Findings that have no relevance to the allegations.

When a child is brought to the emergency department, sexual abuse may not be identified as the chief complaint. The ED nurse must be aware of symptoms or behavior relating to abuse. Some symptoms are specific for the identification of abuse, while others may be from other causes as well as from sexual abuse. These complaints can be either physical or behavioral (Ludwig, 2000):

- Physical complaints or findings specific to sexual abuse:
  - Genital injury
  - Bruises
  - Lacerations
  - Rectal laceration, fissures
  - Sexually transmitted disease
  - Pregnancy
- Physical complaints and findings nonspecific to sexual abuse:
  - Anorexia
  - Abdominal pain
  - Enuresis
  - Dysuria
  - Encopresis
  - Evidence of physical abuse in genital area
  - Vaginal discharge
  - Urethral discharge
  - Rectal pain
- Behavioral complaints or findings specific to sexual abuse:
  - Explicit descriptions of sexual contact

- Inappropriate knowledge of adult sexual behavior
- Compulsive masturbation
- Excessive sexual curiosity, sexual acting out
- Behavioral complaints or findings nonspecific to sexual assault:
  - Excessive fears, phobias
  - Refusal to sleep alone, nightmares
  - Runaways
  - Aggressive behavior
  - Attempted suicide
  - Any abrupt change in behavior

Often sexual abuse does not result in physical injury. Therefore, often there are no physical findings on the medical exam. The child with pain or bleeding has an increased likelihood of showing physical evidence. Several factors influence the existence of physical findings (Finkel, 2000):

- Injuries to the genitalia are infrequent. The perpetrator usually does not intend to cause physical harm. Also, the perpetrator is frequently someone the child knows and trusts, so force is not needed for the child to comply.
- Healing of the genital area is rapid, because of high vascularity. Most injuries to the genital and anal tissue are superficial and heal completely in 96 hours.
- Most children do not disclose until they feel safe, sometimes long after the last contact. When injuries occur in children, they are generally superficial and heal without posttraumatic residue.
- Many injuries will heal, leaving scars or other findings that do not appear to be reflective of the extent of the original injury.
- Estrogen changes the thin mucosa of the pepubertal hymen and vestibular structures to a thickened, redundant, elastic appearance, thus disguising any findings in the prepubescent hymen.

Psychosocial Assessment

When dealing with a suspected victim of sexual abuse, the nurse needs to convey interest, sincerity, and respect. Forensic investigating agencies (Child Protective Service agency and the police agency) will do the detailed interview. The role of the medical provider is to gather and preserve medical evidence and to identify and care for medical needs. Inquiring about the family norms and any change in the child's behavior can be helpful in the assessment process. For example:

- Sleeping arrangements (e.g., everyone sleeps in the same room with the parents)
- Exposure to nudity or pornography
- Sudden appearance of unusual fears; nightmares
- Runaway or suicidal thoughts or gestures
- Nonorganic pain or illness
- School problems
- Eroticized behavior

A list of nursing diagnoses and their expected outcomes is given in Table 47.1.

Triage Decisions

Emergent

- Strangulation injuries, damaging the airway and causing respiratory compromise
- The use of "date rape" drugs (e.g., Rohypnol), causing respiratory depression
- Excessive uncontrolled bleeding from the genital area or rectum or signs of internal bleeding from blunt trauma, causing hypovolemia and its complications

TABLE 47.1
Nursing Diagnoses and Expected Outcomes

Nursing Diagnosis	*Expected Outcomes*
Self-esteem disturbance	Child receives appropriate counseling to help him or her to understand that he or she is not to blame for abuse.
Powerlessness or fear	Child feels safe in the ED environment because of the appropriate use of explanations and involvement throughout the exam; appropriate counseling will help child to feel in control.
Altered family processes relating to sexual abuse	Family and child will receive appropriate counseling.

Urgent

- Sexual contact reportedly occurring in the past 72 hours. (Prompt evidence collection is vital.)
- Current acute medical problems associated with onset of abuse (e.g., vaginal or rectal bleeding or discharge; severe abdominal pain, lacerations; bruising or other anogenital injuries
- Severe emotional distress of child or caregiver (possible threat to self or others)
- Any child for whom safety is a concern (i.e., when there is concern that the caregiver will not comply with coming to the exam or the perpetrator may have access to the child)

Nonurgent (Evaluation needed within one week)

Medical issues that can be referred for assessment by an expert in pediatric sexual abuse within one week include:

- Sexual contact beyond 72 hours and two weeks (too late for evidence collection)
- Nonacute symptoms, possibly related to abuse (vaginal or rectal discharge, nonacute genital pain, blisters in genital or rectal area, enuresis, encopresis)
- Serious behavioral problems (refusing to attend school, nightmares, extreme fears)
- Danger of upcoming contact with alleged perpetrator (such as through a weekend visit or through school attendance)

Inform child protection services of concerns.

Nonurgent (When an appointment is available, and time is not an issue)

Referral to a medical care provider with expertise in child sexual abuse and colposcopy evaluations is appropriate under the following circumstances:

- There has been no possible contact with alleged perpetrator for past two weeks.
- There is no current medical problems relating to abuse (e.g., no genital bleeding, no vaginal or rectal discharge, no continuing abdominal or genital pain).
- The child is adequately protected from ongoing abuse until the exam can be done.

The ED is often the setting where sexual assault is first evaluated. This occurs for several reasons:

- Law enforcement sends victims to the ED for evaluation and evidence collection.
- Emergent and urgent care is best addressed in the ED setting.
- The ED is always open and available to walk-in patients. When disclosure occurs, the caregiver wants to know immediately what happened and if their child is injured in any way.
- Caregivers bring children to the ED for evaluation not knowing where else to go or what else to do.

The ED may not be the ideal setting for a sexual assault exam because of the time required to:

- Get a history from the caregiver and the child.
- Build trust and prepare the child for the exam.
- Perform the exam itself and collect the necessary evidence.
- Preserve the chain of evidence. Once the evidence collection begins, the nurse must maintain physical possession of the evidence until it is dried, packaged, and sealed.

If the child is triaged to another facility for medical care and there is danger of the caretaker not keeping the appointment, the police and child protective services need to be involved prior to the transfer. An escort for the child and family during transfer may be necessary.

Nursing Interventions

The goals of nursing intervention are to assist with the sexual assault exam according to state rules and regulations. The International Association of Forensic Nurses (IAFN) has published Standards of Practice for Sexual Assault Nurse Examiners. The Association recommends that forensic evaluations be performed by registered nurses with advanced educational and clinical preparation who practice nursing within the community framework of agency policies and procedures, and within the legal framework of a medically supervised protocol (IAFN, 1996).

There are many variables in the assessment and diagnosis of pediatric sexual abuse. The pediatric sexual assault exam is different from the adult exam for the following reasons:

- Psychosocial development: Children should not be expected to have an adult understanding of sexual activities (Finkel, 2000).
- Physical development: Before estrogen stimulation, which begins about menarche, the hymen is thin tissue with translucent edges (Girardin, Faugno, Seneski, Slaughter, & Wheelan, 1998).
- The types of abuse perpetrated on children: The perpetrator usually does not have a desire to harm the child physically. This is one aspect that differentiates sexual abuse from classic rape (Finkel & DeJong, 2001).
- The types of forensic evidence to be collected. In the prepubescent girl only the external genitalia need to be examined. Exams requiring internal exploration or

repair are best done under general anesthesia (Ludwig, 2000).

Emergent or urgent nursing intervention of the sexually abused child include:

- Reporting allegations to the proper authorities.
- Recording a complete medical history.
- Performing a complete physical exam, focusing on evidence of trauma, pregnancy, and sexually transmitted diseases.
- Making an assessment of the victim's psychological status.
- Documenting the evidence of trauma, including photographs of physical findings.

The pediatric sexual assault exam is ideally performed by a pediatric expert trained in both the exam and the collection of evidence.

Sexual Assault Exam Goals

The pediatric sexual assault examiner should to the following:

- Diagnose and treat trauma and infection.
- Recognize and refer emotional trauma.
- Initiate social and emotional healing:
  - Honestly reassure the child that his or her body is healthy (or will heal to be normal and healthy).
  - Refer the child to therapeutic modalities.
- Collect and preserve forensic evidence with chain of evidence, following protocols developed by the reporting agencies involved.
- Involve the appropriate reporting and investigative agencies.
- Prevent further trauma. One of the primary goals in managing a child sexual abuse case is to avoid secondary abuse phenomenon. Secondary abuse is caused by a physical exam that is so overzealous that it assumes a rape-like quality in the mind of the child (Ludwig, 2000).

Sexual Assault Exam Steps

Keeping the abovementioned goals in mind, the nurse should include the following steps in the sexual assault exam:

1. Prepare the child and caregiver.
   - The nurse must first develop a rapport and trust with the child and caregiver. This can be accomplished by:
     - Talking directly to the child.
     - Using words and explanations that are understood by the child and caregiver.
     - Giving the child choices whenever possible.
     - Explaining the exam process and show all of the equipment that may be used in the exam.
     - Not forcing the child to have the exam.
     - Truthfully explaining that if anything hurts during the exam, the child can say "ouch" and the nurse or examiner will stop and try to do it differently.
   - If the exam needs to be completed for forensic and/or medical purposes and the child refuses the exam, anesthesia or conscious sedation is a consideration. The need for anesthesia is generally not necessary if there is adequate preparation and skilled examiners and assistants. Table 47.2 describes helpful hints in performing a sexual abuse exam.
2. The genital examination.
   - Most children have not had a genital exam. Often they are afraid of the unknown and afraid of pain.
   - Continue to give choices as much as possible and remind the child they can say "stop" at any time. This allows the child some control.
     - To assess the genital area of a female, have the prepubescent child assume a frog-leg position. This enables the examiner to visualize the genitalia and allows for the labia to separate somewhat and allows for visualization of the outer genitalia.
     - Apply labial traction while the medical exam is taking place, as this allows for the best visualization of the female genitalia.
     - Colposcopic visualization under a 15-power microscope, helps identify any irregularities of the genitalia. Injury can be detected in 87% of the victims presenting within 48 hours of the assault with colposcopic exams (Groleau & Jackson, 2001). Photographs capture what is seen at the time of evaluation, allowing other experts to evaluate the photo documentation rather than having the child examined a second time. If no colposcope is available, an otoscope generally has 10-power microscopic capability and allows the examiner to identify injury in the absence of a colposcope.
3. Evaluation of the anus.
   - The external anal tissue generally has symmetric, circumferentially radiating folds called rugae.
   - There is much disagreement regarding the interpretation of anal findings. Due to several variables a child may or may not have any physical findings after the insertion of a foreign body into the anus. The variables include (Finkel & DeJong, 2001):
     - Size of the object introduced

TABLE 47.2 Helpful Hints in Performing a Sexual Abuse Examination

Explain all aspects of the evaluation.	Use "soft," nonfrightening words and actions.
Offer the child the option of wearing an exam dress or shirt.	This option allows the child to have some control.
Take the child's blood pressure.	Hug the arm while taking the blood pressure.
Do an ophthalmology exam.	Look for sparkles in the child's eyes.
Explain how cultures are done.	Explain use of "baby cotton" (Q-tip). Dip cotton end into saline; ask permission to touch the back of the child's hand to see if the water is hot or cold to provide assurance that the cotton doesn't injure skin.
Describe the culture medium.	Explain that the medium is a "house" for the baby cotton (Q-tip) to touch or the place where it sleeps.
Prepare the child for labial traction or anal traction.	Hold skin on the child's arm or hand and tell him or her that you will pull the skin to help stretch out the wrinkles on their front and back private parts for the examiner to see all the skin parts.
Reassure and comfort child during the exam.	Have interactive toys available (such as song books, audio tapes with accompanying story book, and *I Spy* books). Provide reassurance that the examiner will stop if anything feels uncomfortable and will try something different. (Follow through is imperative!)
Reassure the child after the exam.	Reassure the child that his or her body is healthy; it is healing or not damaged, and that the child is normal.

- Presence of force
- Use of lubricants
- Degree of cooperativeness from the victim
- Number of episodes of penetration
- Time interval since last contact

- Forty to 50% of victims with a history of anal penetration have abnormalities identified on examination (Finkel & DeJong, 2001). Photo documentation (especially under magnification) is helpful for experts to clarify and diagnose injury.
- Venous pooling (circumferential swelling of the vessels around the anus) can occur normally after traction has been applied to the anus during the exam. Irregular pooling can suggest damage or scarring due to the interruption of venous flow.
- The position of irregularities, lines, or scars is vital information when accompanied by the history of sodomy. A variety of perianal findings are seen in both abused and nonabused children. One example is smooth shaped areas in the midline of the verge, which appear to be a congenital anomaly (Finkel & DeJong, 2001).

Evidence Collection

Emergency departments should have a protocol for a standard sexual abuse laboratory evaluation and collection of specimens. The protocol should specify careful labeling of all specimens and documentation of the chain of evidence. Regardless of differences in protocols there are some standards for evidence collection:

- Two pieces of paper are placed on the floor for the victim to stand on while disrobing. The top paper is carefully folded to maintain any debris that falls from the victim or the clothing. The bottom paper is to prevent contamination from the floor of the top evidence paper and can be discarded.
- The victim undresses carefully, to keep any debris in the clothing. Each piece of clothing is placed in a separate paper bag. (Plastic bags are not breathable, and so clothing placed in plastic bags will mold and be useless for forensic evaluation).
- Evidence samples are collected before culture samples.
- A standard is collected to identify the victim and to differentiate the victim from the perpetrator. This can be done with:
    - Hair samples, 15 to 30 pieces of hair including roots.
    - Saliva, on a swab for DNA testing.
    - Pubic hair, which can be cut after careful combing to remove any debris. (The debris from combing is carefully collected for evidence.)
    - Blood, collected for DNA testing.

- Two swabs are done at the same time whenever possible. (One swab is for the prosecution, and one saved for the defense to evaluate.) The swabs are rotated to ensure uniform distribution of the sample. Swabs must be dry and packaged in cardboard or paper to prevent molding.
- A slide is made from the two swabs before they are dried to be examined for sperm. Nonmotile sperm can be detected up to 3 days in samples from the vaginal pool and up to 7 days in the cervix after coitus (Groleau & Jackson, 2001).
- Laboratory tests that are recommended (Groleau & Jackson, 2001):
  - Gonorrhea cultures are collected from the endocervix as a baseline; other STD cultures are obtained as indicated.
  - If sodomy is reported, a gonorrhea culture is collected from the rectum as a baseline, and other STD cultures are collected as indicated.
- Blood tests for the hospital's lab analysis may include:
  - Pregnancy test
  - Alcohol test
  - Syphilis serology
  - Hepatitis panel
  - Baseline HIV testing
  - Blood and urine toxicology screen

Documentation

A check list may be helpful to ensure that all information is properly documented. Table 47.3 lists elements of documentation to be completed after the sexual assault evaluation.

Medications and Follow-up

- The patient is treated for sexually transmitted diseases if indicated.

TABLE 47.3 Documentation Requirements of the Sexual Assault Examination

Include historical data and description of the suspected abuse in the documentation.	Include date, time, referral source, and person(s) accompanying the child to the medical site. Include: ▪ Names of all individuals involved in the evaluation. ▪ The time that the incident reportedly happened and when child initially disclosed. ▪ Child's statement of the abuse, and what questions the interviewer asked to elicit the disclosure. (Document the words of the child within quotes.) ▪ The emotional state of the child at the time of the disclosure.
Document the physical exam.	Include a thorough explanation and drawings of all findings.
Describe the forensic evidence.	Describe what was collected, observing the chain of evidence and the techniques to preserve samples.
Document all diagnostic tests and treatments.	Describe the baseline cultures and blood tests. List all medications for prophylaxis.
Itemize all required reports and referrals.	▪ Document all reports or attempts to report to state reporting agencies. ▪ Document all referrals for ongoing medical care, mental health services, victim advocacy services, and so on.
Document the discharge instructions.	▪ Keep with the medical record a copy of the verbal and written instructions, with a signature of understanding by the caregiver. ▪ Include the recommendations for follow-up care. ▪ Include the names and phone numbers of community resources.
Include photo documentation.	Negatives and photos should be stored in confidential, secure, and separate areas.
Ensure availability of the documentation.	Ensure the chart is complete and available to legally authorized reporting agencies, as required.

- A contraceptive is offered to the postmenarchal adolescent girl who is seen within 72 hours.
- The CDC recommends repeating STD cultures in two weeks, and serology testing in 12 weeks after the last abuse episode (Finkel & DeJong, 2001).
- Referral to a child abuse specialist for counseling should be done within one or two days after the ED visit.

Home Care and Prevention

Prior to discharge the nurse must ensure that:

- The child is medically and psychologically stable.
- The child will be protected from the alleged perpetrator.
- The child and family have received verbal and written instructions for follow up care with:
  - A healthcare practitioner with expertise in child sexual abuse.
  - A mental health agency.
  - A victim advocacy program.
- Complete reports, as mandated, to state reporting agencies.
- Discharge instructions also need to include the following:
  - Telephone numbers for follow-up calls and questions.
  - Instructions for taking medications, follow up tests (such as for HIV).
  - Community resources for crime victims, reparations, counseling, and therapy.
  - Recommendations for follow-up care.

Conclusion

Child abuse is unfortunately not an uncommon chief complaint in the ED. Children are vulnerable and need protection from anyone who may sexually abuse them. Professionals need to have an understanding of their role in reporting sexual abuse. The nurse plays an important role in preventing the exam process from becoming another abusive experience for the child.

Nurses need to promote prevention of sexual abuse and the research that improves its identification and treatment. The goals are to address the medical needs of victims as well as to collect and preserve evidence. Practitioners and nurses need to be educated regarding the signs and symptoms of sexual abuse and to know when to refer to a pediatric expert in sexual assault exams.

References

Becker, J. V. (1994). Offenders: Characteristics and treatment. *Future Child*, *4*(2), pp. 176–197.

Finkel, M. A. & DeJong, A. R. (2001). Medical findings in child sexual abuse. In R. M. Reece & S. Ludwig (Eds.), *Child abuse medical diagnosis and management* (2nd ed., pp. 207–286). Philadelphia: Lippincott Williams & Wilkins.

Finkel, M. A. (2000). Initial medical management of the sexually abused child. In R. M. Reece (Ed.), *Treatment of child abuse* (pp. 3–13). Baltimore, Maryland: The John Hopkins University Press.

Girardin, B. W., Faugno, D. K., Seneski, P. C., Slaughter, L., & Whelan, M. (1998). Normal Anatomy and the Human Sexual Response. In B. W. Girardin, D. K. Faugno, P. C. Seneski, L. Slaughter, & M. Wheelan, *Color Atlas of Sexual Assault* (pp. 1–17). St. Louis: Mosby—Year Book.

Groleau, G. A. & Jackson, M. C. (2001). Forensic examination of victims and perpetrators of sexual assault. In J. S. Olshaker et al. (Eds.), *Forensic emergency medicine* (pp. 85–117). Philadelphia: Lippincott Williams & Wilkins.

International Association of Forensic Nurses. (1996). *A sexual assault nurse examiner standards of practice: SANE Council*. Theofare, NJ: Slack.

Kelley, S. J. (1994). Sexual abuse. In S. J. Kelley (Ed.), *Pediatric emergency nursing* (2nd ed., pp. 109–125). Norwalk, CT: Appleton and Lange.

Ludwig, S. (2000). Child abuse. In G. R. Fleisher & S. Ludwig (Eds.), *Textbook of pediatric emergency medicine* (4th ed., pp. 1669–1704). Philadelphia: Lippincott Williams & Wilkins.

Sedlak, A. & Broadhurst, D. (1996). *Executive summary of the third national incidence study of child abuse and neglect.* Washington, DC: U.S. Government Printing Office.

Reece, R. M. (2000). Preface. In R. M. Reece (Ed.), *Treatment of child abuse* (pp. xiii–xvi). Baltimore: The John Hopkins University Press.

Wang, C. T. & Daro, D. (1998). *Current trends in child abuse reporting and fatalities: The results of the 1997 annual fifty-state survey.* Chicago: National Committee to Prevent Child Abuse.

INDEX

Page numbers followed by t indicate tables

C

S

T

W

X

Y